# Recent Results in Cancer Research 13

Fortschritte der Krebsforschung
Progrès dans les recherches sur le cancer

# Tumours in Children

Edited by

H. B. Marsden and J. K. Steward

Second, Revised and Enlarged Edition

With 295 Figures

Springer-Verlag
Berlin · Heidelberg · New York 1976

HENRY BASIL MARSDEN
University of Manchester, Department of Child Health,
Christie Hospital, Withington, Manchester M20 9BX,
Great Britain

JAMES KENRICK STEWARD †

*Sponsored by the Swiss League against Cancer*

ISBN-13: 978-3-642-81022-0 e-ISBN-13: 978-3-642-81020-6
DOI: 10.1007/978-3-642-81020-6

Library of Congress Cataloging in Publication Data. Marsden, Henry Basil.
Tumours in children. (Recent results in cancer research; 13.)
Bibliography: p. Includes index. 1. Tumours in children. I. Steward, James Kenrick.
Tumours in children. II. Title. III. Series.
DNLM: 1. Neoplasms — In infancy and childhood. W1 RE106P v. 13/
QZ200 T929 RC261.R35 no. 13, 1976 RC281.C4 616.9'94'008s 618.9'29'92
76-6091



Softcover reprint of the hardcover 1st edition 1976

*To the memory of* SAUL KEIDAN, *paediatric oncologist, and* LESLIE WHITE, *paediatric pathologist, who did so much pioneer work in the field of childhood malignancy*

Dr. Steward died on 20th June 1975.
The royalties from this book go to the J. K. Steward Memorial Fund for Children's Cancer

# Foreword

Cancer in childhood is a rare disease, but for many reasons attracts interest out of proportion to its frequency. There is, of course, the parental anguish associated with a catastrophic illness in a son or daughter — anguish shared in large measure by the physician. This aspect no doubt has spurred on clinicians and investigators in their race to develop more effective means of treatment. The rewards are great. Not only is there the human element, but there is also the fact that survival of the successfully treated child is measured in scores of years rather than the ordinary five to ten year survival rates cited for the adult. Associated with this aspect of paediatric oncology is the responsibility to make those many years as trouble-free as possible. The challenge to the team organizing the care of children with cancer is clear. Cure is to be obtained, but not at the cost of progressively more severe somatic or psychic lesions as the child develops through adolescence to maturity. The cured child of today must not become the chronically ill adult of tomorrow.

The spectrum of malignant diseases in childhood is not so varied as that of older patients. The kinds of tumour seen in children are relatively few in number; therefore, concentrated attention can be focussed on each entity, and specific strategies developed for clinical management. It was in the field of paediatrics that the extraordinarily successful and fruitful concept of the oncology team was first developed in full measure. Effective collaboration between surgeons, chemotherapists, radiation therapists, and pathologists has led to gratifying improvements in survival rates for many of the tumour types. In many instances, they are now at levels that were scarcely believable a decade ago. Efforts to go beyond this point continue. Equally important is the increasing, albeit, subtle change in emphasis from improvement in survival rates as an end in itself to the study of the late complications of successful therapy given in childhood. This has led to a search for refinements in treatment. For example, two of the major American clinical trials were designed to test whether routine postoperative radiation therapy is needed for early cases of Wilms' tumour and rhabdomyosarcoma. Treatments not truly essential for improvement in survival rates are being identified, and eliminated from the routine for each specific entity. This entails a greater understanding of the individual malignant diseases of childhood. Proper classification according to histology, extent of disease at diagnosis, age factors, and the like must be and are being defined with greater clarity. Better estimates of prognosis will result. This, in turn, will lead to the abandonment of comprehensive and therefore unnecessarily radical routines of treatment, now too commonly in use without regard to stage and histological discriminants. The happy result will be specific treatment directed to the particular problem of each individual child.

Tumours in Children takes these many factors into consideration. General aspects of the problem, such as aetiology, epidemiology, and the delivery of medical care are first presented. Then, individual chapters pursue treatment recommendations, and include pertinent comments regarding clinical and laboratory investigations underway for the elucidation of each type of cancer discussed.

The authors review the problem of tumours in childhood from a unique standpoint. They have at their disposal one of the few all-inclusive population-based compilations dealing with cancer in children, the justly renowned Manchester Registry. They, therefore, are able to provide data with respect to the frequency with which each type of cancer is found in children. They go beyond this, however, and courageously address themselves to the problem of how best to provide care for these unfortunate children. This is done by first defining the clinical needs, and then evaluating the available resources, including the number of specialists. They then draw logical and provocative conclusions and make recommendations with respect to what is required to provide the specialized care which is essential for these patients. It is to be hoped that governmental and medical authorities in Britain and elsewhere in the world will take notice.

It is a tragedy that Dr. Steward succumbed to a prolonged illness before this volume appeared in press. He leaves a rich legacy in the Registry, to which he gave so many years of devoted service, and in the first and second editions of this work. It remains for clinicians and investigators around the world to continue the advances in which he shared. Surely, the task will not be complete until the causes of malignant disease — be they environmental or genetic — are identified and eliminated, and the harsh note of cancer is no longer heard in the joyous rhapsody that is childhood.

New York G. J. D'Angio

# Preface

The aim of this book is to describe the clinical, epidemiological, and pathological manifestations of tumours in children and to discuss methods which are available for their treatment. Since the first edition was published in 1968, the need for special centres where children with tumours are treated by teams experienced in paediatric oncology has been widely accepted. Furthermore, collaborative therapeutic trials with improved clinical staging and pathological grading have resulted in many better methods of treatment. Consequently the preparation of a second edition has meant virtually rewriting the book.

Much of the material used is included in the files of the Manchester Children's Tumour Registry and most of the chapters have resulted from collaboration between Manchester contributors. In addition, we have been fortunate in drawing on the experience of six other contributors: Dr. R. W. Miller has discussed epidemiology, Professor J. N. P. Davies has described variations of incidence in different parts of the world, Dr. C. H. G. Price has discussed malignant bone tumours, Dr. J. Lindley Smith and Mr. M. A. Bedford have written the chapter on retinoblastomas and Dr. N. J. Brown has discussed testicular tumours.

Many of the chapters can be divided into two parts. Firstly, the pathological, clinical, and prognostic features of each tumour are described from a study of the cases included in the Registry during the 15 years up to the end of 1968 when, in Manchester, surgery and radiotherapy were nearly always the only methods used in trying to cure children with non-leukaemic tumours and chemotherapy was, almost exclusively, reserved for terminal palliation. Secondly, an attempt has been made to review the more important literature and to describe the treatment methods used at the present time. We are very conscious that any literature review must be incomplete and the therapy used while this book is being written will be, to a certain extent, out-of-date by the time it is published. Undoubtedly the great surge forward of that form of children's cancer research which is concerned with the assessment of new therapeutic agents will continue to produce many more effective chemotherapy schedules, but it is to be hoped that the era when reliance is placed mainly on cytotoxic drugs in treatment will only be transitory. Ultimately, there must be a better understanding of the factors which determine the development and progress of tumours in children. So far, much of the knowledge in this field has come from epidemiological studies but many questions can only be solved by bringing together the methods and skills of basic laboratory cancer research and the particular problems of paediatric oncology. In this sense children's cancer research has hardly started. An attempt is made in the first and last chapters of this book to analyse the reasons for this and to suggest ways of overcoming the organizational difficulties.

Although therapeutic improvement must be our main goal, its achievement will bring further problems. For many years a large number of children with retinoblastomas have been cured and some of these survivors have passed the disease on to their progeny. There is now evidence that the retinoblastoma is not the only children's tumour which may be inherited and as therapy improves, an increasing number of other familial neoplasms will be seen in paediatric practice. It is appalling that anyone who has survived cancer as a child should discover, quite unexpectedly after marriage, that the disease was familial. There is an urgent need to start looking now for ways of recognising those survivors who are at risk in this way.

To many people paediatric oncology must appear one of the most disheartening branches of medicine. Admittedly the majority of affected children still die, but an increasing number are being cured, and for the rest much can be achieved by palliation. As one learns more about the natural history of these tumours, many fascinating research problems become apparent. Unless we are prepared to make the effort to tackle them, the future will remain as black as the present — and we shall have nobody to blame but ourselves.

Manchester, March 1975

HENRY BASIL MARSDEN
JAMES KENRICK STEWARD

# Contents

# Acknowledgments

We would like to thank the clinicians and pathologists of the Manchester Region for their ready co-operation, without which this work would have been impossible. The following have been members of the panel of pathologists over the years: Dr. W. A. Aherne, Professor A. C. P. Campbell, Dr. O. G. Dodge, Dr. W. L. Donohue, Professor J. L. Emery, Professor Sidney Farber, Dr. A. M. MacDonald, Dr. Agnes R. Macgregor, Dr. H. B. Marsden, Dr. Helen Russell, Dr. J. P. Smith, Dr. L. L. R. White, and Professor R. A. Willis. We are very grateful for the services which they have so generously given.

Our thanks are due to Miss Linda Hunt for statistical help and to Mr. R. Schofield and his staff in the Medical Illustration Department of the Christie Hospital for drawing the graphs; also to the Department of Medical Illustration and Mr. P. Fletcher, Department of Pathology, Royal Manchester Children's Hospital, and Miss J. Perry, Department of Medical Illustration, Crumpsall Hospital, for their help with the photographs. Mr. G. Landen-Turner has given great help with the photomicrography of Chapter 8.

We are grateful to Dr. Ali Ahmed and Dr. Patricia Kumar for the descriptions and illustrations of the electronmicroscopic appearances of sympathetic and Ewing's tumours. The histological grading of sympathetic tumours was carried out in conjunction with Dr. M. Hughes.

We wish to thank Mrs. N. Rowe and Mrs. C. Christmas for the vast amount of secretarial work which they have undertaken in the preparation of this book.

Grants from the Medical Research Council and Cancer Research Council have from time to time supported the Manchester Children's Tumour Registry. Professor J. N. P. Davies received personal support from the Damon Runyon Memorial Fund for Cancer Research (DRG 1053), from the Brown-Hazen Fund and from N.I.H. contract no. NIH 72-2426 from the National Cancer Institute. The Bristol Bone Tumour Registry, of which Dr. C. H. G. Price is secretary, is supported by grants from the Cancer Research Campaign. Dr. C. B. Freeman is in receipt of a Medical Research Council grant.

We are grateful to Professor Wilfrid Gaisford, Professor A. C. P. Campbell, Professor Eric Easson, and Dr. Edith Paterson for all their help, advice, and encouragement.

Finally, high praise is due to the publishers, Springer-Verlag, for their great efficiency and unfailing courtesy and to the Swiss League against Cancer who have sponsored this series.

# Contributors to the Second Edition


M. A. BEDFORD M.B., B.S., F.R.C.S., Consultant Eye Surgeon, St. Bartholomew's Hospital, London; Consultant Surgeon in charge of the Oncology Clinic, Moorfields Eye Hospital, London

N. J. BROWN M.B., Ch.B., F.R.C.P., F.R.C.Path., Consultant Pathologist, Southmead Hospital, Bristol

J. N. P. DAVIES D.Sc., M.D., F.R.C.Path., Professor of Pathology, Albany Medical College, New York

B. H. DAWSON M.D., F.R.C.S., Consultant Neurosurgeon, Royal Manchester Children's Hospital and Salford Royal Hospital

D. I. K. EVANS M.B., M.R.C.P., D.C.H., Consultant Haematologist, Royal Manchester Children's Hospital, Monsall Hospital and Booth Hall Children's Hospital; Honorary lecturer, Manchester University

C. B. FREEMAN M.A., B.M., Ch.B., M.R.C.P., Research Fellow, Department of Medical Genetics, Manchester University

E. M. HAMMOND B.Sc., Principal Biochemist, Royal Manchester Children's Hospital

A. JOLLEYS M.D., F.R.C.S., Consultant Surgeon, Royal Manchester Children's Hospital; Honorary Lecturer, Manchester University

P. H. M. JONES M.B., M.R.C.P., D.C.H., Senior Lecturer, Department of Child Health, Manchester University; Consultant Paediatrician, Royal Manchester Children's Hospital and the Christie Hospital, Manchester

S. KUMAR Ph.D., M.V.Sc., Immunologist, Christie Hospital, Manchester

F. A. LANGLEY M.Sc., M.D., F.R.C.O.G., F.R.C.Path., Professor of Obstetrical and Gynaecological Pathology, Manchester University

H. B. MARSDEN M.B., Ch.B., F.R.C.Path., D.Path., D.C.H., Consultant Pathologist, Royal Manchester Children's Hospital, Monsall Hospital and Booth Hall Children's Hospital; Honorary Lecturer, Manchester University

R. W. MILLER M.D., Dr.P.H., Chief, Epidemiology Branch, National Cancer Institute, National Institutes of Health, Bethesda

M. K. PALMER B.Sc., M.I.S., F.S.S., Chief Medical Statistician, Christie Hospital

D. PEARSON M.B., Ch.B., D.M.R.T., F.F.R., Consultant Radiotherapist, Christie Hospital, Manchester

C. H. G. PRICE M.D., F.R.C.Path., Research Fellow (Pathology) Bristol University; Honorary Secretary, Bristol Bone Tumour Registry

J. ROLAND M.B., Ch.B., Research Assistant, Manchester Children's Tumour Registry

J. LINDLEY S. SMITH M.D., D.O.M.S., Consultant Pathologist, United Liverpool Hospitals

J. K. STEWARD † M.D., F.R.C.P., D.C.H., Senior Lecturer in charge of the Children's Tumour Registry, Departments of Child Health and Pathology, Manchester University; Honorary Consultant, the Christie Hospital

M. W. P. WADE M.B., Ch.B., Research Assistant, Manchester Children's Tumour Registry

M. WAGHE Ph.D., B.V.Sc. and A.H., Research Fellow, Department of Immunology, Manchester University

P. O. YATES M.D., F.R.C. Path., Professor of Neuropathology, Manchester University

# Chapter 1
# Problems of Children's Tumours in Britain

With the steady improvement in the prevention and treatment of bacterial disease during the past 30 years, their importance as a cause of death in children has greatly diminished. During the same period the practical benefits resulting from cancer research have not been so striking and consequently neoplasms have assumed a relatively greater importance in paediatrics. In 1970 they were the second commonest cause of death between the ages of 1 and 15 years in England and Wales (Registrar-General), being exceeded only by accidents (Table 1).

Table 1. Commonest cause of death in children 1 - 15 years in England and Wales during 1970 (Registrar-General 1972)

| | |
|---|---|
| Accidents | 1526 |
| Tumours | 772 |
| Respiratory diseases | 680 |
| Congenital abnormalities | 610 |

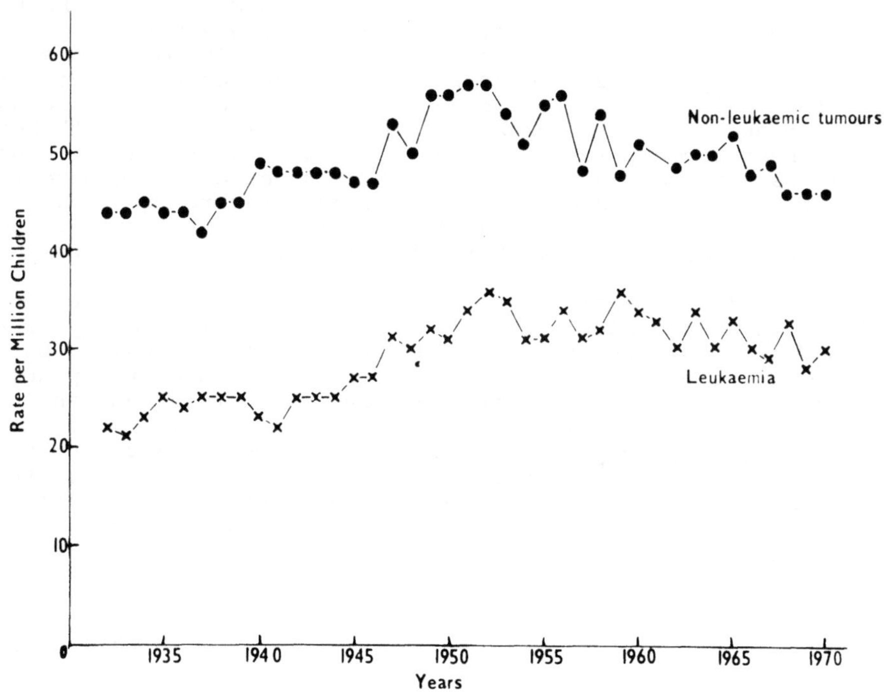


*Fig. 1. Incidence of fatal tumours in children under 15 years in England and Wales 1932 - 1970 (Registrar-General)*

Although it is easy to show that tumours have increased in importance relative to other children's diseases, it is more difficult to be certain whether there has been any absolute alteration in their frequency. The incidence of fatal tumours in children in England and Wales since 1932 is shown in Figure 1. There has been a rise in both leukaemia and non-leukaemic tumours but this was almost entirely confined to the period 1946 - 1953. It will be realised that these figures depend on the accuracy of the diagnoses given in death certificates. The fact that the apparent increase occurred during the time when the paediatric and pathological services in Britain were being greatly improved could easily be explained on the basis of greater diagnostic accuracy. Thus the Registrar-General's figures do not provide incontrovertible evidence that tumours in children have in fact become more frequent. On the other hand, they indicate that there has been no increase during the past 10 years.

Children with tumours are treated in many different centres and the value of reports from individual hospitals is limited by selective factors. To try to overcome this difficulty, information about these patients has been recorded in the Manchester Children's Tumour Register since January 1954. Patients were included in the Register only if the following conditions were fulfilled:

1. They were first seen by a consultant because of their tumour after 1st January 1954.
2. They lived in the Manchester Hospital Region which consisted of considerable portions of Lancashire, Cheshire, Derbyshire, and Westmorland and contained approximately one million children.[1]
3. They were under 15 years old.

The first condition was made because, if any analysis of cases collected during a given period was to be made, some date in the history of each tumour had to be selected to determine whether the patient should be included in that particular analysis. The only date in the clinical history of the disease which could be determined accurately was that on which the child was first seen by a consultant because of the tumour and this date has been used in all analyses. Both benign and malignant tumours were included but frank hamartomas were not. Since it is sometimes difficult to determine exactly the borderline of neoplasia, some diseases of doubtful nature were included. Histiocytosis X, fibroma of bone, granular myoblastoma and calcifying epithelioma were, perhaps rather arbitrarily, regarded as tumours.

In the case of the leukaemias the diagnosis was based on the reports of the hospital pathologists. Sections of the vast majority of non-leukaemic tumours were obtained and submitted to a panel of pathologists, and the diagnoses were assigned on the basis of the panel's reports, the clinical picture, the subsequent progress and any necropsy findings. However, to demand histological evidence in every case before accepting that a patient is suffering from a tumour introduces an element of selection, since in certain situations (e. g., the brain stem) a biopsy is seldom performed. It was considered justifiable, therefore, to include those cases in which the diagnosis appeared practically certain on purely clinical evidence.

---

[1]For purposes of National Health Service administration Britain is divided into a number of regions each containing a complete range of hospital specialist services. Before 1974 there were 16 such Hospital Regions in England and Wales, but with the reorganisation of the National Health Service in April 1974 the boundaries of these regions were altered.

Three tests of the completeness of the survey were carried out:

1. The Medical Officers of Health provided lists of children who had died and on whose death certificates there was mention of neoplasms. According to these returns 284 children who lived in the Manchester Hospital Region died from tumours during the 4 years, 1954 - 1957, i. e., there were 71 fatal cases per year. During the 15 years ending 1968, 1589 cases were included in the Register and an assessment in 1972 showed that 1123 of these patients had died (Table 2), i. e., 74 fatal cases per year.

2. An analysis in 1959 (CAMPBELL et al., 1961), showed that the children in the Register were, on the whole, evenly distributed throughout the Region, indicating that cases were not missed because they were treated in hospitals distant from Manchester.

3. LECK (1974) examined the cases included in the Registry from 1956 to 1968. Ten percent of the Manchester children suffered from conditions (e. g., Histiocytosis X) which are not included in the National Cancer Registration Scheme. After excluding these, he found that the annual incidence of tumours per million children during 1956 - 1968 according to the Manchester Children's Tumour Registry was 91.8, whereas the national incidence for 1968 of cases correctly registered under the National Cancer Registration Scheme was estimated to be 90.5.

These three tests indicate that the great majority of children with potentially fatal tumours were included in the Manchester Children's Tumour Registry, but it must be admitted that many cases of small benign tumours (e. g., fibromas and lipomas) were certainly not included, since the consultants concerned would not have considered them serious enough to notify. Nevertheless, it is probable that the cases in the Register give a fairly true picture of the frequency of children's serious tumours in the Manchester Region (Table 2).

Table 2. Manchester Children's Tumour Registry 1954 - 1968 (assessed 1972)

| | Alive | Dead | Total |
|---|---|---|---|
| Leukaemias | 11 | 454 | 465 |
| Non-leukaemic reticuloendothelial | 59 | 89 | 148 |
| Gliomas | 89 | 196 | 285 |
| Sympathetic | 25 | 89 | 114 |
| Retinoblastomas | 44 | 8 | 52 |
| Connective tissues | 88 | 103 | 191 |
| Renal | 28 | 59 | 87 |
| Gonadal | 8 | 6 | 14 |
| Teratomas | 35 | 16 | 51 |
| Epithelial | 38 | 25 | 63 |
| Ewing's | 2 | 28 | 30 |
| Rare miscellaneous | 31 | 18 | 49 |
| Third ventricular (clinical diagnosis only) | 5 | 4 | 9 |
| Malignant unclassified | 3 | 28 | 31 |
| | 466 (29%) | 1123 (71%) | 1589 |

It will be seen that rather over one-third of all the tumours were reticuloendothelial while a slightly lesser number arose in some part of the nervous system (glia, sympathetic, or retina). Connective tissue tumours accounted for one-eighth of all cases. Other neoplasms were less common. Wilms' tumours made up 5% of the total, being only slightly more frequent than teratomas and epithelial tumours. There were 30 children with Ewing's tumours. In 31 patients it was not possible to make an accurate histogenetic diagnosis and these cases were designated as "malignant unclassified". The miscellaneous group was made up of tumours which were so uncommon that only a few examples of each were included in the Register. The fact that 1589 cases were included in the Register during 15 years indicates that 105 out of a population of a million children develop tumours each year and the frequency of the various neoplasms is most easily expressed as the average annual incidence (Table 3).

Table 3. Manchester Children's Tumour Registry 1954 - 1968 (assessed 1972)

| Average annual incidence of children's tumours in the Manchester Hospital Region. (Total population 5,000,000; population <15 years 1,000,000) | |
|---|---|
| Leukaemia | 31 |
| Non-leukaemic reticuloendothelial | 10 |
| Gliomas | 19 |
| Sympathetic | 8 |
| Retinoblastoma | 3 |
| Connective tissue | 12 |
| Renal | 6 |
| Gonadal | 1 |
| Teratomas | 3 |
| Epithelial | 4 |
| Ewing's | 2 |
| Miscellaneous | 4 |
| Malignant unclassified | 2 |
| | 105 |

## Multiple Primaries

There have been 6 children in the Registry who developed two or more dissimilar tumours.

CTR.67/54. Boy, who had Hodgkin's disease at the age of 8 years in 1954 and then developed a leiomyosarcoma of the iris in 1959. He remained alive and well in 1972 (DUGMORE, 1972).

CTR.94/54. Boy, who had a fibrosarcoma of the scalp in 1947 at the age of 3 years. In 1954 he developed an osteogenic sarcoma of the right fibula and in 1957 an osteogenic sarcoma of the right ulna appeared. Lung secondaries were seen in 1958 and he died in 1959. He had a twin brother who was said to be identical. This brother had a son who presented with an embryonic sarcoma of the nasopharynx in 1972.

CTR.34/54. Girl, who in 1954 at the age of 10 years, had a teratoma of the ovary removed and a year later a mass in the upper lobe of the right lung was noted. This was irradiated without any effect and a benign teratoma of the lung was removed. In 1968 at the age of 24 she developed a carcinoma of the right breast from which she died.

CTR.79/57. A boy, who had a medulloblastoma treated successfully with irradiation in 1957 at the age of 2 years. During the 1960's he developed multiple basal cell carcinomas (naevoid-basal cell carcinoma syndrome). The child's father had a basal cell carcinoma of the neck in 1960 and died from a glioma in 1962.

CTR.33/60. Boy, who in 1960 developed ataxia, headache and squint at the age of 8 years. Ventriculograms showed a filling defect of the fourth ventricle and a diagnosis of a brain stem tumour was made and X-ray treatment was given. In 1969 the child died from a rapidly growing abdominal sarcoma.

CTR.13/61. Boy who had both eyes removed for familial retinoblastoma in January 1961 when he was 5 months old. He remained well up to November 1972 when he developed an osteogenic sarcoma of the upper end of the left tibia. Pulmonary metastases developed in January 1973 and he died in December 1973.

REGELSON et al. (1965) found 8 cases of second primaries amongst 150 children with leukaemia and solid tumours coming to autopsy in a service devoted exclusively to paediatric neoplasms. Their findings cannot be compared with those in the Manchester series in which only a minority had autopsies.

Sex. The proportion of boys and girls who were included in the Registry is shown in Table 4.

Table 4. Manchester Children's Tumour Registry 1954 - 1968

| | Sex | | | |
|---|---|---|---|---|
| | Males | Females | Ratio M : F | P |
| Leukaemias | 253 | 212 | 1.19 | Not significant |
| Lymphosarcomas | 33 | 11 | 3.00 | 0.005 |
| Hodgkin's | 35 | 15 | 2.33 | 0.01 |
| Medulloblastomas | 55 | 20 | 2.70 | 0.001 |
| Neuroblastomas | 66 | 35 | 1.91 | 0.005 |
| Presacral teratomas | 3 | 12 | 0.25 | 0.02 |
| Other tumours | 438 | 401 | 1.08 | Not significant |
| | 883 | 706 | 1.25 | 0.001 |

There was a statistically significant excess of boys over girls who developed either lymphosarcomas, Hodgkin's Disease, medulloblastomas or neuroblastomas. Presacral teratomas were the only tumours which occurred more frequently in girls. In the case of leukaemia there was an excess of boys which was not statistically significant. However, during 1964 - 1966, 561 boys and 457 girls died from leukaemia in England and Wales (Reg. Gen.), giving a statistically significant excess of boys (P = 0.01).

Prognosis. The condition of those patients included up to 31st December 1968 was assessed in 1972. The prognosis of the individual types of tumours is shown in Table 2. The overall mortality was 71%.

## FACTORS INFLUENCING PROGNOSIS

Treatment. In Manchester during the period under review any attempt at radical treatment of children's tumours consisted almost entirely of local therapy, i. e., surgery and/or X-rays. Chemotherapy was usually reserved for the palliative treatment of those children with widespread disease (Table 5).

It will be seen that whereas 922 of the 1124 children with non-leukaemic tumours were given local treatment, only 170 received chemotherapy.

Table 5. Manchester Children's Tumour Registry 1954 - 1968. Treatment given to 1124 children with non-leukaemic tumours in the Manchester Region

| Tumour type | Number given local treatment (Excision and/or irradiation) | | | Number given chemotherapy (with or without local treatment) | | |
|---|---|---|---|---|---|---|
| | Alive | Dead | Total | Alive | Dead | Total |
| Non-leukaemic reticulo-endothelial | 41 | 51 | 92 | 27 | 45 | 72 |
| Gliomas | 88 | 141 | 229 | 0 | 6 | 6 |
| Sympathetic | 25 | 56 | 81 | 1 | 15 | 16 |
| Retinoblastomas | 44 | 8 | 52 | 0 | 0 | 0 |
| Connective tissue | 87 | 87 | 174 | 7 | 23 | 30 |
| Renal | 28 | 55 | 83 | 11 | 12 | 23 |
| Gonadal | 8 | 6 | 14 | 0 | 1 | 1 |
| Teratomas | 34 | 13 | 47 | 0 | 1 | 1 |
| Epithelial | 37 | 17 | 54 | 0 | 1 | 1 |
| Ewing's | 2 | 28 | 30 | 1 | 14 | 15 |
| Miscellaneous | 28 | 9 | 37 | 0 | 1 | 1 |
| Third ventricle (clinical diagnosis only) | 4 | 2 | 6 | 0 | 0 | 0 |
| Malignant unclassified | 3 | 20 | 23 | 0 | 4 | 4 |
| Total | 429 | 493 | 922 | 47 | 123 | 170 |

Chemotherapy, therefore, contributed very little to the cure of Manchester children with tumours before 1968. Out of the 47 survivors who were given chemotherapy, 18 received steroids for Histiocytosis X and 10 were given Actinomycin D for Wilms' tumours.

## Nature, Site, and Presentation of the Tumour (Table 6)

Seventy-two percent of the fatal tumours fell into one of four categories, all of which were difficult or impossible to cure by local means. Those children presenting with generalized disease obviously required generalized treatment. Abdominal tumours usually had grown to a very large size before they were detected; the radiotherapist can rarely give much help with malignant connective tissue tumours and the patient's chances largely depended on whether the surgeon could make a complete excision; surgical and radiological interfer-

Table 6. Manchester Children's Tumour Registry 1954 - 1968 (assessed 1972)

| Fatal cases | | |
|---|---|---|
| Generalised at clinical onset | 497 ) | |
| Abdominal | 120 ) | 811 = 72% |
| Connective tissue | 100 ) | |
| Brain, third ventricle or cord | 94 ) | |
| Others | 312 | = 28% |

ence with lesions of the brain stem, third ventricle and cord is strictly limited due to the danger to vital structures.

Malignancy. Leukaemia, Wilms' tumours, neuroblastomas and embryonic sarcomas progress rapidly in children, but some paediatric neoplasms may grow quite slowly. Hodgkin's disease appears to behave in children as it does in adults. The juvenile astrocytoma is histologically benign and medulloblastomas and Ewing's tumours may grow extremely slowly. Neuroblastomas and presacral teratomas have a better prognosis in infancy than in later childhood, while thyroid carcinomas progress more slowly in children than in adults.

## Speed of Diagnosis

Since success in treatment depends to a certain degree on the extent of the tumour, it is pertinent to ask whether earlier diagnosis is feasible with children's tumours. The time from clinical onset to hospital attendance of the children in the Register is shown in Table 7.

Table 7. Time from clinical onset to hospital consultation

| | |
|---|---|
| Less than one month | 650 |
| 1 - 2 months | 353 |
| 2 - 3 months | 174 |
| 3 - 6 months | 200 |
| Over six months | 182 |
| Not known | 30 |
| | 1589 |

It will be seen that 42% attended within 1 month and 76% within 3 months. Is it reasonable to expect general practitioners to refer children with tumours to hospital any earlier than this? Two factors have to be taken into consideration in answering this question.

1. A general practitioner sees on an average 1 child with a neoplasm every 15 years.
2. The early signs of the disease are usually vague - some pallor, a little unsteadiness, loss of appetite, occasional headaches - all of which are common to less serious diseases.

Might earlier diagnosis be achieved by making the lay public more aware of the possibility of children developing tumours? AITKEN-SWAN and PATERSON (1959), recording the effects of cancer education on the public, showed that women with cancer of the breast or cervix sought medical advice more rapidly if they came from an area which had been subjected to a campaign of cancer education. Their figures are shown in Table 8.

It will be seen that even after cancer education the proportion of women who sought medical advice within 3 months was smaller than the proportion of children who were admitted to hospital within 3 months of the clinical onset of their tumours. AITKEN-SWAN and PATERSON point out that the fear of knowing the truth is a potent cause of delay in seeking treatment. In the case of children this does not apply since the decision to visit a doctor is not taken by the child but by the parents.

Table 8. Percentage seeking medical aid within three months (AITKEN-SWAN and PATERSON, 1959)

| Site of cancer | Women living in area with cancer education | Women living in area without cancer education |
|---|---|---|
| Breast | 56% | 50% |
| Cervix | 59% | 36% |

Table 9. Time interval from clinical onset to hospital consultation

| Mode of presentation | Number of children | Median time interval (weeks) | % cases with over 3 months delay |
|---|---|---|---|
| Brain | 310 | 8.1 | 40 |
| Bone | 115 | 7.3 | 31 |
| Eye | 50 | 6.9 | 9 |
| Subcutaneous lump | 155 | 6.7 | 29 |
| Neck glands | 66 | 6.1 | 33 |
| Chest | 43 | 5.3 | 18 |
| Spinal | 36 | 4.9 | 25 |
| Generalised | 512 | 4.5 | 13 |
| Abdominal | 199 | 3.2 | 17 |
| Others | 73 | 3.2 | 19 |
| Total | [a]1559 | 5.4 | 24 |

[a]In 30 cases the time interval was not known

Table 10. Time interval from hospital consultation to diagnosis

| Mode of presentation | Number of children | Median time interval (weeks) | % cases with over three months delay |
|---|---|---|---|
| Neck glands | 67 | 4.3 | 22 |
| Spinal | 36 | 2.5 | 11 |
| Subcutaneous lump | 166 | 1.7 | 23 |
| Chest | 45 | 1.5 | 1 |
| Bone | 116 | 1.2 | 10 |
| Brain | 316 | 1.1 | 16 |
| Others | 74 | 1.1 | 13 |
| Generalised | 513 | <0.5 | 6 |
| Abdominal | 202 | <0.5 | 2 |
| Eye | 53 | <0.5 | 1 |
| | [a]1588 | 0.5 | 11 |

[a]In one case the time interval was not known

The speed with which children with tumours were referred to hospital depended to a certain extent on the mode of presentation. This is shown in Table 9 in which the cases in the Registry are divided into ten groups depending on the way the tumour presented.

The greatest delay in hospital referral was in children with brain or bone tumours. In 40% of the children with brain tumours and in 31% of those with bone tumours the delay was over 3 months.

Once the child was seen by a consultant there was usually little delay in making a diagnosis, but, here again, the time interval depended on the mode of presentation (Table 10).

After hospital consultation the greatest delay in diagnosis occurred in those children who presented with enlarged neck glands.

Thus it seems that there are two main areas where there could be improvement - parents and general practitioners often fail to realise the significance of the early manifestations of brain tumours and consultants may be reluctant to suspect that enlarged neck glands may be neoplastic. Probably one reason why brain tumours are missed is that the symptoms may be intermittent - a child may have headache and vomiting for a few days and then be symptom-free for several months. The reason why neoplastic neck glands may be misdiagnosed by consultants is their rarity compared with all the cases of infected neck glands which are seen in hospital outpatient departments. However, consultants might be more aware of the possibility of enlarged neck glands having a neoplastic cause and be more ready to do a biopsy in any suspicious case.

## Conclusion

During the period of this survey surgery and irradiation were considered by most clinicians to be virtually the only effective methods of curing children with cancer. An examination of the factors which influenced the prognosis of patients included in the Manchester Children's Tumour Registry up to the end of 1968 indicates that there was a high mortality mainly because children's neoplasms do not usually cause impressive signs or symptoms until the disease is incurable by local treatment alone. Although speedier diagnosis might have been achieved in some cases, avoidable diagnostic delay was a relatively minor cause of the high mortality compared with the frequent ineffectiveness of purely local treatment. In other words, combined treatment using chemotherapy, often given in dosages to the limit of the patient's tolerance, together with local treatment, must be employed to produce any significant reduction in the mortality. Immunotherapy could be incorporated in this combined treatment.

The use of combined therapy immediately presents organisational problems - treatment strategy must be decided upon by a group of specialists as soon as the clinical diagnosis is made; children on high doses of anti-cancer drugs need special supportive care which is not available in most hospitals; therapy assessment can only be done by statistical analysis of large series of cases. It is obvious, therefore, that children with tumours need to be treated in an organisation which is planned for their special needs.

## THE ORGANISATION OF A SERVICE FOR CHILDREN WITH TUMOURS

There are three aims in the design of a service for children with tumours.

1. To ensure that existing forms of treatment are used as effectively as possible.
2. To assess and develop new therapeutic methods as quickly as possible.
3. To attract research workers to the problems of paediatric oncology and provide them with the opportunities to solve these problems.

These aims will be considered in further detail.

## The Use of Existing Therapeutic Methods

The institution of the National Health Service was followed by an enormous improvement in the standard of paediatric care in Britain, but there was little decrease in the number of children who died from tumours up to 1970 (see Figure 1). In general there has been a policy of decentralisation of specialist services - every town has its paediatrician, surgeon and pathologist. This policy has been right for the treatment of the great majority of diseases, but it does not take into account the requirements of children with cancer.

In the Manchester Region each year 105 children develop tumours which can be divided into at least 12 main groups. A comparison of the incidence of these tumours with the number of consultants shows that, if there was no centralization, nobody would be able to become experienced in paediatric oncology. This may be illustrated with leukaemia, Wilms' tumours and Ewing's tumours. The Manchester Region contains 34 paediatricians, 87 general surgeons, 2 paediatric surgeons and 54 orthopaedic surgeons. If the leukaemias were evenly distributed amongst the paediatricians, each would see one case per year; if the Wilms' tumours were evenly distributed amongst the general and paediatric surgeons, each would see one case every 15 years, and if the Ewing's tumours were evenly distributed amongst the orthopaedic surgeons each would see one case every 27 years. It is no slur on the general ability of these consultants to say that, under such circumstances, existing forms of treatment would not be used to the best advantage. A surgeon, who may be extremely skilled at performing a gastrectomy or thyroidectomy, cannot be an expert at removing a Wilms' tumour if he only sees one case in 15 years. Furthermore, it is not just a matter of technical skill. Since a combination of surgery, radiotherapy and chemotherapy often needs to be employed, treatment strategy has to be decided as soon as possible after the clinical diagnosis has been made. This can only be done by a team of specialists who have the opportunity of treating many children with tumours.

## The Assessment and Development of New Therapeutic Methods

It is obviously a waste of time and effort for research workers to produce new methods of treatment if clinicians are not able to assess these methods and learn how to use them. The following example shows that there is a very real danger of failing to use new methods when children with tumours are scattered amongst many hospitals and treated by many doctors. By 1953 the antifolics (FARBER, 1949), steroids (PEARSON and ELIEL, 1950), and 6-mercaptopurine (BURCHENAL et al., 1953) had all been shown to have an established place in the treatment of children with leukaemia. However, an analysis of 87 cases in the Manchester Region between 1953 and 1957 showed that the advent of these drugs had caused practically no improvement in the survival time compared with that of children who had leukaemia prior to 1950 (TIVEY, 1952). This was due to the fact that no paediatrician in the region saw enough children with this disease to be able to gain sufficient experience in the effective use of these drugs. In order to work out a satisfactory treatment technique these patients were to a certain extent centralized during 1957 - 58. After this the survival time was doubled.

The assessment of new methods of treatment can only be done in properly designed trials in which enough cases are included to provide results which are statistically significant. It is far easier to carry out these trials if the children are treated in a few large centres staffed by doctors experienced in paediatric oncology. In the Medical Research Council leukaemia trials it was found that children treated outside large centres often had to be excluded from the final analyses because the clinicians had not kept to the treatment protocols.

## Attraction of Research Workers to the Problems of Children's Tumours

Although there are many unsolved problems in children's cancer, few research workers are attracted to these problems and, in Britain at least, children have derived very little benefit from the vast amount of effort and expenditure which has been put into cancer research. There are two main reasons for this.

1. Children with tumours have been scattered throughout so many hospitals that material for research has been extremely difficult to obtain. No research worker is going to undertake a project unless he can be assured of obtaining the material to carry it through.

2. Research in paediatric oncology is essentially applied - in other words it seeks to solve practical problems by using methods which have been developed by basic cancer research workers. Since paediatrics and cancer research have developed separately there has been a great gulf between them and this has prevented the problems of paediatric oncology being brought together with the research techniques which might be used to solve them.

There can be no doubt, therefore, that in the past the service for children with tumours has had one fundamental defect. These patients have been treated in so many hospitals by so many doctors that existing therapeutic methods have not been used skilfully, new methods have not been assessed quickly and research in paediatric oncology has been completely inadequate.

The only reasonable solution is for children with tumours to be treated by paediatric teams working in specialist oncological centres to which patients are referred as soon after clinical diagnosis as possible. The size of these centres would, of course, be determined by geographical considerations, but the progress which could be made would be directly related to the number of children treated. For a centre to work efficiently it would need to drain a population which would provide at least 100 new cases of children's tumours each year. The paediatric team would contain some (e. g., radiotherapists, neurosurgeons and orthopaedic surgeons) who treat patients of all ages. However, the team needs to be given a cohesion by a paediatric oncologist, who would give all, or nearly all, of his time to the problems of children's cancer. This paediatric oncologist should be experienced in general paediatrics and have had several years training in oncology. His presence is necessary not only to act as the focal point of the team, but also to be the link in the management of the patient throughout all stages of his illness. This continuity of clinical care is important to provide psychological support for the children and their parents and also to ensure that experience of the value of new therapy given initially to patients with widespread disease is subsequently used for the benefit of children with early tumours. Not only is the paediatric oncologist an essential member of the team but his appointment can be used as a starting point for a children's tumour centre. Experience in Manchester indicates that at least two paediatric oncologists are required to cope with the clinical work load provided by a population of one million children. In some large cities there may have been for a variety of historical reasons a separation of the responsibility for children with leukaemia on the one hand and solid tumours on the other. Such a separation should be avoided whenever possible.

The establishment of special centres for the treatment of children with malignant disease is the first and most important step to improve the care of these patients, but for children with two types of neoplasm - retinoblastomas and malignant bone tumours - these regional centres need to be supplemented by national centres.

1. Approximately 50 children develop retinoblastomas in Britain each year. More than half of these tumours are unilateral and any ophthalmologist can treat them effectively by unilateral enucleation. Since there are no more than 25 children each year with bilateral disease, the very special ophthalmological techniques described in Chapter 8 to treat their less affected eyes conservatively, can only be applied efficiently if all these children with bilateral retinoblastoma in Britain are treated in one national centre.

2. There are approximately 150 patients of all ages who develop osteosarcomas (in the absence of Paget's disease) in Britain each year and only one-third of these are under 15 years old. The results of the treatment of malignant bone tumours are extremely bad (see chapters 9 and 13) but the problem of these tumours in children should not be considered separately from that in adults. The establishment of a national centre for the treatment of malignant bone tumours in patients of all ages would be the best way of allowing the development of better treatment techniques. Children with these tumours in the regional children's centres would receive treatment based on the experience gained in the national centre.

## Research in Paediatric Oncology

Although the first essential is to provide an efficient clinical service, it must be remembered that the main problem of paediatric oncology is that even if existing therapy was always applied with maximum skill and minimum delay, many of the children with tumours would still die. Therefore it is necessary to link clinical centres to cancer research institutes in such a way that research workers are attracted to the problems of paediatric oncology. In order to achieve this end, two facts have to be taken into consideration.

1. Children cannot give informed consent to any procedure which is carried out purely for research purposes and even venepunctures are often distressing for them. Therefore any project involving children can only be undertaken by a partnership between research workers and clinicians who must take into account their moral and humane responsibilities to the patients.

2. Research workers can only survive if they maintain a reasonable output of scientific papers and therefore they naturally prefer projects for which material is easily available. Even when clinical centralisation of children's tumours has been achieved, it is still more difficult to obtain material from these children than from adult

patients, or from animals. In the case of children's non-leukaemic tumours it is usually necessary to build up a store of frozen material collected over several years before undertaking a paediatric project. Thus, research in paediatric oncology presents special problems which cannot be satisfactorily solved by those who only have a passing or part-time interest in this field. In any centre where a serious effort at children's cancer research is made, there must be a small group of research workers who are occupied full-time in paediatric oncology. Therefore there should be career projects not only for those who wish to be clinical paediatric oncologists but also those who have proven laboratory or epidemiological research ability and wish to devote their skills to the problems of children's cancer.

One thing must be accepted. It is the joint responsibility of paediatricians, radiotherapists, surgeons, pathologists and medical administrators to ensure that children with cancer are given the best available treatment and that better therapeutic methods are provided for future generations. This cannot be achieved while these patients are treated in many different hospitals by doctors who can never become experienced in paediatric oncology. Improvement will only come when children with cancer are treated in centres by specialist teams who are able to develop new methods and take advantage of the great research potential which is available.

## REFERENCES


AITKEN-SWAN, J., PATERSON, R.: Br. Med. J. 1, 708 (1959)

BURCHENAL, J. H., MURPHY, M. L., ELLISON, R. R., SYKES, M. P., TAN, T. C., LEONE, L. A., KARNOFSKY, D. A., CRAVER, L. F., DARGEON, H. W., RHOADS, C. P.: Blood 8, 965 (1953)

CAMPBELL, A. C. P., GAISFORD, W. F., PATERSON, E., STEWARD, J. K.: Br. Med. J. 1, 448 (1961)

DUGMORE, W. N.: Br. J. Ophthalmol. 56, 366 (1972)

FARBER, S.: Blood 4, 160 (1949)

LECK, I.: Paediatric aspects of epidemiology - the frequency of disorders of early life. In: Scientific Foundations of Paediatrics. DAVIS, J. A., DOBBING, J. (eds.). London: Heinemann Medical, 1974, p. 705

PEARSON, O. H., ELIEL, L. P.: J. A. M. A. 144, 1349 (1950)

REGELSON, W., BROSS, I. D. J., HANANIAN, J., NAGOGOSYAN, G.: Cancer 18, 58 (1965)

Registrar-General: Statistical Reviews for England and Wales for the years 1932-1970. Tables Medical, H. M. S. O. London

TIVEY, H.: Pediatrics (Springfield) 10, 48 (1952)

Chapter 2

# Aetiology of Childhood Cancer: Epidemiological Approach

ROBERT W. MILLER

Epidemiology is an important source of clues to the origins of cancer. Until recently, this research approach has been focussed on the more numerous cancers of adults. The epidemiology of childhood cancer received little attention, because paediatricians were mainly concerned with diagnosis, pathological physiology, and therapy.

Cancers that occur in large numbers are, of course, of great public health importance. Peculiarities in the occurrence of specific rare cancers, including those of children, may be more easily detected than in the more numerous cancers of adults. These peculiarities may point the way to causality.

## Descriptive Studies

The simplest approach is to describe the frequency of cancers by cell type in hospital series or in tumour registries. The ideal source of such data is a population-based registry (so rates may be calculated) with excellent pathology, as in Manchester, England (1). But even the very simple enumeration of cases according to cell type in one clinical series when compared with another may show an excess or deficiency of cases, perhaps related to the sex or ages of the children. It was in this way that Burkitt's lymphoma was first recognized as peculiar to central Africa. Care must be taken not to ascribe an excess or deficiency in relative frequency (percentage of the total) of a disease to genetic or environmental influences, when selective referral to a hospital may be the true explanation. Thus, data from Columbia University would suggest a marked excess of retinoblastoma in New York, when in fact the University's famous treatment centre for that neoplasm attracted cases far beyond the hospital's locale.

One need not be an epidemiologist to make important contributions through its methods. Quite the contrary - alert practitioners have provided new insight to aetiology by noting an excess of pre-existent disease with certain forms of cancer; e. g., nephroblastoma (Wilms' tumour) with congenital hemihypertrophy (reviewed by FRAUMENI et al. (2) ) or leukaemia in children with Down's syndrome (reviewed by MILLER (3) ).

Alert practitioners have also been the first to recognize some of the environmental causes of cancer, as for example radiation-induced leukaemia (reviewed by DUNLAP (4) ), and the manufacturing of mustard gas as a cause of an epidemic of respiratory-tract cancer in Japan (5). These insights occurred when the physicians looked back into the histories of the patients and learned of heavy environmental (in these instances occupational) exposures.

## Testing Hypotheses

Epidemiology is not only a source of hypotheses on oncogenesis; it can also test hypotheses generated by clinical observations, laboratory research, or other epidemiological studies. Tests of hypotheses may involve looking back into the histories of persons with a given form of cancer in search of the factor under suspicion. In other instances, it may be feasible and appropriate to study a cohort of persons with exposure to the agent in question to determine if rates for specific neoplasms exceed those of a non-exposed but otherwise similar group. Cohort studies can refine the magnitude of the risk with respect to such variables as age, sex, exposure dose, and cell type. Thus, cohort study of Japanese survivors of the atomic bomb revealed that acute leukaemias (AL) and chronic myelogenous leukaemia (CML) were induced by irradiation, but the chronic lymphocytic form of the disease was not (6). Also, the effect was greater when exposure occurred under 10 years of age than in later life, and a peak in frequency, greater for AL than for CML, was observed in 1951, 6 years after the explosion. It is apparent that radiation can induce some forms of leukaemia, but not all forms, and that host factors affect susceptibility.

Technically, studies of case histories are called "retrospective" and cohort studies are called "prospective". It seems logical that there be an approach designated "laterospective", in which one looks sideways for collateral disease. Indeed, this technique has proved particularly effective in relating specific congenital malformations to certain forms of cancer. When pre-existent diseases are found excessively with specific neoplasms, one can evaluate the origins of the neoplasm in terms of what is already known about the aetiology of the diseases with which it is associated. Thus, new avenues of research are open for the study of neoplasia. Recognition of such associations is also of clinical benefit: the clinician who sees a child with a disorder known to carry a high risk of a neoplasm can be alert for the earliest detectable evidence of the neoplasm, prompt treatment of which may be life-saving.

## Environmental Causes of Childhood Cancer

Ionizing Radiation. The only environmental exposure thus far proven to cause cancer before 14 years of age is ionizing radiation. Acute leukaemia was the sole neoplasm noted in excess before this age among Japanese atomic-bomb survivors (7, 8). The latent period for cancer may, of course, extend beyond the paediatric years. Indeed, from 16 - 31 years of age the heavily exposed children experienced 8 deaths from cancers other than leukaemia (no specificity as to cell type) as compared with 1.1 expected (8). This result was supported by a morbidity survey which revealed that 6 other children had cancer as compared with 1.3 expected (8). These observations may portend a larger difference to come as the cohort ages.

Prenatal Exposures. A stunning development in 1971 was the discovery that a drug, stilbestrol, given in heavy doses to mothers during pregnancy, caused adenocarcinoma of the vagina in their daughters 14 - 22 years later (9). In this instance the role of the drug was quickly recognized because it induced a cluster of 7 cases of a rare cancer in one city - 6 in one hospital - in only 4 years. A similar increase in a more frequent neoplasm, such as leukaemia or lymphoma, would have gone unnoticed. This first evidence of transplacental chemical carcinogenesis in man raises the possibility that other cancers may be induced by this or other drugs used in pregnancy. One might, for example, look for an excess of Hodgkin's disease among children whose mothers received diphenylhydantoin (DPH) during pregnancy for epilepsy. DPH is suspect because several persons on the drug have developed a lymphoreticular hyperplasia resembling Hodgkin's disease. The process was apparently reversible in its early stages, but was lethal in some instances (10).

Several studies have shown that diagnostic abdominal X-ray exposure during pregnancy (very low doses) was associated with an increase of about 50% in the relative risk of each category of cancer in children under 10 years of age (11, 12). One study reported a response in proportion to dose (number of films taken (13) ). The causal relationship, however, has come into question because (1) the increase in deaths expected on the basis of hospital exposures in the above-mentioned studies was not found among Japanese survivors exposed in utero to the atomic bomb (14), (2) the dissimilar epidemiology of each form of childhood cancer (see below) makes it seem biologically implausible that each category of childhood cancer would be equally induced by X-ray, as found in the hospital-based studies (11, 12), and (3) unpublished data on about 7000 mice irradiated in utero revealed no increase in cancer occurrence during their life span (15).

Viruses. The viral aetiology of cancer has received immense attention in recent years. Yet the same epidemiological methods that readily revealed the carcinogenicity of certain chemicals, ionizing radiation, and genetic influences, have not to date implicated any virus in human carcinogenesis. A major function of epidemiology in this regard is to test hypotheses concerning possible viral modes of spread from one person to another. To date, Burkitt's lymphoma is the childhood cancer that exhibits characteristics most suggestive of a viral aetiology. The rates for the disease change rather quickly over time in a given locale, time-space clustering has been observed, and the distribution of the disease is confined to a climate that favours the proliferation of certain microbial agents (16). A chemical carcinogen would have some of these characteristics, but would be unlikely to move across a geographical area, as Burkitt's lymphoma has. Kaposi's sarcoma also appears to have this trait, unlike other childhood cancers.

Leukaemia is the only other paediatric neoplasm as yet extensively studied for time-space clustering. There is no doubt that individual clusters can be found of events having the same low frequency as leukaemia. The question is not whether clusters occur, but whether they occur excessively. To make this evaluation one must dispassionately define units of time and space before examining the distribution of cases in an area. Several statistical procedures have been devised to determine if the number of clusters observed significantly exceeds that expected by chance (17, 18). The results have shown either no excess (17), or (in 2 studies) weak clustering of acute lymphocytic leukaemia under 6 years of age (19, 20).

If leukaemia were infectious in the usual sense, one might expect a concentration of cases among persons heavily exposed to present or future victims of disease. No excess of cases has been found among persons whose marital partners developed leukaemia (21), in children whose mothers had leukaemia during pregnancy or subsequently (22), or in persons who received blood transfusions from donors who later developed leukaemia (a preliminary study (23) ), and the small extent to which childhood leukaemia affects sibs in a family can readily be explained on a genetic basis (24, 25). Other hypotheses about viral leukaemogenesis have also been tested epidemiologically. The disease does not show patterns of spread suggestive of a slow virus (as in kuru); is apparently not related to breast-feeding or to exchange-transfusions in the neonatal period, when the child's immunological defenses are low (23).

Table 1. Hereditary Neoplasms [a]

| Syndrome | Inheritance [b] | Major Features | Associated Disorders |
|---|---|---|---|
| Retinoblastoma | AD | Retinoblastoma | D-deletion syndrome in small proportion of cases |
| Naevoid basal-cell carcinoma syndrome | AD | Multiple basal-cell cancers of skin, with various developmental defects | Defects include jaw cysts, skeletal deformities, skin pits on palms and soles, soft-tissue calcifications, & hypertelorism. Ovarian fibromas, medulloblastoma |
| Multiple endocrine adenomatosis | AD | Adenomas of anterior pituitary parathyroid, & pancreatic islet cells | Adenomas of thyroid & adrenal cortex. Carcinoid tumours of intestine & bronchus. Ulcerogenic islet-cell tumours of pancreas predominate in some cases (Zollinger-Ellison syndrome) |
| Phaeochromocytoma with medullary thyroid carcinoma | AD | Phaeochromocytoma & medullary thyroid carcinoma | Multiple neurofibromas & mucosal neuromas. Parathyroid hyperplasia & neoplasia |
| Chemodectomas | AD | Paragangliomas of chemoreceptor system in major blood vessels | - |
| Polyposis coli | AD | Multiple adenomatous polyps & adenocarcinomas of large bowel | Some families feature osteomas, fibromas, lipomas, & epidermal cysts (Gardner's syndrome) |
| Tylosis with oesophageal carcinoma | AD | Squamous-cell carcinoma of oesophagus, with keratosis of palms and soles | - |

[a] Adapted from FRAUMENI (29)
[b] AD = autosomal dominant

Table 2. Hereditary Pre-Neoplastic Syndromes

| Hamartomatous Syndromes | Inheritance | Major Features | Neoplasms |
|---|---|---|---|
| Neurofibromatosis (von Recklinghausen's syndrome) | AD | Multiple neurofibromas and café-au-lait spots. Various hamartomatous growths, mental retardation, & bone defects are common | Neurofibrosarcoma in 10% of patients. Gliomas of brain & optic nerve, acoustic neuromas, meningiomas, & phaeochromocytoma |
| Tuberous sclerosis | AD | Adenoma sebaceum, epilepsy, & mental retardation. Characteristic hamartomas in brain, retina, heart, lungs, & kidneys | Brain tumours, chiefly, giant-cell astrocytoma, in 1-3% of patients |
| Von Hippel-Lindau syndrome | AD | Angiomatosis of retina & cerebellum. Cysts & angiomas often present in viscera | Hypernephroma, phaeochromocytoma, ependymomas in several reported cases |
| Multiple exostoses (diaphysial aclasia) | AD | Osteochondromas with severe bone deformities | Chrondrosarcoma in 5-11% of patients |
| Peutz-Jeghers syndrome | AD | Hamartomatous gastrointestinal polyps with melanin spots on buccal mucosa, lips, & digits | Ovarian neoplasms in 5% of female patients. Gastrointestinal carcinoma reported rarely |
| Genodermatoses | | | |
| Xeroderma pigmentosa | AR | Progressive sun-sensitive dermatosis, often with ocular complications | Basal-cell & squamous-cell carcinomas, melanomas, or sarcomas of skin in nearly all patients exposed to sun |
| Albinism | AR | Absence of melanin pigmentation, with extreme sensitivity to light | Skin cancers, chiefly squamous-cell type, in sun-exposed areas |
| Epidermodysplasia verruciformis | AR | Multiple virus-induced warty lesions | Basal-cell & squamous-cell carcinomas, particularly in sun-exposed areas |
| Polydysplastic epidermolysis bullosa | AR | Extensive bullae, atrophy, scars of skin & membranes, & nail dystrophy | Skin cancers, chiefly squamous-cell type, in scars |
| Dyskeratosis congenita | AR | Skin pigmentation & atrophy, nail dysplasia, & leucoplakia of mucous membranes. Features of Fanconi's anaemia often reported | Squamous-cell carcinomas of skin & mucous membranes |
| Werner's syndrome | AR | Scleroderma-like skin, soft-tissue calcification, growth retardation, cataracts, & shortened life span due to early atherosclerosis or cancer | Soft-tissue sarcomas |

Table 2 (continued)

| Syndromes with Chromosome Instability | Inheritance | Major Features | Neoplasms |
|---|---|---|---|
| Bloom's syndrome | AR | Dwarfism, characteristic facies, & photosensitive telangiectatic erythema on face | Acute leukaemia in 10% of patients |
| Fanconi's syndrome | AR | Constitutional aplastic anaemia & various anomalies (retarded growth, skeletal defects, hyperpigmentation, genitourinary defects, ear deformities) | Acute monocytic or myelomonocytic leukaemia in 10% of patients |
| Syndromes with Immune Deficiency [a] | | | |
| Ataxia-telangiectasia | AR | Cerebellar ataxia telangiectasia of skin & conjunctivae, & recurrent sinopulmonary infections | Cancers, chiefly lymphoreticular tumours, in 10% of patients |
| Wiskott-Aldrich syndrome | SLR | Eczema, thrombocytopenic purpura, & marked susceptibility to infection | Cancers, chiefly lymphoreticular tumours, in 10% of patients |
| Common variable immunodeficiency | ? | Heterogeneous, ill-defined category | Cancers, chiefly lymphoreticular tumors, in 10% of patients |

[a] GATTI and GOOD (37)
AD = autosomal dominant
AR = autosomal recessive
SLR = sex-linked recessive

A new hypothesis about viral spread of a childhood cancer was suggested by the observation in Albany, New York, that Hodgkin's disease appeared to pass not directly from person to person, but through an asymptomatic intermediary (carrier) (26). A scientific design must now be developed to assure that the linking of cases is not attributable to a selective reporting of occurrences in support of the concept.

Opportunities to seek human oncogenic viruses arise when a marked excess is observed in a particular form of cancer in a localized area. An episode of this nature occurred recently in Ankara, Turkey, where 40% of childhood leukaemia was of the acute monomyelogenous type, often associated with chloroma of the eye (27). Normally this cell type accounts for only 5% of leukaemia in children (28). Special virological studies are being made of the affected children in Ankara.

The failure of epidemiological studies to identify human oncogenic viruses does not, of course, signify that they do not exist. The findings indicate that if viruses do play a role, it is too subtle to be detected by the usual methods of epidemiology. Special laboratory screening may be needed. Identification of oncogenic viruses may be easiest in persons at exceptionally high risk of cancer, such as those exposed to known environmental carcinogens, or persons with inborn high risk of specific neoplasms. This thought brings us to the subject of genetic determinants in childhood cancer.

## GENETICS

The inheritance of human cancer has recently been clarified by FRAUMENI (29). A small proportion of cancers may be genetically induced in Mendelian patterns. The mutant gene may be expressed either directly as a hereditary neoplasm (Table 1) or in consequence of a preneoplastic state which carries a high risk of cancer (Table 2) (29).

Hereditary neoplasms. Some cancers are transmitted as autosomal dominant traits. They may be the only manifestation of genetic defect (e.g., bilateral retinoblastoma or intestinal polyposis) or may be part of a systemic disorder with multiple neoplasms or developmental defects (e. g., multiple basal-cell naevoid syndrome or medullary thyroid carcinoma with amyloid struma and phaeochromocytoma). Persons with the abnormal gene usually develop neoplasms (30).

KNUDSON (31) has developed a hypothesis that retinoblastoma, when unilateral and sporadic, involves two events (somatic mutations) after conception, whereas bilateral or familial cases involve only one. This concept derives from his demonstration of a linear decline with age in the percentage of bilateral cases remaining undiagnosed, as compared with a curvilinear decline for unilateral cases. Applying the same rationale to Wilms' tumour, KNUDSON and STRONG (32) found the same relationships. SORSBY (33) has recently published further data on the low frequency (5 - 10%) with which unilateral sporadic retinoblastoma occurs in parent and child as contrasted with the high frequency with which bilateral retinoblastoma is so transmitted. This difference is of importance in genetic counselling.

Hamartomatous Syndromes. Hereditary preneoplastic syndromes may be classified into four categories (Table 2). Hamartomatous syndromes, transmitted as autosomal dominant traits, involve tumour-like malformations in several organs which exhibit faulty differentiation (e. g., tuberous sclerosis). Up to 10% of affected persons develop neoplasms which vary in site with the particular hamartomatous syndrome, brain tumours being the most frequent in multiple neurofibromatosis and in tuberous sclerosis.

Genodermatoses. The genodermatoses are disorders of the skin (e. g., xeroderma pigmentosum) induced by the action of autosomal recessive genes, in which malignant neoplasms of the skin commonly develop. In some of these syndromes, exposure to sunlight increases the risk of skin neoplasia, a circumstance which illustrates an interaction of genetic and environmental determinants of human cancer.

Syndromes With Chromosomal Fragility. Autosomal recessive genes also induce Bloom's syndrome and Fanconi's aplastic anaemia, in each of which there are multiple but dissimilar congenital anomalies. Both, however, are characterized by a marked fragility of chromosomes of lymphocytes in cultures, and a predisposition to leukaemia - acute myelogenous in Bloom's syndrome (34), and acute monomyelocytic in Fanconi's aplastic anaemia (35). Skin fibroblasts from persons with Fanconi's anaemia or from their heterozygous relatives (carriers of the trait) also exhibit increased "malignant" transformation in culture when infected with Simian virus 40 (SV40), a microorganism which induces cancer in certain newborn laboratory animals (36). Results of the transformation test in Bloom's syndrome have not yet been reported, due in part to the difficulty of growing skin fibroblasts in culture from persons with this disorder.

Immunodeficiency Syndromes. Genetically-induced immunodeficiency syndromes predispose principally to lymphoreticular neoplasia, although other neoplasms occasionally have been observed (37). Wiskott-Aldrich syndrome is transmitted as a sex-linked recessive trait, whereas ataxia-telangiectasia (AT) is induced by an autosomal recessive gene. Fibroblasts from some children with AT have exhibited chromosomal fragility on culture (38). About 10% of affected persons develop neoplasia (37), but the frequency must be substantially higher among survivors of the heavy early mortality from infection.

Other categories of immunodeficiency are being defined as laboratory procedures for differentiating them become more sophisticated (39). Some disorders are acquired, either spontaneously or through the use of immunosuppressive drugs after organ transplantation. Again, predisposition to lymphoreticular neoplasia in particular has been observed (39).

Persons with immunodeficiency and high risk of lymphoma are generally not at high risk of leukaemia, although some small overlap does occur (e. g., acute lymphocytic leukaemia has been reported in 5 children with AT including two pairs of sibs (38) ). Skin fibroblasts from patients with inborn immunodeficiency do not show increased transformation by SV40 in culture, as in Fanconi's anaemia (40).

Consanguinity Effect. The influence of rare recessive genes on the occurrence of specific neoplasms can be evaluated by determining if cousin marriage is more frequent than usual among parents of persons with a specific neoplasm. In Japan, where 7% of marriages involve second cousins or closer relationships, a consanguinity effect was found when leukaemia affected sibs (nine of 18 sets of parents were cousins), but not when leukaemia occurred sporadically (41). It would be useful to study other childhood cancers in the same way in Japan.

Twins. A higher concordance rate for a specific neoplasm in monozygotic (MZ) than in dizygotic (DZ) twins may be evidence of a genetic influence. The only childhood cancer with this characteristic, known to date, is leukaemia early in life. The concordance rate is virtually 100% when one of a pair of MZ twins develops leukaemia before his first birthday. As the age at onset in the first twin increases, the co-twin becomes progressively less likely to develop leukaemia. No increase in risk has been detected after about 6 years of age (42, 43). DZ twins, similarly studied, showed essentially no concordance for leukaemia. The disappearance of the effect in MZ twins and its absence in DZ twins suggests that the mechanism was transplantation of leukaemic cells from one MZ twin to the other, while they shared the placental circulation during intrauterine life (44).

Ethnicity. Ethnic differences which persist after migration from one environment to another, suggest genetic influences. Ewing's tumour has a very low frequency in U. S. Blacks (45), and apparently also in African Blacks (46). The difference in rates as compared with U. S. Whites or Europeans suggests that Blacks have a genetic resistance to this form. The same explanation may apply to the absence of a childhood peak in mortality from acute lymphocytic leukaemia among U. S. Blacks, as contrasted with a marked peak among Whites (47). In Japan, pineal tumours have a much greater frequency than is found elsewhere in the world (48). Variations in rates of specific neoplasms in other areas may be due to environmental factors; e. g., high rates of Burkitt's lymphoma and Kaposi's sarcoma in Africa (see Chapter 3), the increased frequency of acute monomyelogenous leukaemia in Ankara, Turkey (27), and low rates of neuroblastoma in Africa (46).

## FAMILIAL CANCER

The clustering of cancer in families, if not due to chance, may be heritable, environmentally induced, or a combination of the two. This section, as distinguished from the preceding one, concerns familial childhood cancer not yet proven to be genetic.

Review of death certificates for 33,437 children who died of cancer in the United States, 1960 - 67, revealed (by matching initially on mother's maiden name) that 8 pairs had brain tumours as compared with 0.9 expected. Genetic disorders which predispose to such neoplasia (e. g., multiple neurofibromatosis or tuberous sclerosis) may have been present but not recorded on the death certificates. One family has been reported in which 8 of 17 members developed brain tumours, possibly due to subclinical multiple neurofibromatosis (49). The death certificates also revealed that in eight families versus 0.9 expected, one child had died of brain tumour and another had succumbed to cancer of bone or muscle. Again, hamartomatous syndromes are suspect, and indeed one of the pairs were known to have tuberous sclerosis.

When soft-tissue cancers occur in siblings, which they do more often than can be attributed to chance, cancer of the breast appears to be more frequent than usual in the mother and other young female relatives (50, 51).

Despite the rarity of adrenocortical neoplasms, they have occurred twice in children whose sibs had rhabdomyosarcoma, and 4 times in children whose close relatives had brain cancer (43). In 4 children, adrenocortical neoplasia and independent brain tumours have occurred as double primaries. These concurrences in the same person or the same family suggest a factor in common in the genesis of the neoplasms involved.

Case reports indicate that Wilms' tumour clusters in some families (52), as does osteosarcoma (53). Neuroblastoma seems less often to be familial (54), although one family has been reported in which 3 children had gross tumours and a fourth had an in situ (microscopic) neuroblastoma (55).

In caring for members of cancer families, the clinician should search more frequently than usual for neoplasms among persons in the line of descent. At research centres, newly developed laboratory procedures can be applied to seek subclinical abnormalities in members of cancer families which may portend predisposition to neoplasia. An example concerns a family in which six members had acute myelogenous leukaemia (AML) and two had malignant reticuloendotheliosis (56). When skin fibroblasts were cultured and infected with the oncogenic virus, SV40, increased transformation was found among fibroblasts from the only survivor with AML, his healthy sib, and mother, but transformation rates were normal for two other sibs and the father. Thus, both the propensity to leukaemia and the susceptibility to transformation of fibroblasts were transmitted through the maternal line. One would want to recommend to the healthy sib with the abnormal skin transformation test that he avoid unnecessary exposure to known leukaemogens, such as ionizing radiation.

## CANCER-MALFORMATION SYNDROMES

In addition to the malformation in hereditary cancer syndromes already discussed, certain nonfamilial malformations carry a high risk of cancer. Some of these are characterized by chromosomal abnormality that arises before conception or soon thereafter. In Down's syndrome (trisomy 21), leukaemia occurs ten or more times more often than usual (3). The childhood peak occurs at 1 year of age, 3 years earlier than the peak in the general population. D- and E-trisomy usually cause early death, yet two children with D-trisomy and leukaemia have been described (47). D-deletion syndrome carries an increased risk of retinoblastoma (57).

Dysgenetic gonads, excluding those in XO Turner's syndrome, are prerequisite for gonadoblastoma (58). Sex chromosome anomalies have not been shown conclusively to predispose to specific neoplasms.

Children with congenital aniridia (bilateral absence of the iris) have about 1000 times the normal risk of Wilms' tumour (52). By 1968, 28 cases had been described in the literature, in all but one of which aniridia was sporadic (59). Usually aniridia is not sporadic; it is inherited as an autosomal dominant trait, and two out of three cases have affected parents. Thus, the aniridia-Wilms' tumour syndrome must be due either to a new mutation or to an environmental agent that mimics the action of a gene. The syndrome also includes cataracts, small head circumference, mental retardation, genitourinary anomalies, and a folding-over of the upper pinnae.

Wilms' tumour is also associated with diverse pre-existent abnormalities of growth: congenital hemihypertrophy in which there is general overgrowth of half of the body or a segment of it; congenital visceral cytomegaly (Beckwith-Wiedemann syndrome), in which the cells of the abdominal viscera are much larger than usual; and hamartomas, a form of benign tumours (47). Apparently, during development different tissues respond in diverse ways to some growth stimulant.

Leukaemia, as already noted, occurs excessively in persons with congenital chromosomal anomalies. The neoplasm is also induced by ionizing radiation (62), and probably by benzene (60), both of which produce long-persisting chromosomal breakage (61, 62). Lymphoma, in contrast, is associated with immunosuppression, either inborn or iatrogenic (37). Neuroblastoma, studied in similar fashion, showed no association with specific malformations or environmental circumstances (54). Thus, each of these major categories of childhood cancer has its own pattern of relationships with congenital anomalies - patterns which suggest that dissimilar processes are involved. Whether the same is true of these neoplasms when not associated with malformations, remains to be determined.

## PERSPECTIVE

This presentation has sought to show the wide spectrum of aetiological information concerning cancer that has been revealed through epidemiological research. Important clues to aetiology, which can be tested epidemiologically, have come from observations made by alert practitioners. The opportunities today in this regard are as great as they have ever been.

Progress in cancer aetiology would be aided if physicians at the bedside would take note of the cancer patient's environmental exposures or family history, and refer unusual findings to an appropriate research centre for assistance in evaluation.

## REFERENCES


1. PEARSON, D., STEWARD, J. K.: Malignant disease in juveniles. Proc. R. Soc. Med. 62, 17-20 (1969)
2. FRAUMENI, J. F., Jr., GEISER, C. F., MANNING, M. D.: Wilms' tumour and congenital hemihypertrophy: report of five new cases and review of literature. Pediatrics 40, 886-899 (1967)
3. MILLER, R. W.: Neoplasia and Down's syndrome. Ann. N. Y. Acad. Sci. 171, 637-644 (1970)
4. DUNLAP, C. E.: Effects of radiation on blood and hemopoietic tissues, including spleen, thymus and lymph nodes. Arch. Pathol. 34, 562-608 (1942)
5. WADA, S., MIYANISHI, M., NISHIMOTO, Y., KAMBE, S., MILLER, R. W.: Mustard gas as a cause of respiratory neoplasia in man. Lancet 1, 1161-1163 (1968)
6. ISHIMARU, T., HOSHINO, T., ICHIMARU, M., et al.: Leukaemia in atomic bomb survivors, Hiroshima and Nagasaki, 1 October 1950 - 30 September 1966. Radiat. Res. 45, 216 - 233 (1971)
7. MILLER, R. W.: Delayed effects occurring within the first decade after exposure of young individuals to the Hiroshima atomic bomb. Pediatrics 18, 1-18 (1956)
8. JABLON, S., TACHIKAWA, K., BELSKY, J. L., et al.: Cancer in Japanese exposed as children to atomic bombs. Lancet 1, 927-931 (1971)
9. HERBST, A. L., ULFELDER, H., POSKANZER, D. C.: Adenocarcinoma of the vagina: association of maternal stilbestrol therapy with tumour appearance in young women. N. Engl. J. Med. 284, 878-881 (1971)

10. ANTHONY, J. J.: Malignant lymphoma associated with hydantoin drugs. Arch. Neurol. 22, 450-454 (1970)

11. STEWART, A., KNEALE, G. W.: Changes in the cancer risk associated with obstetric radiography. Lancet 1, 104-107 (1968)

12. MacMAHON, B.: Prenatal X-ray exposure and childhood cancer. J. Natl. Cancer Inst. 28, 1173-1191 (1962)

13. STEWART, A., KNEALE, G. W.: Radiation dose effects in relation to obstetric X-rays and childhood cancers. Lancet 1, 1185-1188 (1970)

14. JABLON, S., KATO, H.: Childhood cancer in relation to prenatal exposure to atomic-bomb radiation. Lancet 2, 1000-1003 (1970)

15. BRENT, R. L.: Personal communication

16. PIKE, M. C., WILLIAMS, E. H., WRIGHT, B.: Burkitt's tumour in the West Nile District of Uganda. 1961-5. Br. Med. J. 2, 395-399 (1967)

17. MANTEL, N.: The detection of disease clustering and a generalized regression approach. Cancer Res. 27, 209-220 (1967)

18. GLASS, A. G., MANTEL, N., GUNZ, F. W., et al.: Time-space clustering of childhood leukaemia in New Zealand. J. Natl. Cancer Inst. 47, 329-336 (1971)

19. KNOX, G.: Epidemiology of childhood leukaemia in Northumberland and Durham. Br. J. Prev. Soc. Med. 18, 17-24 (1964)

20. TILL, M. M., HARDISTY, R. M., PIKE, M. C., DOLL, R.: Childhood leukaemia in Greater London: a search for evidence of clustering Br. Med. J. 3, 755-758 (1967)

21. MILHAM, S. Jr.: Leukaemia in husbands and wives. Science 148, 98-100 (1965)

22. FRAUMENI, J. F. Jr.: Sex ratio of children born of leukaemic mothers. Pediatrics 33, 587-589 (1964)

23. MILLER, R. W.: The viral etiology of leukaemia: an epidemiologic evaluation. In: Zarafonetis, C. J. D. Proceedings of the International Conference on Leukaemia-Lymphoma. Philadelphia: Lea & Febiger, 1968, pp. 23-29

24. MILLER, R. W.: Down's syndrome (mongolism), other congenital malformations, and cancers among the sibs of leukaemic children. N. Engl. J. Med. 268, 393-401 (1963)

25. HECHT, F., KOLAR, R. D., RIGAS, G. S., et al.: Leukaemia and lymphocytes in ataxia-telangiectasia. Lancet 2, 1193 (1966)

26. VIANNA, N. J., GREENWALD, P., DAVIES, J. N. P.: Extended epidemic of Hodgkin's disease in high-school students. Lancet 1, 1209-1211 (1971)

27. ÇAVDAR, A.O., ARCASOY, A., GÖZDAŞOĞLU, S., DEMIRAĞ, B.: Chloroma-like ocular manifestations in Turkish children with acute myelomonocytic leukaemia. Lancet 1, 680-682 (1971)

28. FRAUMENI, J. F., Jr., MANNING, M. D., MITUS, W. J.: Acute childhood leukaemia: epidemiologic study by cell type of 1,263 cases at the Children's Cancer Research Foundation in Boston, 1947-65. J. Natl. Cancer Inst. 46, 461-470 (1971)

29. FRAUMENI, J. F., Jr.: Genetic factors in the etiology of cancer. In: Cancer Medicine. HOLLAND, J. F., FREI, E. (eds.). Philadelphia: Lea & Febiger, In press

30. ANDERSON, D. E.: Genetic varieties of neoplasia. In: Genetic Concepts and Neoplasia. Baltimore: Williams and Wilkins, 1970, pp. 85-104

31. KNUDSON, A. G., Jr.: Mutation and cancer: statistical study of retinoblastoma. Proc. Natl. Acad. Sci. USA 68, 820-823 (1971)

32. KNUDSON, A. G. Jr., STRONG, L. C.: Mutation and cancer: a model for Wilms' tumour of the kidney. J. Natl. Cancer Inst. 48, 313-324 (1972)

33. SORSBY, A.: Bilateral retinoblastoma: a dominantly inherited affection. Br. Med. J. 2, 580-583 (1972)

34. GERMAN, J.: Bloom's syndrome. 1. Genetical and clinical observations in the first twenty-seven patients. Am. J. Hum. Genet. 21, 196-227 (1969)

35. DOSIK, H., HSU, L. Y., TODARO, G. J., et al.: Leukaemia in Fanconi's anemia: cytogenetic and tumour virus susceptibility studies. Blood 36, 341-352 (1970)

36. TODARO, G. J.: Variable susceptibility of human cell strains to SV40 transformation. Natl. Cancer Inst. Monogr. 29, 271-275 (1968)

37. GATTI, R. A., GOOD, R. A.: Occurrence of malignancy in immunodeficiency diseases. A literature review. Cancer 28, 89-98 (1971)

38. GERMAN, J.: Genes which increase chromosomal instability in somatic cells and predispose to cancer. Prog. Med. Genet. 8, 61-101 (1972)

39. SPECTOR, B. D.: Personal communication

40. KERSEY, J. H., GATTI, R. A., GOOD, R. A., et al.: Susceptibility of cells from patients with primary immunodeficiency diseases to transformation by Simian Virus 40. Proc. Natl. Acad. Sci. USA 69, 980-982 (1972)

41. KURITA, S., KAMAI, Y.: Genetics of familial leukaemia. Jap. J. Hum. Genet. 14, 163-179 (1969)

42. ZUELZER, W. W., COX, D. E.: Genetic aspects of leukaemia. Semin. Hematol. 6, 228-249 (1969)

43. MILLER, R. W.: Deaths from childhood leukaemia and solid tumours among twins and other sibs in the United States, 1960-67. J. Natl. Cancer Inst. 46, 203-209 (1971)

44. CLARKSON, B. D., BOYSE, E. A.: Possible explanation of the high concordance for acute leukaemia in monozygotic twins. Lancet 1, 699-701 (1971)

45. JENSEN, R. D., DRAKE, R. M.: Rarity of Ewing's tumour in Negroes. Lancet 1, 777 (1970)

46. International Union Against Cancer, Committee on Cancer in Children. Unpublished data

47. MILLER, R. W.: Relation between cancer and congenital defects: an epidemiologic evaluation. J. Natl. Cancer Inst. 40, 1079-1085 (1968)

48. ARAKI, C., MATSUMOTO, S.: Statistical re-evaluation of pinealoma and related tumours in Japan. J. Neurosurg. 30, 146-149 (1969)

49. LEE, D. K., ABBOTT, N. L.: Familial central nervous system neoplasia. Case report of a family with von Recklinghausen's neurofibromatosis. Arch. Neurol. 20, 154-160 (1969)

50. LI, F. P., FRAUMENI, J. F. Jr.: Soft-tissue sarcomas, breast cancer and other neoplasms. A familial syndrome. Ann. Intern. Med. 71, 747-752 (1969)

51. LI, F. P., FRAUMENI, J. F. Jr.: Rhabdomyosarcoma in children, epidemiologic study and identification of a familial cancer syndrome. J. Natl. Cancer Inst. 43, 1365-1373 (1969)

52. MILLER, R. W., FRAUMENI, J. F. Jr.. MANNING, M. D.: Association of Wilms' tumour with aniridia, hemihypertrophy and other congenital malformations. N. Engl. J. Med. 270, 922-927 (1964)

53. EPSTEIN, L. I., BIXLER, D., BENNETT, J. E.: An incident of familial cancer. Including 3 cases of osteogenic sarcoma. Cancer 25, 889-891 (1970)

54. MILLER, R. W., FRAUMENI, J. F. Jr., HILL, J. A.: Neuroblastoma: epidemiologic approach to its origins. Am. J. Dis. Child. 115, 253-261 (1968)

55. CHATTEN, J., VOORHESS, M. L.: Familial neuroblastoma. Report of a kindred with multiple disorders, including neuroblastomas in four siblings. N. Engl. J. Med. 227, 1230-1236 (1967)

56. SNYDER, A. L., LI, F. P., HENDERSON, E. S. et al.: Familial acute myelogenous leukaemia: identification of possible inherited leukaemogenic factors in a kindred. Lancet 1, 586-589 (1970)

57. JENSEN, R. D., MILLER, R. W.: Retinoblastoma: epidemiologic characteristics. N. Engl. J. Med. 285, 307-311 (1971)

58. MELICOW, M. M.: Tumours of dysgenetic gonads in intersexes: case reports and discussion regarding their place in gonadal oncology. Bull. N. Y. Acad. Med. 42, 3-20 (1966)

59. FRAUMENI, J. F. Fr., GLASS, A. G.: Wilms' tumour and congenital aniridia. JAMA 206, 825-828 (1968)

60. AKSOY, M., DINCOL, K., ERDEM, S. et al.: Acute leukaemia due to chronic exposure to benzene. Am. J. Med. 52, 160-166 (1972)

61. AWA, A. A., NERIISHI, S., HONDA, T., et al.: Chromosome-aberration frequency in cultured blood-cells in relation to radiation dose of A-Bomb survivors. Lancet 2, 903-905 (1971)

62. FORNI, A., PACIFICO, E., LIMONTA, A.: Chromosome studies in workers exposed to benzene or toluene or both. Arch. Environ. Health 22, 373-378 (1971)

# Chapter 3
# Some Variations in Childhood Cancers Throughout the World
J. N. P. DAVIES

Since 1968 a very marked series of changes have occurred in every aspect of childhood neoplasia. From a rather neglected field (1) it has become one of greatly increased interest. From one of therapeutic depression it has become one of hope as therapeutic success after success is reported, each one bringing calls for earlier diagnosis, centralization of facilities, and controlled trials to improve treatment still further. Indeed, some of these successes have affected the death rates of some cancers (2). International societies of paediatric oncologists have been formed to advance our knowledge by co-operative studies. New cancer entities (3, 4) and syndromes (5, 6) have been described and more details of syndromes of congenital defects and anomalies conducive to cancer have been detected enabling more and more groups of children at especially high risk of developing cancer to be identified (7, 8). The role of irradiation (9, 10) and of drugs administered to the mother in the gestational period producing cancer in the offspring (11, 12) has concentrated attention on the environmental determinants of childhood cancer and led to the recognition of the need for the monitoring of cancer in childhood and early adult life. With the realisation that, in an increasing number of countries childhood cancer is the second commonest cause of death of children over 1 year of age, there is every justification for extending studies of the epidemiology of cancer throughout the world. This is essential for two immediate reasons, firstly to provide that basic information on which childhood cancer can be monitored and secondly because children in different countries and even in different communities in the same country have very different cancer problems. Thus Negro children in the U. S. rarely develop Ewing's sarcoma, in contrast to their white compatriots (13). Indeed, there seems no norm of childhood cancer anywhere.

These differences may provide us with the opportunity of recognizing causative factors in the environment and international studies are being developed by the International Union against Cancer (14) in cooperation with other international agencies and these have evoked a most generous response from collaborators in many countries (16). Much new and important information can be found in Cancer Incidence in Five Continents (15) Vol. II which complements the information in Volume I (16, 1). Many published papers, with increasingly comparable data, have added useful knowledge, and analyses of such data on the worldwide distribution of cancers has provided new insights, as for example into the epidemiology of Hodgkin's disease which in many parts of the world is primarily a paediatric problem (17). Despite this, vast gaps in our knowledge exist and in the majority of the world's children paediatric cancer problems are minuscule compared with those of infection, infestation, and malnutrition. Shortages of facilities, physicians and hospitals, travel difficulties and apathy, indifference and poverty must prevent the majority of childhood neoplasms from coming to medical attention. In less developed communities no demographic baselines exist by which incidence rates can be calculated. Happily, as will be seen, some of these difficulties can be overcome, at least in respect of childhood cancers. But still today a review of the variations of childhood cancer throughout the world can only be tentative and exploratory.

With increasing information however, the difficulties of interpretation also increase. Does an increase or a decrease in cancer, or in a particular type of cancer reported from an area or a community, indicate a change in the pattern, past failure of diagnosis, or a change in histological fashion or terminology? These questions are often difficult if not impossible to answer. No one would contend that vaginal adenosis and adenocarcinoma in young girls in the U. S. had been underestimated or misdiagnosed just because a large series of such cases has been reported recently (12). Indeed, it was precisely because large numbers were suddenly recognized, that an unusual situation was revealed and the cause identified as a synthetic chemical of known historical development and usage. But when such reports come from an underdoctored area the evidence is often ambiguous, in need of most careful interpretation, and should not necessarily be taken at its face value. Leukaemia in African children is a case in point. Initial observations (1, 18, 19) and subsequent studies (20, 21) failed to show that leukaemia occurred in African children with a frequency proportional to that with which it occurs in white children in the U. S. and U. K. The deficiency was solely in children, no comparable lack of cases being detected in adults (22). Later, when it was reported from Uganda that as a result of special investigations more cases had come to be diagnosed in numbers comparable to those seen in white children (23, 24), some instantly deduced that underdiagnosis was responsible for the previously reported deficiencies without considering the numerous discrepancies between the African reports and those from the U. S. and U. K. There were differences in the types of leukaemia and the age and sex of the children. Furthermore, it needed to be realised that the local environment was changing and that Negro children in the U. S. and Japanese children in Japan also showed deficiencies (25, 26, 27, 28, 29, 30) in leukaemia. Similar considerations apply to gliomas in Africa which have long appeared deficient in both adults and children (31, 32, 33). The opening of a neurosurgical service for the Bantu population of Johannesburg led to a vast increase in the neurosurgical work (31) but to no more gliomas being found. As all cases dying at home in cerebral coma were autopsied by the medico-legal services it was possible to confirm that a remarkable deficiency in intracranial tumours did, in fact, exist in the Bantu. When any specialised service opens in an area where it was previously lacking a flush of appropriate cases is seen but it is important to determine if these come from defined areas or are cases harvested from a wide area (32, 33).

## Measurements of the Impact of Childhood Cancer

The annual average incidence rate data from many countries in the world as compiled in cancer registries is documented in the two volumes of Cancer Incidence in Five Continents (15, 16) but the new information does not substantially modify the situation as it was reviewed in 1968 (1). The separation of the 0-1 age group by some registries is advantageous in drawing attention to the special cancer problems of the first year of life. The figures show (Table 1) that the overall highest incidence rates are not necessarily seen in countries in which the other lethal diseases of childhood have been eliminated or controlled. Thus Nigeria (15, 19) and Mozambique (16, 34) have very high rates due to the Burkitt's lymphoma and primary hepatocellular carcinoma which can be hardly other than environmentally determined cancers. Since both tumours develop in the later years of childhood the excess in the

Table 1. Childhood cancers: Average annual incidence rates/100,000 modified from refs. 15, 16

| Area | Ages Males | | | Females | | |
|---|---|---|---|---|---|---|
| | 0- | 5- | 10- | 0- | 5- | 10- |
| Mozambique | 8.3 | 11.1 | 63.8 | 15.6 | 3.6 | 23.5 |
| Nigeria | 13.0 | 30.6 | 24.7 | 6.1 | 13.3 | 13.3 |
| Uganda | 8.8 | 13.6 | 9.7 | 5.1 | 10.4 | 4.8 |
| Rhodesia | 16.2 | 2.1 | 2.8 | 13.6 | 4.4 | 6.0 |
| Jamaica | 13.0 | 13.2 | 9.1 | 11.3 | 9.4 | 7.3 |
| Connecticut | 18.8 | 12.0 | 11.1 | 15.6 | 10.2 | 10.9 |
| Bombay | 6.9 | 6.8 | 6.6 | 5.5 | 4.2 | 5.2 |
| Japan. Miyagi | 13.8 | 7.0 | 8.9 | 10.7 | 3.6 | 6.1 |
| Denmark | 15.6 | 11.7 | 10.2 | 16.0 | 9.5 | 7.5 |
| Sweden | 16.9 | 9.1 | 9.7 | 18.0 | 8.5 | 10.9 |
| Chile | 6.4 | 6.5 | 7.7 | 5.4 | 8.3 | 8.8 |
| Puerto Rico | 12.0 | 8.4 | 8.6 | 9.5 | 5.9 | 5.7 |

first childhood quinquennium which occurs in Western Countries, and is very largely due to acute lymphatic leukaemia, is not seen in these African series where there is an excess, including leukaemia (21), in the third quinquennium.

In the light of the very apparent differences in childhood cancers between countries and communities, the problem of establishing baselines for comparative purposes becomes important and difficult. The modern tendency for children with cancer to be referred to special centres is to be encouraged but it may mean that such children escape the registration network set up in their home areas, even if death ensues, while the centre has much material which is not demographically based.

It is particularly fortunate that this bias has been avoided in the Manchester Children's Tumour Registry and that we have, from a carefully defined population in a single geographical area as complete a collection of childhood neoplasms as can probably be secured from a population of children. Very importantly it has been found that in this locale containing one million children aged under 15 years, 100 childhood neoplasms develop each year with a known distribution of cell types. Where we have defined populations of children, these can be assessed against the Manchester experience. If the population is not so exactly defined, we may use proportional rates for specific tumours (14, 35). Unhappily, but as might be expected, it is those countries without the necessary basic demographic data that seem to provide the most interesting and enlightening comparisons. We could however, gain much insight if there existed an Index Reference tumour which did not vary from community to community in incidence and was uninfluenced by race, sex, climate, or geography. Such a cancer has long been sought and at one time it seemed that retinoblastoma might be such an index cancer occurring as it does in a relatively fixed proportion of the recorded live births (1 to 23-25,000) (36). Unhappily it is now clear that retinoblastoma development is influenced by environmental factors (37) and that in some countries its incidence is increasing rapidly. However, the evidence from Cancer Incidence in Five Continents showed that the Wilms' tumour (14, 38) was occurring in many countries, with children of different races and under very variable climatic conditions, with remarkably constant incidence and it is the only childhood cancer in which such a constancy can be detected. These results have been confirmed in the UICC survey. It might seem strange that the Wilms' tumour which is known to be associated with aniridia, hemihypertrophy, and other defects (39) should have such a constant frequency throughout the world but it seems that such associations are found in only a small minority of those affected (40). Thus it seems that from about each 250,000 children at risk each year, one nephroblastoma will develop. This information can be used as a basis for comparisons within a country, to attempt perhaps to assess the degree of under-reporting (29) or it can be used for intercountry or intercommunity comparisons.

When the ratios of each type of childhood neoplasm to the Wilms' tumour are calculated, remarkable differences are found from country to country in respect of all other childhood tumours (14). The most extreme fluctuations are noted in the leukaemias and these are difficult to assess because of the known diagnostic difficulties, the fact that the diagnosis is often made in haematology departments, and their greater tendency to escape registration. But even if the leukaemias are excluded, the discrepancies are very evident (see Table 2). These are often in

Table 2. Childhood cancers: Average annual incidence rates/100,000 comparisons between selected populations in different areas (16)

| Area | Group | Ages Males | | | | Females | | | |
|---|---|---|---|---|---|---|---|---|---|
| | | 0- | 1- | 5- | 10- | 0- | 1- | 5- | 10- |
| S. Africa | Natal African | 10.0 | 14.2 | 11.7 | 13.8 | 15.6 | 5.7 | 9.1 | 8.7 |
| S. Africa | Natal Indian | 22.8 | 12.1 | 11.4 | 15.8 | 7.7 | 4.0 | 4.7 | 1.7 |
| Canada | Quebec | - | 13.9 | 10.8 | 9.9 | - | 10.1 | 7.0 | 7.5 |
| Canada | Newfoundland | - | 18.2 | 11.5 | 20.1 | - | 19.2 | 9.4 | 15.2 |
| California | White | - | 18.0 | 9.5 | 8.6 | - | 10.4 | 8.1 | 9.3 |
| California | Negro | - | 12.6 | 5.0 | 10.0 | - | 2.5 | 7.9 | 5.4 |
| Texas | Latin | 10.5 | 18.9 | 13.0 | 13.9 | 5.3 | 16.3 | 17.5 | 13.8 |
| Texas | Non-Latin | 0.0 | 16.3 | 6.0 | 16.1 | 4.6 | 5.1 | 5.1 | 8.1 |
| Israel | Israel born | - | 14.6 | 14.4 | 11.9 | - | 12.6 | 9.6 | 11.4 |
| Israel | Africa/Asia born | - | 30.5 | 22.6 | 15.1 | - | 23.0 | 25.0 | 19.5 |
| Israel | Europe/Am. born | - | 40.8 | 28.5 | 19.4 | - | 42.1 | 21.0 | 9.4 |
| Israel | Non-Jews | - | 17.9 | 18.3 | 18.8 | - | 6.7 | 10.3 | 11.3 |
| New Zealand | Europe | - | 17.3 | 11.1 | 10.8 | - | 13.9 | 9.8 | 9.5 |
| | Maori | - | 17.1 | 8.9 | 7.8 | - | 19.9 | 10.3 | 9.8 |
| Hawaii | Hawaiian | - | 23.9 | 7.4 | 11.5 | - | 13.5 | 5.2 | 14.9 |
| Hawaii | Caucasian | - | 15.3 | 11.6 | 14.0 | - | 20.5 | 6.0 | 7.4 |
| Hawaii | Chinese | - | 27.7 | 0.0 | 0.0 | - | 9.9 | 0.0 | 9.7 |
| Hawaii | Filipino | - | 8.7 | 4.9 | 0.0 | - | 4.5 | 21.3 | 0.0 |
| Hawaii | Japanese | - | 11.0 | 8.8 | 12.9 | - | 3.9 | 5.5 | 7.6 |

previously recognised directions as in the excess of lymphomas in African children or of leukaemias in Caucasian children, but a great many previously unsuspected variations are coming to light as in the distribution of neuroblastomas which in Europe shows differences between Eastern and Western countries (14).

## The Leukaemia-Lymphoma-Glioma Complex

In 1968 (1) the disparities reported in the distribution of the leukaemias, lymphomas, and gliomas were discussed at some length. On the then available evidence it seemed that the gliomas and leukaemias, which together make up more than half the childhood cancers in Western countries, were both singularly deficient in other countries and that they appeared to be related in that both seemed either very common, or very deficient, or occurred roughly equivalently and intermediately. Conversely where they were both common, solid lymphomas occurred infrequently; where they were both uncommon, lymphomas were very frequent and where both were intermediate, lymphomas also occurred intermediately. Nothing has really emerged to render these concepts invalid but important developments have taken place in our knowledge of the distribution of these types of childhood neoplasias which warrant their separate consideration.

## Intracranial Tumours and Gliomas

As stated above, a gross deficiency of gliomas and intracranial tumours was noted in the Johannesburg Bantu (31) and the deficiency covered every type of glioma including those seen predominantly in childhood. Examples of all types of tumour have been seen but they occur comparatively infrequently in Africans. The situation in India is not altogether clear. One interesting finding from Israel is that there is a remarkable difference in the incidence of gliomas according to the place of birth (41). Thus in European-born Israelis the average annual incidence of gliomas is 15.6 per 100,000 per annum whereas it is 7.3 per 100,000 for the African-born. Conversely with the lymphomas it is the Africa-born who are at considerably greater risk.

But while the deficiencies reported seem to be in all types of intracranial tumour, there is one which appears in Japanese in remarkably high frequency (42). This is the pinealoma which, in Japanese children, seems to occur at eleven times the incidence that it has in U.S. children. The initial report (42) roused the usual scepticism but this phenomenon is not confined to Japanese in their homeland for of 18 intracranial neoplasms reported in Japanese children in Hawaii 2 were pinealomas which, as MILLER (43) says, shows the value of even small series. The reasons for this remarkable frequency of such an unusual tumour are quite obscure and the geographical and racial limits of the situation have to be explored. Other than this, no specific situations in regard to childhood intracranial tumours seem to be recorded. Attention has recently been drawn to apparent clustering of brain tumours in Kentucky (44).

## Leukaemias and Lymphomas

It is more than ever necessary to consider these separately and together. Both categories comprise numerous and often very dissimilar entities, almost certainly of separate and different aetiologies yet all are linked by an increasingly recognised series of common factors. In all, the histological or the cytological diagnosis can be extremely difficult and often no final conclusion is reached. In tropical regions, infections and infestations, particularly if they are multiple, can cause changes in lymph nodes which are extremely difficult to interpret, particularly as excess of melanin pigment or of fat may be present especially in inguinal nodes. Changes in the bone marrow may be extremely difficult to interpret especially as malnutrition, malaria, infection, and haemoglobinopathies may combine to produce extraordinary leukaemoid reactions. Malnutrition (45, 46) itself may have profound effects on the whole lymphoid system and the body's immune defences. Above all, the enormous pressure on the available paediatric services all too often prevents adequate attention being given to the affected child.

## Childhood Leukaemia

Leukaemia is the major paediatric oncological problem in many economically developed countries and as therapy has improved, larger and larger series of cases are being studied. In all these, there is an immense peak of cases in the 2-4 year age group and it is generally agreed that this is due mostly to acute lymphatic leukaemia or to an undifferentiated type which is probably closely related to it. A series of 1263 cases of acute childhood leukaemia in Boston (47) consisted of 4.0 % acute lymphatic, 24.6% undifferentiated, 23.8% myelogenous, and 7.8% monocytic and this was roughly comparable to a larger series of U. S. children previously analysed though the latter had more undifferentiated and fewer myelogenous cases (48). In the Boston series a difference was noted between the undifferentiated and the acute lymphatic in that the former did not exhibit the gross excess age peak in the young and the survival pattern was intermediate between that of the acute lymphatic and the acute myelogenous. While this Boston series was overwhelmingly composed of children of Caucasian extraction, both the age distribution and the type pattern corresponded closely with that described in Jamaica in children of Negro extraction (49). However, in 1965 (25) the young age peak was not evident in Negro children in the U. S. nor in Japanese children in Japan or the U. S. though in both it is evidently now emerging. There are signs that the pattern of childhood leukaemia in developed countries has been altering in recent times and the incidence rates, at least in Caucasian children, seem to have ceased to rise and may actually have fallen.

Comparison with series in other "Western" countries shows that they conform reasonably well with these American series, as do series from Jamaica (49) and some other countries. But with series in other countries there are considerable differences both in respect of age and type as well as incidence. Thus in Nigeria the incidence rate is estimated at 0.19 per 100,000 per annum (21) and of 89 carefully studied cases of acute leukaemia only 5 were under 5 years of age and the bulk of childhood cases were aged between 10 and 14 years, as had been previously noted (19). In Uganda the incidence rate of leukaemia in children was estimated at 0.5 per 100,000 per annum (30). As in the Nigerian series there were distinct type differences from the American series (Table 2). In Kenya (28) of 19 carefully studied cases of acute childhood leukaemia (Table 3) 12 were acute lymphocytic. The authors noted, as have nearly all who have studied childhood leukaemia in Africa a much greater proportion of myelogenous cases (51), a fair number of which were of the chronic variety and indeed there are quite a number of cases of chronic lymphatic leukaemia. They also noted, as have others (52, 21), the frequency of solid tumour masses in African children with leukaemia. Thus of the 19 Kenya cases (28), 4 had proptosis, 3 of these being due to orbital chloromas; 12 were febrile; 9 had severe anaemia; 3 had

Table 3. The relative frequency of different types of cancer in African and European children (136)

| Diagnosis | Age at notification in years: 0 - 4 A | 0 - 4 B | 0 - 4 (SIR) | 5 - 9 A | 5 - 9 B | 5 - 9 (SIR) | 10 - 14 A | 10 - 14 B | 10 - 14 (SIR) | All ages A | All ages B | All ages (SIR) |
|---|---|---|---|---|---|---|---|---|---|---|---|---|
| Leukaemia | 23 | 671 | (7) | 37 | 375 | (19) | 38 | 258 | (29) | 98 | 1304 | (15) |
| Lymphomas | 131 | 137 | (186) | 493 | 156 | (614) | 288 | 221 | (253) | 912 | 514 | (345) |
| Neural tumours | 36 | 629 | (10) | 27 | 404 | (13) | 16 | 314 | (10) | 75 | 1347 | (11) |
| Other cancers | 302 | 640 | (92) | 142 | 231 | (119) | 185 | 352 | (102) | 629 | 1223 | (100) |
| Leukaemia + lymphomas | 143 | 808 | (37) | 530 | 531 | (194) | 326 | 479 | (132) | 1010 | 1810 | (108) |
| Neural and others | 334 | 1269 | (51) | 169 | 635 | (52) | 201 | 666 | (59) | 704 | 2570 | (53) |
| Total | 488 | 2077 | (46) | 699 | 1166 | (117) | 527 | 1145 | (89) | 1714 | 4388 | (76) |

A. A consecutive series of cancer notifications from Ibadan, Kampala, and Nairobi Cancer Registries (1966-1969)

B. Cancer notifications, England and Wales. The Registrar General's Cancer Supplement 1962-1965

The Standardized Incidence Ratios are shown in parentheses. Standard equals 100

The slight excess (8%) of lymphatic tumours in Series A was accompanied by an 85% deficit in leukaemias, and an 89% deficit of neural tumours. For children under 5 years of age the corresponding figures were 93% and 90% and for children over 10 years they were 71% and 90%. See Ref. 136.

purpura; 5 had bone pains, and 5 had severe renal or intracranial bleeding. The majority of cases had severe lesions which required hospitalisation beyond those of symptomatic anaemia.

However, some have suggested that, among the large number of very anaemic children in Africa, leukaemia is seriously underdiagnosed and that the true incidence approximates to that seen in Western countries (23, 24, 50). Thus in Uganda, VANIER and PIKE (23), by outpatient marrow examinations of children not admitted to hospital diagnosed 9 cases of acute leukaemia in as many months. However, these cases comprised 3 acute lymphatic, 3 acute myeloid, 2 undifferentiated, and 1 lymphosarcoma cell leukaemia. Whatever the time frequency may be, these cell types are not consonant with Western experience.

There is, however, a distinct impression amongst clinicians in tropical Africa that they are now seeing more cases of acute leukaemia and this is especially marked in areas where malaria has been reduced in childhood chiefly by the administration of antimalarial drugs (26). It was long ago suggested that Burkitt's lymphoma might be the biological equivalent in African children of the missing acute lymphatic or undifferentiated childhood leukaemia (51). Some now consider malaria a predominating factor in the development of Burkitt's lymphoma (53, 54) and if it were eliminated the expected result, which seems to have been observed in New Guinea (55), would be a decline in the incidence of the lymphoma. The question has been raised as to whether this would also result in an increase in acute lymphatic leukaemia

(26). The difficulties to be faced in investigating this possibility are great and recent publications suggest that when leukaemia does develop in a Burkitt's lymphoma, as rarely it does, it is of a specific Burkitt's cell type (56, 57). However, with improvement in the paediatric services in Africa we can certainly expect, by European experience, that acute leukaemia will become more common. In England, STEWART and KNEALE (58) showed that children in the pre leukaemia state are particularly liable to die from infection and that reduction in the childhood deaths from pneumonia following the introduction of antibiotics may have been the factor responsible for half the rise in the leukaemia incidence in England in recent decades. In most tropical countries the death rates from infections in childhood are appallingly high. It is thus possible that the apparent deficiency in African children of leukaemias, gliomas, and neuroblastomas is due to the susceptibility of these children in the induction phase to death from infections, or perhaps, in the tropics, malaria may be a major factor. All this increases the urgency of the establishment of baselines.

STEWART and KNEALE (9, 10) have extended their views to other childhood neoplasms. The Oxford Survey of Childhood Cancers produced evidence that gestational irradiation of the foetus not only increased the incidence of childhood leukaemia but of childhood cancer generally, at least of the more specific childhood cancers, and that in Britain they estimated that maternal irradiation produced 6-7% of all childhood cancers. This could not be established for foetuses irradiated by atom bombs in Japan (59) and controversy has ensued over the findings. Indeed, BURCH (60) claims that irradiation in utero may actually reduce the frequency of one type of leukaemia and one type of cerebral tumour. But if the conclusions of STEWART and KNEALE (9, 10) are confirmed, it means that, since the radiogenically produced neoplasms had a later childhood age peak than the non-radiogenically induced and since virtually all in-utero irradiation is given in the last trimester of pregnancy, all non-radiogenic cancers are induced in the first and second trimesters. Therefore they may have relatively long induction periods during which, if leukaemia is a guide, the children may be unduly susceptible to death from infections, and perhaps from infestations such as malaria. If this is so, we may expect the childhood cancer pattern as a whole in tropical countries to change as the general health of children improves and it will be important to watch for these changes.

Turning from the more controversial aspects of childhood leukaemia in the tropics to other aspects of leukaemia, one that has continued to excite attention is the distribution of chloroma and chloroma-like lesions. Since attention was first drawn to the remarkable frequency of chloromas in Uganda (52) they have been reported from many African centres, from Middle Eastern countries (61, 62) and also from India (63). In Nigeria (21) 7% of acute leukaemias had chloromas but these developed in all instances as deposits intracranially or in the spinal meningeal membranes and not in the orbits where they are commonly seen in children in East Africa. In Uganda 8 chloromas were found in 60 orbital tumours of childhood (64). It should be noted that the chloroma may develop as long as a year before there are marrow or blood changes diagnosable as leukaemia (65) and it is by no means uncommon for there to be no blood changes when the tumour develops even if there are changes in the marrow. The reasons why chloromas are so frequently seen in some populations are obscure, but are probably connected with socioeconomic factors. However, they must also be related to biological factors since in African children with acute lymphatic leukaemia orbital masses may develop; 1 in 11 such cases in Kenya (28).

This tendency is not restricted to Africa. The largest series of chloroma-like ocular lesions in association with leukaemia has been reported from Turkey by ÇAVDAR et al. (61) who, in children under 14 years of age, recorded 84 cases of acute leukaemia; 34 were of the acute myelomonocytic type, 12 (35%) of whom had ocular lesions which included orbital tumours, exophthalmic proptosis, chemosis, corneal opacities, and swollen eyelids. The lesions were not true chloromas as they lacked the typical green colouration but in all there was tissue swelling due to leukaemic infiltration. Again the reasons why this particular type of leukaemia and this association with tumour lesions should be so common in Turkish children awaits explanation; indeed it has yet to be established that it is peculiar to Turkey and is not present in neighbouring countries. However, the myelomonocytic type of leukaemia has been increasingly recognised in recent years and has peculiarities. It is claimed to be the commonest form of leukaemia seen at the Mayo Clinic in recent years (66). It has been seen in children with Bloom's syndrome and Fanconi's anaemia (67). In myelo-monocytic leukaemia, tumourous lesions may be due to xanthomatous masses (6). This type of leukaemia has a tendency to develop in adults as a complication of multiple myeloma and other neoplastic conditions and the existence of a pre-leukaemic phase, detectable both clinically and haematologically and possibly lasting for many years, has been recognised (68). It is now evident that an unusual situation exists in children in Turkey and probably in other Middle Eastern countries and the time is ripe for a thorough exploration of childhood leukaemia in these regions.

Beyond the association with irradiation the other causes of acute leukaemia in childhood remain obscure. A statistical association with maternal influenza has been reported (69) and there is a known association with a number of chromosome abnormalities in children, congenital or acquired (70). The association with Down's syndrome has been much studied, with some conflicting results (71). It seems undisputed that the leukaemias that do develop in Down's syndrome involve all types and are comparable with those which develop in unaffected children. In Manchester the incidence of leukaemia in Down's syndrome is 10-18 times greater than in the normal child population and acute lymphatic leukaemia is the most common type (72). Elsewhere it is claimed that the incidence is no higher and that the main difference between the normal and affected children lies not in the incidence of leukaemia but that children with Down's syndrome develop a transient myeloid leukaemoid reaction rarely seen in normal children (71). Clearly until these differences are sorted out in developed countries little progress can be expected. But this controversy reminds us of the importance of leukaemoid reactions which are so common in African children.

The world distribution of leukaemia is a subject which needs looking into again, including countries in which there has been much past investigation. The re-examination requires both clinical and pathological scrutiny of the incidence. In Africa there have been reports, not only of the greater frequency of chronic leukaemias and of tumourous leukaemic manifestations but also marked differences in the clinical features. Thus in lymphatic leukaemia attention (27) has been drawn to the greater degree of splenomegaly and the lesser degree of lymphadenopathy as well as the tendency to form extra osseous and extra nodal masses.

## Childhood Lymphomas

In 1968 (1) many aspects of Burkitt's lymphoma were discussed in detail but in view of the many published accounts of this cancer such detailed consideration is no longer required and only certain aspects will be discussed. This disease continues to occur in many parts of Africa with remarkable frequency. It would seem that a number of tumour hot spots occur, e. g., round Ilesha in Nigeria. The recognition of the Epstein-Barr virus and the evidence that continues to incriminate further herpes viruses as oncogenic agents gave hope that the aetiological importance of the E. B. virus would be speedily established

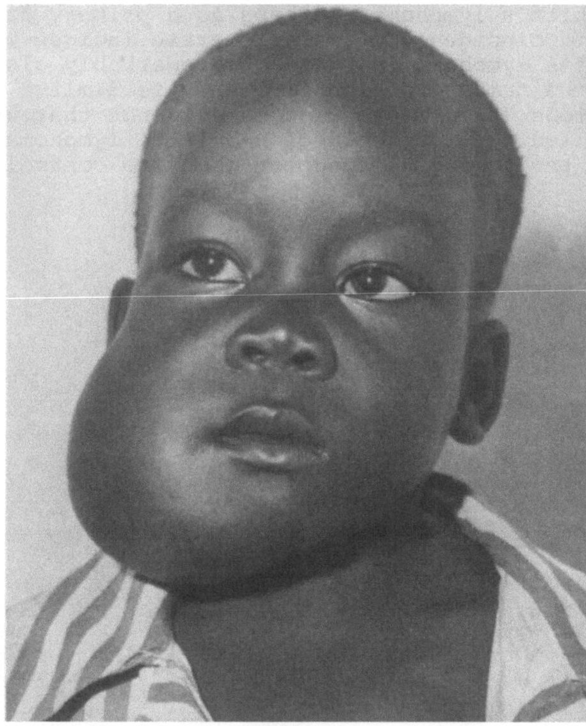

*Fig. 1. African child. Burkitt's lymphoma involving maxilla and mandible*

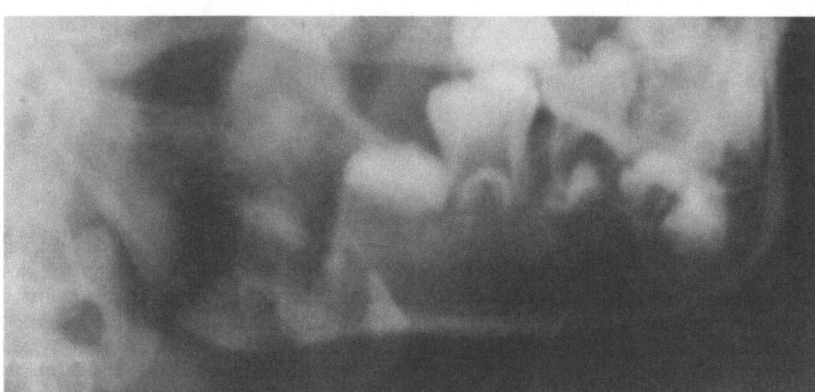

*Fig. 2. X-ray of mandible showing radiolucencies. Burkitt's lymphoma*

and its role is strengthened by the serological evidence of its presence in every North American case of Burkitt's lymphoma (74). It is established that the E. B. virus can produce cell transformation. However, it is also closely associated, perhaps causally, with infectious mononucleosis and nasopharyngeal carcinoma, while it seems that its association with Hodgkin's disease, chronic lymphocytic leukaemia, sarcoidosis and lupus erythematosus is less close and may only represent reactivation of latent E. B. virus due to the depression of cell-mediated immunity which is seen in all those states (75). The other factor suspected of playing a part in the pathogenesis of Burkitt's lymphoma, perhaps as a primary factor, is malaria (53, 54, 76). Coincidence of malariometric indices with the incidence of Burkitt's lymphoma in Uganda is remarkably close (77) and the occurrence of the tumour in high frequency is limited to holoendemic malarial regions (53). There is some evidence that where malaria has been controlled the incidence of Burkitt's lymphoma has rapidly fallen only for the tumour to reappear when the control has lapsed (94).

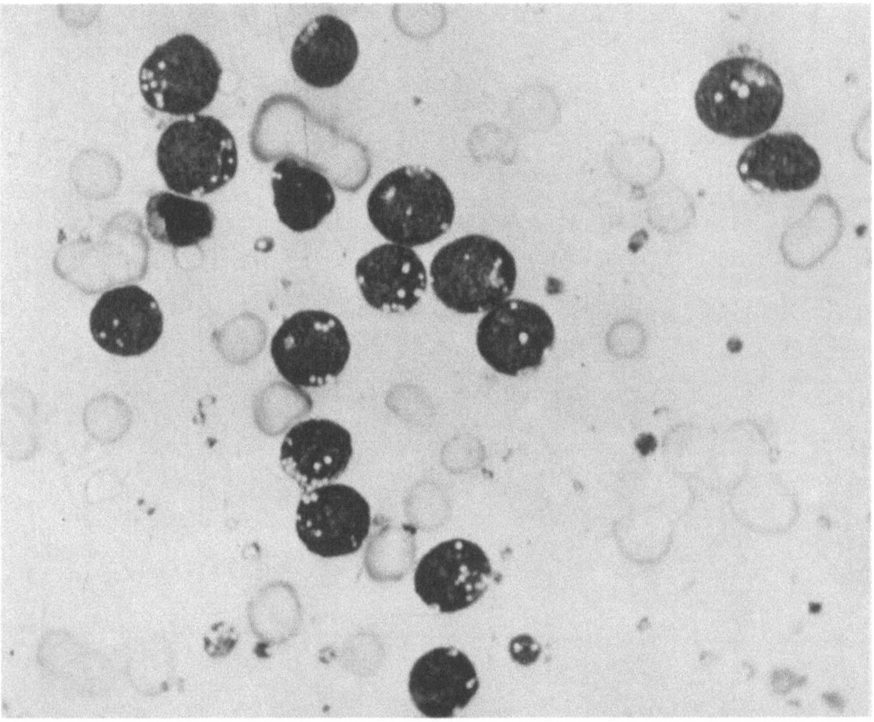

*Fig. 3. Burkitt's lymphoma. Imprint preparation. Stained Giemsa to show fine cytoplasmic fatty vacuolation. Courtesy Dr. D. H. WRIGHT, Kampala and Mr. R. TUNNICLIFFE, F.I.M.L.T.*

In the W. Nile district of Uganda virtually all children have positive E. B. antibody titres by the age of 2 years (83), though some may lose these later. However, the suggestion that Burkitt's lymphoma, which is a rare phenomenon, is due to the conjunction of two common factors, malaria and the E. B. virus, is difficult to square with other epidemiological evidence. In both the W. Nile and the Bwamba districts of Uganda, Burkitt's lymphoma has behaved in epidemic fashion occurring in a relatively brief outbreak in the Bwamba region, and showing "epidemic drift" over several years in the W. Nile district with local outbreaks occurring at a few months interval between successive clus-

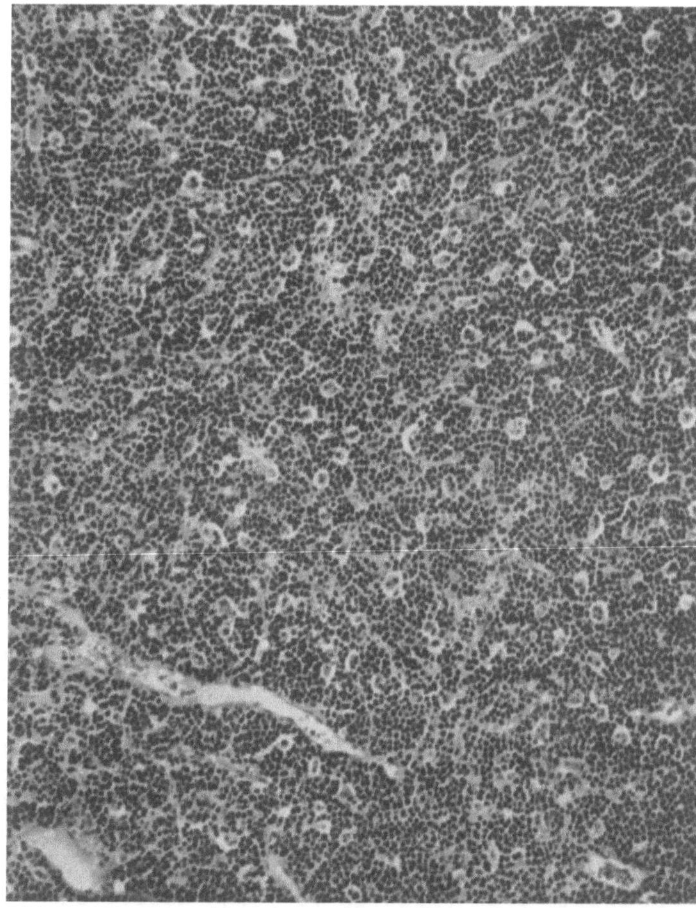

*Fig. 4. Histological appearance of Burkitt's lymphoma in African child showing marked "starry sky" effect. H. & E. Magn. approx. x 65 Courtesy of Dr. D. H. WRIGHT of Kampala and Mr. R. TUNNICLIFFE, F.I.M.L.T.*

tered cases (78). However, in other areas these time-space clusters have not been observed. All this would suggest that some additional factor is necessary to trigger off lymphoma development in children who may be infected with the E. B. virus and have malaria, or whose R. E. system may have been conditioned by some other factor in non-malarial areas. Cyto- and histo-logically Burkitt's lymphomas in non-malarial areas (79) are similar to those in malarial areas but there is a lesser tendency to develop jaw tumours and a greater tendency to develop diffuse marrow involvement with a leukaemic termination which may be of Burkitt's lymphoma-like cells (56, 57). The remarkable therapeutic successes of chemotherapy in this condition are, however, the most happy features of this disease.

## Hodgkin's Disease

In Western countries Hodgkin's disease has long been known to exhibit a bi-modal age peak, one in young adults and the other in old people. In pointing this out MacMAHON (80) noted that reports from some countries suggested that they might have a further peak in childhood. He further suggested that under the term Hodgkin's disease perhaps two or three aetiologically different entities were being concealed. Attempts to probe further into the fruitful suggestions of MacMAHON have enormously increased our knowledge of Hodgkin's disease. Reports from many countries (17) have shown that often many cases occur in children, and indeed the disease in these countries may be mainly a paediatric problem. Clinical studies have shown that in countries where the disease is common it is more advanced on presentation, even though diagnosis had not been delayed, and it behaves more aggressively than in countries where the disease is uncommon in childhood (81). Correspondingly histological studies showed that the more disseminated aggressive disease showed a far higher proportion of the prognostically less favourable RYE classification subtypes (82).

Hodgkin's disease thus varies, in both adults and children, from country to country and one determinant of this is the socioeconomic level. Where this is low, as in many African and S. American countries, the disease peaks in children and the young adult age peak is missing but in countries with high socioeconomic development the disease in children is uncommon and there is a pronounced young adult age peak (17). In such countries an intermediate pattern may occur in rural areas and this is seen in Southern states of the U. S. In such an advanced community the disease is most likely to affect members of the most affluent sections of society.

It is evident that, in these manifestations, Hodgkin's disease is different from all other childhood cancers although some parallels can be found with Burkitt's lymphoma and the leukaemias. The suggestion of MacMAHON (80) that there might be two or more distinct entities cannot be ruled out but the fact that the same range of histological types is found at all ages and all areas suggests that the differing manifestations of the disease are related to the resistance of the affected patient rather than to different aetiological factors and that these may be related to HLA type, to sex and to other unknown factors. With economic and social improvement the major impact of the disease shifts from children to young adults and there is a shift in the histological subtypes to those of more favourable prognosis especially in the females who so often develop the nodular sclerosing type. The unfavourable male sex differential obtains under all circumstances, so far known, in children (84) as in adults but MILLER (85) noted in the U. S. a more abrupt increase in the number of females affected in the later years of childhood which reduced but did not eliminate the male excess since the incidence rates for both sexes were increasing rapidly in this age group. It was suggested that this might be related to the normal involution of the lymphoid apparatus of Waldeyer's Ring which is a feature of late childhood. There are indications that surgically induced lymphoid tissue involution, as by tonsillectomy and appendectomy, results in an increased liability to develop Hodgkin's disease (86). Evidence has been produced that the disease may produce a long lasting epidemic (87). In such epidemics both case-to-case and case-to-contact-to-case spread seem to occur with an incubation period of over 3 years. Contacts, who remain healthy, seem more important than cases in spreading the disease. This is a feature of infectious mononucleosis, which seems to have some obscure connection with Hodgkin's disease (and of some other virus diseases). Thus with this very cosmopolitan disease, the paediatric oncologist may expect to see startling differences in frequency and in manifestations and behaviour from country to country. Happily, even with advanced progressive histologically unfavourable disease the response to adequate chemotherapy alone may be remarkably good. The 5 year survival of 24 Uganda children so treated projected actuarily was 89% and the 2 children who died did not die of Hodgkin's disease (81).

## Lymphosarcoma and Histiocytic Sarcomas

Compared with the increased information on the epidemiology of Burkitt's lymphoma and Hodgkin's disease, little information has come forward on the epidemiology of the lympho- and histiocytic sarcomas. Certainly the latter, in children as in adults, can be divided into the more uniform histioblastic type, with its tendency to develop . leukaemic manifestations, and the histiocytic of less uniform cytology and of different behaviour. It seems to be well appreciated that there occurs, albeit uncommonly in children, lymphosarcomas arising in nodal tissues which remain localised without leukaemic manifestations developing even till death ensues.

For some years reports have been coming from the Arab world and from Israel (88) of a high frequency of abdominal lymphomas, variously diagnosed as lympho- or reticulum cell-sarcomas, developing in children and young adults often in association with malabsorption states. In Western countries, primary gastrointestinal lymphomas are found as solitary masses usually in the terminal ileum of children or as diffuse widespread multifocal deposits in elderly adults many of whom have suffered for years from a sprue-like condition. For such a diffuse lymphomatous pattern to be seen in a child in a Western country is very unusual but it is by no means uncommon in children living in Eastern Mediterranean regions and in some other parts of the world where children are poor and ill-nourished and liable to repeated intestinal infections. RAMOT (88) summarises it by saying that the diffuse intestinal lymphoma in Israel affects chiefly teenagers and young adults, without any sex preponderance and with involvement of the proximal rather than the distal small intestine. It is not associated with a long antecedent sprue-like condition though clinically cases often present as a malabsorption syndrome and in the early stages there is a marked plasma cell infiltration of the gut and a heavy chain IgA paraproteinaemia. However, the morphology of the lymphomas that develop is very variable, in contrast to the uniformity of Burkitt's lymphoma, and includes Hodgkin's disease, lymphosarcoma and histiocytic sarcoma. Little is so far known about the world-wide distribution of this interesting syndrome or of the aetiological factors that produce it.

Much recent study has tended to show the importance of the extranodal accumulations of lymphoproliferative cells in neoplastic development, no matter how these are produced or maintained. By and large in children, the neoplasms of the reticuloendothelial system seem to be largely of nodal development, the great exception being Burkitt's lymphoma.

## The Progressive and Non-progressive Histiocytoses

No very satisfactory system of nomenclature is at present applied to this rather disparate group of conditions which are not easily identified and distinguished either histologically or clinically. Nor are the boundaries which separate reaction from neoplasia clearly defined. In some of these conditions the histiocytes phagocytose some abnormal product that is being stored in the body and several of these entities have been distinguished. In one such condition, or group of conditions, a variety of names have been applied and identifications made which may be premature (89). This is the condition which, in young children, is a progressive lethal histiocytosis with skin lesions and termed Letterer Siwe disease and in older children is called Hand-Schuller-Christian disease especially when it produces all the major components of the classic syndrome. It has also been identified as the same condition described as eosinophilic granuloma of bone. This identification has never been satisfactory to some and has recently been severely criticised (89). An alternative name applied to the lymph node lesions is histiocytosis X. While detailed consideration of this condition is not called for, it would appear that there are very considerable geographic differences in the frequency with which histiocytosis X is diagnosed in children.

In histiocytosis X the material phagocytosed is lipid. There are a number of conditions described in which, for unknown reasons, the histiocytes phagocytose cells or red blood corpuscles or both with resultant lymphadenopathy and perhaps hepatosplenomegaly which may be massive. ROSAI and DORFMAN (90) have described a febrile benign lymphoma, in which the lymphadenopathy is massive and the sinus histiocytes engulf lymphocytes, plasma cells, and red blood corpuscles. The histiocytes may be large, multinucleated, and show various changes of atypia but mitoses are not seen and after some years of progression or stability the glands slowly subside. The cause is unknown and the disease seems to have a special predilection for the cervical nodes and for Negro children. It is an uncommon disease, or so it appears, but it may be more common in Africa for TEMPLETON recorded 4 cases in 6 months in Uganda (90).

Obviously this is quite different from the well-recognised condition of histiocytic medullary reticulosis which also occurs in Negro children in Uganda with some frequency since 5 children were included in a report of 14 cases (91). It is often mistakenly diagnosed as acute Hodgkin's disease and it pursues a rapid relentless course with fever, lymphadenopathy, hepatosplenomegaly, and with the histiocytes actively phagocytosing and destroying red blood corpuscles. It may follow acute leukaemia (92). It does not respond to any therapy and the late stages are dominated by extreme anaemia. The cause is unknown. It is especially curious that whereas in the benign condition described by ROSAI and DORFMAN (90) the phagocytosed cells are of varied type, the red cells alone are engulfed in histiocytic medullary reticulosis. In addition, to complicate matters still further there are other histiocytic proliferative conditions in which erythrophagocytosis is seen but which do not behave in the malignant manner of histiocytic medullary reticulosis (89). Until we have much more information on all these conditions and they are more widely recognised we cannot say much about their geographical distribution except that they seem to be more common in tropical regions.

## Kaposi's Sarcoma

In children in Africa the polylymphadenopathic form of Kaposi's sarcoma can mimic Hodgkin's disease to perfection, producing soft rubbery elastic lymph nodes together with obstructive and compression syndromes from enlargement of internal lymph nodes (1). In African children about 20% of children presenting with generalised lymphadenopathy turn out to be cases of Kaposi's sarcoma and these form about 3 % of all childhood cancers. SLAVIN et al. (93) were able to report on no less than 53 cases in East African children alone. In general their experience was similar to that of previous workers except that they considered that salivary and lacrimal gland involvement producing a Mikulicz syndrome was more likely to be due to involvement of the lymphoid tissue in the neighbourhood of the glands than of the secretory gland parenchyma. They noted how the mode of presentation varied with age, the younger the child the greater the tendency both to lymphadenopathy and to absent or sparse and usually oddly distributed, skin lesions. The lymph nodes in the young children continuously enlarge

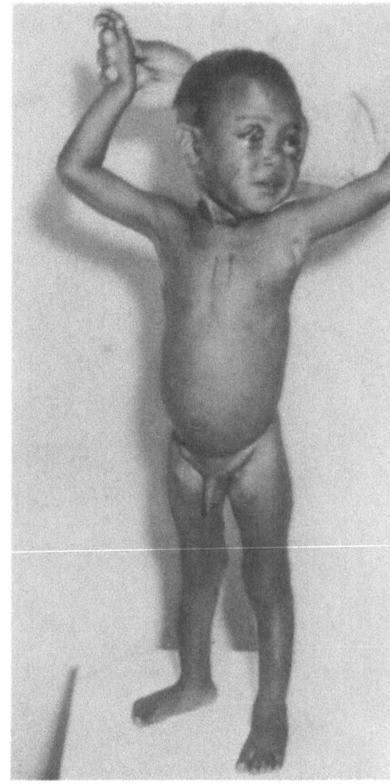

*Fig. 5. Kaposi's sarcoma in Uganda child aged 2 years (KCR 462/58), showing generalised lymphadenopathy and involvement of eyelids*

and later become matted, adherent, and haemorrhagic; but, in older children, progression is often much more limited and nodal lesions may regress. In older children too the distribution of skin lesions corresponds to that seen in adults. If a typical skin lesion is present, even in an unusual site, a clinical diagnosis can be made but more commonly biopsy of an enlarged node shows that the gland is replaced by the angiomatous and spindle-cell components of Kaposi's tissue. No specific histological differences can be seen between adult or childhood Kaposi's tissue or between those pursuing a fulminant or an indolent course. In the more aggressive type of lesion a greater degree of cellular pleomorphism and more mitoses are seen (95). Nor can any histological differences be recognised between different racial groups in their response. However, in childhood the male to female ratio is only about 3 : 1 as opposed to about 20 : 1 in adults. In females, particularly if young, the disease tends to run a very fulminant course. A detailed study of the pathology of Kaposi's sarcoma largely based on African experience has been made by TEMPLETON (95).

The nodal form of Kaposi's sarcoma is being increasingly recognised in African children while the frequency with which it affects children in other tropical countries is not fully known because it may well be underdiagnosed. Cases, in Africa and elsewhere, have been found under the labels of angiofibromas, metastasising angiomas, and even fibrosarcoma. It is a tumour in which both adults and children develop identical histological lesions but with very different bio-

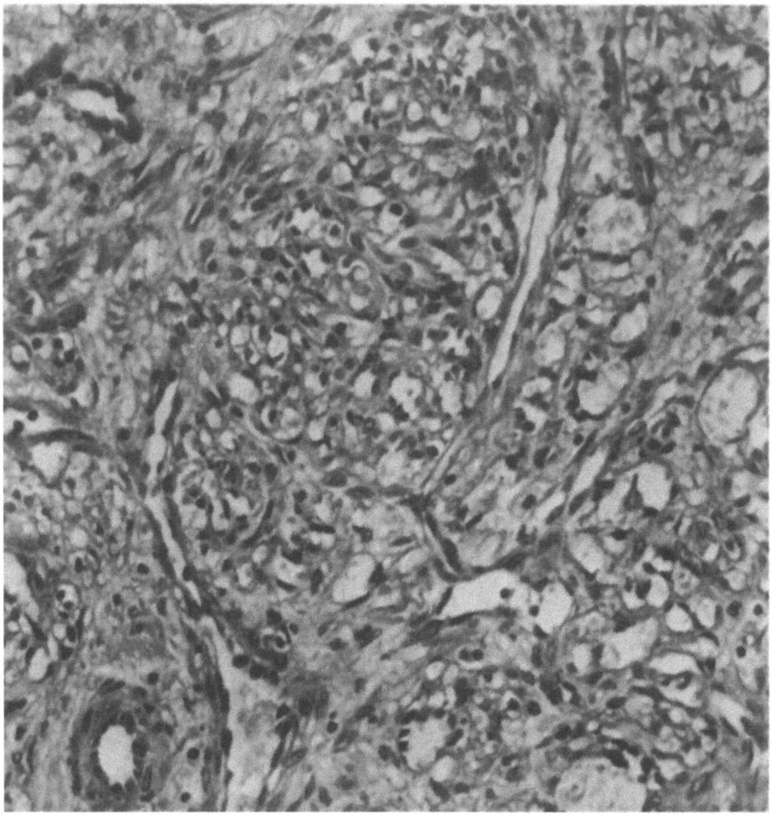

*Fig. 6. Histologic appearance of lymph gland from child shown in Fig. V. Gland entirely replaced by Kaposi tissue. H. & E. stain. Magn. x 65 approx.*

logical behaviour. No genetic causes have been identified and the uneven distribution in Africa points to the importance of environmental factors, none of which have as yet been identified. There seems a tendency in Africa for the more atypical cases to appear in areas where the disease is less common in the community. At the same time there is a lesser tendency for the African patient with Kaposi's sarcoma to develop any second primary neoplasm, especially of the reticuloendothelial system (95, 96), such as Hodgkin's disease, as is common elsewhere. It is debatable whether Kaposi's sarcoma itself causes a state of immunodepression which can render sufferers liable to develop another cancer or some lethal infection but it has developed in a renal transplant patient who was immunodepressed (97). The cell of origin is disputed; cell cultures show predominant growth of fibroblastoid and epithelioid cells and recent evidence has indicated the possible importance of a herpes-type virus (98). Again this is a tumour in which radiotherapy and chemotherapy are remarkably effective. Many have argued that Kaposi's sarcoma is a disease of reticuloendothelial system origin and this recent evidence perhaps strengthens the case.

The lymphomas cannot as yet be aetiologically defined but more and more evidence points in childhood to the importance of immune deficiency states, congenital and acquired, and to the oncogenic importance of the herpes-type viruses that are increasingly being identified. There is evidence to suggest that malaria can produce a state of acquired partial immune deficiency and again it is suggested that malaria may play a role in the distribution of Kaposi's sarcoma in Africa as it may do with Burkitt's lymphoma.

## Neuroblastomas

Neuroblastomas have attracted much attention especially since their elaboration of a number of catecholamines and their derivatives has been recognised. In contrast to the many clinical and chemical studies is the paucity of epidemiological studies (99). It is now evident that geographical variations are very significant though the high proportion of cases misdiagnosed, in the absence of chemical confirmation, can obscure this. Thus at one time neuroblastomas were believed to be very common in African children but with the recognition of Burkitt's lymphoma they were found to be very uncommon cancers in Africa and every series has confirmed this (14). There is an even greater paucity of ganglioneuroblastomas and ganglioneuromas which are accepted as differentiated neoplasms developing from neuroblastomas under circumstances not yet defined. In Asian series the frequencies of these tumours is above that of African series but well below those recorded in Western countries. Even in Europe there seem differences for, while the Manchester experience of 101 neuroblastomas (111 if ganglio-neuromas are included) to 82 nephroblastomas corresponds with experience in other Western European countries, there is an excess, often considerable, of nephroblastomas over neuroblastomas in Eastern Europe as in Africa and parts of South America.

No reasons for these discrepancies can be adduced but there are some very unusual features of neuroblastomas which are being studied and deserve further study in different communities. At autopsy in many children dying before 3 months of age small, *in situ* foci of neuroblastomas can be identified but thereafter they can rarely be found (100). Children who develop clinically recognisable neuroblastomas in the first year of life have an appreciable rate of spontaneous regression and a much better prognosis for those that do not regress spontaneously and it has been suggested that in situ neuroblastomas are probably present in many children but the majority regress. The causes of regression are not known but do not seem to involve the nerve-growth factor of LEVI-MONTALCINI.

An epidemiological study of 1535 children dying from neuroblastomas and of 504 clinical cases in the U. S. was reported by MILLER et al. (99). There was a greater frequency in whites than in non-whites which might reflect differences in diagnostic accuracy or be due to a racial factor in view of the infrequency of neuroblastomas in African children. Only 27 neonatal deaths from neuroblastoma were found, 13 of which occurred on the first day of life. In sharp contra-distinction to other types of childhood neoplasia common in the first year of life there was no significant association with specific congenital defects or anomalies. There was a suggestion of a link with skull and brain defects but no relationship to cardiac, gastrointestinal, genitourinary or skeletal malformations or to other types of neoplasms in siblings, or in the family concurrently or sequentially. No excess of summer deaths was found but there were year to year variations in deaths in some groups of states. This was not a local phenomenon in a state but occurred in a group of states. Another finding was a fall in the male preponderance in children under 5 years of age in successive years in 1960-1964.

We thus require much more information on the epidemiology of neuroblastomas which seem to be conditioned by undetermined prenatally acting environmental factors. No group of survivors seems to have been followed into child-bearing age. It would seem that, without chemical confirmation the disease should be diagnosed with hesitation (101) especially in persons of African descent.

## Retinoblastomas

Contrasted with the paucity of neuroblastomas in many series from less developed parts of the world, especially from India and Africa, are the seeming plethora of retinoblastomas but this requires caution in interpretation because of the likelihood that retinoblastomas are brought comparatively more frequently to medical attention because of the unpleasant lesions of the late stages when the eye is fungating and destroyed. In most countries facilities for expert radiotherapeutic help are lacking, the disease is usually lethal within a few months and none survive to have children of their own. But where these patients are cured the frequency with which survivors produce affected children is only about 15% and it therefore follows that the sporadic non-familial retinoblastomas are not the result of new mutations producing autosomal dominant genes, as had been supposed, but must be due to some other factor in the environment (37).

In many countries the tumour develops in about one in every 23 - 25,000 live births. There is an impression that it occurs more commonly in some racial groups but in no instance does this seem to be adequately established statistically. The fact that there is a very much greater mortality peak for Negro children as compared to white in the U. S. (2.5 times) seems to be mainly due to delayed diagnosis (102) since fewer diagnoses in Negro children were made in the first year of life and more in the 1-4 year age group (37). Study of a large series of 1578 cases in the U. S. (37) showed that only a very small minority of cases had congenital anomalies or major malformations, the latter only occurring in 53 children. Of the children without major malformations 57% had bilateral retinoblastomas. A total of 6 children had the malformations described in the D-deletion syndrome but only one defect, severe mental retardation not secondarily related to the tumour or its treatment, significantly exceeded expectation. Others have commented on the high mental status of some retinoblastoma victims.

It is a tragedy if delayed diagnosis is the cause of the excess Negro mortality in the U. S. because with early diagnosis, treatment is happily highly effective - thus it was estimated that nationally in the U. S. 81% of retinoblastoma victims survived. But in some cases there may be a histological reason for radio-resistance and considering how long and how much attention has been given to retinoblastomas it is astonishing that only in 1968 did TS'O et al. (103) show that there were photo-receptor element cells present in some retinoblastomas (found in 18 of 300 retinoblastomas examined) which differed histologically both from the undifferentiated retinoblastoma cells and from the cells in the various types of rosettes. These photo-receptor cells which seemed less anaplastic and more differentiated were found to be more resistant to radiotherapy and their presence explained the greater degree of resistance to irradiation in some retinoblastomas (104). The distribution of the photoreceptor cells in retinoblastomas throughout the world needs to be assessed.

Retinoblastomas are notoriously associated with other malignant neoplasms developing in the irradiated areas. Thus SAGERMAN et al. reported 21 such cases including several osteosarcomas and other sarcomas and some carcinomas (105). JENSEN and MILLER (37) reported a further 9 but also noted 11 other children with retinoblastomas in whom further neoplasms developed in areas that had not been irradiated or in children who never received radiotherapy. These included three osteosarcomas of the femur and three brain tumours and raised the question as to some innate susceptibility of patients with retinoblastomas to develop other cancers, notably osteosarcomas, irrespective of irradiation.

In many less developed countries, not only retinoblastomas but also other orbital tumours are often brought to clinical attention in a very advanced state. The differential diagnosis needs to be established as rapidly as possible and presents considerable difficulties. However, the need has become even greater as chemotherapy has proved extremely successful with some orbital tumours but much less so with others. A series of papers from various African centres (64, 106, 107, 108) on oculo-orbital tumours have enormously clarified the situation on that continent and similar series need to be studied in other areas. All the African studies emphasise the high local frequency of oculo-orbital tumours compared with intracranial ones and stress the predominance of limbal carcinomas, retinoblastomas, lymphomas, and in some areas leukaemic tumour masses. In all series there is a great infrequency of intra-ocular melanomas. TEMPLETON (64) studied 60 orbital tumours in children in Uganda of which 28 were Burkitt's lymphomas and 8 were chloromas and provided details for their histological differentiation. The diagnosis of a chloroma by histology alone may be extremely difficult as it may closely resemble a histiocytic lymphoma and blood and bone marrow changes may in some cases not have developed. To separate Burkitt's lymphoma and retinoblastoma may only be possible in advanced cases by the fine dystrophic calcification seen only in retinoblastomas. Curiously, TEMPLETON encountered only one orbital rhabdomyosarcoma, so common in children in Western countries (109) and in Nigeria (107) in a large series of oculo-orbital tumours no chloromas were seen, all being intracranial (21).

## Nephroblastomas

We have now, as mentioned above, most important information on the epidemiology of nephroblastomas, namely, that of all childhood cancers these show the least variation in frequency from country to country, continent to continent and this constancy is a feature of all racial groups (14, 38). A minority of cases only, but a very interesting one, are associated with congenital defects, aniridia, hemi-hypertrophy, hypospadias, cryptorchidism, and horseshoe kidney (39). No features of birth characteristics were found which seemed to influence nephroblastoma formation and very few cases have occurred in identical twins. Any associations can but affect a minority of cases and this tumour arises, for unknown reasons, with such a remarkably constancy over all the world that it can be used as an Index Cancer to which all other neoplasms are related.

This, and the excellent response to therapy, increases the need for accuracy of diagnosis. In early life it must be differentiated from the benign renal tumour (3) to which a variety of names have been given, "Fibrosing Hamartoma" being the most popular. At the other extreme of childhood, sarcomas of the kidney are reported in some numbers in some countries in the third quinquennium (41) and there is dispute as to whether these are nephroblastomas or more closely related to the carcinosarcomas of the kidney occasionally seen in adults. Similarly, distinction must be made between nephroblastomas and the renal tumours, often bilateral and massive, which develop from leukaemic or lymphomatous renal involvement, as well as from the true renal carcinomas (110) which occur with some frequency in some countries.

## Connective Tissue Tumours and Non-Embryonal Childhood Sarcomas

There is no doubt that connective tissue tumours occur in children with a fairly high frequency, perhaps 10% in most series. However, they consist of a large number of different types and with greater subdivision both classification and comparison become more difficult and discussions degenerate into anecdotal pathology. Even in adults these tumours present great difficulty in diagnosis and classification. Far too little has so far been published on the epidemiology of most of these types. It seems that the fibromatous tumours of childhood are more commonly seen in centres in less developed countries but whether this is due to culling or to a genuine increase in frequency is uncertain. The microepidemiology of rhabdomyosarcomas has been explored especially in relation to the so-called familial sarcoma syndrome (111) and the recognition of a rhabdomyosarcoma in a young child should alert the clinician to the likelihood that cancers, especially breast cancer, may develop in other family members at unusually young ages. An association between familial sarcomas and multiple polyposis of the colon has been noted and soft tissue sarcomas have developed in children in association with congenital anomalies (112).

## Bone Tumours

With bone cancers it is possible to be more specific. In a series of 1532 deaths from primary bone cancers in U. S. children (113) it was found that though 1199 died before their 15th birthday, very few died in the first quinquennium. A sex differential was noted - for boys with osteosarcoma the incidence continued to rise to past 19 years of age and similarly, but at a lower level, did Ewing's sarcoma in white males. Girls showed a rapid incidence rate rise for osteosarcoma after 10 years of age, and for the 12-16 year age group the rate exceeded that of boys but the female rate for Ewing's sarcoma declined after the age of 16 years. No seasonal, geographical, or space-time clustering variations could be detected. Almost the only agreed features of the distribution of osteosarcomas (114) are that they are affected by general skeletal growth both in humans and animals resulting in a close relationship with age curves and body size in children and that there is a tendency for sarcomas to develop in some rare familial bone diseases. In animals there is some indication of a virus aetiology of osteosarcomas and some evidence supports such an effect in humans. A small outbreak of osteosarcoma in a school in Wales has been reported in which a possible relationship to pet birds was postulated (115). Osteosarcomas also are concerned in the familial sarcoma syndrome noted above (111). Beyond this, uncertainty prevails and we know very little of the international or racial distribution of bone tumours.

There is one notable exception to this and that is in the distribution of Ewing's sarcoma (113). In the U. S. there was found to be a remarkably low frequency of Ewing's sarcoma in Negro children. It is very difficult to ascribe this to delays or to deficiencies in diagnosis and it seems to correspond to the situation in Africa where this cancer seems rarely to be encountered. In India (116) there does not seem to be any such deficiency and in the rest of the world there is too little information. The situation is even more complicated because of the anomalous status of Ewing's sarcoma which is usually classified as a bone tumour but develops in the marrow and does not involve bone cells. For long, controversy raged over its very existence as a specific entity but MARSDEN and STEWARD (117) showed clearly the gross, microscopic, behavioural, and chemical differences between Ewing's sarcoma and neuroblastoma and the distinction can now be clearly made. We need more studies of the epidemiology of all types of soft tissue and bone tumours.

Epithelial Cancers of Non-endocrine Organs

The importance of the study of the epithelial cancers of childhood for the light they may throw on similar tumours in adults has been much emphasised but has evoked little response probably because of the rarity of such cancers and the difficulty of collecting an adequate number of cases. It is evident from existing data, however inadequate, that differences exist in the distribution of carcinomas in childhood as remarkable as the differences in adults and some of these are discussed in more detail elsewhere.

There is one complicating factor which should be borne in mind and which should both caution and encourage investigators. Many carcinomas in childhood arise on the basis of some inherited metabolic defect. Thus xeroderma pigmentosum (118) is responsible for the early development of squamous carcinomas of the skin in African children and for at least some of the cases of squamous carcinomas of the penis and of the tongue that occasionally are seen in them. Similarly tyrosinosis is a factor in the precocious development of hepatocellular carcinoma in children and other metabolic hepatic lesions operate similarly (119). Ataxia-telangiectasia has been at the base of the development of some gastric carcinomas in children (120) and congenital polyposis at the base of some childhood colonic carcinomas (121). Once such metabolically determined carcinomas are excluded the causes of the remaining carcinomas need to be determined and short of evidence to the contrary can be assumed to be similar to the causes of adult carcinomas in the same organs but acting prematurely. We can thus assume that the carcinomas of the adult colon that arise in connection with ulcerative colitis are similar in causation to the childhood colon carcinomas arising on the same basis (122).

In general, four situations seem to obtain but can only be tentatively indicated in view of present lack of knowledge:

1. An adult carcinoma may occur with great frequency and this is reflected by such carcinomas occurring prematurely in childhood. This seems to be the situation as regards hepatocellular carcinoma in Mozambique (34) and other parts of Africa, of nasopharyngeal carcinomas in Northern Uganda (123, 124), other parts of Africa and of Hong Kong Chinese (125) and may be true of papillary carcinoma of the thyroid in several countries. It may be true of gallbladder cancer in American Indians (126, 127).

2. A particular carcinoma may be common in adults but is not seen in children. This appears to be a very common situation - it is notable in areas where oesophageal cancer in adults occurs in very high frequency (35) and where oropharyngeal cancer associated with betel chewing is common (this may not be the case) (128). In no country where gastric carcinoma is common does this cancer seem to occur in childhood and this seems true too of bronchogenic, breast, and cervical carcinomas in all areas. Notable exceptions seem unreported but would be of immense interest if discovered.

3. Intermediate uncertain situations. There are several of these of which colonic cancer is the most interesting. It is uncertain if

carcinoma of the colon occurs any more commonly in children in areas where it is a common adult cancer than it does in areas where it is uncommon in adults. The fact that colon carcinomas occur in childhood under three circumstances, with congenital polyposis, with ulcerative colitis, and with no obvious cause (122) should encourage the search for the antecedent factors in the latter. This is the situation with many other cancers. It seems that the known cancer-associated parasites, Schistosoma haematobium with bladder cancer and Clonorchis sinensis with biliary duct carcinomas never produce cancers in children under 15 years of age.

4. A particular form of carcinoma may be unduly common in children but these carcinomas are not frequent in adults. Although statistics are not yet adequate to be certain about this situation, renal carcinomas appear to occur relatively frequently in children but to be relatively uncommon in adults in some African and South American series. This may also be the case with adrenal cortical carcinomas in Brazil and perhaps other parts of South America (129).

It would appear most unlikely that, save in extreme situations such as with liver carcinoma in Mozambique, any single centre will see a sufficient number of cases to enable adequate collection of data to be made and co-operative efforts are needed.

As discussed previously in connection with leukaemia, it may be in the case of carcinomas too that prenatal influences are decisive and that it is useless looking for postnatal environmental factors. While experimental study in animals of prenatal carcinogeneses has not had much effect on paediatric oncology a recent discovery has had a decisive impact.

## Adenocarcinoma of the Vagina (12)

Much attention has been paid to cases of adenocarcinoma of the vagina occurring with vaginal adenosis since it was recognised in Boston to be associated with the administration of the synthetic steroidal drug - diethylstilbestrol - to the mother during the pregnancy (12). After a gap of up to 24 years or more the daughter resulting from the pregnancy may develop adenosis and adenocarcinoma of the vagina, the onset signified by a bloodstained vaginal discharge and often a negative cytology screening test. The tumour is a carcinoma to be distinguished from the benign and malignant mesonephric and polypoid tumours that are known to occur very rarely in the cervix and vagina of girls.

The long latent period is of interest as many of the exposed girls do not develop vaginal adenocarcinoma till the late teens or twenties though others have developed it by the age of 12 years. While the maternal dosage of diethylstilbestrol may have been very high, cases have been reported in the daughters of mothers who received only very low doses and the precise timing and the factors necessary to produce this tumour have to be elucidated. The use of this drug for practical purposes ceased some years ago, leaving a considerable if unknown number of young females at risk and the level of risk may possibly be ascertained. However, this episode has concentrated attention once more on pre-natal carcinogenesis and this time of an epithelial carcinoma (12).

## Gonadal and Endocrine Tumours

Increasing attention has been paid to gonadal and endocrine tumours in childhood in recent years. Attention was previously drawn to significant differences in European, East African, and Brazilian experience (1). There seems to be a variation in papillary carcinomas of the thyroid in children reflecting the situation in adults and associated with iodine deficient goiters though not necessarily directly. Again comparative and epidemiological studies have been much hampered by basic information deficiencies and when studies that remedy this are reported they are of great value. NORRIS and JENSEN (130) have now broken down 353 ovarian neoplasms according to cell type and age at diagnosis; 40% were seen in consultation and 55% were malignant. Only 18 occurred in the first quinquennium, 36 in the second, 82 in the third, and no less than 217 between 13 and 19 years of age. This increase in the late teens continued into later life being largely due to a great increase in epithelial tumours following the menarche. No carcinoma was seen in this series before 15 years of age. Ovarian tumours are so uncommon that attempts to base international comparisons on registry based material have been difficult (131, 132) save in respect of the large number of ovarian lymphomas seen in Nigeria. However, collected cases from three East African registries differ from the NORRIS-JENSEN series (133) in containing fewer malignant teratomas but relatively many more gonadal tumours (especially dysgerminomas) and stromal tumours (especially granulosa cell tumours) and a higher proportion of embryonal cell carcinomas. Clearly further studies are needed where adequate series exist. Similarly studies of other gonadal and endocrine tumours on an epidemiological basis are required.

There are also differences in testicular tumours. Overall in Africans, testicular tumours are rarely seen due mainly to a gross deficiency in seminomas and embryonal carcinomas. These are apparently rare tumours in the Negro population of the U. S. (134). American Negro children very rarely seem to develop testicular tumours of any type. However, in Uganda (135) though the shortage of adults with testicular tumours is established, there appears to be no shortage of orchioblastomas. The clear cell adenocarcinoma of the infant testis occurs commonly and forms 20% of all testicular tumours seen. But whether the actual incidence is increased is uncertain.

## The Future Needs

This essay can still only be tentative and exploratory despite the great increases in our knowledge in the last few years. It is to be hoped that there will be rapid future gains. We need much more information, put forward in a standardised fashion with histological control and agreed terminology and international attention is being devoted to this need. A handicap is the International Classification of Disease code which needs, especially for childhood cancers, to be supplemented with a histological code. It cannot be assumed that all renal tumours are carcinomas in adults and nephroblastomas in childhood. Too many series are being published which do not include all tumours occurring before the 15th birthday, or do not include haematological malignancies or specify the benign or malignant nature of the tumours.

But deficient as is our information, great advances have been made. We have now identified groups of children at special risk of cancer, we have more clearly recognised the role of congenital defects and transplacental carcinogenesis, we have begun to see the child with cancer as a possible example of carcinogenesis signalling to us about environmental carcinogens of interest to the community at large. While the interests of the child must be paramount, these wider interests should not be overlooked. And while we can all rejoice in the enormous improvements in the therapy of childhood tumours and hope for even greater triumphs, we should not forget that the goal should be, not the cure of cancer, however desirable this be, but that children should not develop cancer.

Acknowledgement

Personal Research Support has come from the Damon Runyon Memorial Fund for Cancer Research (DRG1053), from the Brown-Hazen Fund, and from N.I.H. Contract No. NIH 72-2426 from the National Cancer Institute. This support is gratefully acknowledged.

## REFERENCES

1. DAVIES, J. N. P.: Some Variations in Childhood Cancers Throughout the World. In: Tumours in Children. MARSDEN, H. B., STEWARD, J. K. (eds.). Berlin: Springer-Verlag, 1968, Chap. 2
2. FRAUMENI, J. F. Jr., EVERSON, R. B., DALAGER, N. Y.: Declining mortality from Wilms' tumour in the United States. Lancet 2, 48 (1972)
3. FAVARA, B. E., JOHNSON, W., ITO, J.: Renal tumors in the neonatal period. Cancer 22, 845-855 (1968)
4. BANNAYAN, G. A.: Lipomatosis, angiomatosis and macrencephalia. A previously undescribed congenital syndrome. Arch. Path. 92, 1-5 (1971)
5. MOE, P. G., NELLHAUS, G.: Infantile polymyoclonia-opsoclonus syndrome and neural crest tumors. Neurology 20, 756-764 (1970)
6. SCHAISON, G., WEISGERBER, C., SELIGMAN, M., BERNARD, J.: Les leucemies myelo-monocytaires avec xanthomes. Nouv. Rev. Franc. Hemat. 10, 284-288 (1970)
7. MILLER, R. W.: Childhood cancer and congenital defects. A study of U.S. death certificates during the period 1960-1966. Pediat. Res. 3, 389-397 (1969)
8. MILLER, R. W.: Relation between cancer and congenital defects: an epidemiological evaluation. J. Natl. Cancer Inst. 40, 1079-1085 (1968)
9. STEWART, A., KNEALE, G. W.: Changes in the cancer risk associated with obstetric radiography. Lancet 1, 104-107 (1968)
10. STEWART, A. M., KNEALE, G. W.: Age-distribution of cancers caused by obstetric X-rays and their relevance to cancer latent periods. Lancet 2, 4-8 (1970)
11. SCHWEISGUTH, O., GERARD-MARCHANT, R., PLAINFOSSE, B., LEMERLE, J., WATCHI, J. M., SERINGE, P.: Bilateral non functioning thecoma of the ovary in epileptic children under anticonvulsant therapy. Acta Pediat. 60, 6-10 (1971)
12. HERBST, A. L., ULFELDER, H., POSKANZER, D. C.: Adenocarcinoma of the vagina. Association of maternal stilbestrol therapy with tumor appearance in young women. N. Eng. Med. J. 284, 878-881 (1971)
13. FRAUMENI, J. F. Jr., GLASS, A. G.: Rarity of Ewing's sarcoma among U. S. negro children. Lancet 1, 366-367 (1970)
14. MILLER, R. W.: Interim Report: UICC International study of childhood cancer. Int. J. Cancer 10, 675-677 (1972)

15. U.I.C.C. Cancer incidence in five continents. DOLL, R., MUIR, C. S., WATERHOUSE, J. A. H. (eds.). Geneva UICC, 1970, Vol. II

16. U.I.C.C. Cancer incidence in five continents. DOLL, R., PAYNE, P., WATERHOUSE, J. A. H. (eds.). Geneva UICC, 1966, Vol. I

17. CORREA, P., O'CONOR, G. T.: Epidemiologic patterns of Hodgkin's disease. Int. J. Cancer 8, 192-201 (1971)

18. DAVIES, J. N. P.: Leukaemia in children in Tropical Africa. Lancet 2, 65-67 (1965)

19. EDINGTON, G. M., MacLEAN, C. M. U.: A cancer rate survey in Ibadan, Western Nigeria. 1960-1963. Br. J. Cancer 19, 471-481 (1965)

20. SONNET, J., MICHAUX, J. L., HEKSTER, C.: Incidence and forms of leukaemia among the Congolese Bantus. Trop. Geog. Med. 18, 272-286 (1966)

21. ESSIEN, E. M.: Leukaemia in Nigerians, Part 1: The acute leukaemias. Afr. J. Med. Sci. 3, 117-130 (1972)

22. DAVIES, J. N. P., KNOWELDEN, J., WILSON, B. A.: Incidence rates of cancer in Kyadondo county, Uganda 1954-1960. J. Natl. Cancer Inst. 35, 789-821 (1965)

23. VANIER, T. M., PIKE, M. C.: Leukaemia incidence in tropical Africa. Lancet 1, 512-513 (1967)

24. LOTHE, F.: Leukaemia in Uganda. Trop. Geog. Med. 19, 163-171 (1967)

25. MILLER, R. W.: Childhood cancer mortality in USA and Japan. Tohoku J. Exp. Med. 91, 103-107 (1967)

26. DALLDORF, G., BARNHART, F. E.: Childhood leukemia, malaria, and Burkitt's lymphoma. N. Eng. Med. J. 286, 1216 (1972)

27. HADDOCK, D. R. W.: The pattern of leukaemia in Accra, Ghana. J. Trop. Med. Hyg. 70, 60-62 (1967)

28. BARR, R. D., MacCULLOCH, P. B., SUDHA, MEHTA and KENDALL, A. G.: Acute leukaemia in Kenya. Scot. Med. J. 17, 330-333 (1972)

29. TEMPLETON, A. C., BIANCHI, A.: Bias in an African cancer registry. Int. J. Cancer 10, 186-193 (1972)

30. TEMPLETON, A. C., VIEGAS, O. A. C.: Racial variations in tumour incidence in Uganda. Trop. Geog. Med. 22, 431-438 (1970)

31. FROMAN, C., LIPSCHITZ, R.: Demography of tumours of the central nervous system among the Bantu (African) population of the Transvaal South Africa. J. Neurosurg. 32, 660-664 (1970)

32. BAILEY, I. C.: The pattern and presentation of intracranial tumours in Uganda. E. Afr. Med. J. 48, 565-575 (1971)

33. RUBERTI, R. F., POPPI, M.: Tumours of the central nervous system in the African. E. Afr. Med. J. 48, 576-584 (1971)

34. PRATES, M. D., TORRES, F. O.: A cancer survey in Lourenço Marques Portugese East Africa. J. Natl. Cancer Inst. 35, 729-757 (1965)

35. COOK, P.: Cancer of the oesophagus in Africa. Br. J. Cancer 25, 853-880 (1971)

36. DAVIES, J. N. P.: Retinoblastoma as a possible index cancer. Lancet 2, 1039 (1967)

37. JENSEN, R. D., MILLER, R. W.: Retinoblastoma: Epidemiological characteristics. N. Eng. Med. J. 285, 307-311 (1971)

38. INNIS, M. D.: Nephroblastoma: Possible index cancer of childhood. Med. J. Aust. 1, 18-20 (1972)

39. MILLER, R. W., FRAUMENI, J. F., MANNING, M. D.: Association of Wilms' tumor with aniridia, hemihypertrophy and other congenital malformations. N. Eng. Med. J. 270, 922-927 (1964)

40. LEDLIE, E. M., MYNORS, L. S., DRAPER, G. J., GORBACH, P. D.: Natural history and treatment of Wilms's tumour: An analysis of 335 cases occurring in England and Wales 1962-1966. Br. Med. J. 4, 195-201 (1970)

41. VIRAG, I., MODAN, B.: Epidemiologic aspects of neoplastic diseases in Israeli immigrant population. II. Malignant neoplasms in childhood. Cancer 23, 137-141 (1969)

42. ARAKI, C., MATSUMOTO, S.: Statistical reevaluation of pinealoma and related tumors in Japan. J. Neurosurg. 30, 140-149 (1969)

43. MILLER, R. W.: Relation between cancer and congenital malformations. Israel. J. Med. Sci. 7, 1461-1464 (1971)

44. BROOKS, W. H.: Geographic clustering of brain tumors in Kentucky. Cancer 30, 923-926 (1972)

45. SMYTHE, P. H., SCHONLAND, M., BRERETON-STILES, G. G., COOVADIA, H. M. et al.: Thymolymphatic deficiency and depression of cell-mediated immunity in protein-calorie malnutrition. Lancet 2, 939-943 (1971)

46. MUGERWA, J. W.: The lymphoreticular system in Kwashiorkor. J. Path. 105, 105-109 (1971)

47. FRAUMENI, J. F. Jr., MITUS, W. J., MANNING, M. D.: Acute childhood leukemia. Epidemiologic study by cell type of 1263 cases at the Children's Cancer Research Foundation in Boston, 1947-1965. J. Natl. Cancer Inst. 46, 461-470 (1971)

48. PIERCE, M. I., BORGES, W. H., HEYN, R., WOLFF, J. A., GILBERT, E.S.: Epidemiological factors and survival experience in 1770 children with acute leukemia. Cancer 23, 1296-1304 (1969)

49. BRAS, G., COLE, H., ASHMEADE-DYER, A., WATLER, D. C.: Report on 151 childhood malignancies observed in Jamaica. J. Natl. Cancer Inst. 43, 417-421 (1969)

50. PIKE, M.C., SMITH, P.G.: Epidemiology of Burkitt's lymphoma. N. Eng. Med. J. 287, 934 (1972)

51. O'CONOR, G. T., DAVIES, J. N. P.: Malignant tumors in African children. With special reference to malignant lymphoma. J. Pediat. 56, 526-535 (1960)

52. DAVIES, J. N. P., OWOR, R.: Chloromatous tumours in African children in Uganda. Br. Med. J. 2, 405-407 (1965)

53. O'CONOR, G. T.: Persistent immunologic stimulation as a factor in oncogenesis with special reference to Burkitt's tumor. Am. J. Med. 48, 279-285 (1970)

54. BURKITT, D. P.: Etiology of Burkitt's lymphoma - an alternative hypothesis to a vectored virus. J. Natl. Cancer Inst. 42, 19-28 (1969)

55. BOOTH, K., BURKITT, D. P., BASSETT, D. J., COOKE, R. A., BIDDULPH, J.: Burkitt lymphoma in Papua, New Guinea. Br. J. Cancer 21, 657-664 (1967)

56. JAMRA, M., CARVALHO, R. P. S., DALLDORF, G.: Evolution of an atypical case of Burkitt lymphoma. Lancet 2, 672 (1970)

57. STEVENS, D. A., O'CONOR, G. T., LEVINE, P. H., ROSEN, R. B.: Acute leukemia with "Burkitt's lymphoma cells" and Burkitt's lymphoma. Simultaneous onset in American siblings; description of a new entity Ann. Int. Med. 76, 967-973 (1972)

58. STEWART, A., KNEALE, G. W.: Role of local infections in the recognition of haemopoetic neoplasms. Nature 223, 741-742 (1969)

59. JABLON, S., KATO, H.: Childhood cancer in relation to prenatal exposure to atomic bomb radiation. Lancet 2, 1000-1003 (1970)

60. BURCH, P. R. J.: Prenatal radiation exposure and childhood cancer. Lancet 2, 1189 (1970)

61. ÇAVDAR, A. O., ARCASOY, A., GÜZDAŞOĞLU, S., DEMIRAĞ, B.: Chloroma-like ocular manifestations in Turkish children with acute myelomonocytic leukaemia. Lancet 1, 680-682 (1971)

62. MORTADA, A.: Orbital reticulum-cell sarcoma with monocytic leukemia. Report of two cases. Arch. Ophthal. 67, 572-577 (1962)

63. GUPTA, S. P., AGARWAL, P. K., PRATAP, V. B.: Proptosis - a manifestation of acute myelogenous leukaemia. Orient. Arch. Ophthal. 8, 94-97 (1970)

64. TEMPLETON, A. C.: Orbital tumours in African children. Brit. J. Ophthal. 55, 254-261 (1971)

65. HURWITZ, B. S., SUTHERLAND, J. C., WALKER, M. D.: Central nervous system chloromas preceding acute leukemia by one year. Neurology 20, 771-775 (1970)

66. SAARNI, M. I., LINMAN, J. W.: Myelomonocytic leukemia: Disorderly proliferation of all marrow cells. Cancer 27, 1221-1230 (1971)

67. BENNETT, J. M.: Myelomonocytic leukemias: A historical review and perspectives. Cancer 27, 1218-1220 (1971)

68. LINMAN, J. W.: Myelomonocytic leukemia and its preleukemic phase. J. Chronic Dis. 22, 713-716 (1970)

69. FEDRICK, J., ALBERMAN, E. D.: Reported influenza in pregnancy and subsequent cancer in the child. Br. Med. J. 2, 485-488 (1972)

70. MILLER, R. W.: Persons with exceptionally high risk of leukemia. Cancer Res. 27, 2420-2423 (1967)

71. ROSNER, F., LEE, S. L.: Down's syndrome and acute leukemia. Myeloblastic or lymphoblastic. Am. J. Med. 53, 203-218 (1972)

72. EVANS, D. I. K., STEWARD, J. K.: Down's syndrome and leukaemia. Lancet 2, 1322 (1972)

73. BURKITT, D. P., WRIGHT, D. H.: Burkitt's lymphoma. London: Livingstone, 1970

74. LEVINE, P. H., O'CONOR, G. T., BERARD, C. W.: Antibodies to Epstein-Barr Virus (EBV) in American patients with Burkitt's lymphoma. Cancer 30, 610-615 (1972)

75. HENLE, W.: Role of Epstein-Barr Virus in infectious mononucleosis and malignant lymphomas in man. Fed. Proc. 31, 1674 (1972)

76. GREENWOOD, B. M., PLAYFAIR, J. H. L., TORRIGIANI, G.: Burkitt lymphoma and malaria. Lancet 2, 418 (1970)

77. KAFUKO, G. W., BURKITT, D. P.: Burkitt's lymphoma and malaria. Int. J. Cancer 6, 1-9 (1970)

78. MORROW, R. H., PIKE, M. C., SMITH, P. G., ZIEGLER, J. L., KISUULE, A.: Burkitt's lymphoma: A time space cluster of cases in Bwamba County of Uganda. Br. Med. J. 2, 491-492 (1971)

79. CARBONE, P. P., BERARD, C. W., BENNETT, J. M., ZIEGLER, J. L., COHEN, M. H., GERBER, P.: Burkitt's tumour. Ann. Int. Med. 70, 817-832 (1969)

80. MacMAHON, B.: Epidemiology of Hodgkin's disease. Cancer Res. 26, 1189-1200 (1966)

81. ZIEGLER, J. L., BLUMING, A. Z., FASS, L., MAGRATH, I. T., TEMPLETON, A. C.: Chemotherapy of childhood Hodgkin's disease in Uganda. Lancet 2, 679-682 (1972)

82. BURN, C., DAVIES, J. N. P., DODGE, O. G., NIAS, B.C.: Hodgkin's disease in English and African children. J. Natl. Cancer Inst. 46, 37-41 (1971)

83. KAFUKO, G. W. et al.: Epstein-Barr Virus antibody levels in children from the West Nile district of Uganda. Lancet 1, 706-709 (1972)

84. FRAUMENI, J. F., LI, F. P.: Hodgkin's disease in childhood. An epidemiologic study. J. Natl. Cancer Inst. 42, 681-691 (1969)

85. MILLER, R. W.: Mortality in childhood Hodgkin's disease: An etiologic clue. JAMA 198, 1216-1217 (1960)

86. VIANNA, N. J., GREENWALD, P., DAVIES, J. N. P.: Tonsillectomy and Hodgkin's disease: The lymphoid tissue barrier. Lancet 1, 431-432 (1971)

87. VIANNA, N. J., GREENWALD, P., BRADY, J., POLAN, A. K., DWORK, A., MAURO, J., DAVIES, J. N. P.: Hodgkin's disease: Cases with features of a community outbreak. Ann. Int. Med. 77, 169-180 (1972)

88. RAMOT, B., MANY, A.: Primary intestinal lymphoma: Clinical manifestations and possible effect of environmental factors. Current Problems in the Epidemiology of Cancer and Lymphomas. GRUNDMANN, E., TULINIUS, H. (eds.). Berlin: Springer-Verlag, 1972, 193-199

89. VOGEL, J. M., VOGEL, P.: Idiopathic histiocytosis: A discussion of eosinophilic granuloma, the Hand-Schuller-Christian Syndrome and Letterer-Siwe Syndrome. Seminars Hematol. 9, 464-469 (1972)

90. ROSAI, J., DORFMAN, R. F.: Sinus histiocytosis with massive lymphadenopathy: A pseudolymphomatous benign disorder. Analysis of 34 cases. Cancer 30, 1174-1188 (1972)

91. SERCK-HANSSEN, A., PURCHIT, G. P.: Histiocytic medullary reticulosis. Report of 14 cases from Uganda. Br. J. Cancer 22, 506-516 (1968)

92. SKARIN, A. T., KARB, K., REYNOLDS, E. S.: Acute leukaemia terminating in histiocytic medullary reticulosis. Arch. Path. 93, 256-260 (1972)

93. SLAVIN, G., CAMERON, H. Mc D., FORBES, C., MITCHELL, R. M.: Kaposi's sarcoma in East African children: a report of 51 cases. J. Path. 100, 187-199 (1970)

94. OLSON, C. W., SMITH, J. H., TESTERMAN, N., BASTIN, J. P., FRAZER, H.: Burkitt's tumor in the democratic republic of the Congo. Cancer 23, 740-746 (1969)

95. TEMPLETON, A. C.: Studies in Kaposi's sarcoma. Cancer 30, 854-867 (1972)

96. GOMES D'OLIVEIRA, J. J., TORRES, F. O.: Kaposi's sarcoma in the Bantu of Mozambique. Cancer 30, 553-561 (1972)

97. SIEGEL, J. H., JANIS, R., ALPER, J. C., SCHUTTE, H., ROBBINS, L., BLAUFOX, M. D.: Disseminated visceral Kaposi's sarcoma. Appearance after human renal homograft operation. J.A.M.A. 207, 1493-1496 (1969)

98. GIRALDO, G., BETH, E., HAGUENAU, F.: Herpes-type virus particles in tissue culture of Kaposi's sarcoma from different geographic regions. J. Natl. Cancer Inst. 49, 1509-1526 (1972)

99. MILLER, R. W., FRAUMENI, J. F. Jr., HILL, J. A.: Neuroblastoma. Epidemiologic approach to its origin. Am.J. Dis. Child. 115, 253-261 (1968)

100. BECKWITH, J. B., PERRIN, E. V.: In situ neuroblastomas: A contribution to the natural history of neural crest tumors. Am. J. Path. 43, 1089-1104 (1963)

101. VOORHESS, M. L.: Neuroblastoma with normal urinary catecholamine excretion. J. Pediat. 78, 680-683 (1971)

102. NEWELL, G. R., ROBERTS, J. D., BARANOVSKY, A.: Retinoblastoma; presentation and survival in negro children compared with whites. J. Natl. Cancer Inst. 49, 989-992 (1972)

103. T'SO, M. O. M., ZIMMERMAN, L. E., FINE, B. S.: The Nature of Retinoblastoma I. Photoreceptor differentiation. A clinical and histopathologic study. Am. J. Ophthal. 69, 339-349 (1970). II. Photoreceptor differentiation: an electron microscopic study ibid 69, 350-359 (1970)

104. T'SO, M. O. M., ZIMMERMAN, L. E., FINE, B. S., ELLSWORTH, R. M.: A cause of radioresistance in retinoblastoma: photoreceptor differentiation. Trans. Am. Acad. Ophth. Otol. 74, 959-969 (1970)

105. SAGERMAN, R. H., CASSADY, J. R., TRETTER, P., ELLSWORTH, R. M.: Radiation induced neoplasia following external beam therapy for children with retinoblastoma. Am. J. Roentgenol. Rad. Ther. Nucl. Med. 105, 529-535 (1969)

106. QUERE, M. A., CAMAIN, R., LAMBERT, D.: The pathology of orbito-ocular tumours in tropical Africa. Klin. Mbl. Augenheil. 149, 829-840 (1964) (in German)

107. OLURIN, O., WILLIAMS, A. O.: Orbito-ocular tumors in Nigeria. Cancer 30, 580-587 (1972)

108. TEMPLETON, A. C.: Tumors of the eye and adnexa in Africans of Uganda. Cancer 20, 1689-1698 (1967)

109. PORTERFIELD, J. F., ZIMMERMAN, L. E.: Rhabdomyosarcoma of the orbit. Virchow's Arch. Path. Anat. 335, 329-344 (1962)

110. DEHNER, L. P., LEESTMA, J. E., PRICE, E. B.: Renal cell carcinoma in children: a clinicopathologic study of 15 cases and review of the literature. J. Pediat. 76, 358-368 (1970)

111. LI, F. P., FRAUMENI, J. F. Jr.: Rhabdomyosarcoma in children. epidermologic study and identification of a familial cancer syndrome. J. Natl. Cancer Inst. 43, 1365-1373 (1969)

112. SLOANE, J. A., HUBBELL, M. M.: Soft tissue sarcomas in children associated with congenital anomalies. Cancer 23, 175-182 (1969)

113. GLASS, A. G., FRAUMENI, J. F.: Epidemiology of bone cancer in children. J. Natl. Cancer Inst. 44, 187-199 (1970)

114. HEMS, G.: Aetiology of bone cancer and some other cancers in the young. Br. J. Cancer 24, 208-214 (1970)

115. TURNER, R. C.: Unusual group of tumours among schoolgirls. Br. J. Cancer 21, 17-26 (1967)

116. SIRSAT, M. V.: Sarcoma of bone. Ind. J. Surgery 18, 1-30 (1956)

117. MARSDEN, H. B., STEWARD, J. K.: Ewing's tumours and neuroblastomas. J. Clin. Path. 17, 411-417 (1964)

118. CLEAVER, J. E.: Xeroderma Pigmentosum: a human disease in which an initial stage of DNA repair is defective. Proc. Nat. Acad. Sci. (US) 63, 428-435 (1969)

119. KEELING, J. W.: Liver tumours in infancy and childhood. J. Path. 103, 69-85 (1971)

120. HAERER, A. F., JACKSON, J. F., EVERS, C. G.: Ataxia-telangiectasia with gastric adenocarcinoma. J. Am. med. Ass. 210, 1884-1887 (1969)

121. KOTTMEIER, P. K., CLATWORTHY, H. W.: Intestinal polyps and associated carcinoma in childhood. Am. J. Surg. 110, 709-716 (1965)

122. PEMBERTON, H.: Carcinoma of the large intestine with survival in a child of nine and his father. A study of carcinoma of the colon with particular reference to children. Br. J. Surg. 57, 841-846 (1970)

123. SCHMAUZ, R., TEMPLETON, A. C.: Nasopharyngeal carcinoma in Uganda. Cancer 29, 610-621 (1972)

124. TEMPLETON, A. C., SCHMAUZ, R.: Cervical lymphadenopathy in Ugandans. E. Afr. Med. J. 47, 582-587 (1970)

125. BELAMARIC, H.: Malignant tumors in Chinese. Int. J. Cancer 4, 560-573 (1969)

126. RUDOLPH, R., COHEN, J. J.: Cancer of the gall bladder in an 11 year old Navajo girl. J. Pediat. Surg. 7, 66-67 (1972)

127. CREAGAN, E. T., FRAUMENI, J. F. Jr.: Cancer mortality among American Indians, 1950-67 J. Natl. Cancer Inst. 49, 953-958 (1972)

128. GROVER, S., HARDAS, U. D.: Childhood malignancies in central India. J. Natl. Cancer Inst. 49, 953-958 (1972)

129. MARIGO, C., MULLER, H., DAVIES, J. N. P.: Survey of cancer in children admitted to a Brazilian Charity Hospital. J. Natl. Cancer Inst. 43, 1231-1240 (1969)

130. JENSEN, R. D., NORRIS, H. J.: Epithelial tumours of the ovary. Occurrence in children and adolescents less than 20 years of age. Arch. Path. 94, 29-34 (1972)

131. LINDFORS, O.: Primary ovarian neoplasms in infants and children. A study of 81 cases diagnosed in Finland and Sweden. Ann. Chir. Gynae. Fenn. Supp. 177, 1-66 (1971)

132. EIN, S. H., DARTE, J. M. M., STEPHENS, C. A.: Cystic and solid ovarian tumors in children. A 44 year review. J. Pediat. Surg. 5, 148-156 (1970)

133. GINSBERG, R., DAVIES, J. N. P.: Unpublished work, 1972

134. LI, F. P., FRAUMENI, J. F. Jr.: Testicular cancers in children: Epidemiological characteristics. J. Natl. Cancer Inst. 48, 1575-1582 (1972)

135. TEMPLETON, A. C.: Testicular neoplasms in Ugandan Africans. Afr. J. Med. Sci. 3, 157-161 (1972)

136. STEWART, A., DAVIES, J. N. P., DALLDORF, G., BARNHART, F.: Malignant lymphomas of African children. Proc. Nat. Acad. Sci. U. S. A. 70, 15-17 (1973)

# Chapter 4
# Leukaemia

During the period 1954 - 1968, 465 patients with leukaemia were included in the Manchester Children's Tumour Registry. The frequency of the various types is shown in Table 1.

The number of new cases in the Manchester Region varied between 24 and 41 per year with a mean of 31 (Fig. 1). These patients were drawn from a total population of five million containing approximately one million children under 15 years. Thus there was an annual incidence of 31 per

Table 1. Manchester Children's Tumóur Registry. Leukaemia 1954 - 1968

| | |
|---|---|
| Acute lymphoblastic (ALL) | 251 |
| Acute stem cell (ASC) | 125 |
| Acute myeloid (AML) | 60 |
| Acute monocytic | 14 |
| Acute myelomonocytic | 9 |
| Acute erythroleukaemia | 2 |
| Chronic myeloid leukaemia (adult type) | 3 |
| Chronic myeloid leukaemia (juvenile type) | 1 |
| | 465 |

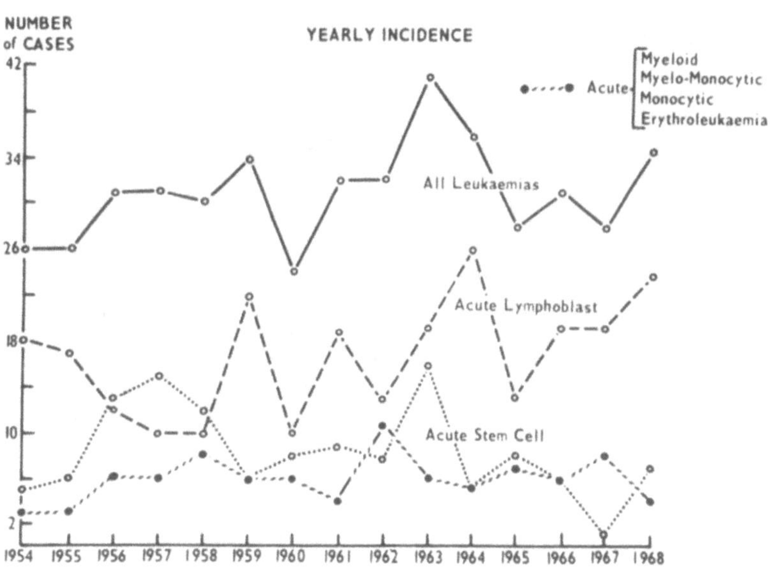


*Fig. 1. Annual incidence of leukaemia in Manchester Region, 1954-1968*

million compared with figures for England and Wales (1950 - 59) showing a mortality of 32.5 per million (1).

The commonest type of leukaemia was acute lymphoblastic, which was found in 251 Manchester children (54%). Chronic lymphatic leukaemia is virtually unknown in paediatric practice and no case was seen in the Manchester series. The acute leukaemia of adults is usually myeloid (granulocytic), but this is not the case in children : only 60 of the 465 Manchester cases (13%) were classified as acute myeloid and if the other varieties of monocytic, myelomonocytic and erythroleukaemia were added, there was a total of only 85 cases (18%). Chronic myeloid leukaemia is rare: the adult type occurs in older children, and the disease found in younger children and referred to as juvenile chronic myeloid leukaemia (2) is a very different disorder from the disease found in adults and older children. Only one case was diagnosed in Manchester during the 15-year period compared with three of the adult type.

Stem cell leukaemia was diagnosed in 125 children (27%). This group includes not only patients in whom a positive diagnosis was made on the basis of a blast cell morphology which was poorly differentiated, with scanty cytoplasm and indistinct nuclear detail, but also those children in whom the information available was inadequate for accurate typing. Many of these latter cases were probably lymphoid in origin, since they responded to treatment with steroids and anti-metabolites, but the survival of children with stem cell leukaemia was worse than of those with pure lymphoblastic leukaemia (see Fig. 2). The information available to the Registry has improved over the years, with the result that fewer cases are classified as stem cell leukaemia in successive quinquennia: there were 51 cases in 1954 - 1958, 47 cases in 1959 - 1963 and 27 in 1964 - 1968. While the number of myeloid cases showed only a slight increase of doubtful significance, the number of lymphoblastic cases rose considerably as the number of stem cell leukaemias fell. As

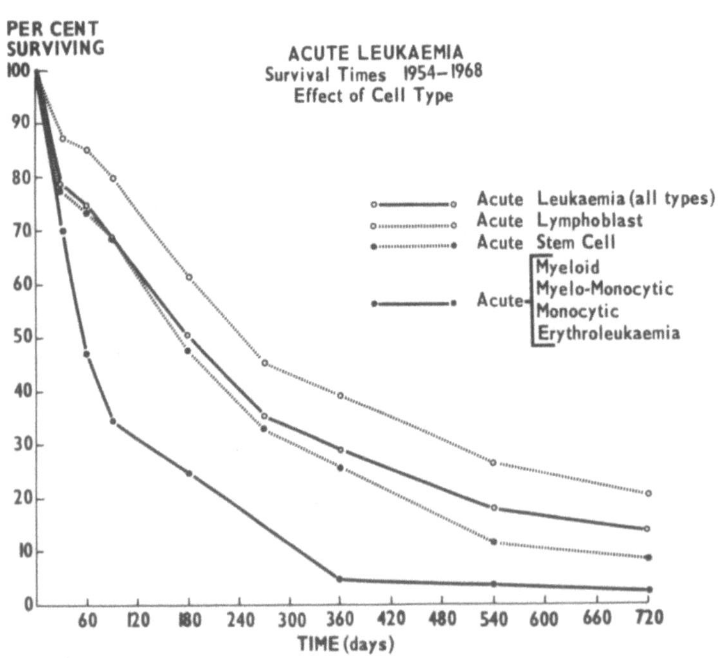


*Fig. 2. Effect of cell type on survival in leukaemia*

Table 2. Incidence of types of acute leukaemia by five-year periods

| | 1954-1958 | | 1959-1963 | | 1964-1968 | |
|---|---|---|---|---|---|---|
| Acute lymphoblastic | 67) | 118 | 83) | 130 | 101) | 128 |
| Acute stem cell | 51) | | 47) | | 27) | |
| Myeloid, monocytic, and other types | 26 | | 33 | | 30 | |
| | 144 | | 163 | | 158 | |

a result, the combined figure for lymphoblastic and stem cell leukaemias is almost constant (Table 2), suggesting that most of the cases diagnosed as stem cell leukaemia in the early years would have been classed as lymphoblastic leukaemia in the last quinquennium. Consequently these two types have been grouped together in some of the analyses of results.

For the period 1969 - 1972, a considerable proportion of new cases has been seen at one Manchester hospital and bone marrows have been reviewed from other cases. The distribution of types is shown in Table 3. A diagnosis of acute lymphoblastic leukaemia was made in 120 cases, an incidence of 79%.

Table 3. Manchester Children's Tumour Registry

| Leukaemias 1969-1972 | |
|---|---|
| Acute lymphoblastic | 120 |
| Acute myeloid | 17 |
| Acute myelomonocytic | 2 |
| Acute monocytic | 1 |
| Erythroleukaemia | 2 |
| Acute undifferentiated | 5 |
| Acute stem cell | 3 |
| Chronic myeloid < juvenile | 1 |
| Chronic myeloid < adult | 1 |
| | 152 |

There are variations in the diagnosis of leukaemia types in different series: FRAUMENI et al. (1971) (3) found 43.9% lymphocytic, 24.6% undifferentiated, and 31.6% myeloid and monocytic in a study of 1263 cases seen at the Children's Cancer Research Foundation in Boston; PIERCE et al. (1969) (4) studying the 1770 cases treated by Children's Cancer Group A in the U.S.A. concluded that reliable criteria do not exist for morphological delineation of lymphoblastic from undifferentiated cell types. They classed the two together, finding 77.9% of cases to be acute lymphoid leukaemia, with only 16.6% coming into the acute myeloid and monocytic types. In Manchester, up to 1968, the acute lymphoblastic and stem cell leukaemias together accounted for 81% of all cases, which is near the figure reported by PIERCE et al. in their multicentre trials and contrasts with the figure of 68.5% for combined lymphoblastic and undifferentiated types in Boston. BROWNING and GROSS (1968) (5), studying 168 children with leukaemia in Cuyahoga County, Ohio, representing 96% of leukaemia deaths for the period 1955 - 1965, found 92.9% had acute lymphocytic leukaemia and only 7.1% had acute myelogenous leukaemia. Fifty-three percent of their cases were seen personally. The differences in these series may reflect environmental or racial factors, but they may be explicable, partly at least, by differences in diagnosis and haematological opinion or by the selection occurring when patients are referred to special centres.

The disease is commonest among young children, with a peak incidence between the ages of 2 and 3 years, due mainly to an increased incidence of acute lymphoblastic leukaemia at this time. There is a second small peak at the age of 12 (Fig. 3). The non-lymphoid leukaemias show a peak

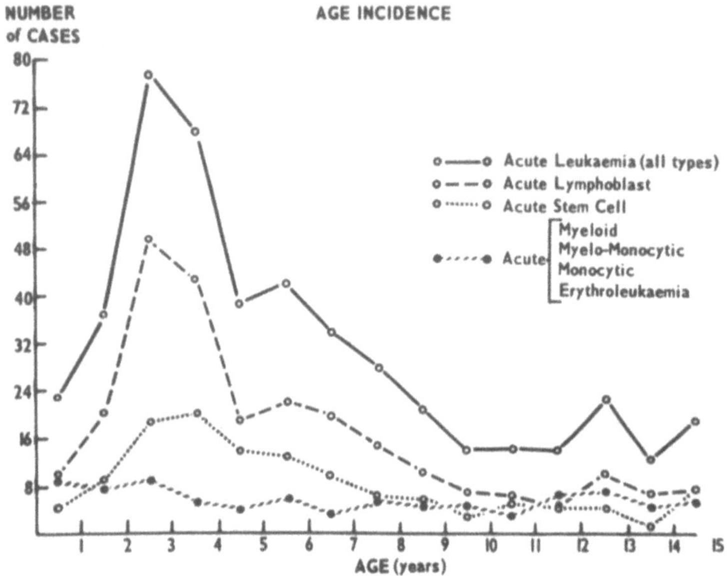


*Fig. 3. Age incidence of leukaemia in Manchester Region, 1954-1968*

incidence during the first year of life: of 23 infants presenting with leukaemia at this time, 9 (39%) had acute myeloid or monocytic leukaemia (6 acute myeloblastic leukaemia and 3 acute monocytic leukaemia). Thereafter, the incidence of the non-lymphoid leukaemias declines and from the age of 4 there is little variation in the incidence of these leukaemias throughout childhood. This early peak of non-lymphoid leukaemias appears to be due, firstly, to the increase of acute monocytic leukaemia in the first 3 years of life when 7 cases of the 14 were recorded, and secondly, to an increased incidence of acute myeloblastic leukaemia in the early years, with a slight trough between the ages of 8 and 11. After the first 3 years, the incidence of acute monocytic leukaemia has been only one or none for each year of life, and this difference is significant ($P < 0.01$). Although there are only a few cases in these groups, the trough for acute myeloid leukaemia for a similar age was also shown by LEE (1961) (9) studying a large number of cases from England and Wales, Scotland, Canada and the United States.

These facts are not entirely in accordance with other large series. For instance, PIERCE et al. (1969) (4), in their study of 1770 children with leukaemia found a peak incidence of acute granulocytic leukaemia at 2 years, but confirmed that monocytic leukaemia occurred most commonly in children under 3 years. Their data were collected from 11 paediatric centres dealing with childhood leukaemia and may therefore be selective. It is generally agreed that the peak incidence in the third year is due to acute lymphoblastic leukaemia, and that this disease is the commonest type of malignancy in childhood (3, 4, 5, 6). However, this applies to white populations in Western societies, and not to non-whites in the U.S.A. and Japan (1, 7, 8). The non-white population in the Manchester Region is increasing, but was small during the time of study and no specific information about the ethnic origin of all the children at risk is available. It is unlikely that ethnic factors affect the incidence of leukaemia in the Manchester children.

Boys were slightly more commonly affected than girls: 253 boys were diagnosed compared with 212 girls. Studies of leukaemia death rates for England and Wales confirm the increased incidence for boys compared with girls at all ages (1). However, the Manchester data also showed an unexpected increase of monocytic leukaemia in girls, particularly after the age of 3. It has already been mentioned that acute monocytic leukaemia appears with a significantly greater frequency in the first 3 years of life, but after this age there has been only one boy diagnosed with the disease whereas 6 girls have been diagnosed. These differences do not quite reach statistically significant levels, owing to the small numbers. There is no sex difference in the first three years (3 boys, 4 girls). The data for acute myelomonocytic leukaemia were examined in view of the fact that, although there is seldom any doubt about diagnosing monocytic elements in a leukaemia, there is often a hazy boundary between pure monocytic and myelomonocytic leukaemias. There were no boys under three years with this diagnosis, but three girls, and after this age there were three children of each sex with the disease. If the cases of monocytic and myelomonocytic leukaemia are combined there is a total of 7 boys and 16 girls, with 3 boys under three and 4 boys over three, compared with 7 girls under three and 9 girls over three. Data from other series are scarce, but FRAUMENI et al. (1971) (3) showed very little difference between boys and girls for monocytic leukaemia and did not give figures for the ages of individual groups. There was an increase of myelogenous leukaemia in boys. A peak incidence of this disease has also been reported for boys in later adolescence (9), but PIERCE et al. (1969) (4) found more acute myeloid leukaemia in girls than boys, and no difference in the incidence of monocytic leukaemia.

These features suggest that childhood leukaemia is not a homogenous disease, and hence the aetiological factors may differ for the various types. It has been suggested that the peak incidence of leukaemia, due to acute lymphoblastic leukaemia occurring between the ages of 2 and 4 years, is due to antenatal influences on the foetus, such as a viral infection. The recent discovery that mothers of these children have high levels of IgM (10, 11), is evidence in favour of this theory. In Manchester high levels of IgM in a group of mothers of leukaemic children have been found, but levels in the fathers and siblings were normal (12).

## CLINICAL MANIFESTATION OF ACUTE LEUKAEMIA

The clinical picture of acute leukaemia is fairly constant. Pallor and lassitude of recent onset are the commonest symptoms: many parents date the onset of symptoms from an upper respiratory infection several weeks previously from which the child has failed to make the expected recovery. Other forms of presentation include pyrexia of unknown origin, headache, or sore throat. Bone pain occurred in approximately one quarter of the

Table 4. Signs or symptoms at diagnosis in cases of acute leukaemia presenting between 1964 and 1968. The figures are calculated from the cases in which a definite annotation was made. Cases where there was no definite annotation were ignored

| Sign or symptom | Positive | Negative | Total | % positive |
|---|---|---|---|---|
| Glands + | 93 | 51 | 144 | 64 |
| Spleen + | 83 | 59 | 142 | 58 |
| Liver + | 81 | 62 | 143 | 57 |
| Bruising + | 63 | 73 | 136 | 46 |
| Bone pain | 25 | 81 | 106 | 24 |

Manchester cases. Glandular enlargement is the commonest finding on clinical examination, followed by hepato-splenomegaly and bruising. The incidence of these clinical features is shown in Table 4, based on an analysis of the 158 cases presenting between 1964 and 1968. Skin infiltration is rarely found after the first year of life, but may occur in infants. Oral ulceration is rare, due to the small number of monocytic and allied leukaemias in childhood.

Laboratory examination reveals anaemia. The red cells usually show anisocytosis and poikilocytosis even when anaemia is not very advanced. The sedimentation rate is high. The haemoglobin levels at diagnosis in 154 cases presenting between 1964 and 1968 are shown in Table 5. Ninety-five percent of the cases had haemoglobin levels below 10.5 g per 100 ml.

Table 5. Haemoglobin levels at diagnosis in 154 cases of acute leukaemia presenting between 1964 and 1968

| Haemoglobin g per 100 ml | No. of cases | % |
|---|---|---|
| 10.5 or more (> 75%) | 8 | 5 |
| 7.3-10.4 (50-75%) | 59 | 38 |
| 3.7- 7.2 (25-50%) | 75 | 49 |
| 3.6 or less (< 25%) | 12 | 8 |
| | 154 | 100 |

The total leucocyte count may be low, normal or high in approximately equal proportions of patients, although the distribution of the white cells is abnormal. There is usually an absolute neutropenia, and a careful search may reveal blast cells in cases even where the total leucocyte count is low or normal.

The platelet count is commonly reduced. Analysis of 131 cases presenting between 1964 and 1968 shows that 17% of cases had platelet counts over 150,000/μl, whereas 65% had platelet counts of less than 50,000 μl (Table 6).

In about 20% of cases, the presence of massive enlargement of liver, spleen and lymph nodes together with anaemia, thrombocytopenia and a high white cell count with blast cells in the blood make possible an immediate diagnosis of acute leukaemia; but in most children examination of the marrow is necessary. This should be obtained by aspiration of the posterior iliac crest. Other sites, including the sternum,

Table 6. Platelet counts in 131 cases of acute leukaemia presenting between 1964 and 1968 for whom the platelet count was recorded at initial diagnosis

| Platelets (thousands per μl) | No. of cases | % |
|---|---|---|
| over 200 | 15 | 11 |
| 150-200 | 8 | 6 |
| 100-150 | 9 | 7 |
| 50-100 | 14 | 11 |
| Less than 50 | 85 | 65 |
| Total | 131 | 100 |

tibia, vertebral spine and anterior iliac crest are rarely used and reserved for cases when the initial posterior crest aspirate is not diagnostic.

In almost every case of acute lymphoblastic leukaemia the marrow shows extensive involvement with the leukaemic process and 70% or more of the marrow cells are malignant. Normal elements are usually reduced. Erythropoiesis may be megaloblastic; more commonly the scanty erythroid cells are normoblastic or show minor dysplastic changes. In the non-lymphoid leukaemias the changes may be less distinct. In any case where the diagnosis is not instantly clear a repeat examination from another site is advisable. This may be necessary when the first aspirate is diluted with blood, or because only a very poorly cellular sample of inadequate volume could be aspirated. In a small number of cases the percentage of blast cells is low and the characteristic changes may take time to appear. Ten percent of blast cells is suspicious of a malignant process, but to make a diagnosis of acute leukaemia at least 40% of blasts should be present.

## Atypical Presentation of Leukaemia

Leukaemia sometimes presents in an unusual way, and three presentations are of particular interest: congenital and infantile leukaemia, leukaemia with Down's syndrome, and the leukaemia which presents with bone marrow aplasia. In the Manchester series no cases of leukaemia arising in other rare preleukaemic conditions such as Bloom's syndrome or Fanconi's anaemia have been encountered.

1. Congenital and Infantile Leukaemia. Although there is no excess of leukaemia in children born of mothers who were leukaemic during pregnancy (13), the disease may present in the newborn or within the first 3 months of life and is then referred to as congenital leukaemia. The infants are found to have anaemia and hepatosplenomegaly, and there is a marked leucocytosis due to increase of blast-cells and early granulocytes with extensive involvement in non-haemopoietic organs as well as the customary extramedullary sites of haemopoiesis.

Twenty-two Manchester children with leukaemia were under the age of 1 year at diagnosis, five being under 3 months. The distribution of cell types for the group was: lymphoblastic 9 cases (41%), stem cell 4 cases (18%), myeloblastic 6 cases (27%), and monocytic 3 cases (14%), giving a higher proportion of myeloblastic and monocytic cases than is seen in later childhood. There were 14 boys and 8 girls, a male/female ratio of 1.75 : 1.

Hepatosplenomegaly at presentation was common and occurred in 17 (77%) of the infants. In one case there was splenic enlargement only and in four cases neither the spleen nor the liver was enlarged. Ten infants were recorded as having lymph node enlargement, in 7 cases this feature was not present, and in the remaining 5 cases details were not recorded. These features contrast with the findings in children of all ages with leukaemia in whom hepatosplenomegaly is present in approximately 60%, and the commonest feature is glandular enlargement (see Table 4). In 6 infants there were skin nodules due to local infiltration of the skin with leukaemic cells, an unusual finding in older children (MARSDEN, 1974) (17). Two of these cases were lymphoblastic, 3 were monocytic, and 1 was myeloblastic.

The infants received a variety of treatments, mainly corticosteroids and 6-mercaptopurine, but fared badly. Although one survived 41 months and another 15 months, 17 (68%) survived only 2 months or less and the median survival was only 1 month.

None of these infants was diagnosed as having juvenile chronic myeloid leukaemia, although WEISGERBER and SCHAISON (1970) (14) using a broader classification for this disease which they referred to as myelomonocytic leukaemia, included 10 children under 1 year in their group of 25 cases. Three of the Manchester infants (CTR 59/59, 11/60 and 91/62) showed hepatosplenomegaly and a high white cell count with relatively few blast cells, thought to be myeloid or monocytic in origin. Although they showed some features reminiscent of juvenile chronic myeloid leukaemia by the criteria of BERNARD and SELIGMANN (1968) (15), they have been classified as cases of acute leukaemia.

2. Leukaemia in Down's Syndrome. Many authors have commented upon the increased incidence of leukaemia in Down's syndrome. Five of the 465 Manchester cases had Down's syndrome. Four were lymphoblastic and one was acute myeloid. The patient's ages were 1, 1 1/2, and three of 2 1/2 years. The youngest child had acute myeloid leukaemia with 80% blasts in the marrow. All the children died. The incidence of leukaemia in Down's syndrome is said to be increased about twenty times (16).

ROSNER et al. (1972) (18) have pointed out that a syndrome of ineffective granulopoiesis masquerading as acute myeloblastic leukaemia occurs in Down's syndrome; they believe that because the children may recover, the disease is in fact not leukaemia. This syndrome accounts for the commonly held misconception that leukaemia in Down's syndrome is myeloid in origin. In their review of the world literature they found that leukaemia in Down's syndrome is commonly lymphoblastic. The Manchester figures support their argument.

3. Aplastic Presentation of Leukaemia. In 6 of the 465 cases the initial diagnosis was of bone marrow hypoplasia; aplastic anaemia in 5 cases and agranulocytosis in 1 case. For the 5 cases diagnosed initially as aplastic anaemia the interval until the diagnosis of leukaemia was made was 12 days, 5 weeks, 4 months and 8 months (two cases). For the case of agranulocytosis it was 9 months.

It is not uncommon for leukaemia to present with peripheral pancytopenia and for bone marrow aspirates to produce only hypocellular films, but usually the nucleated cells are seen to be blast cells and the diagnosis is not in doubt. Poor cellularity of the aspirate may be due to fibrosis in the marrow. Less often, as in these 5 children, there is pancytopenia with most cells appearing to be mature lymphocytes and blast cells being scanty, while in the sixth child there was depression of only the granulocyte series. It is difficult to decide whether the initial aplasia is a part of, or a prelude to, the leukaemic process. Furthermore, antileukaemic

Table 7. Leukaemia preceded by marrow hypoplasia

| CTR. No. | Sex | Age (years) | Signs (apart from pallor) | Initial blood picture | Initial marrow | Clinical onset to diagnosis of hypo-plasia | Hypoplasia to leukaemia | Leukaemia to death | Type of leukaemia |
|---|---|---|---|---|---|---|---|---|---|
| 82/55 | M | 11 | Liver +<br>Spleen + | Hb. 20%<br>WBC. 2000/μl<br>P.57%,L.40%<br>M. 3% | Hypocellular<br>Blasts 2%<br>"No evidence of leukaemia" | 7 weeks | 8 months | 4 months | A.S.C. |
| 85/60 | F | 1 | Bruising<br>Spleen + | Hb. 42%<br>WBC.3000/μl<br>Platelets 50,000/μl | Hypoplastic | 8 days | 12 days | 2 weeks | A.M.L. |
| 79/62 | M | 4 | Tonsils +<br>Neck glands+<br>Liver + | Hb. 46%<br>WBC.1500/μl<br>P.4%, L.89%,<br>M. 6%<br>Platelets plentiful | Hypoplastic with lympho-cytes predominating. No increase in blasts | 2 days | 5 weeks | 3 months | A.L.L. |
| 62/63 | F | 9 | Liver +<br>Spleen +<br>Neck glands+ | Hb. 29%<br>WBC.2500/μl<br>P.8%, L.92%<br>Platelets 50,000/μl | Hypoplastic | 5 months | 4 months | 18 months | A.S.C. |
| 73/63 | F | 1 | Bruising | Hb. 25%<br>WBC.3000/μl<br>Platelets 105,000/μl | Aplastic | ? | 8 months | 4 months | A.L.L. |
| 124/66 | F | 11 | Skin rash | Hb. 83%<br>WBC.1250/μl<br>P. 5%<br>Platelets plentiful | Agranulo-cytosis | 7 months | 9 months | 10 months | A.M.L. |

therapy may be difficult to maintain in the face of a persistent tendency to aplasia, yet it may result not only in full remission, but also in restoration of the marrow to normal cellularity. Details of these cases are shown in Table 7. There are few constant features: age of onset, interval between initial aplasia and diagnosis of leukaemia, and subsequent survival show no consistent pattern. There were 4 girls and 2 boys; 2 cases proved to be acute myeloblastic leukaemia, 2 were stem cell and 2 were lymphoblastic, which is approximately the sort of distribution to be expected from the incidence of the different leukaemias in the series. Certainly there is no indication that any one type of leukaemia presents more commonly in this way.

Clear demonstration of initial hypoplasia of the bone marrow requires more than one aspiration, and from different sites, together with trephine biopsy, conditions which may not have been met in some early cases in this group. However the interval between the initial and the final diagnoses was substantial in most cases, and this favours an atypical leukaemic presentation. Perhaps case CTR.85/60, with an interval of only 12 days between the two bone marrows is an exception, but the possibility of very rapid transition is not excluded. A more typical case, seen in 1971, is presented:
CTR.167/71. A girl, 22 months, had 3 months' malaise and pyrexia, with no lymph node enlargement or hepatosplenomegaly. Tests showed pancytopenia; bone marrow from sternum and both iliac crests was hypocellular with 50-70% lymphocytes and 5-20% blast cells. A trephine biopsy showed patchy cellularity with some hyperplastic areas. Her condition improved with blood transfusion. Three months later she had a cytomegalovirus infection and the next month, with bone pain and persisting pancytopenia, leukaemia was apparent with 98% lymphoblasts in iliac crest and tibia. The subsequent course of the disease was unusual, as relapse was preceded by return of bone marrow hypoplasia, with normal cellularity after induction of remission.

## Classification of Acute Leukaemia

At one time classification of the acute leukaemias was a matter of academic interest. Now that a remission can be obtained in the majority of cases, and since the treatment used for each type of leukaemia will differ considerably, an attempt at classification is essential.

Occasionally, oral ulceration is associated with myeloid or monocytic leukaemia. Thymic enlargement, lymphadenopathy or gross hepatosplenomegaly tend to favour a diagnosis of lymphoblastic leukaemia, but usually clinical symptoms are not helpful.

Even after bone marrow examination there is a minority of cases which are difficult to classify. They are characterised by the presence of small, poorly differentiated blast cells, with scanty cytoplasm showing no distinguishing features. Some may be identified by cytochemical tests described below; those which are not must be classified as undifferentiated acute leukaemia. In many other retrospective series (1, 3, 4), such a group has been included. Many of those in the Manchester series were probably lymphoid in origin, since they responded to treatment with steroids and antimetabolites, but in Figure 2 they have been included in the stem cell group which has a worse prognosis.

The fact that acute leukaemias may be difficult to classify by Romanowsky stains has led to the greater use of cytochemical tests. Following the lead of HAYHOE et al. (1964) (19), who reported on 140 acute leukaemias studied by cytochemical means, it is common practice to use the periodic acid-Schiff reaction (PAS), peroxidase reaction, and staining with Sudan black to attempt to differentiate the leukaemias. With PAS a variable number of cells in lymphoblastic leukaemias may show coarse granules or large blocks and this feature can be regarded as diagnostic of lymphoblastic leukaemia. Fine granules may also be seen but are not diagnostic of a lymphoid origin. Variable reactions are given by monocytic and myeloid leukaemias. Lymphoblasts are negative with peroxidase and Sudan black, which may reveal large numbers of positive granules in myeloblasts, particularly in those acute myeloid leukaemias where some granulation is already apparent with the Romanowsky stains. They are helpful in distinguishing the occasional lymphoblast or prolymphocyte with cytoplasmic granules. Other tests used in differentiating the acute leukaemias include the serum and urinary muramidase and the neutrophil alkaline phosphatase reaction. Muramidase levels are high in the monocytic leukaemias (20, 21).

Enzyme cytochemistry of leukaemic blast cells has given variable results with a variety of enzyme studies, including esterases, dehydrogenases and aryl sulphatase (22, 23). In spite of periodic claims of the value of such tests, it appears that cases which are poorly differentiated by the usual morphological criteria may also be the most difficult to differentiate by special stains and enzyme cytochemistry.

Leucocyte alkaline phosphatase (L.A.P.) scores have been reported to be helpful in distinguishing the acute leukaemias. The normal range by the method of HAYHOE and QUAGLINO (1958) (24) is 14-60, and the score is said to be high in lymphoblastic leukaemia and low in myeloblastic leukaemia. However, in the Manchester material this test has given variable results. In a small group of 18 children with lymphoblastic leukaemia one case scored only 4/400, and two further cases gave normal scores of 18 and 38. Thirteen cases scored from 52 to 270 with a mean of 122, and in two further cases individual cells showed high activity but insufficient neutrophils were present for scoring.

The recent demonstration that a small number of lymphoid leukaemias can be classified as T-cell leukaemias while most show no surface markers promises to be a useful indication of a group with a poor prognosis (91, 92). CATOVSKY et al. (93) have shown that the blasts in T-cell acute leukaemia show strong acid phosphatase activity. Preliminary results in Manchester confirm these reports. The patients are usually boys in the older age group, often have a thymic mass and a high white cell count, and respond poorly to treatment.

## Chronic Myeloid Leukaemia in Childhood

Four of the 465 leukaemic cases reviewed up to 1968 were chronic myeloid in type. By 1973, two further cases had presented. Four have been the adult type of disease; two have had a disorder characteristic of early childhood, which, although known as juvenile chronic myeloid leukaemia (2) has no Philadelphia (Ph') chromosome, and bears little relationship to the adult disease. French haematologists, because of the frequent prominence of monocytes, refer to it as myelomonocytic leukaemia (15), but this description may lead to confusion with the more common acute myelomonocytic leukaemia. The disease is not chronic and the two Manchester cases died in 3 and 6 months.

The children with chronic myeloid leukaemia usually presented with pallor, loss of weight, bruising and bone pain. All had splenomegaly, four had lymph node enlargement and three hepatomegaly. Results of initial laboratory tests (Table 8) show distinct differences between the adult and juvenile types of disease. The adult type usually affects older children, but this is by no means invariable.

Table 8. Features of the two varieties of chronic myeloid leukaemia of childhood

| CTR. No. | Type | Sex | Age at onset | Initial WBC. (per µl) | Percentages myelocytes | Platelets (per µl) | Survival | Mode of death |
|---|---|---|---|---|---|---|---|---|
| 126/56 | Adult | M | 13 years | 81,900 | 21.5% | 480,000 | 4 3/4 years | Generalised disease |
| 26/61 | Adult | F | 12 years | 310,000 | 27% | 615,000 | 3 years | Blast transf. |
| 92/64 | Adult | F | 12 years | 540,000 | 20% | 300,000 | 22 months | Blast transf. |
| 50/72 | Adult | F | 11 years | 420,000 | 30% | 234,000 | - | Still alive |
| 34/62 | Juvenile | F | 7 years | 39,000 | 5% | 12,000 | 6 months | Pneumonia |
| 106/70 | Juvenile | M | 2 years | 91,000 | 7% | 76,000 | 3 months | Pneumonia, haemorrhage |

CTR.36/75. A boy presenting with pyrexia and abdominal distension at the age of thirteen months. There was marked hepatosplenomegaly and the blood showed Hb 6.4 g%. WBC 539,000/μl (neutrophils 20%, lymphocytes 11%, monocytes 4%, eosinophils 14%, metamyelocytes 17%, myelocytes 20%, promyelocytes 9%, blasts 5%) platelets 95,000/μl. Ph' chromosome was present in blood and marrow.

Of the four adult type in the 20-year review, one was Ph' positive, in two cases the cultures failed to grow and in the fourth case chromosome studies were not done. The younger children with the juvenile type were aged 2 and 7 years: chromosome analysis was Ph' negative in one and not carried out in the other.

The blood picture of the older children was typical of adult chronic myeloid leukaemia, with myelocytes often prominent in blood and bone marrow; all cases showed at least 20% myelocytes. Platelet counts were high or normal. The children were treated with busulphan, three had splenic irradiation, and one received radiophosphorus. The outcome is shown in Table 8. The three who died had 6-mercaptopurine and prednisone for the terminal illness but showed no response. The report of the Medical Research Council (1968) (25) showed that in chronic myeloid leukaemia survival rates were better with busulphan than with irradiation of the spleen, which also carried the risk of earlier development of blast cell transformation.

The Ph' negative juvenile type of the disease was found in the two young children who presented with pallor, malaise and purpura. The blood count showed a leucocytosis due mainly to an increase of mature neutrophils with less than 10% myelocytes in the peripheral blood. Platelets were reduced. There was a poor response to both busulphan and 6-mercaptopurine, and the patients died from infection with pneumonia. In young children the disorder is characterised by increased levels of foetal haemoglobin in the red cells, changes in red cell antigens and enzymes, and many other features suggesting a persistence of, or a reversion to, a primitive type of foetal blood cell formation (26). These features are illustrated by the following case report:
CTR.106/70. P. A. presented at the age of 26 months with a history of 3 months' malaise followed by bruising, pallor and the development of generalised petechiae. He had hepatosplenomegaly and generalised lymphadenopathy. The blood count showed Hb. 9.0 g per 100 ml, white cells 91,000/μl (neutrophils 30%, lymphocytes 10%, basophils 2%, monocytes 8%, staff cells 20%, metamyelocytes 15%, myelocytes 7%, promyelocytes 2% and myeloblasts 6%) platelets 76,000/μl. The bone marrow reflected the changes in the peripheral blood, with 10% myeloblasts, and bone marrow culture gave a moderate number of metaphases with counts ranging from 40 to 48 chromosomes. Those with 46 chromosomes had normal morphology; no Ph' chromosome was seen. The leucocyte alkaline phosphatase score was normal (23/400), which differs from the adult form (22). Thirty percent alkali resistant haemoglobin was detected by alkali denaturation. No HbH inclusions were present. Acid elution of blood films showed positive HbF cells or negative cells with no intermediate staining. Electrophoresis of the haemolysate showed no abnormal bands, but no $HbA_2$ was demonstrated and carbonic anhydrase B and C were very low. Studies of the red cell antigens showed blood group $OR_1R_1$. Both the patient and his father were $Fy^{a+}$, the father's blood showing a stronger reaction; the H antigen was present but reacted more weakly than with 2 adult bloods and 2 cord blood cells. Testing with anti-I gave a weaker reaction than cord blood cells and there was no reaction with anti-i.

Weak antigenicity of the red cells, deficiency of $HbA_2$, low carbonic anhydrase, and raised levels of HbF are all features of haemopoiesis in the perinatal period and are characteristic of this disease. Although capable of a good delayed hypersensitivity reaction to candida, and of producing normal immunoglobulins, the patient was troubled by severe oral candidiasis. The disease showed no convincing response to busulphan or 6-mercaptopurine, and death occurred 3 months later with haemorrhage, pneumonia, perinephric abscess, subdural haematoma, and candidiasis.

## PROGNOSIS

Up to a few years ago leukaemia in children was regarded as a uniformly fatal disease. However, in 1968 BURCHENAL (27) reported 157 long-term survivors, including 103 patients from different centres who had had acute leukaemia and remained alive and in remission 5 to 17 years after diagnosis. In the Manchester Tumour Registry there are 4 children who developed leukaemia before 1964 who are well over 10 years later. During the past 5 years, intensive chemotherapy has been used for all cases, and at the time of writing 5-year survival rates for acute lymphoblastic leukaemia are over 50%. Ten of the 21 cases diagnosed 5 years ago are in continuous complete remission and off treatment.

The treatment given to the 465 children during the first 15 years of the Registry must be regarded as incomplete by modern standards. It falls into three 5-year periods. During 1954 - 1958 comparatively few children were given effective specific treatment. Between 1959 and 1963 it was usual to induce remissions with steroids and to maintain them with 6-mercaptopurine or methotrexate in low dosage. During 1964 - 1968 other drugs such as vincristine and cyclophosphamide were increasingly added to this regime (Table 9). Although the survival of the earlier cases might have been improved by more effective treatment, the presenting features have not changed and assessment of results can be made in this context.

The survival times of the Manchester children with acute leukaemia varied with the following factors:

1. Cell type
2. Age of patient
3. Initial white cell count
4. Sex
5. Year of registration
6. Number of drugs used
7. Hospital where patient was treated

The statistical significance of these factors is indicated below:

1. Cell Type (Fig. 2). Children with lymphoblastic leukaemia survived longer than those with stem cell leukaemia. Acute myeloid, myelomonocytic and erythroleukaemia had the worst prognosis. These differences were significant.

2. Age of Patient (Figs. 4, 5, 6, and 7). Children between the ages of 2 and 10 years survived the longest and those under 2 the shortest. The good prognosis in the 2 - 10 year-olds was made up of two peaks - one at age 2-6 and the other at 10 years. The effect of age on prognosis was significant only in the lymphoblastic and stem cell leukaemias. Very similar results were reported in the national study of acute lymphoblastic leukaemia, 1963 - 1967 (28).

Table 9. Treatment used in acute leukaemia 1954 - 1968

| Period | No drugs | Steroids only | Steroids and antimetabolites only | Steroids and antimetabolites plus one or more of the following: vincristine, cyclophosphamide, asparaginase, cytosine arabinoside | Other chemotherapy |
|---|---|---|---|---|---|
| 1954-1958 | 48 (34%) | 43 (30%) | 48 (33%) | 0 (0%) | 4 (3%) |
| 1959-1963 | 29 (18%) | 17 (11%) | 101 (63%) | 12 (7%) | 2 (1%) |
| 1964-1968 | 20 (13%) | 9 (6%) | 58 (37%) | 65 (41%) | 5 (3%) |

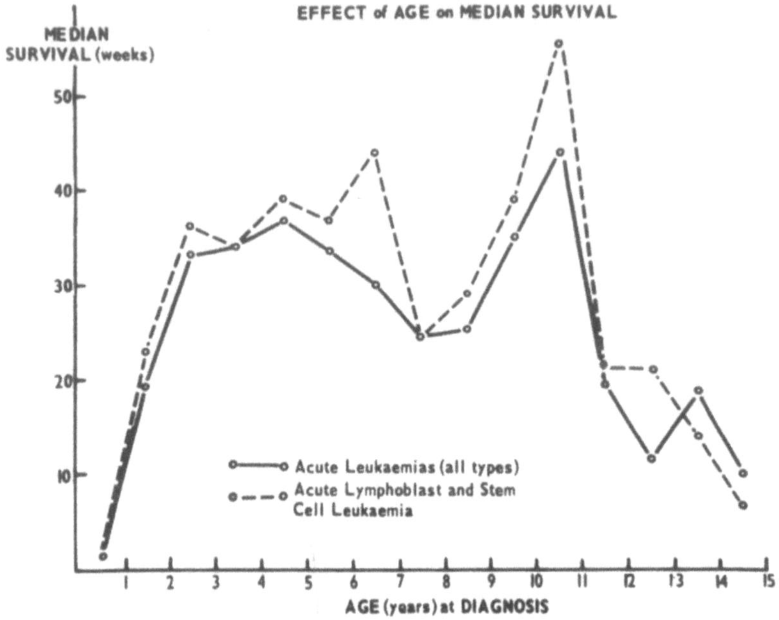


*Fig. 4. Effect of age on median survival*

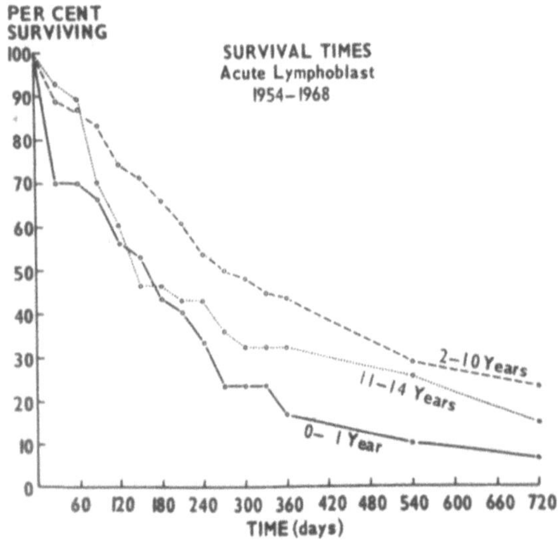


*Fig. 5. Survival time by age groups (acute lymphoblastic leukaemia)*

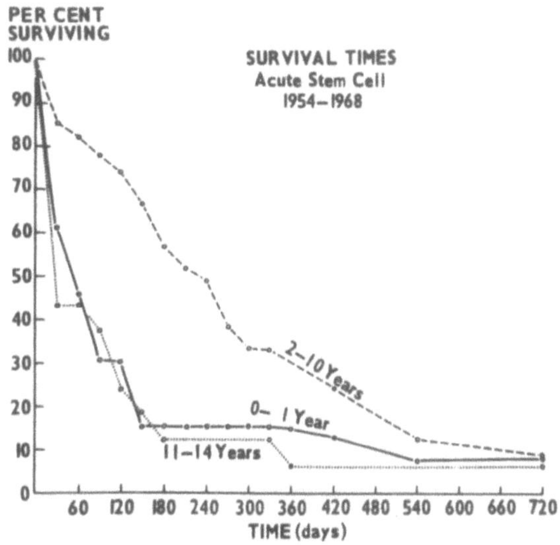


*Fig. 6. Survival time by age groups (acute stem cell leukaemia)*

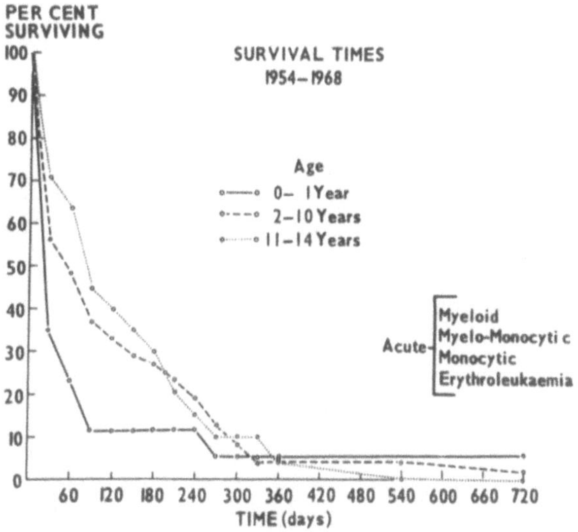


*Fig. 7. Survival time by age groups (acute myeloblastic, monocytic and other leukaemias)*

3. Initial White Cell Count. Cases with counts over 15,000 µl had a significantly worse prognosis in acute lymphoblastic and stem cell, but not other leukaemias (Figs. 8 and 9). Similar observations were made by HARDISTY and TILL (1968) (29).

4. Sex. There appeared to be very little difference in the survival times of boys and girls if all the cases were grouped together (Fig. 10), but girls with acute lymphoblastic leukaemia had significantly longer survivals than boys with the same disease (Fig. 11).

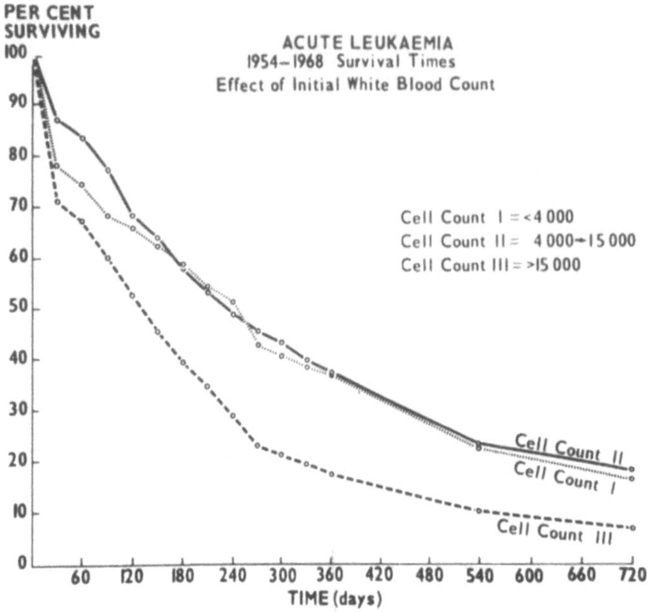


*Fig. 8. Survival time. Effect of initial white cell count*

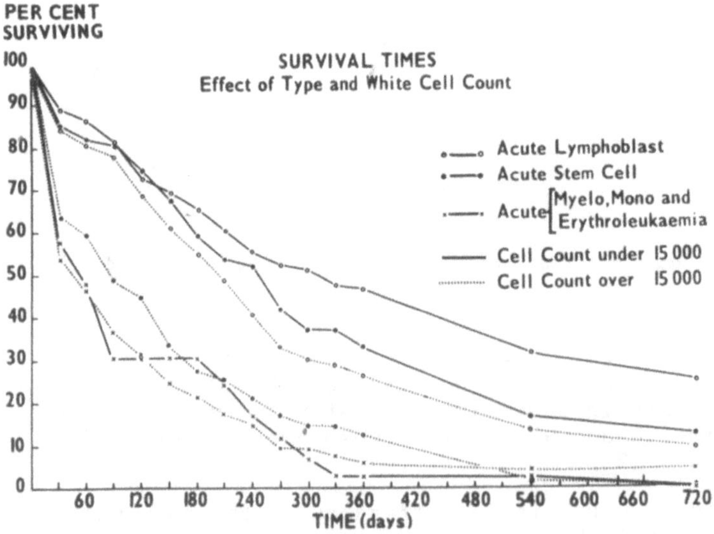


*Fig. 9. Survival time. Effect of initial white cell count and type of leukaemia*

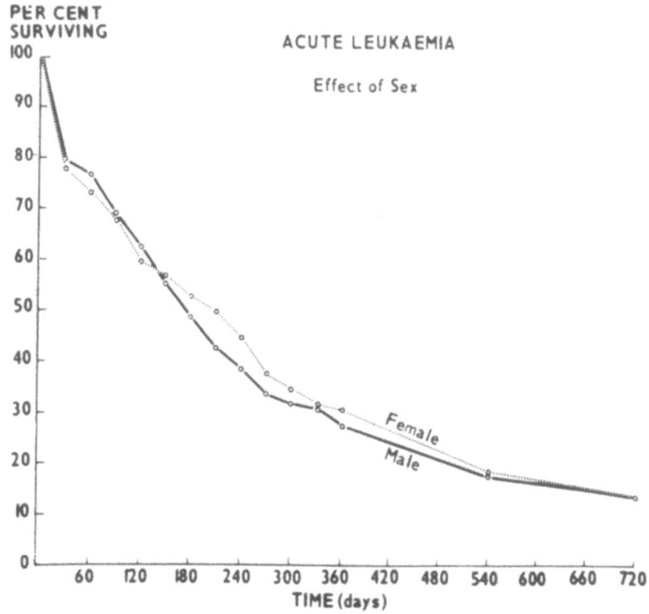


*Fig. 10. Acute leukaemia. Effect of sex on survival*

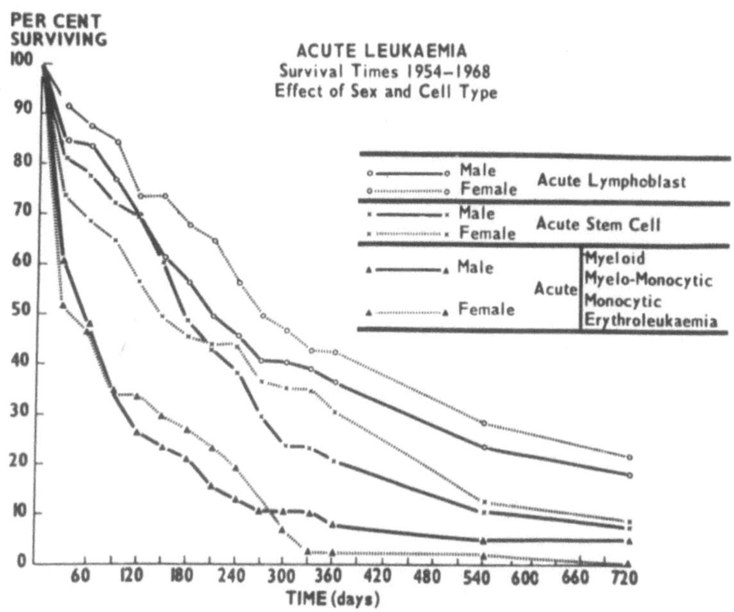


*Fig. 11. Acute leukaemia. Effect of sex and type of leukaemia on survival*

5. Year of Registration. Analysis of the data by 5-year periods, 1954 - 1958, 1959 - 1963, and 1964 - 1968, showed a progressive, significant improvement (Fig. 12), which occurred in children of all ages (Figs. 13 - 15). The improvement in the 2-10 age group started at the end of the first quinquennium and in the 11-14 age group at the end of the second quinquennium.

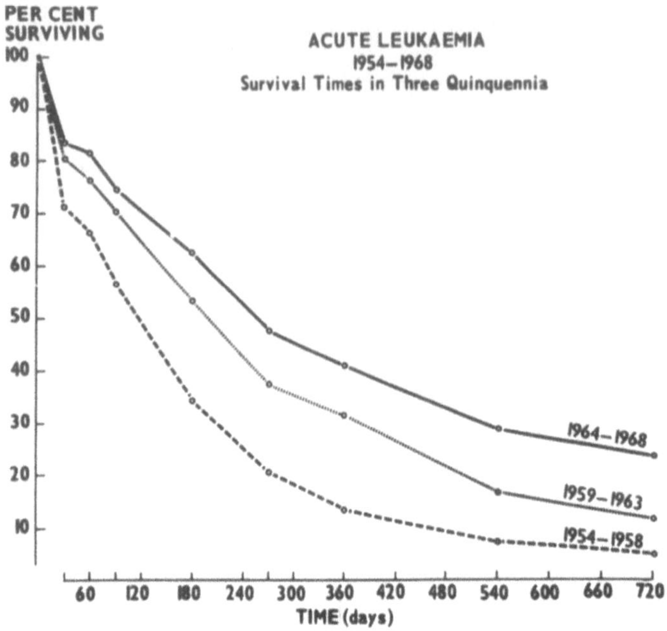


*Fig. 12. Acute leukaemia. Survival times by quinquennia*

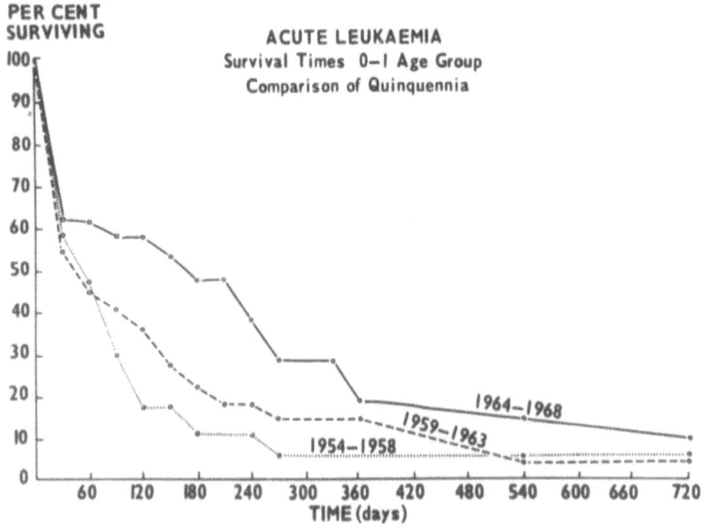


*Fig. 13. Acute leukaemia. Survival times by quinquennia, age 0–1 years*

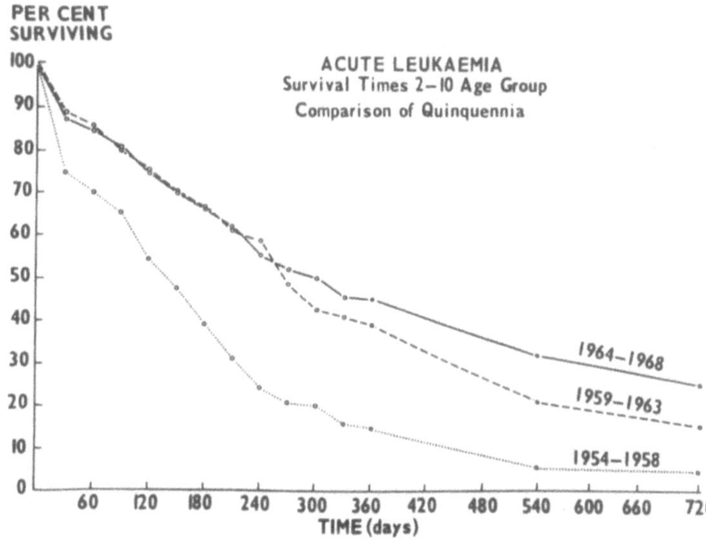


*Fig. 14. Acute leukaemia. Survival times by quinquennia, age 2-10 years*

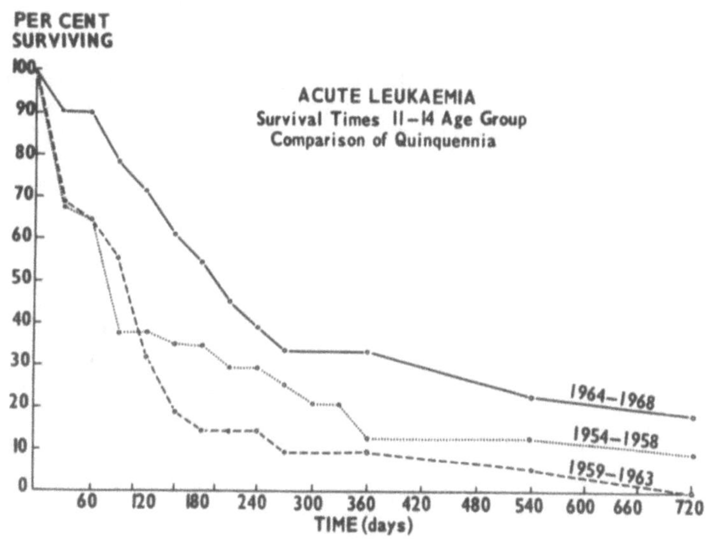


*Fig. 15. Acute leukaemia. Survival times by quinquennia, age 11-14 years*

Table 10. Extramedullary involvement in leukaemia

| Period | C.N.S. | Testicular | Parotid | Renal |
|---|---|---|---|---|
| 1954-1958 | 4 | 0 | 2 | 0 |
| 1959-1963 | 15 | 3 | 0 | 1 |
| 1964-1968 | 34 | 2 | 1 | 3 |

6. The Number of Drugs Used. The improvement in survival times of the children corresponded with an increase in the number of antileukaemic drugs used (Table 10). During 1954 - 1958 one-third of the children were given steroids only, another third were given steroids and antimetabolites and the remainder were given no specific treatment, or doses of drugs unlikely to affect the course of the disease. During 1959 - 1963 the majority were given steroids and antimetabolites, while after 1963 many of the children were given other drugs in addition.

7. The Hospitals Where the Patients were Treated. A comparison was made between the survival times of those children treated in the paediatric units or adult wards of the general hospitals of the region and those children treated in the two large, purely paediatric hospitals - the Royal Manchester Children's Hospital or Booth Hall Children's Hospital. In each quinquennium those treated in the large paediatric hospitals did significantly better (Fig. 16). This could have been partly due to the fact that a higher proportion of children between 2 and 10 years (i. e. those with a better prognosis) were treated in the paediatric than in the general hospitals. However, even when this difference in the children's ages was taken into account, those treated in the large paediatric hospitals survived significantly longer than those in general hospitals (Fig. 17).

It was not possible to demonstrate from the Manchester data the importance of other factors which have been reported to influence the prognosis. Mediastinal lymph node enlargement, gross hepatosplenomegaly, central nervous system involvement at onset and poor nutrition usually associated with low socioeconomic status have all been found to indicate poor prognosis (4, 30). WALTERS et al. (1972) (31) have shown that remission is less likely to be obtained and is shorter in Negro than in Caucasian children. The number of Negro children in the Manchester series does not allow for similar observations to be made, but in recent years there has been an increasing number of Asian children and preliminary studies indicate a worse prognosis in this group.

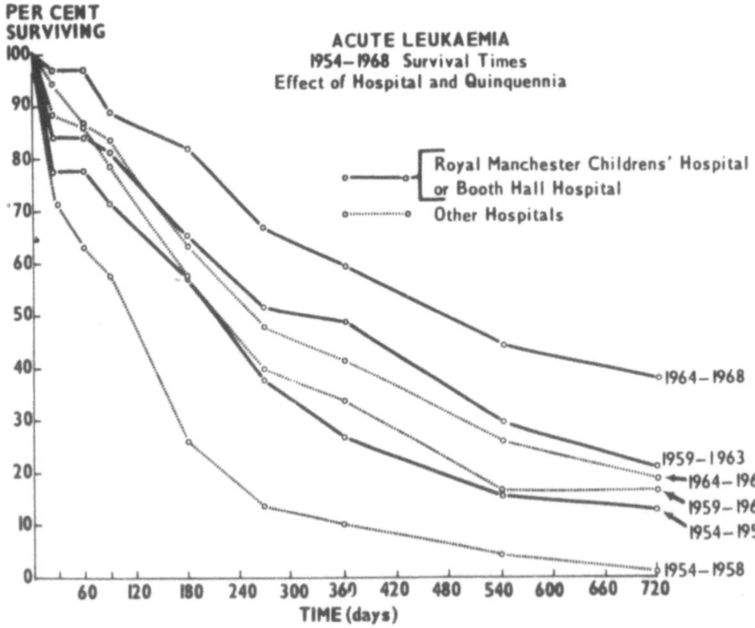


*Fig. 16. Acute leukaemia. Effect of hospital on survival by quinquennia*

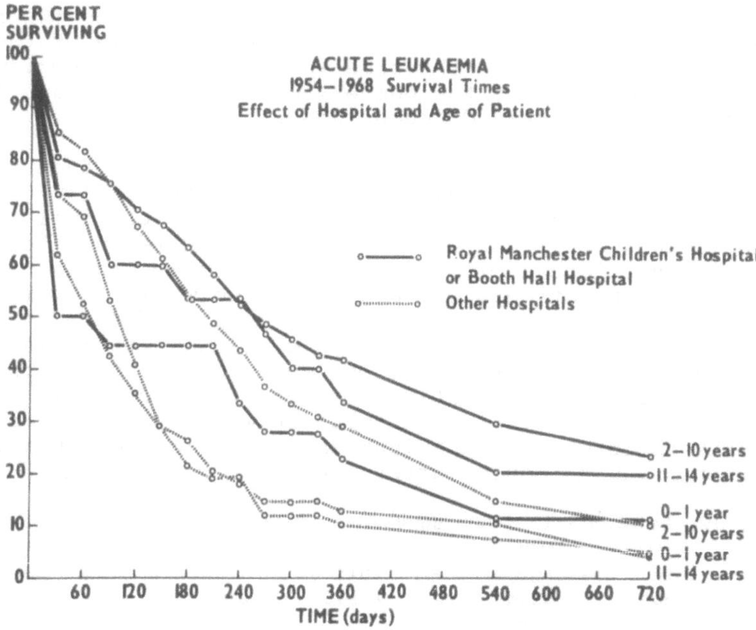


*Fig. 17. Acute leukaemia. Effect of hospital and age of patient on survival*

## Extramedullary Complications

An increase in the number of patients with extramedullary complications of leukaemia has followed the increase in survival times. These complications are not confined to periods of haematological relapse but they clearly represent spread of the leukaemic process. The principal involvement is in the central nervous system but other sites include the testes, parotid glands and kidneys (Table 10).

1. Central Nervous System Leukaemia. Fifty-three of the 465 cases developed central nervous system leukaemia, an overall incidence of 11.5%. This incidence is lower than many recent series (32) because the survival of the children in the earlier quinquennia was too short for this complication to have arisen. As the survival times increased there was a rise in the number of children who developed signs of central nervous system involvement - 3% in 1954 - 1958, 9% in 1959 - 1963, and 22% in 1964 - 1968. Most cases occurred within 18 months of diagnosis (Table 11) and the incidence fell off after this time. There was no sex difference. The majority had ALL (77.5%), while 19% had ASC and 3.5% had AML.

MELHORN et al. (1970) (33) showed that the incidence of C.N.S. leukaemia was higher in those children who had an initial white cell count of over 10,000 μl. WEST et al. (1972) (34) suggested that the leukae-

Table 11. C.N.S. involvement in acute leukaemia, 1954-1968

| Period after diagnosis (months) | -6 | -12 | -18 | -24 | -30 | -36 | -42 | -48 | -54 | -60 | -66 |
|---|---|---|---|---|---|---|---|---|---|---|---|
| No. of cases | 12 | 12 | 11 | 5 | 5 | 3 | 2 | 0 | 2 | 0 | 1 |

mic cells may enter the central nervous system as the result of an intracranial petechial haemorrhage around the time of the initial diagnosis of leukaemia and the time when the C.N.S. symptoms develop is largely determined by the number and replication rate of the leukaemic cells which have gained access there.

2. Testicular, Parotid and Renal Involvement. Other sites are much less frequently involved. Although MATHÉ et al. (1966) (35) in an extensive investigation of patients in apparently full remission were able to show small numbers of leukaemic cells in sites such as liver, spleen and kidneys, it is unusual for these organs to be involved clinically in patients who are otherwise well. In only 4 children was palpable renal enlargement detected during life, and in each case this was found at diagnosis. Five boys developed testicular involvement, an incidence of 2%. Ovarian lesions were not detected. Three children, all boys, developed parotid enlargement. In contrast to renal involvement, parotid or testicular invasion was not seen in any of the Manchester children when the leukaemia was first diagnosed but appeared between 3 and 42 months after treatment was commenced.

Table 12. Leukaemia 1954-68; survivors 1973

| CTR. No. | Date diagnosis | Sex | Age at diagnosis (years) | Cell type | Initial W.B.C. | Initial platelets | Treatment | Date treatment stopped | Comments |
|---|---|---|---|---|---|---|---|---|---|
| 121/59 | Nov. 1959 | M | 10 | ALL | 4800 | 81000 | Steroids; 6-M.P. | May 1969 | Very sensitive to 6-M.P. |
| 2/60 | Jan. 1960 | M | 2 | ALL | 58000 | 160000 | Steroids, 6-MP; Mtx. | Oct. 1962 | Vegetarian diet |
| 70/61 | June 1961 | M | 5 | ALL | 9400 | 60000 | Steroids; 6-MP. | Feb. 1963 | Primary Tb. in 1963 |
| 1/62 | Jan. 1962 | M | 7 | ALL | 3200 | 400000 | Steroids, 6-MP. | April 1965 | |
| 27/64 | March 1964 | M | 7 | ASC | 4700 | 270000 | Steroids, 6-MP. | Feb. 1972 | |
| 68/65 | May 1965 | M | 3 | ALL | 5400 | 140000 | Steroids, 6-MP, Mtx. Vcr. | July 1972 | C.N.S. symptoms Dec.67 No cells in CSF. |
| 85/68 | Dec. 1967 | F | 2 | ALL | 3000 | 229000 | Steroids, 6-MP; Mtx; Cyclo; Vcr. | Still on treatment | Very sensitive to Mtx. |
| 62/68 | June 1968 | M | 4 | ALL | 4600 | 300000 | Steroids; 6-MP; Mtx; Aspar; BCG. | June 1971 | Marrow relapse Feb. 1970 probably due to undertreatment (see text) |
| 89/68 | Sept. 1968 | F | 4 | ASC | 2000 | 5000 | Steroids; 6-MP. | March 1972 | |

## Long-term Survival in Childhood Leukaemia

Details of the children who are still alive are shown in Table 12 and those who died more than 4 years after diagnosis are shown in Table 13. Of the children who presented between 1954 and 1968 9 are alive, an incidence of 1.94%. Four are well more than 10 years after diagnosis (0.86%). Six children died after surviving for over 4 years, C.N.S. disease developing in each case. All of these long-term survivors suffered from either ALL or stem cell leukaemia; no child who had any of the varieties of acute myeloid leukaemia was alive in 1973. Seven of the 9 surviving children are boys, but a larger series of cases from all over the British Isles, including the cases described here, showed that a significantly higher proportion of girls survived more than 4 years, and there was no sex difference for 10-year survivors (36).

The treatment given to the long-term survivors in Manchester would by modern standards be regarded as inadequate to eliminate the disease, since it consisted of using steroids to induce remissions which were then maintained with antimetabolites in low dosage. 6-mercaptopurine

Table 13. Leukaemia 1954-1968; children who died more than four years after diagnosis

| CTR. No. | Date diag-nosis | Sex | Age at diag-nosis (years) | Cell type | Initial W.B.C. | Initial plate-lets | Treatment | Diagnosis to death (years) | Comment |
|---|---|---|---|---|---|---|---|---|---|
| 69/62 | Sept. 1962 | M | 3 | ALL | 7600 | 73000 | Steroids 6-MP; Mtx. | 4 1/2 | CNS. in-volvement Nov. 1965 |
| 95/64 | Oct. 1964 | M | 5 | ALL | 2000 | 85000 | Steroids 6-MP; Cyclo., Arab. C., | 5 3/4 | Appendicitis June 1967; CNS. in-volement April 1970 |
| 4/65 | Jan. 1965 | F | 4 | ALL | 6700 | 98000 | Steroids 6-MP; Mtx. & Vinc., Cyclo., Arab. C. | 6 | CNS. in-volvement Feb. 1969 |
| 87/65 | Oct. 1965 | M | 7 | ALL | 15000 | not done | Steroids 6-MP; Mtx. & Cyclo. | 4 | CNS. in-volvement April 1967 |
| 84/66 | Sept. 1966 | M | 1 | ALL | 11800 | 18000 | Steroids 6-MP; Mtx. & Vinc. | 6 | Haematolog-ical relapse, Dec. 1967 & Jan. 1972. CNS. in-volvement June 1972 |
| 131/68 | March 1968 | M | 3 | ALL | 6300 | 45000 | Steroids 6-MP., Vinc., Arab. C., Aspar. | 4 | CNS. and testicular involvement Jan. 1972 |

and steroids were the sole drugs used in 5 cases. In one child, aged 10 years (CTR.121/59) the disease appeared to be very sensitive to 6-mercaptopurine: a dose of 50 mg per day resulted in a persistent white cell count of 3,000 µl.

Only one child had a high white cell count. In 4 of the 9 survivors the initial platelet count was normal and it was moderately reduced in two others. These features imply a good prognosis and were noted in the series of TILL et al. (1973) (36). The fact that only 7 of the children treated for leukaemia in the Manchester region between 1959 and 1968 were surviving in 1973 suggests that with low-dose treatment less than 3% will be cured. These figures resemble those reported for Los Angeles Children's Hospital by WILLIAMS et al. (1972) (37), who found 1.3% long-term survivals in a study between 1956 and 1967 of 681 cases in which intensive treatment was not used, and of Children's Study Group A who found 0.8% 5-year survivors in 1770 cases treated from 1957 to 1964 (4).

TILL et al. (1973) (36) in an analysis of 100 long-term survivors from acute leukaemia showed that there were no recurrences more than ten years after diagnosis. Patients who had had no relapse during the 4 years after ALL was diagnosed, had a 70% chance of prolonged survival ("cure"), but those who relapsed during that period had only about a 17% chance of prolonged survival. Eight of the 9 Manchester children who are still alive have never had any sign of recurrence since diagnosis, but one of the survivors (CTR.85/68) had a marrow relapse 1 1/2 years after diagnosis. By contrast 4 of the 6 patients who died more than 4 years after diagnosis (Table 13) had relapsed during the initial 4-year period, and all of them had extramedullary involvement at some time during their illness. TILL et al. found that the proportion of patients diagnosed during 1963 - 1967 who survived for 4 years was three times that of those diagnosed during the previous decade but the numbers of very long-term survivors had only increased by 50%.

## THE MANAGEMENT OF ACUTE LEUKAEMIA IN CHILDHOOD

It is no longer acceptable to consider acute leukaemia in childhood as an inevitably fatal disease. Although the number of cures has been small in the past (27), it is reasonable to believe that the continuing improvement in the median survival and disease-free interval due to improved therapy will lead to an increase in the number of children cured.

### Acute Lymphoblastic Leukaemia

Because of the much greater frequency of acute lymphoblastic leukaemia in childhood most experience has been gained in this field and the majority of reports relate to the therapy of this type of leukaemia. The improved results with therapy available during recent years and the knowledge that early treatment is important in obtaining these results make it imperative that the children are admitted at the time of diagnosis to a centre where facilities are available for appropriate supportive therapy and where sufficient experience has been gained in management (28, 38). In these circumstances between 20% and 50% of the children can be expected to live for 5 years without evidence of the disease (39, 40). If the children achieve this prolonged disease-free interval, the chances of later relapse diminish; for example, PINKEL (1971) (41) has shown that in a group of 26 children none of those

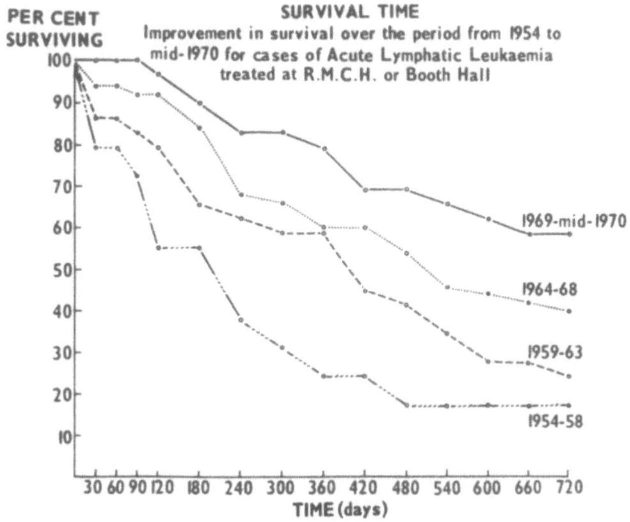


*Fig. 18. Acute leukaemia. Improvement in survival from 1954 to mid-1970 for cases of acute lymphoblastic leukaemia treated at Royal Manchester Children's Hospital or Booth Hall Children's Hospital, Manchester*

remaining in complete remission for 28 months subsequently relapsed and that continuous treatment for 24 - 33 months was sufficient to obtain a 5-year disease-free period in 20% of cases. LAMPKIN et al. (1969) (42) showed a 13% 5-year disease-free rate and KRIVIT et al. (1970) (43) a 6.5% 5-year disease-free rate following a much less intensive treatment programme.

Certain factors are essential in achieving these results:

1. The induction of complete remission following diagnosis. This implies the return of the bone marrow to M 1 Status - a cellular marrow demonstrating satisfactory haematopoiesis and containing 5% or less of lymphoblasts and stem cells and 40% or less lymphocytes plus lymphoblasts plus stem cells. There may be changes in the marrow secondary to therapy. The child must be free of symptoms and signs attributable to leukaemia but may have symptoms associated with therapy.

2. The maintenance of complete remission with the associated prevention of the spread of the disease to the central nervous system.

3. Because these more intensive programmes are associated with an increased mortality in remission the early use of supportive measures such as platelet and white cell transfusions becomes important and in some circumstances sterile rooms and reversed barrier nursing are indicated (44, 45, 46).

## Anti-Leukaemic Drugs

In 1948 SIDNEY FARBER (47) and his colleagues introduced the folic acid antagonists and were able to demonstrate that remission could be obtained in acute lymphoblastic leukaemia. Since that time several other drugs have been used but it has been the combinations of these drugs rather than a single new agent which have achieved the high remission rates now expected. The use of these combinations exploits the different biochemical effects of the agents and gives additive or synergistic results.

Details of the commonly used drugs are outlined below along with the reported remission rates when used alone and in combination (Tables 14 and 15).

Table 14. Anti-Leukaemic drugs

| Drug | Route of Administration | Dose and Interval | Toxicity to marrow | Other side effects | Principal use |
|---|---|---|---|---|---|
| Prednisolone | P.O. or I. V. | 40-60 mgs/$M^2$ daily. Some regimes 200 mgm daily for 5-7 days | O | Hypertension Hyperuricaemia Metabolic | Induction of remission |
| 6-Mercaptopurine | P.O. or I.V. | 50-75 mgs/$M^2$ daily. Some regimes 500 mgs per day in short courses | + | Nausea and vomiting. Hepatotoxicity Skin photosensitivity | Maintenance |
| Methotrexate | P.O., I.M., I.V. or I.T. | 2.5 mgs/$M^2$ daily. 10-20 mgs/$M^2$ in 5 day courses; 100-200 mgs/$M^2$ IV once in 14 days and several other regimes. I.T. 10 mgs/$M^2$. Alt. days or weekly for several courses | + | Gastro-intestinal ulceration. Pneumonitis. Osteoporosis | Maintenance. C.N.S. prophylaxis and treatment of C.N.S. disease |
| Cyclophosphamide | P.O. or I.V. | 50-100 mgs/$M^2$ daily 300-600 mgs/$M^2$ every 7-14 days | + | Alopecia. Nausea and vomiting. Haemorrhagic cystitis and bladder fibrosis | Maintenance |
| Vincristine | I.V. | 1.5 mgs/$M^2$ | + — | Alopecia. Neurotoxicity giving muscle weakness. Sensory and motor changes. Constipation. Jaw pain. Hyponatraemia | Induction |
| Cytosine Arabinoside | I.V., I.M. or I.T. | 80-100 mgs/$M^2$ in various different regimes I.T. 20 mgs/$M^2$ | + | Nausea and vomiting. Mouth ulcers. Anorexia Alopecia | Induction and maintenance |
| Rubidomycin | I.V. | 25-60 mgs/$M^2$ in short and repeated courses. 1-5 days with 14-28 days intervals | + + | Nausea and vomiting. Cardiotoxicity | Induction |
| L. Asparaginase | I.V. or I.M. | 3000-10000 units at variable intervals | + — | Nausea and vomiting. Allergic reactions. Anaphylaxis. Liver toxicity | Induction |

Table 15. Remission rates in acute lymphoblastic leukaemia

| Drug | % Complete remission | Reference |
|---|---|---|
| Methotrexate | 22 | 77 |
| 6-Mercaptopurine | 27 | 77 |
| 6-Mercaptopurine and Methotrexate | 39 | 77 |
| Prednisone | 57 and 63 | 78, 79 |
| Vincristine | 57 | 80 |
| Prednisone and Vincristine | 83 - 90 | 81, 82, 59, 64 |
| Rubidomycin | 38 | 83 |
| Prednisone, Vincristine and Rubidomycin | 94 - 100 | 63, 83, 46, 54 |
| Asparaginase | 55 and 76 | 84, 85 |
| Cytosine Arabinoside | 30 | 86 |
| Asparaginase and Cytosine Arabinoside | 89 | 87 |
| Prednisone, Vincristine, Rubidomycin and Asparaginase | 100 | 50 |
| Cyclophosphamide | 18 and 40 | 88, 89 |
| Cyclophosphamide and Prednisolone | 76 | 90 |

## Corticosteroids

Prednisolone is the most commonly used steroid in this country and is preferred to prednisone as the latter requires to be metabolised in the liver before becoming fully active. It is of particular value in induction because it does not cause marrow depression. High doses of prednisolone have not been shown to increase the incidence of remission (48) though it has been used in very high dosage in the P.O.M.P. and C.O.A.P. regimes.

## Methotrexate

A folic acid antagonist which acts by inhibition of the enzyme dihydrofolic acid reductase and thus prevents the conversion of folic acid to tetrahydro-folic acid. The reduced form is necessary for the synthesis of DNA and RNA. The schedule of administration is very important in respect of remission duration.

## 6-Mercaptopurine

A purine analogue which inhibits purine synthesis and hence DNA formation.

## Cyclophosphamide

A synthetic alkylating agent, i. e. it causes the replacement of a hydrogen ion by an alkyl group and therefore reacts with many cell components including nucleoprotein.

Vincristine

A salt of a natural alkaloid derived from the periwinkle plant. Although there have been detailed studies on the biochemical action (CREASEY, 1968) (95), the exact mode of action is not known. In vitro experiments suggest that it arrests mitotic division at the stage of metaphase.

Cytosine arabinoside

A synthetic nucleoside which differs from the nucleosides, cytidine and deoxycytidine in the replacement of ribose and deoxyribose respectively by arabinose. Its mode of action appears to be that of inhibition of deoxycytidine synthesis, and of cytidylic acid kinases. It also causes chromosome breaks in human leucocytes in vitro. DNA synthesis is inhibited in cell culture after exposure to cytosine arabinoside.

Daunorubicin (Rubidomycin)

An antibiotic of the anthracycline group isolated from streptomyces peucetius, and caeruleorubidus. Its mode of action is directly upon the nucleic acids of the cell, particularly on DNA, probably by inhibition of polymerases, so that the drug forms a complex with DNA which is thereby prevented from acting as a primer in duplication and transcription reactions.

Asparaginase

A protein of undetermined structure usually obtained from Escherichia coli. It catalyses the hydrolysis of L-asparagine to L-aspartic acid and ammonia and its action is dependent on the inability of some leukaemic cell lines to synthesise their own L-asparagine and the need for it to be provided by extracellular sources. This is due to a lack of the enzyme asparagine synthetase. By depleting extracellular sources the sensitive cells cannot function and thus asparaginase utilizes a specific metabolic defect in certain malignant cells.

Most of these agents kill leukaemic cells by interfering with a particular phase of the mitotic cycle, and with this in mind a combination of drugs will produce the best results. There are, however, serious obstacles to the complete elimination of leukaemic blast cells because of the pool of quiescent cells which are resistant to chemotherapy but nevertheless appear to be capable of active proliferation after long periods of rest (49).

Treatment of Acute Lymphoblastic Leukaemia

Once the diagnosis of ALL has been made treatment should begin without delay. It is necessary, however, to bear in mind that at this time there is severe marrow failure and supportive therapy is particularly important (see below). Baseline investigations are necessary before treatment begins and should include:

1. F.B.C. with differential and platelets
2. Bone marrow examination
3. Skeletal survey and chest X-ray
4. Single film I.V.P.
5. Blood cultures

6. Blood urea
7. Serum uric acid
8. Liver function tests
9. Immunoglobulins
10. Swabs and cultures of urine, faeces, nose, throat and any septic skin lesions

Other investigations which may be included where facilities allow are chromosome studies on blood and bone marrow.

The combination of vincristine and prednisolone has the least depressant effect on the normal bone marrow and allows for the induction of remission in the majority of children with minimal toxic effects. The addition of other drugs such as daunorubicin, asparaginase, and cytosine arabinoside will increase the percentage of remission inductions but will also increase the danger of early death due to haemorrhage and infection and should therefore probably be reserved for cases in which there are specific indications (50). Those features which indicate that the disease may be difficult to treat have been discussed in the section on prognosis. They include a high initial white count, the presence of mediastinal lymph node enlargement, gross hepatosplenomegaly, central nervous system disease at the onset, and poor nutrition - usually associated with the lower socioeconomic status. Age of onset is also important - the outlook being less satisfactory in children under the age of 2 years or greater than 10 years. Remissions in Negro children are more difficult to obtain than in Caucasians.

Once complete remission has been obtained the object of ongoing therapy is to maintain this state for as long as possible, as the length of remission is directly correlated with the overall length of survival and it is extremely rare for any long-term survivors to have shown evidence of relapse at any time. The drugs most commonly used in induction programmes tend to be less satisfactory in maintaining remission and also have undesirable side effects (Table 14).

For some years after anti-leukaemic drugs became available the tendency was to use, as maintenance therapy, a lower dose of the drug which had achieved remission and to continue its use until relapse occurred. This has been shown to impair the chance of long-term survival (51), and has therefore been superseded by the cyclical use of a number of agents in as high a dose as possible and in combinations tailored to make most effective use of their specific effects while minimising toxicity. There are no advantages in using reduced dosages during remission as one of the aims of continued therapy is to obtain further cytoreduction and more effective elimination of leukaemic cells. In addition, once the marrow has returned to a normal state following remission it is better able to tolerate high dose therapy than at the time of diagnosis when there is hypoplasia of normal cells. Most protocols therefore cite an optimum dose which should be aimed for but altered to allow for different host tolerance and rate of drug metabolism. The direct effects on hepatic and renal function by the drugs may induce impaired tolerance with prolonged use and require alterations in dosage. It is probably better, however, to give the drugs in high dose less frequently than to maintain the original interval between courses and reduce dose.

Two different principles of maintenance are at present in use:

1. Continuous maintenance with one or more drugs with or without the superimposition of reinduction courses (39, 52, 54).
2. Pulses of combination therapy without continuous maintenance (55 - 59).

It would appear that both types of maintenance therapy need to be continued for at least 2 years to achieve appreciable long-term survival rates.

## Central Nervous System Leukaemia

No programme of therapy for ALL would now be considered complete without some attempt being made to prevent the development of overt disease in the central nervous system. This complication has been shown to interrupt complete remission with an increasing frequency directly related to the length of remission (60, 61, 32). Intensive systemic chemotherapy does not prevent this. The signs are those of raised intracranial pressure with morning headache, vomiting and sometimes photophobia. Examination of the retina reveals papilloedema and occasionally white plaque-like deposits alongside the vessels. Lumbar puncture shows the fluid to be under raised pressure with a pleocytosis and a variable rise in protein levels. There is usually no change in other parameters. The cytocentrifuge may be of considerable help in diagnosing C.N.S. disease (97).

A proportion of children with C.N.S. involvement develop a "hypothalamic syndrome" with very rapid weight gain and a voracious appetite. When florid signs and symptoms are present the diagnosis does not give rise to difficulties but it has been shown that the total cell count in the C.S.F. may be normal even when leukaemic cells are present and therefore it is necessary to have special methods of examination (62). It is particularly important in programmes involving the prophylactic therapy to the C.N.S. to know whether or not leukaemic cells can be detected before the start of treatment in order to assess the effect of therapy. Treatment of C.N.S. involvement has consisted of craniospinal irradiation (63) or intrathecal drugs or a combination of the two methods. Intrathecal methotrexate 10 mg/$m^2$ at twice weekly or weekly intervals is the commonest drug used and may be given by the lumbar route (64) or through an Ommaya reservoir into the ventricles (56). None of these procedures is without risk. Irradiation will cause temporary alopecia, bone marrow depression, and in some patients transient headache and vomiting. Intrathecal methotrexate can give rise to a chemical arachnoiditis. Rarely encephalopathy (65), paralysis (66) and death (67) have been reported.

There have been three phases in the use of irradiation to all or part of the central nervous system.

The first group of patients treated had cranial and spinal irradiation but at different dose and time levels. The cranial irradiation covered the whole of the brain and the retro-orbital tissues. The dose delivered was 2400 rads in the midplane from two parallel opposed megavoltage or cobalt fields, in 2 1/2 - 3 weeks. In the Manchester cases the time was 2 1/2 weeks, using 4 fractions per week. To this was added spinal irradiation, using straight on spinal fields 5 cm wide with gaps at 4 MeV of 1.5 cm between contiguous fields and taking a dose of 1000 rads on the posterior surface of the vertebral bodies in 4 fractions over 5 - 6 days. Intrathecal methotrexate was given after the completion of therapy.

The second group of children was treated with craniospinal irradiation, the same dose being delivered throughout. The lateral fields to the cranium were extended to take in the cervical spine down to the shoulder level and the spinal fields matched on at this level, the gap calculated to be necessary on the skin to give reasonable homogeneity at depth being 1.5 cm. The spinal dose was again that at the posterior surface of the spinal bodies. The dose delivered here and in the mid-plane of the head was 2400 rads in 4 weeks, treating 5 fractions per week. No intrathecal methotrexate was used in this group.

The third group had cranial irradiation alone as described for group one and the dose was again 2400 rads in 2 1/2 weeks, given in 4 fractions per week. Five doses of intrathecal methotrexate were given over this period at weekly intervals.

At the present time there seems to be no significant difference between the efficacy of the different programmes but some early evidence suggests a higher morbidity in those protocols which include craniospinal irradiation.

In Manchester 81 children with leukaemia received craniospinal irradiation between June 1970 and December 1972. Seven of these were irradiated after the first sign of C.N.S. involvement and in every case the disease recurred within the nervous system. Forty-five children are still in complete continuous remission; 15 have developed haematological relapse without evidence of C.N.S. leukaemia; 8 at the time of relapse had disease both in the marrow and C.N.S. and in only six children has there been C.N.S. disease as the first sign of relapse. In other words, in 74 children given prophylactic C.N.S. irradiation (some of whom had intrathecal methotrexate as well) only 14 have so far developed signs of nervous system involvement.

Since March 1973 cranial irradiation with intrathecal methotrexate have been used for C.N.S. prophylaxis but it is too early to assess the result.

## Gonadal and Renal Leukaemia

Involvement of the gonads is a much less common overt complication and apparently is of less sinister significance (68). Radiotherapy is the treatment of choice.

Renal infiltration causing enlargement of the kidneys may be present at the time of diagnosis and can be associated with hypertension. Radiotherapy is probably indicated in addition to chemotherapy as the kidneys may well act as sanctuaries for residual leukaemic cells.

## Bone Lesions

It has already been stated that bone pain is a common presenting feature of acute leukaemia. Associated radiological lesions are often demonstrable (69) and range from generalised osteoporosis to circumscribed osteolytic lesions, metaphyseal translucent bands, and periosteal reaction with elevation (70, 71). Some of the more florid lesions may resemble the metastatic lesions of neuroblastoma or primary Ewing's tumours of bone. The bone pain usually settles satisfactorily when remission is induced but severe local pain will respond readily to a low dose of irradiation.

## Infection

Infection is the major cause of death in children with leukaemia. A small percentage of children die in the initial induction phase before remission can be achieved. This group usually has a gram-negative septicaemia but a very wide variety of different organisms has been incriminated. During relapse and in the terminal phase of the disease infections are again common, since granulocytopenia is usual and response to infection is impaired at these times. Every effort should be made to isolate the organism concerned but in our experience the most efficacious combination of drugs to use until the organism has been isolated is cloxacillin 250-500 mg 6-hourly and gentamycin 1 mg/kg 6-hourly, both drugs being given by the intravenous route. Once the organism has been identified and sensitivities known, changes in antibiotics may be necessary.

Some centres have advocated the use of a larger number of antibiotics to cover a wider spectrum of organisms (56). In the paediatric field this does not appear to be necessary and in the last 5 years only two deaths have occurred in Manchester in the induction phase due to infection in a total of approximately 200 children treated.

The use of granulocyte transfusions can be of great value. Normal donors can be used and transfusions of $0.5 \times 10^{10}$ cells will usually produce significant improvement in otherwise unresponsive patients. In Manchester three or four leucocyte transfusions are usually given to treat an infection.

Viral infections may be prolonged and troublesome and are often associated with bone marrow depression, so that chemotherapy may have to be stopped for a time. Varicella and zoster should be treated either with gamma globulin 1 mg/kg or with cytosine arabinoside 100 mg/m$^2$ daily for 3 days and the latter has also been reported to be useful in herpes simplex infection. Cytomegalovirus infection is not uncommon but should not be considered the cause of problems unless a rising titre can be demonstrated. Idoxuridine may be helpful in its treatment.

Pneumocystis carinii is an increasing hazard in patients in remission (72, 73). It can only be diagnosed with certainty by lung or bronchial brush biopsy. The treatment is pentamidine isothionate (4 mg/kg per day).

Fungal infections - systemic candidiasis being the most common - should be treated with amphotericin B and oral and intestinal lesions usually respond to nystatin.

## Hyperuricaemia

Even before the commencement of induction therapy many patients have a raised serum uric acid level and this often rises further due to rapid turnover of nucleic acids and destruction of a large tumour cell mass. The condition is often worse in patients with evidence of leukaemic infiltration of the kidneys. The development of uric acid nephropathy can be prevented by the use of allopurinol (10 mg/kg) daily in three divided doses for 5 - 7 days during induction. Allopurinol should not be used in conjunction with 6-mercaptopurine as it acts by preventing the action of xanthine oxidase which is the enzyme concerned in conversion of xanthine to uric acid and also in 6-MP degradation.

## Acute Myeloid Leukaemia

Until fairly recently the incidence of complete remission in acute leukaemia of the myelogenous group was uncommon. PIERCE et al. (1969) (4) reported a 20% remission rate with a median survival of 1 month in 1967. The introduction of rubidomycin and cytosine arabinoside has made a considerable difference, however, and this is probably enhanced by the addition of thioguanine which has been shown to have a synergistic effect with cytosine arabinoside.

In Manchester since 1970 18 children with acute myeloid leukaemia have been treated with a 4-drug protocol using cytosine arabinoside, daunorubicin, prednisolone and 6-mercaptopurine or 6-thioguanine. The initial remission rate overall was 78%. Median survival was 5 months and the median survival for those entering remission was 8 1/2 months (EVANS et al., 1975) (96).

Multiple drug chemotherapy has been used with some success in the treatment of acute transformation of chronic granulocytic leukaemia in adults (SPIERS et al., 1974) (94).

It seems reasonable to assume, therefore, that increasingly effective regimes of treatment will be developed for this disease and that there will be improvement in survival.

### Immunotherapy

The role of immunotherapy in the treatment of acute leukaemia has still to be evaluated. MATHE et al. (1969) (74) have shown prolonged disease-free periods in patients treated with BCG, pooled irradiated leukaemic cells, or both. All these patients had received previous intensive chemotherapy. BCG was also used in a Medical Research Council study (75) which showed no difference between controls and immunized patients. Another study involved the use of pertussis antigen (76). A group with lymphoblastic leukaemia has been treated in Manchester with irradiated blasts and BCG after 2 years' chemotherapy. No significant effect has appeared.

The evidence for the efficacy of active immunotherapy in acute myeloid leukaemia is at present being studied in a trial sponsored by the Medical Research Council in this country and early results are encouraging.

## OTHER CONSIDERATIONS

Evaluation of success in the management of treatment of children with leukaemia needs to take into account the quality of their survival and the stress on the family as a whole. In order to enhance the former and minimise the latter there is a need for the close co-operation of a dedicated group of people including nurses, technicians, pharmacists, clerks and medical social workers as well as the doctors and research workers, parents and patient. The prime object of therapy must be to co-ordinate in minimizing mental and physical trauma while in no way impairing chances of cure. There is a need to establish a mutual trust between parents, patient and doctor, and for this to be possible, adequate time must be given to explanation and discussion, and the parents and patient should feel able to call on an individual doctor at all times. Experience shows that this arrangement does not lead to advantage being taken or excessive demands being made as the parents have confidence in the arrangement and find their worries are minimized.

Once a child becomes resistant to therapy, having had treatment with a variety of drugs, further aggressive attempts at treatment are not undertaken. In the light of present knowledge there is no evidence that prolonged remission can then be achieved. The period of time waiting for a child to die is a far greater strain on the family than the actual event of death. For this reason, in addition to ensuring that the child's immediate needs are being dealt with, the doctors and nursing staff must devote much of their time to supporting the family during the final illness and after death. There is often a need to explain to parents their reactions, which may include anger towards the child, doctors and nurses, blame of themselves and each other, as well as guilt, depression and sadness.

After the death of the child the doctor's job is not complete. There is a need to take time to sit and talk with the parents both immediately and after a few weeks in order to help the family to live and grow without bitterness and with a sense of gain as well as loss.

## REFERENCES


1. COURT BROWN, W. M., DOLL, R.: Br. Med. J. I, 981-988 (1961)
2. HARDISTY, R. M., SPEED, D. E., TILL, M.: Br. J. Haemat. 10, 551-566 (1964)
3. FRAUMENI, J. F., MANNING, M. D., MITUS, W. J.: J. Nat. Cancer Inst. 46, 461-470 (1971)
4. PIERCE, M. I., BORGES, W. H., HEYN, R., WOLFF, J. A., GILBERT, E. S.: Cancer 23, 1296-1304 (1969)
5. BROWNING, D., GROSS, S.: Amer. J. Dis. Child 116, 576-585 (1968)
6. CUTLER, S. J., AXTELL, L., HEISE, H.: J. Nat. Cancer Inst. 39, 993-1026 (1967)
7. FRAUMENI, J. F., MILLER, R. W.: J. Nat. Cancer Inst. 38, 593-603 (1967)
8. STARK, C. R., CLEINICK, A.: J. Nat. Cancer Inst. 37, 369-379 (1966)
9. LEE, J. A. H.: Brit. Med. J. I, 988-992 (1961)
10. SUTTON, R. N. P., BISHUN, N. P., SOOTHILL, J. F.: Brit. J. Haem. 17, 113-119 (1969)
11. CHANDRA, R. K.: Arch. Dis. Childh. 47, 618-620 (1972)
12. EVANS, D. I. K.: Arch. Dis. Childh. 48, 441-445 (1973)
13. FRAUMENI, J. F.: Seminars in Haematology 6, 250-260 (1969)
14. WEISGERBER, C., SCHAISON, G.: Actualités, Hemat. 4, 47-58 (1970)
15. BERNARD, J., SELIGMANN, M.: Nouvelle Rev. Fr. hématol. 8, 759 (1968)
16. STEWART, A., WEBB, J., HEWITT, D.: Brit. Med. J. I, 1495 (1958)
17. MARSDEN, H. B.: In: Scientific Foundations of Paediatrics, Lymphoma and Leukaemia. DAVIS, J. A., DOBBING, J. (eds.). London: W. Heinemann Medical Books Ltd., 1974, p. 785
18. ROSNER, F., LEE, S. L., and Acute Leukaemia Group B: Am. J. Med. 53, 203-218 (1972)
19. HAYHOE, F. G., QUAGLINO, D., DOLL, R.: The Cytology and Cytochemistry of Acute Leukaemias. A study of 140 cases. London, Her Majesty's Stationery Office, 1964. Medical Research Council Special Report series No. 304
20. JOLLES, P., STERNBERG, M., MATHÉ, G.: Israel J. med. Sci. 1, 445 (1965)
21. OSSERMAN, E. F., LAWLOR, D. P.: J. exp. Med. 124, 921 (1966)
22. HAYHOE, F. G.: Seminars in Haematology 6, 261-270 (1969)

23. HAYHOE, F. G., CAWLEY, J. C.: Clinics in Haematology 1, 49 (1972)
24. HAYHOE, F. G., QUAGLINO, D.: Brit. J. Haem. 4, 375-389 (1958)
25. Medical Research Council: Brit. Med. J. I, 201-208 (1968)
26. MAURER, H. S., VIDA, L. N., HONIG, G. R.: Blood 39, 778 (1972)
27. BURCHENAL, J. A.: Cancer 21, 595-9 (1968)
28. Medical Research Council: Brit. Med. J. 4, 7-9 (1971)
29. HARDISTY, R. M., TILL, M. M.: Arch. Dis. Child. 43, 107-115 (1968)
30. LIPWORTH, L., ABELIN, T., CONNELLY, R. R.: J. of Chronic Disease 23, 105-116 (1970)
31. WALTERS, T. R., BUSHORE, M., SIMONE, J.: Cancer 29, 210-214 (1972)
32. BRODER, L. E., CARTER, S. K.: Meningeal Leukaemia, Plenum Press New York - London: Plenum Press, 1972
33. MELHORN, D. K., GROSS, S., FISHER, B. J., NEWMAN, A. J.: Blood 36, 55-60 (1970)
34. WEST, R. J., GRAHAM-POLE, J., HARDISTY, R. M., PIKE, M. C.: Br. Med. J. 3, 311-314 (1972)
35. MATHÉ, G., SCHWARZENBERG, L., MERY, A. M., CATTAN, A., SCHNEIDER, M., AMIEL, J. L., SCHLUMBERGER, J. R., POISSON, J., WAJCNER, G.: Brit. Med. J. I, 640-642 (1966)
36. TILL, M., HARDISTY, R. M., PIKE, M. C.: Lancet I, 534-538 (1973)
37. WILLIAMS, K., HYMAN, C., HIGGINS, G., SHORÉ, N., ORTEGA, J., HAMMOND, D., KARON, M.: Blood 40, 973 (1972)
38. HOLLAND, J. F.: J.A.M.A. 209, 1511-1515 (1969)
39. PINKEL, D., SIMONE, J., HUSTU, O., AUR, R.J.A.: Pediatrics 50, 246-251 (1972)
40. SINKS, L. S.: Archives of Dis. Childhood 47, 811-813 (1972)
41. PINKEL, D.: J.A.M.A. 216, 648-652 (1971)
42. LAMPKIN, B.: Pediatric Clinics of North America 19, 1123-40 (1969)
43. KRIVIT, W., BEATTY, E. C., GILCHRIST, G.: J. of Pediatrics 76, 138-141 (1970)
44. JAMESON, B., GAMBLE, D. R., LYNCH, J., KAY, H.E.M.: Lancet I, 1034-1040 (1971)
45. BODEY, G. P., FREIREICH, E. J., FREI, E. III: Cancer 24, 972-980 (1969)
46. MATHÉ, G., SCHWARZENBERG, L., SCHNEIDER, M., SCHLUMBERGER, J., HAYAT, M., AMIEL, J. L., CATTAN, A., JASMIN, C.: Lancet 2, 380-382 (1967)
47. FARBER, S., DIAMOND, L. K., MERCER, R. D., SYLVESTER, R. F. Jr., WOLFF, J. A.: New Eng. J. Med. 238, 787 (1948)
48. LEIKIN, S. L., BRUBAKER, C., HARTMANN, J. R., MURPHY, M. L., WOLFF, J. A., PERRIN, E.: Cancer 21, 346-351 (1968)
49. KILLMAN, S. A.: Clinics in Haematology 1, 95 (1972)
50. AUR, R. J. A., SIMONE, J. V., HUSTU, H. O., PRATT, C. B., PINKEL, D.: Cancer 27, 1332-1336 (1971)
51. PINKEL, D., HERNANDEZ, K., BORELLA, L., HOLTEN, C., AUR, R., SAMOY, G., PRATT, C.: Cancer 27, 247-256 (1971)
52. Report to the Medical Research Council by the Leukaemia Committee and the Working Party on Leukaemia in Childhood: Brit. Med. J. 2, 381-384 (1973)

53. Australian Cancer Societies Children's Leukaemia Study Group: Lancet I, 313-318 (1968)

54. BERNARD, J.: Cancer Research 27, 2565-69 (1967)

55. FREI, E. III, KARON, M., LEVIN, R. H., FREIREICH, E. J., TAYLOR, R. J., HANANIAN, J., SELAWRY, O., HOLLAND, J. F., HOOGSTRATEN, B., WOLMAN, I. J., ABIR, E., SAWITSKY, A., LEE, S., MILLS, S. D., BURGERT, E. O. Jr., SPURR, C. L., PATTERSON, R. B., EBAUGH, F. G., JAMES, G. W. III, MOON, J. H.: Blood 26, 642-656 (1965)

56. SPIERS, A. S. D.: Clinics in Haematology 1, 127 (1972)

57. HENDERSON, E. J.: Cancer Research 27, 2570-2572 (1967)

58. WHITECAR, J. P., BODEY, G. P., FREIREICH, E. J.: Proc. Am. Assoc. Cancer Res. 11, 83 (1970)

59. SELAWRY, O. S., HANANIAN, J., WOLMAN, I. J., ABIR, E., CHEVALIER, L., GOURDEAU, R., DENTON, R., GUSSOFF, B. D., LEVY, R., BURGERT, O. Jr.: J.A.M.A. 194, 75-81 (1965)

60. EVANS, A. E., GILBERT, E. S., ZANDASTRA, R.: Cancer 26, 404-409 (1970)

61. HARDISTY, R. M., NORMAN, P. H.: Arch. Dis. Childh. 42, 441-447 (1967)

62. KOMP, D. M., COX, B. J.: J. Ped. 81, 992-994 (1972)

63. AUR, R. J. A., SIMONE, J. V., HUSTU, H. O., VERZOSA, M. S.: Cancer 29, 381-391 (1972)

64. AUR, R. J. A., SIMONE, J. V., HUSTU, H. O., WALTERS, T., BORELLA, L., PRATT, C., PINKEL, D.: Blood 37, 272-281 (1971)

65. KAY, H. E. M., KNAPTON, P. J., O'SULLIVAN, T. J., WELLS, D. G., HARRIS, R. F., INNES, E. M., STUART, J., SCHWARTZ, F. C. M., THOMPSON, E. N.: Arch. Dis. Childh. 47, 344-354 (1972)

66. BAUM, E. S., KOCH, H. F., CORBY, D. G., PLUNKETT, D. C.: Lancet I, 649 (1971)

67. BACK, E. H.: Lancet II, 1005 (1969)

68. FINKELSTEIN, J. Z.: Pediatrics 43, 1042 (1969)

69. SILVERMAN, S. N.: Am. J. Roentgenol. 59, 819-844 (1948)

70. THOMAS, L. B., FORKNER, C. E. Jr., FREI, E. III, BESSE, R. E., STABENAU, J. R.: Cancer 14, 608-621 (1961)

71. SIMMONS, C. R., HARLE, T. S., SINGLETON, E. B.: Radiol. Clin. of N. America 1, 115-130 (1968)

72. HUGHES, W. T.: Am. J. Dis. Child. 122, 283 (1971)

73. SIMONE, J. V., HOLLAND, E., JOHNSON, W.: Blood 39, 759-770 (1972)

74. MATHÉ, G., AMIEL, J. L., SCHWARZENBERG, L., SCHNEIDER, M., CATTAN, A., SCHLUMBERGER, J. R., HAYAT, M., VASSAL, F.: Lancet I, 697-699 (1969)

75. Preliminary report to the Medical Research Council by the Leukaemia Committee and Working Party on Leukaemia in Childhood: Brit. Med. J. 4, 189-194 (1971)

76. GUYER, R. J., CROWTHER, D.: Brit. Med. J. 4, 406-407 (1969)

77. FREI, E. III, FREIREICH, E. J., GEHAN, E., PINKEL, D., HOLLAND, J. F., SELAWRY, O., HAURANI, F., SPURR, C. L., HAYES, D. M., JAMES, G. W., ROTHBERG, H., SODEE, D. B., RUNDLES, R. W., SCHROEDER, L. R., HOOGSTRATEN, B., WOLMAN, I. J., TRAGGIS, D. G., COOPER, T., GENDEL, B. R., EBAUGH, F., TAYLOR, R.: Blood 18, 431-454 (1961)

78. FREIREICH, E. J., GEHAN, E., FREI, E. III, SCHROEDER, L. R., WOLMAN, I. J., ANABARI, R., BURGERT, E. O., MILLS, S. D., PINKEL, D., SELAWRY, O. S., MOON, J. H., GENDEL, B. R., SPURR, C. L., STORRS, R., HAURANI, F., HOOGSTRATEN, B., LEE, S.: Blood 21, 699-716 (1963)

79. WOLFF, J., BRUBAKER, C. A., MURPHY, M. L., PIERCE, M. I., SEVARO, N.: J. of Paediatrics 70, 626-631 (1967)

80. KARON, M., FREIREICH, E. J., FREI, E. III, TAYLOR, R., WOLMAN, I. J., DJERASSI, I., LEE, S., SAWITSKY, A., HANANIAN, J., SELAWRY, O., JAMES, D., GEORGE, P., PATTERSON, R. B., BURGERT, O., HAURANI, F. I., OBERFIELD, R. A., MACY, C. T., HOOGSTRATEN, B., BLOM, J.: Clin. Pharm. and Therap. 7, 332-339 (1966)

81. STORRS, R. C., WOLMAN, I. J., GUSSOF, B. D., HANANIAN, J.: Cancer Res. 26, 241-244 (1966)

82. HOLLAND, J. F., GLIDEWELL, O.: XII. Congress Int. Soc. Haemat. p. 9 1968

83. BERNARD, J.: XII. Congress Int. Soc, Haemat. p. 5, 1968

84. TAILAL, L., TAN, C., CETTGEN, H., WOLLNER, N., McCARTHY, M., HELSEN, L., BURCHENAL, J., KARNOFSKY, D., MURPHY, M. L.: Cancer 25, 306-320 (1970)

85. OETTGEN, H., OLD, L. J., BOYSE, E. A., CAMPBELL, H. A., PHILIPS, F. S., CLARKSON, B. D., TALLAL, L., LEEPER, R. D., SCHWARTZ, M. K., KIM, J. H.: Cancer Res. 27, 2619-2631 (1967)

86. HOWARD, J. P., ALBO, V., NEWTON, W. A.: Cancer 21, 341-345 (1968)

87. McELWAIN, T. J., HARDISTY, R. M.: Brit. Med. J. 4, 596-598 (1969)

88. FERNBACH, D. J., SUTOW, W. W., THURMAN, W. G., VIETTI, T. J.: J.A.M.A. 182, 30-37 (1962)

89. HOLCOMBE, T. M.: Cancer Chemotherapy Report 51, 389-392 (1967)

90. FERNBACH, D. J.: New Eng. J. Med. 275, 451-456 (1966)

91. SEN, L., BORELLA, L.: New Engl. J. Med. 292, 828-832 (1975)

92. BROWN, G., GREAVES, M. F., LISTER, T. A., RAPSON, N., PAPAMICHAIL, M.: Lancet 2, 753-755 (1974)

93. CATOVSKY, D., GOLDMAN, J. M., OKOS, A., FRISCH, B., GALTON, D.A.G.: Brit. Me.d J. 2, 643-646 (1974)

94. SPIERS, A.S.D., COSTELLO, C., CATOVSKY, D., GALTON, D.A.G., GOLDMAN, J. M.: Brit. Med. J. 3, 77-80 (1974)

95. CREASEY, W. A.: Cancer Chemotherapy Report 52, 501-507 (1968)

96. EVANS, D.I.K., JONES, P.H.M., MORLEY, C.J.: Cancer 36, 1547-1551 (1975)

97. EVANS, D.I.K., O'ROURKE, C., JONES, P.H.M.: J. Clin. Path. 27, 226-230 (1974)

# Chapter 5
# Non-Leukaemic Reticuloendothelial Tumours and Leucosarcomas

During the past 10 years there has been a great change in the clinical management of patients with non-leukaemic reticuloendothelial tumours. Three factors have contributed to this: firstly, the greater use of chemotherapy; secondly, greater precision in assessing the extent of the disease so that both local and general treatment can be planned more rationally and, thirdly, the classification of these tumours in histological subgroups which reflect more closely their natural history.

In children there are three tumours which are sometimes mistaken for reticuloendothelial neoplasms

1. Neuroblastomas. On purely histological grounds the distinction between lymphosarcomas and neuroblastomas may be difficult. However, the demonstration that nearly all patients with neuroblastomas excrete abnormal amounts of catecholamines or their metabolites, has practically eliminated this difficulty (Chapter 7). The characteristic behaviour of neuroblastomas in tissue culture (Chapter 14) may provide valuable diagnostic help when the catecholamine excretion is not increased. Widespread neuroblastoma may present with anaemia and lymphadenopathy. The bone marrow in such cases contains cells resembling reticulum cells which may lead the unwary into making a diagnosis of "an unusual form of reticulosis". This diagnosis should never be made in a child unless the possibility of neuroblastoma has been eliminated.

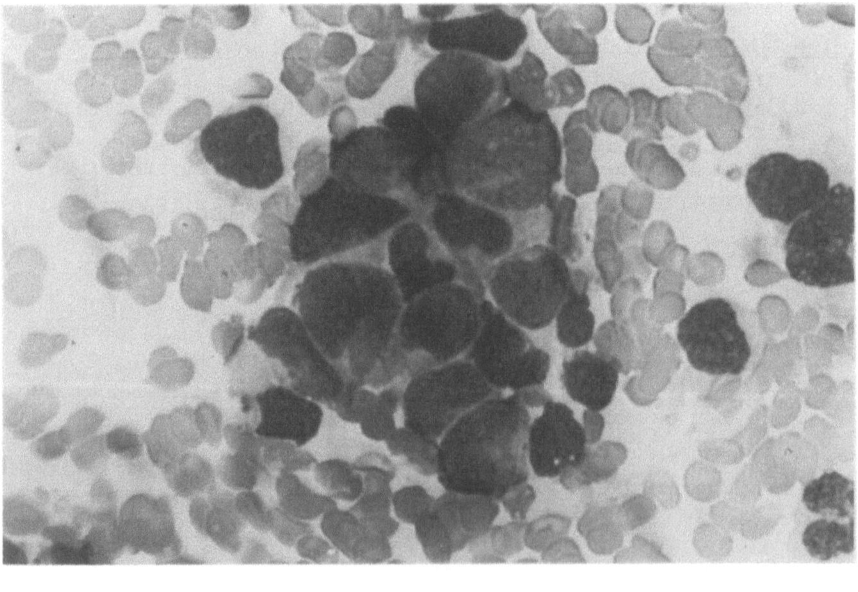

*Fig. 1. Clumps of neuroblasts in bone marrow smear (Jenner-Giemsa X625)*

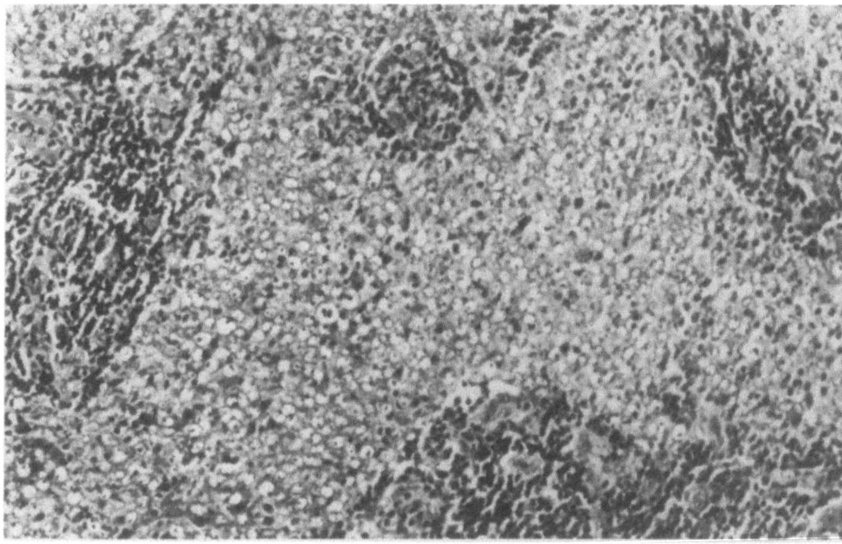

*Fig. 2a. Epithelial cords and lymphocytes in lymphoepithelioma (H. & E. X250)*

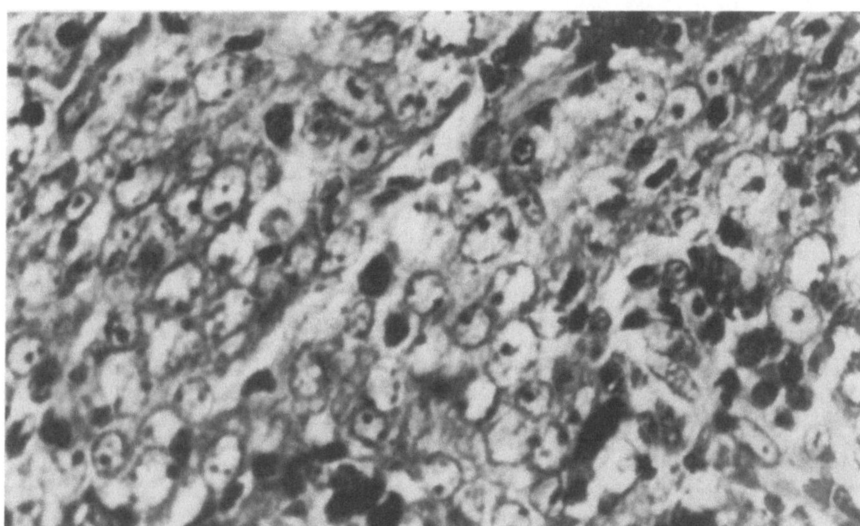

*Fig. 2b. Detail of Fig. 2a (H. & E. X625)*

2. Carcinoma in lymphoid tissue ("pharyngeal lymphoepithelioma") may be confused with reticulosarcoma. This tumour is considered in Chapter 12.

3. An embryonic sarcoma may be mistaken for a reticuloendothelial tumour, particularly if only a small biopsy is taken, since embryonic sarcomas contain areas of large spheroidal or polygonal cells (see Chapter 9).

It was pointed out in Chapter 1 that in Manchester prior to 1968 attempts at the radical treatment of children with tumours consisted very largely of local therapy, while chemotherapy was mainly used for terminal palliation. Thus, the reticuloendothelial tumours included in the Registry during this period were, by modern standards, neither investigated nor treated adequately. While certain conclusions can be drawn about the natural histories of these tumours from the Manchester Registry, the principles underlying the clinical management are largely derived from the literature and our experience since 1968.

During the 15 years 1954-1968, 148 children with non-leukaemic reticuloendothelial tumours were included in the Registry. In addition 13 children with tumours (11 lymphosarcomas, one myelosarcoma and one erythraemic myelosis) which were initially non-leukaemic but became leukaemic later, are considered. Children with Ewing's tumour or reticulosarcoma of bone are excluded since they are discussed separately in Chapter 13. There are thus 161 cases for review. The frequency and prognosis of the various types are shown in Table 1.

Table 1. Non-leukaemic reticuloendothelial tumours and leucosarcomas 1954 - 1968 (assessed 1972)

| | Alive | Dead | Total |
|---|---|---|---|
| Hodgkin's disease | 20 | 30 | 50 |
| Histiocytosis X | 27 | 18 | 45 |
| Lymphosarcoma (non-leukaemic) | 10 | 34 | 44 |
| Leucosarcoma | 0 | 11 | 11 |
| Reticulosarcoma | 1 | 3 | 4 |
| Erythraemic myelosis | 1 | 2 | 3 |
| Microgliomatosis | 0 | 1 | 1 |
| Mycosis fungoides | 0 | 1 | 1 |
| Myelosarcoma (chloroma) | 0 | 1 | 1 |
| Atypical | 0 | 1 | 1 |
| | 59 | 102 | 161 |

## HODGKIN'S DISEASE

During the 15 years up to the end of 1968, 50 children with Hodgkin's disease were included in the Registry, making it the most common non-leukaemic reticuloendothelial tumour in children.

Age of Patients. Hodgkin's disease tends to present in the second half of childhood (see Table 2) and is rare under the age of 5 years. However, 2 children in the Manchester series developed the disease at the age of 2 years.

Progress of the Disease. This is much slower than lymphosarcoma or histiocytosis X. EASSON and RUSSELL (1963) reviewed 822 patients of all ages treated for Hodgkin's disease at the Christie Hospital between 1934 and 1956 and showed that the mortality rate was greatest in the first 5 years after treatment, but thereafter fewer and fewer patients died from recurrence of the tumour, until between the tenth and fifteenth year after treatment the mortality rate no longer exceeded that of a comparable population group.

The time from diagnosis to death of the Manchester children who died from Hodgkin's disease is shown in Table 3. Five children died more than 5 years and one child more than 10 years after diagnosis.

Table 2. Age incidence 1954 - 1968

| Age (years) | -1 | -2 | -3 | -4 | -5 | -6 | -7 | -8 | -9 | -10 | -11 | -12 | -13 | -14 | -15 |
|---|---|---|---|---|---|---|---|---|---|---|---|---|---|---|---|
| Lymphosarcoma (non-leukaemic) | 1 | 0 | 6 | 3 | 4 | 4 | 5 | 7 | 3 | 2 | 3 | 2 | 2 | 1 | 1 |
| Leukaemia | 23 | 37 | 78 | 68 | 38 | 42 | 34 | 28 | 21 | 14 | 14 | 14 | 23 | 12 | 19 |
| Hodgkin's | 0 | 0 | 2 | 3 | 4 | 1 | 1 | 6 | 2 | 2 | 6 | 5 | 6 | 5 | 7 |
| Histiocytosis X | 16 | 12 | 6 | 3 | 1 | 0 | 2 | 2 | 1 | 1 | 0 | 0 | 0 | 1 | 0 |

Table 3. Fatal cases - Time from diagnosis to death 1954 - 1968 (assessed 1972)

| Time (years) | -1/2 | -1 | -2 | -3 | -4 | -5 | -6 | -7 | -8 | -9 | -10 | -11 |
|---|---|---|---|---|---|---|---|---|---|---|---|---|
| Lymphosarcoma (non-leukaemic) | 30 | 1 | 1 | 0 | 2 | 0 | 0 | 0 | 0 | 0 | 0 | 0 |
| Hodgkin's disease | 6 | 5 | 5 | 3 | 3 | 3 | 1 | 1 | 2 | 0 | 0 | 1 |
| Histiocytosis X | 10 | 5 | 3 | 0 | 0 | 0 | 0 | 0 | 0 | 0 | 0 | 0 |

Table 4. Sex (1954 - 1968)

| | Male | Female |
|---|---|---|
| Lymphosarcoma (non-leukaemic) | 33 | 11 |
| Histiocytosis X | 25 | 20 |
| Hodgkin's | 35 | 15 |
| Leukaemia | 253 | 212 |

Sex. Like lymphosarcoma, more boys than girls developed Hodgkin's disease in the Manchester series (see Table 4).

The Fluctuating Clinical Course of Hodgkin's Disease. Characteristically, the clinical course of Hodgkin's disease is not steady but may be marked by alternating periods of progression and regression. This is illustrated by the following case.
CTR.83/54. A girl, aged 13 years, was well up to October 1954 when quite suddenly a lump appeared on the left side of her neck. Over a period of 1 month the lump got much smaller, but then got bigger again. After a biopsy revealed the diagnosis of Hodgkin's disease, irradiation of the neck resulted in the swelling disappearing and the patient remained well for 18 months, when she rapidly developed signs of generalised disease with itching, sweating, pallor and splenomegaly. She was treated with abdominal irradiation and, later, chemotherapy and died 15 months later.

Histological Classification of Hodgkin's Disease. The value of any histological classification depends on whether it reflects the natural history of the disease. The division of Hodgkin's disease into paragranuloma, granuloma and sarcoma (JACKSON and PARKER, 1947) did this to a certain extent, but such a large proportion fell into the granuloma group that the value of this classification was limited. At the Rye Conference, LUKES et al. (1966) produced a classification based on a correlation between the histological appearance of 377 cases of Hodg-

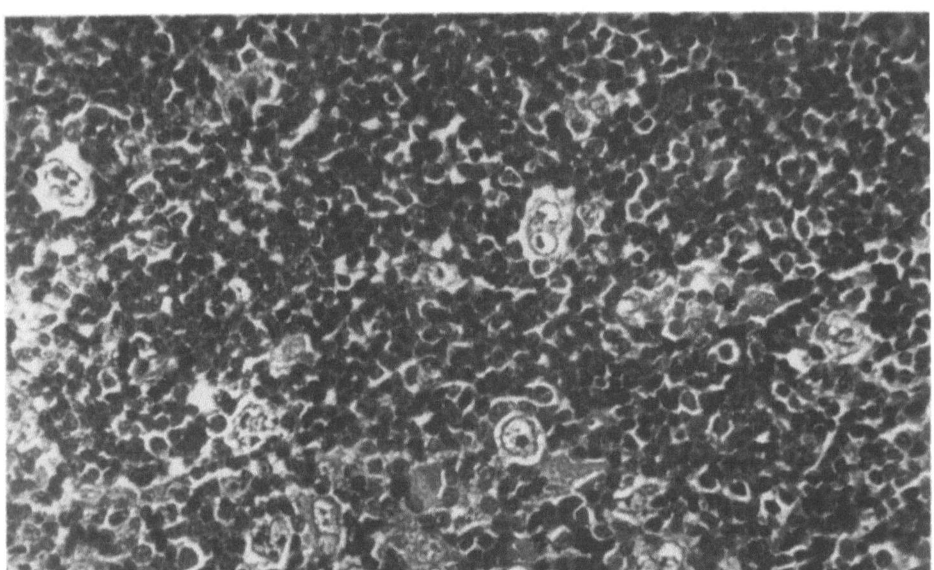

*Fig. 3. Hodgkin's disease, lymphocyte predominance. Scattered isolated cells of Sternberg-Reed type and many lymphocytes (H. & E. X450)*

kin's disease in U.S. Army personnel and the clinical staging and progress of the patients. This is known as the Rye Conference classification and consists of four histological types.

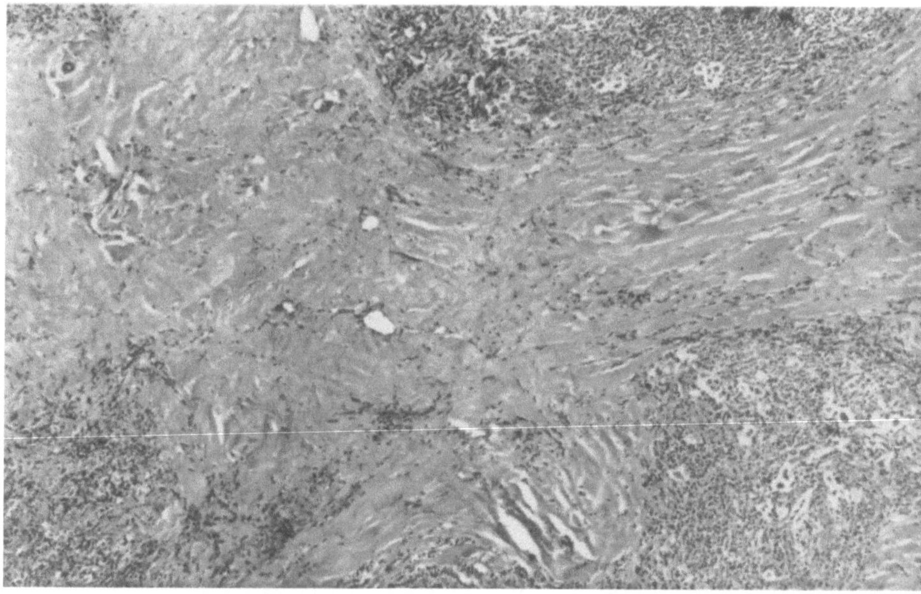

*Fig. 4 a & b. Hodgkin's disease, nodular sclerosis*
*a) Islands of tumour tissue separated by broad sclerotic bands (H. & E. X75)*

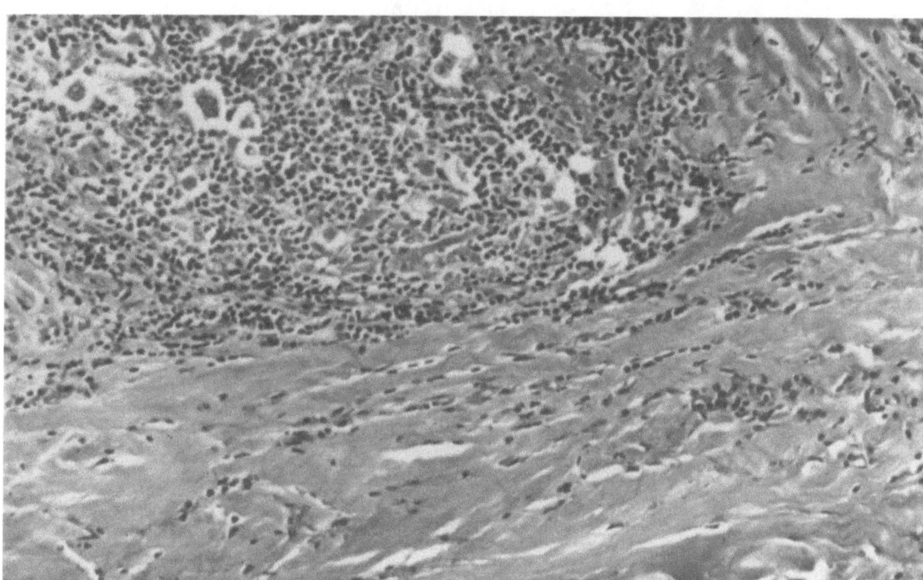

*b) Detail of Fig. 4a (H. & E. X175)*

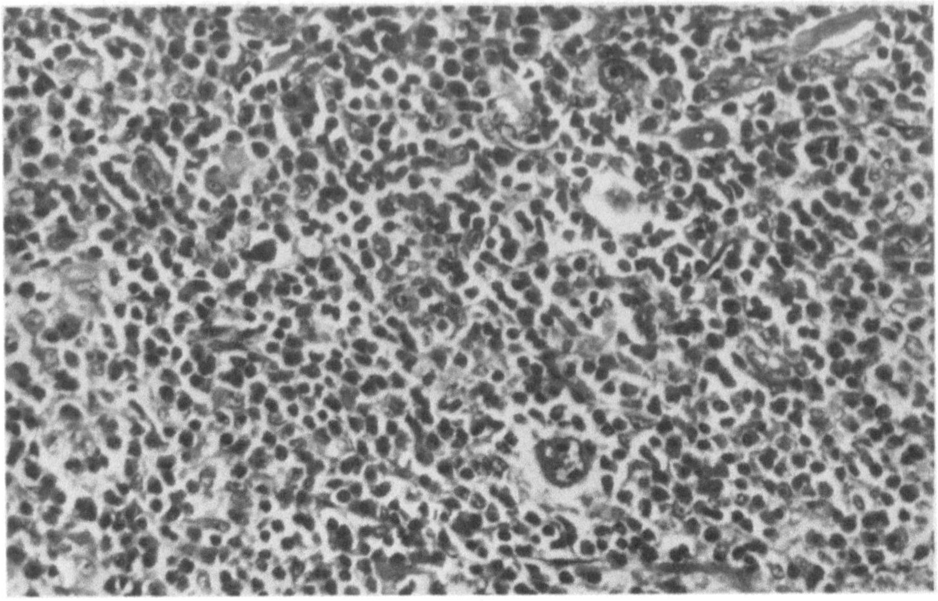

*Fig. 5. Hodgkin's disease mixed cellularity. A variety of cells including plasma cells and eosinophils in addition to those of Sternberg-Reed type (H. & E. X350)*

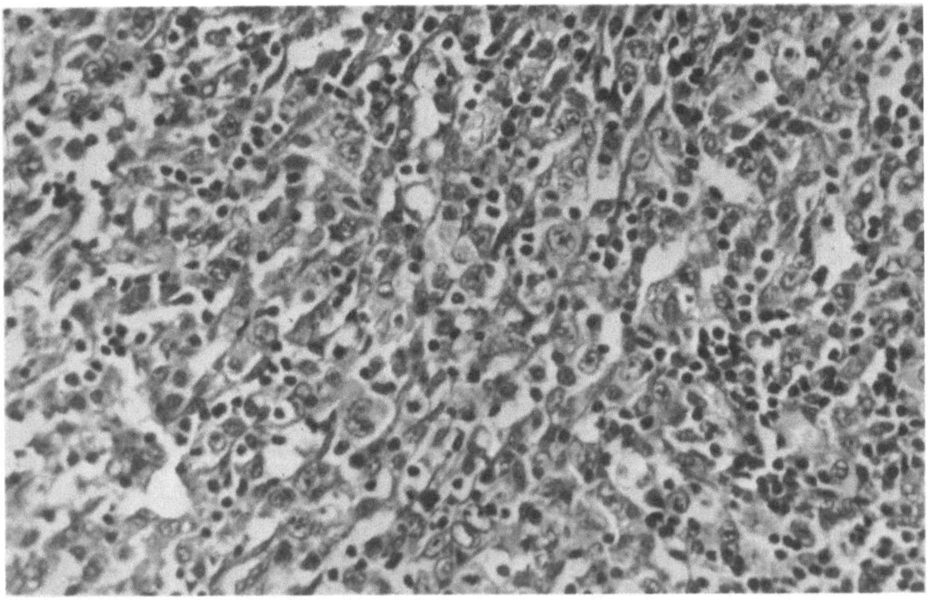

*Fig. 6. Hodgkin's disease, lymphocyte depleted. Numerous pleomorphic reticulum cells, some of Sternberg-Reed type. Few lymphocytes (H. & E. X350)*

1. Lymphocyte predominance
2. Nodular sclerosis
3. Mixed cellularity
4. Lymphocyte depleted

LUKES et al. (1966) showed that these types were in ascending order of malignancy, the lymphocyte predominance type tending to present as a localised glandular enlargement and to have the longest survival time, and the lymphocyte depleted type tending to present as more widespread disease and to have a short survival time.

The division of the cases in the Manchester Children's Tumour Registry according to this classification is shown in Table 5.

Table 5. Hodgkin's disease (1954 - 1968)

| | Alive | Dead | Total | Median survival (months) |
|---|---|---|---|---|
| Lymphocyte predominance | 12 | 8 | 20 | 66 |
| Nodular sclerosis | 5 | 0 | 5 | - |
| Mixed cellularity | 3 | 19 | 22 | 18 |
| Lymphocyte depleted | 0 | 3 | 3 | 3 |

Nodular sclerosis was rare in the Manchester series, contrasting with other series from Europe and America (CORREA and O'CONOR, 1971).

## Epidemiological Pattern

BURN et al. (1971), using the Rye Conference classification showed that the proportion of the various types of Hodgkin's disease in Manchester children differed from that in East African children, the latter having many more lesions of the lymphocyte depleted type with a poor prognosis. CORREA and O'CONOR (1971) extended this observation to series of Hodgkin's disease in a number of different countries and concluded that there were several epidemiological patterns. Pattern I is characterised by high rates in children and a predominance of histological subtypes associated with a poor prognosis. Pattern III is characterised by high rates in young adults and a predominance of subtypes with a better prognosis. Pattern II is intermediate. These patterns are related to the socioeconomic stratification of the communities studied, suggesting that the variation in Hodgkin's disease may be influenced by environmental conditions.

Table 6. Hodgkin's disease 1954 - 1968 (assessed 1972)

| Site of presentation | Alive | Dead | Total |
|---|---|---|---|
| Neck | 16 | 24 | 40 |
| Neck, groin and axilla | 1 | 0 | 1 |
| Groin | 1 | 0 | 1 |
| Sternum | 1 | 0 | 1 |
| Abdomen | 1 | 0 | 1 |
| Generalised | 0 | 6 | 6 |
| | 20 | 30 | 50 |

Clinical Presentation. Hodgkin's disease has a much more constant site of presentation than other reticuloendothelial tumours (Table 6). Most cases present with enlarged cervical nodes.

Speed of Diagnosis. It was pointed out previously (Table 10 of Chapter 1) that after attendance at hospital, there tended to be delay in diagnosing children with neoplastic cervical glands. It is paradoxical, however, that children with Hodgkin's disease presenting as enlarged neck nodes had the highest survival rate when the delay was longest (Table 7).

Table 7. Hodgkin's disease presenting as enlarged neck nodes
40 children. 1954 - 1968 (assessed 1972)

| Time from first hospital attendance to diagnosis | < 2 weeks | 2-8 weeks | 8 weeks + |
|---|---|---|---|
| 3-year survival rate | 54% | 64% | 77% |

It should not be concluded from this that delay in diagnosis and treatment is in any way beneficial to the patient. The most likely explanation can be seen in Table 8.

Table 8. Hodgkin's disease presenting as enlarged neck nodes
40 children 1954 - 1968 (assessed 1972)

Diagnostic delay after hospital consultation and survival rate

| Type | Median diagnostic delay (weeks) | 3 years survival rate |
|---|---|---|
| Lymphocyte predominance + Nodular sclerosis | 7.5 | 90% |
| Mixed cellularity + Lymphocyte depleted | 3.3 | 35% |

There is less delay in the diagnosis of the more malignant forms of Hodgkin's disease because in those cases the lymph nodes grow very quickly and their neoplastic nature is suspected earlier than in those children with the less malignant forms. Consequently, if all types of Hodgkin's disease are considered together, there is a positive correlation between diagnostic delay and survival rate. Therefore, in analysing factors influencing the prognosis, the histological types must be considered separately.

Staging. The division of Hodgkin's disease into four histological types was not the only advance made at the Rye Conference. In addition a system of clinical staging of the disease was described which enabled better planning of treatment (ROSENBURG, 1966). Since its inception, however, it became clear that the Rye Conference system was inadequate in certain respects. At that time it was not clear that with a particular stage the site of the disease had a prognostic significance and a relevance to the likely mode of spread. This has now been demonstrated (PETERS, 1971; TEILLET et al., 1971). Similarly it has been shown that the different histological types are associated with different stages of presentation and in the case of nodular sclerosis with a distinctive anatomical distribution and a predilection for the female sex. (BERARD et al., 1971; DORFMAN, 1971).

Prognosis is related not only to histological type and clinical staging, but also to the presence or absence of systemic symptoms, especially significant weight loss. The modified staging recommended by the Ann Arbor Conference (CARBONE et al., 1971) is outlined below and should be employed whenever possible. Each stage is subdivided into A and B categories, the latter indicating unexplained weight loss, fever or night sweats.

Stage I. Involvement of a single lymph node region (I) or of a single extralymphatic organ or site ($I_E$).

Stage II. Involvement of two or more lymph node regions on the same side of the diaphragm (II) or localised involvement of extra-lymphatic organ or site and of one or more lymph node regions on the same side of the diaphragm ($II_E$). The number of lymph node regions involved may be indicated by a subscript e. g. $II_3$.

Stage III. Involvement of lymph node regions on both sides of the diaphragm (III) which may also be accompanied by localised involvement of extra lymphatic organ or site ($III_E$) or involvement of spleen ($III_S$) or both ($III_{SE}$).

Stage IV. Diffuse or disseminated involvement of one or more extralymphatic organs or tissues with or without associated lymph node enlargement. The reason for classifying the patient as Stage IV should be identified further by defining site by symbols.

## Clinical Management

As information on the pattern of disease emerges through accurate staging and correlation with histological type, it becomes increasingly important to consider carefully and individually the management of new cases of Hodgkin's disease. Evidence is accumulating that site and mode of presentation are also important diagnostic factors. (PETERS, 1971). Although it has been suggested that Hodgkin's disease in childhood tends to have a higher proportion of the favourable histological types (NEWELL et al., 1970), there have been reports that survival in the young is less prolonged irrespective of other parameters (STRUM and RAPPAPORT, 1970; DE VITA et al., 1972; JENKIN et al., 1967). However, this is not borne out with respect to the Manchester children, whose survival compares favourably with other series despite the fact that therapy would not be considered optimal by modern standards.

Accurate evaluation of treatment in past series of cases of Hodgkin's disease has been hampered by the inability to assess the extent of disease. It is essential, therefore, that every effort should be made to record all parameters and to stage the disease accurately. The following investigations should be carried out.

1. An adequate node biopsy, reviewed preferably by a pathologist attached to an oncological centre.

2. A detailed history with specific reference to fever, sweating, pruritus and weight loss.

3. A careful examination carried out by a physician experienced in the evaluation of Hodgkin's disease; with special attention paid to the areas where lymphadenopathy usually occurs; assessment of the

lymphoid tissue of Waldeyer's ring, the size of the liver and spleen, and specific examination for areas of bony tenderness.

4. Laboratory investigations:
a) Full blood count, Hb, W.B.C. and differential, platelet count and E.S.R.
b) Liver function tests including serum alkaline phosphatase
c) Blood urea
d) Serum calcium
e) Bone marrow biopsy

5. Radiological studies:
a) Chest X-rays, P. A., and lateral views
b) Skeletal survey
c) I.V.P. - This is abnormal in 30% of a reported series of children with Hodgkin's disease (GROSSMAN et al., 1970).
d) Lymphangiography may be of more use than pyelography, but in children it presents problems both of technique and interpretation and is unlikely to be successful in those under 6 years old. The interpretative difficulties are usually those of false negatives. In those with suspected involvement below the diaphragm a lymphangiogram may provide confirmation of a clinical impression, but in those with unsuspected subdiaphragmatic disease a negative lymphangiogram is not conclusive (GROSSMAN et al., 1970).

6. Exploratory laparotomy with splenectomy and liver biopsy are more often indicated in children than in adults because of the frequent inconclusiveness of lymphangiography. It is advisable to carry this out in all children except those with proven stage IV disease. A standard technique should be employed (HAYES et al., 1972).

7. The following investigations are necessary in some cases.
a) Tomography of lungs and bones
b) Inferior vena cavagrams
c) Gastrointestinal series
d) Scans of liver and spleen

## TREATMENT

When the patient has been investigated it is possible to embark upon a considered plan of therapy adapted to the individual patient and best able in the light of present knowledge to achieve cure or a prolonged disease-free interval.

The treatment of choice in stage $I_A$ or $II_A$ disease is radiotherapy and it has always been accepted in Manchester that the volume to be irradiated in these patients should be of the so-called wide field type. In the days before megavoltage X-rays made it possible to treat all lymph node areas from the base of the skull to the dome of the diaphragm, and even include the axillae whilst at the same time being able to protect the lungs, it was felt that when one lymph node region was involved, the groups of nodes on each side should be included in the treatment, and that at worst a minimum of 5 cm of normal tissues should be included all round the clinically abnormal nodes. In the past few years there has been a world-wide move to use even wider fields, so that even with disease confined to the neck nodes, the volume to be irradiated extends from the base of the skull to the dome of the diaphragm, and laterally to take in the axillae: the mantle technique. Megavoltage radiation in the range 4-8 MeV is used. The fields to be irradiated are checked by X-ray films so that care can be taken to ensure that the lungs and the epiphyses of long bones such as the humerus are completely shielded. Treatment is given from anterior and posterior fields on alternate days, there being 16 exposures. The dose delivered to this volume differs somewhat in different centres, but our experience is that in 3 weeks, which is our normal treatment time, it can rarely exceed 2750 rads and often has to be only 2500 rads. This would correspond with a dose of 3500 rads in 5 weeks which is more the order of time chosen in other centres.

In some instances with nodes high in the neck, a more restricted volume may be considered to be adequate, in which the lower edge is the lower limit of the manubrium sternii and the axillae are not included. This volume will tolerate 3000 rads in 3 weeks. In both techniques the lips are shielded from the anterior field throughout. No attempt is made to shield the spinal cord and therefore, the doses described are the limit that can be given. If higher doses are considered necessary, shielding of the spinal cord will be needed.

The X-ray technique used for disease below the diaphragm has commonly been the technique known as an inverted Y. This takes in the upper abdominal para-aortic nodes in the leg of the Y and the iliac, inguinal and groin nodes in both arms of the Y. Again megavoltage X-rays in the same range are used, and anterior and posterior fields are treated on alternate days, to a total of 16 exposures. The dose is of the same order, 2500-2750 rads in 3 weeks. This treatment is used when, rarely, disease presents primarily below the diaphragm, but mostly for Stage III disease, when it is matched on to the lower edge of the mantle technique at the dome of the diaphragm. We have been able in children to complete both courses with a gap of 10 days to 2 weeks between them.

Whilst this treatment is taking place regular blood counts are required, and are usually obtained bi-weekly. Depression of white cells and platelets may occur, especially in trying to do the two courses of treatment, and adjustments may have to be made in dosage and time if this is severe. With only one course of treatment, it is unusual to have problems with marrow depression during treatment. Nausea and occasionally vomiting may occur, but are less of a problem in children than in adults. They may be controlled by chlorpromazine. At the end of treatment epilation of the hair occurs where the lower part of the scalp was included in treatment, but is temporary. The mouth, pharynx and larynx develop a radiation reaction, so that eating and swallowing may be painful and hoarseness often occurs. These are temporary and settle in 2 to 3 weeks.

This irradiation is given initially to those patients in whom all investigations, <u>except laparotomy</u>, indicate Stage $I_A$ or $II_A$ disease above the diaphragm. Three to four weeks after it is completed a laparotomy with splenectomy and liver biopsy is carried out. Those who in the light of the laparotomy findings are shown to have Stage III disease, then have X.R.T. to the abdomen. The prior splenectomy allows for more adequate screening of the left kidney and left lower lobe of the lung and radiotherapy is better tolerated (SALZMAN and KAPLAN, 1971). Children with Stage $I_B$ and $II_B$ and Stage III disease diagnosed at the outset are considered better managed by having laparotomy before the start of any treatment and their therapy planned on the basis of the findings at that time.

At the present time we believe that Stage III disease in childhood should be treated by extended field radiotherapy in association with a set number of courses of chemotherapy. Since 1970 we have employed the drugs of the M.O.P.P. programme in a modified regime.

| | Day 1 | 15 | 29 | 43 | 57 | 71 |
|---|---|---|---|---|---|---|
| Nitrogen Mustard | 6 $mg/m^2$ | 6 $mg/m^2$ | 6 $mg/m^2$ | 6 $mg/m^2$ | 6 $mg/m^2$ | 6 $mg/m^2$ |
| Vin-cristine | 1.5 $mg/m^2$ | 1.5 $mg/m^2$ | 1.5 $mg/m^2$ | 1.5 $mg/m^2$ | 1.5 $mg/m^2$ | 1.5 $mg/m^2$ |

| | Day 1-10 | 15-24 | 29-38 | 43-52 | 57-66 | 71-80 |
|---|---|---|---|---|---|---|
| Pro-carbazine | 100 $mg/m^2$ | 100 $mg/m^2$ | 100 $mg/m^2$ | 100 $mg/m^2$ | 100 $mg/m^2$ | 100 $mg/m^2$ |
| Predni-solone | 40 $mg/m^2$ daily for 80 days | | | | | |

In certain instances it has been possible to reduce the interval between the injections of nitrogen mustard and vincristine to 7 days, in which case both procarbazine and prednisolone have been given continuously and the whole course completed in 35 days. In others, delay has been necessary with a wider gap between injections. The 14-day course is then repeated every 28 days for 3 courses and then every 56 days for 3 courses so completing a year's therapy.

This programme of chemotherapy is also used in children with Stage IV disease and if remission is maintained a further four courses have been given at 12-week intervals in the second year. So a total of 16 courses is given over the 2-year period. In Manchester this has not proved unacceptably toxic. There has been no evidence of sustained bone marrow depression and where the regimen has been used in conjunction with X.R.T. in Stage III cases it has only occasionally been necessary to delay chemotherapy because of a low W.B.C. No interruptions in X.R.T. have been required.

The absolute exclusion of X.R.T. in Stage IV disease is not recommended as it can often produce significant and rapid reduction in size of painful gland masses and lasting relief of localised bone pain.

## Treatment of Recurrent and Extending Disease

In cases where radical treatment of Stage I - III disease achieves the expected remission but where relapse occurs, the plan of treatment must depend on the site of recurrence. Where disease manifests in previously irradiated areas an intensive chemotherapy programme as outlined for Stage IV disease is indicated. If disease occurs below the diaphragm a combination of X.R.T. and chemotherapy as for initial Stage III disease would be our treatment of choice.

The treatment of recurrence of generalised disease will depend on whether or not the patient is on chemotherapy at the time. If not, the programme outlined above can be re-introduced. In patients relapsing on chemotherapy other programmes involving different drugs such as B.C.N.U. (MARSH et al., 1971), vinblastine, cyclophosphamide and adriamycin will sometimes prove to be efficacious in achieving further remission.

## Treatment of Special Problems

C.N.S. Disease. Involvement of the central nervous system is a rare complication which is best treated with irradiation of the whole C.N.S. Modifications of field will be dependent on previous irradiation.

Splenomegaly. In Stages III and IV the amount of chemotherapy which can safely be administered may be limited by the cytopenic effects of hypersplenism. There is evidence that splenectomy may be beneficial in such cases (LOWENSTEIN et al., 1971).

Infection. Patients with Hodgkin's disease may have defective immunity due not only to the disease but also to the treatment which they are having and they may suffer from bacterial, fungal or viral infections which rarely cause trouble in normal individuals. Thus a deterioration in the patient's condition may be due to infection and not necessarily to progression of the neoplasm. Aggressive treatment of any invading organisms is required in such cases.

## LYMPHOSARCOMA AND LEUCOSARCOMA

Fifty-five children with histologically proven lymphosarcoma were included in the Register. Eleven of these subsequently showed evidence of leukaemia (leucosarcomas). In all the children with leucosarcoma the pre-leukaemic phase was short, varying between 1 and 11 weeks. It is not possible to estimate accurately the proportion of lymphosarcomas which may become leukaemic, since both in those patients who were cured and in those who died, the leukaemic potentialities of the tumour may not have had time to be realised.

Lymphosarcoma and Burkitt's Lymphoma. The most striking difference between lymphosarcomas in patients living in temperate climates and Burkitt's lymphoma is that the former usually start in lymph nodes, whereas the latter is mainly extranodal. Histologically the presence of macrophages in Burkitt's lymphoma, giving it a "starry sky" appearance, has often been reported. However, DIAMANDOPOULOS and SMITH (1964) and DORFMAN (1965) point out that the "starry sky" appearance is not pathognomonic of the African lymphoma and may be seen in lymphosarcomas in

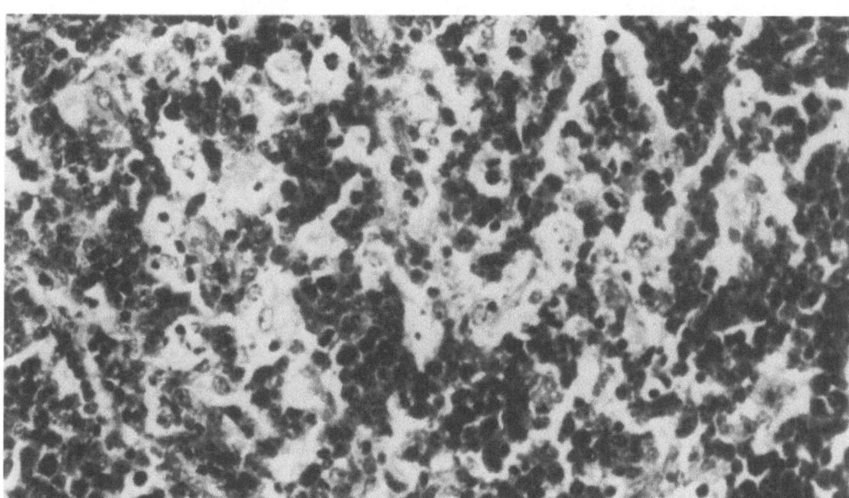

*Fig. 7. Scattered macrophages giving a "starry-sky" appearance in lymphosarcoma (H. & E. X500)*

Table 9. Manchester children with lymphosarcomas showing a "starry sky" appearance (1954 - 1968)

| Sex | Age (years) | Site of tumour |
|---|---|---|
| M | 7 | Nasopharynx |
| M | 6 | Abdomen - large diffuse tumour |
| M | 10 | Ileocaecal region |
| M | 7 | Abdomen - large diffuse tumour |
| F | 2 | Neck glands |
| M | 2 | Neck glands |
| M | 2 | Neck glands ) |
| M | 2 | Neck glands ) Became leukaemic |
| M | 7 | Neck glands ) |
| M | 3 | Tonsil |

patients living in temperate climates. The presence of macrophages was a marked feature of ten of the Manchester children, none of whom had the clinical features of Burkitt's lymphoma (Table 9).

<u>Granuloma Formation in Lymphosarcoma, Reticulosarcoma and Hodgkin's Disease.</u> An unusual feature in one case of lymphosarcoma in the Register was the presence of granuloma formation with giant cells giving the appearance of sarcoid.

<u>CTR.68/55</u>. Boy, aged 8 years, developed a lump in the left side of the neck, which varied in size over a period of 3 months. At this time a biopsy was taken and showed non-caseating granulomata with many giant cells. W.B.C. 24,000 c.mm. with a normal differential. After the biopsy, the nodes rapidly increased in size and a second biopsy a month later showed the appearance of lymphoblastic lymphosarcoma. The child died one month later with widespread metastases. There was no evidence of sarcoid at autopsy.

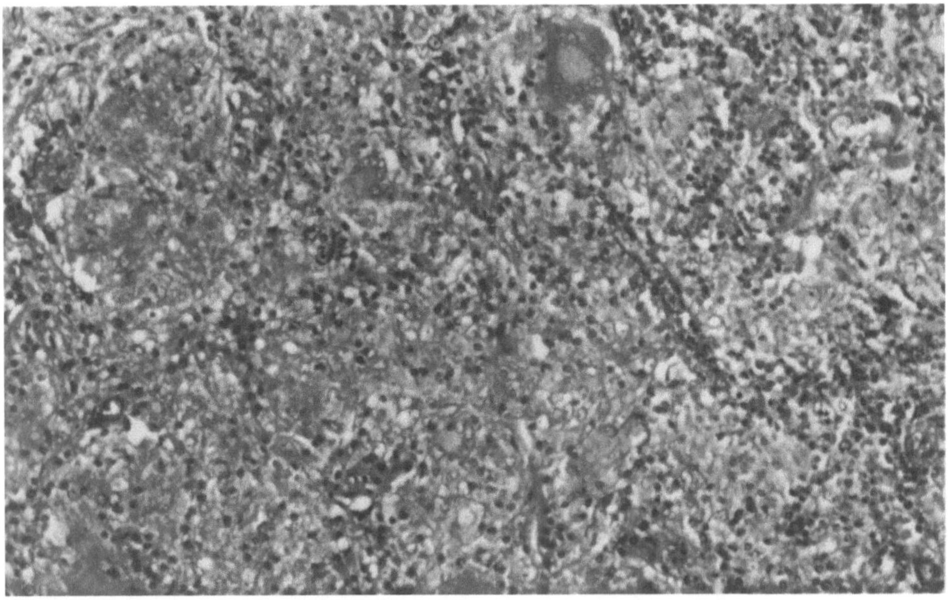

*Fig. 8. Sarcoid lesion in lymphosarcoma (H. & E. X200)*

The presence of sarcoid features in Hodgkin's disease has been reported by STOKER (1971), in reticulosarcoma by ATWOOD et al. (1966) and by GOLDFARB and COHEN (1970), and in carcinoma by GRESHAM and ACKERLEY (1958). In the reports a positive Kveim reaction has been noted and generalised sarcoidosis may be found.

The case underlines the necessity of doing repeat lymph node biopsies in doubtful cases.

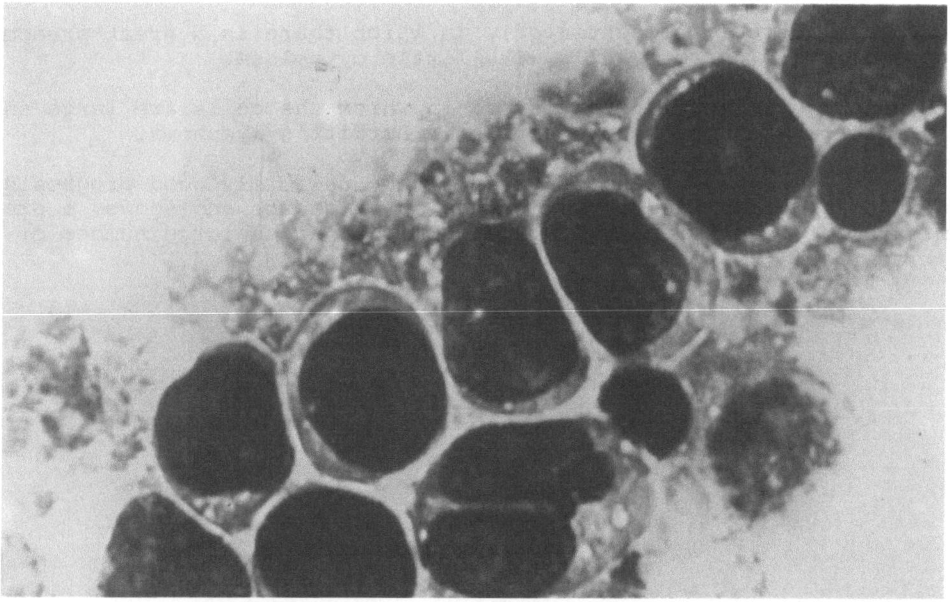

*Fig. 9. Lymphosarcoma. Imprint preparation (Jenner-Giemsa. Original magnification X1200)*

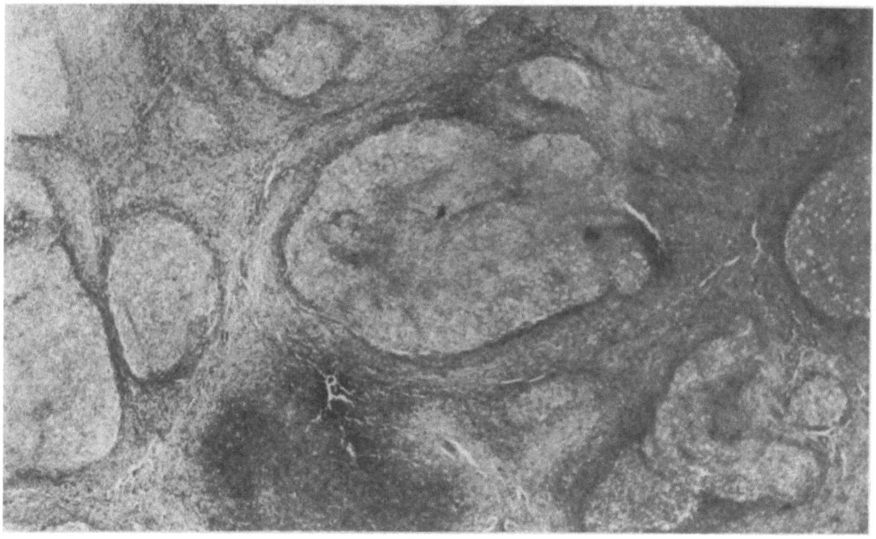

*Fig. 10. Nodular lymphosarcoma (Brill Symmers') showing islands of lymphoblasts without macrophages (H. & E. X60)*

## Histological Types of Lymphosarcoma

In lymphosarcomas, as in other reticuloendothelial tumours, cytology is as important as histology and greater cell detail may be obtained by making imprint preparations from the lymph node.

The following classification was used in the Manchester cases.

a) A nodular type with false follicles ("Brill Symmers" disease).

b) Lymphoblastic (differentiated), in which there is a great predominance of small uniform cells with little cytoplasm.

c) Lymphoblastic (undifferentiated) in which the cells are large and pale. Macrophages may be present as in Burkitt's lymphoma.

d) Atypical. A small group of cases with a uniformly good prognosis could not be classified in any of the above groups and showed a predominance of greatly enlarged true follicles and a large number of histiocytes.

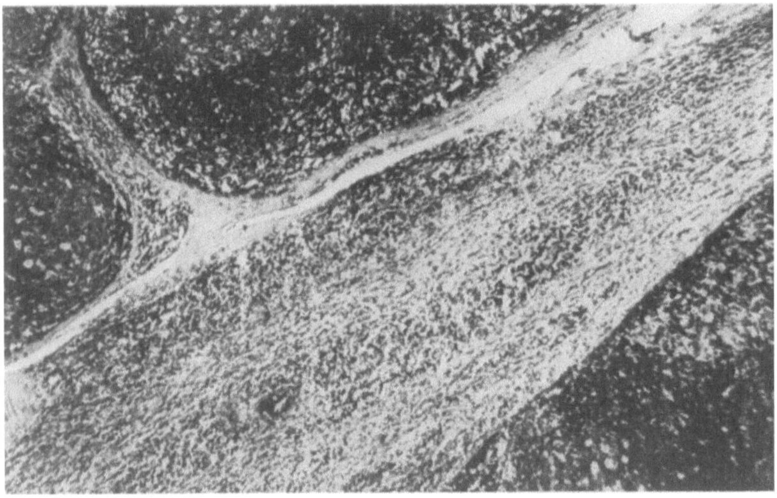

*Fig. 11. Lymphosarcoma invading the gland capsule. Prominent follicles (?non-neoplastic) with macrophages can be seen (H. & E. X60)*

Table 10. Types of lymphosarcoma 1954 - 1968 (assessed 1972)

| | Non-leukaemic | | Leucosarcoma | Total |
|---|---|---|---|---|
| | Alive | Dead | (all dead) | |
| Brill Symmers' | 1 | 1 | 0 | 2 |
| Lymphocytic | 4 | 25 | 4 | 33 |
| Lymphoblastic (differentiated) | 2 | 8 | 7 | 17 |
| Atypical | 3 | 0 | 0 | 3 |
| | 10 | 34 | 11 | 55 |

The frequency of the types of lymphosarcoma in the Manchester series is shown in Table 10. The rarity of the nodular form (Brill Symmers' disease) is seen.

Lymphoblastic lymphosarcoma appeared to have a greater tendency to become leukaemic than did other varieties of lymphosarcoma.

Age of Patients. Lymphosarcomas affect children of all ages (Table 2). Although the Manchester cases showed a predominance in younger children, there was not the peak between the ages of 2 and 6 years which is seen in childhood leukaemia (COOKE, 1942).

Sex. There was a preponderance of boys amongst the patients who developed lymphosarcoma, Hodgkin's disease and leukaemia in the Manchester Region (Table 4).

Progress of the Disease. Lymphosarcoma is a rapidly progressive disease with a natural tendency to become leukaemic or kill the patient within a few months of onset. Thirty of the 34 children with fatal disease lived for less than 6 months after diagnosis (Table 3). Only two children, who eventually died, survived for over 2 years - one had the nodular type of lymphosarcoma and the other had prolonged treatment with vincristine and cyclophosphamide.

Presenting (?Primary) Sites. These were extremely varied - almost any part of the body might be the primary site (Table 11).

Table 11. Primary sites of lymphosarcoma 1954 - 1968 (assessed in 1972)

| | Alive | | Dead |
|---|---|---|---|
| Neck glands | 6 | Abdominal | 11 |
| Ileocaecal | 1 | Multiple | 8 |
| Ileal | 1 | Neck glands | 4 |
| Groin gland | 1 | Mediastinum | 4 |
| Elbow region | 1 | Nasopharynx | 3 |
| | | Paravertebral | 2 |
| | | Orbits | 1 |
| | | Axilla | 1 |
| | 10 | | 34 |

Prognosis. It is seen in Table 11 that the prognosis of lymphosarcoma in the Manchester children who were treated largely by surgery and/or irradiation depended on the presenting site. If the tumour arose in a superficial gland or in the intestine, causing an intussusception, it tended to be diagnosed early and the child could be cured by local means. Unfortunately, most lymphosarcomas arise in situations where they can only be cured by general therapy. A mediastinal lymphosarcoma may be very rapidly fatal, causing the death of a previously healthy child within a few hours. It is important, however, not to subject the child to unnecessary treatment by confusing a benign lymphoid polyp of the intestine with lymphosarcoma.

## RETICULOSARCOMA (HISTIOCYTIC LYMPHOMA)

Four children with reticulosarcoma were included in the Registry. One child, who presented with enlarged cervical nodes, remains well 10 years after being treated by a block dissection of the cervical nodes without irradiation or chemotherapy.

In two cases the disease was rapidly fatal, the children dying within six weeks of diagnosis. In one case the child died 15 months after clinical onset.

The reticulosarcoma has sheets of large cells up to 20 μ diameter, sometimes forming a syncytial mass. The nuclei contain prominent eosinophilic nucleoli and the cytoplasm is palely eosinophilic. Reticulin

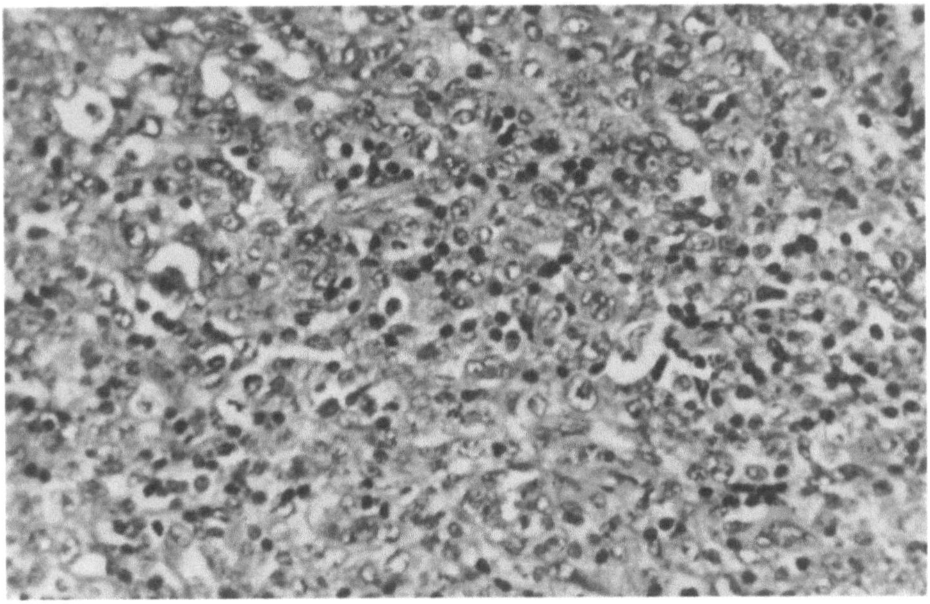

*Fig. 12. Reticulosarcoma. Sheets of pleomorphic reticulum cells with some areas having a syncytial appearance (H. & E. X350)*

fibres between the individual cells may be shown by silver impregnation. It may be difficult to distinguish a reticulosarcoma from lymphocyte-depleted Hodgkin's disease, the diagnosis resting on the presence of Sternberg-Reed cells in the latter condition.

## Clinical Management of Children with Non-Hodgkin's Lymphoma

From a clinical point of view, lymphosarcoma and reticulosarcoma present similar problems and therefore they may be conveniently grouped together under the title of Non-Hodgkin's lymphoma. The clinical staging of these cases is not so easily defined as in Hodgkin's disease because they are less frequently nodal in origin and in those cases which are nodal, spread to contiguous nodes is less common. The majority of patients present with disease comparable to Stage IV. Even without the objective evidence of accurate staging there is little doubt that there is a correlation between the extent of disease and prognosis. This is supported by the fact that the 10 Manchester children who were cured of lymphosarcoma prior to 1969 had tumours which presented early because they were either subcutaneous or arose in the ileocaecal region, causing an intussusception (Table 11). Therefore in every case, clinical staging should be attempted in the hope that combined with histological typing, a pattern of behaviour will be apparent in the future. Although lymphosarcomas which become leukaemic have features in common with acute lymphatic leukaemia, their response to treatment is, on the whole, much less satisfactory.

Investigations. Once a gland biopsy has established the diagnosis and type, a full history and examination as outlined for Hodgkin's disease should be undertaken. The following investigations are obligatory:

Full blood count and marrow examination.

E.S.R. Lumbar puncture for examination for abnormal cells (the use of the cytocentrifuge is advised as abnormal cells may be present in the absence of a raised cell count).

Liver function tests.

Renal function tests.

Chest X-rays.

I.V.P. (Retroperitoneal gland masses are more common in non-Hodgkin's lymphoma than in Hodgkin's disease and they may cause displacement and distortion of the kidneys and ureters).

Lymphangiography.

Staging laparotomy is indicated where I.V.P. and lymphangiography are negative and there is no other positive evidence of disease below the diaphragm.

Treatment. In Stage I and II disease of all histological types confined to the peripheral nodes or gastrointestinal tract, the main line of attack should be surgery and radiotherapy. It is difficult at present to be sure whether the addition of chemotherapy would be valuable in these cases, but the Manchester cases indicate that strictly localised disease is curable without it. There is no reported information of the value of block dissection, but in gastrointestinal tumours wide excision should be the aim.

It has been reported (WANTANABE et al., 1973; JENKIN et al., 1967; SULLIVAN, 1962; JONES and KLINGBERG, 1963) that tumours of the mediastinum, particularly of the lymphoblastic variety, are prone to become leukaemic and therefore it would seem wise to give chemotherapy similar to that used in A.L.L. to these children (AUR et al., 1971). Indeed, it is reasonable to suggest that all lymphosarcomas of lymphoblastic type irrespective of stage should be treated with a 2-3 year chemotherapy programme as discussed in the therapy of A.L.L. The possibility of C.N.S. involvement raises the question of whether prophylactic irradiation of the C.N.S. or intrathecal methotrexate should be given, since once the disease becomes manifest in the nervous system it appears to be incurable by presently available methods.

Stages III and IV disease should be treated by chemotherapy similar to that used in Hodgkin's disease or A.L.L. These programmes have already been shown to improve the prognosis in adults with non-Hodgkin's lymphoma (CARBONE, 1972). Radiotherapy should be introduced for the treatment of residual disease and the prophylactic treatment of the C.N.S.

According to the figures of the Manchester Children's Tumour Registry, histiocytosis X is less common than Hodgkin's disease, but slightly more common than non-leukaemic lymphosarcoma. This may not reflect the true incidence, since it is likely that there is an element of under-

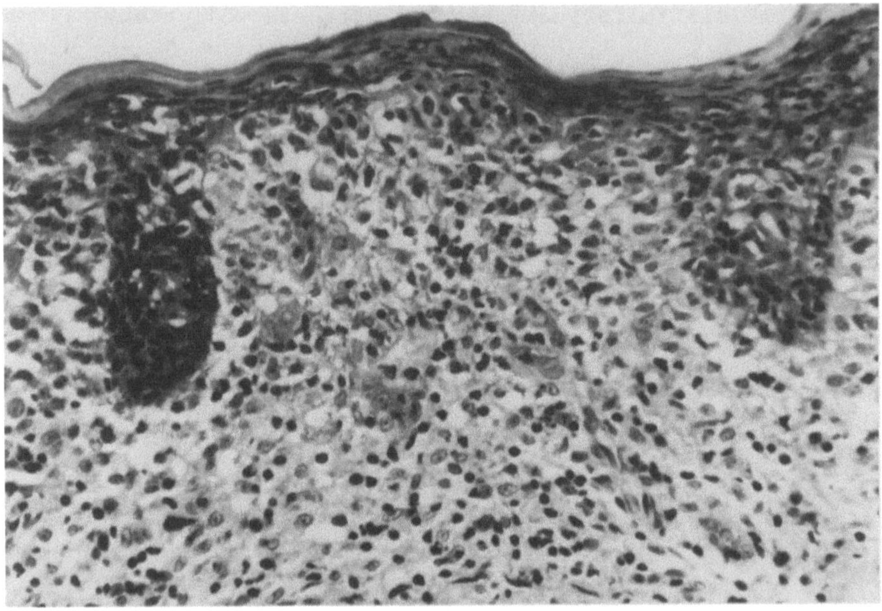

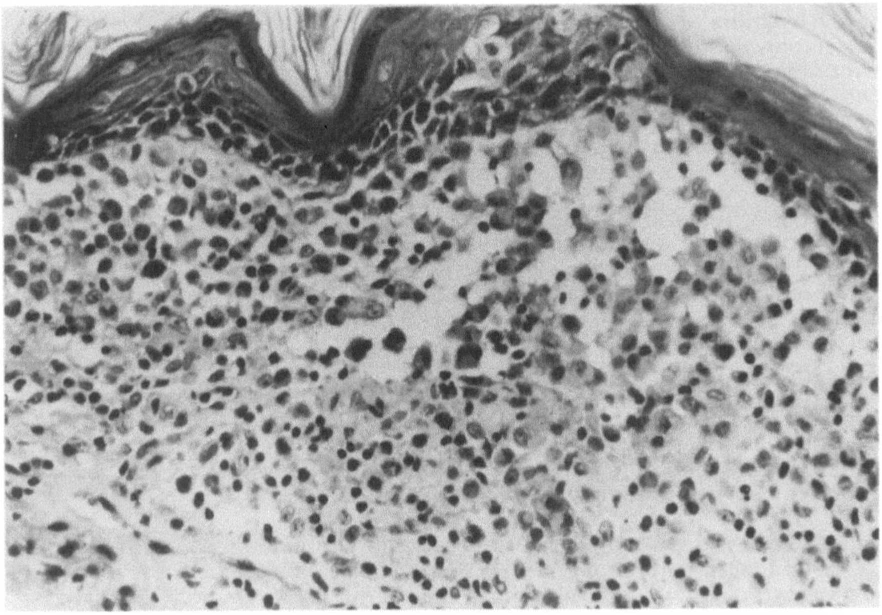

*Fig. 13 a & b. Skin infiltration in histiocytosis X with predominance of mononuclear cells (H. & E. X250 and X625)*

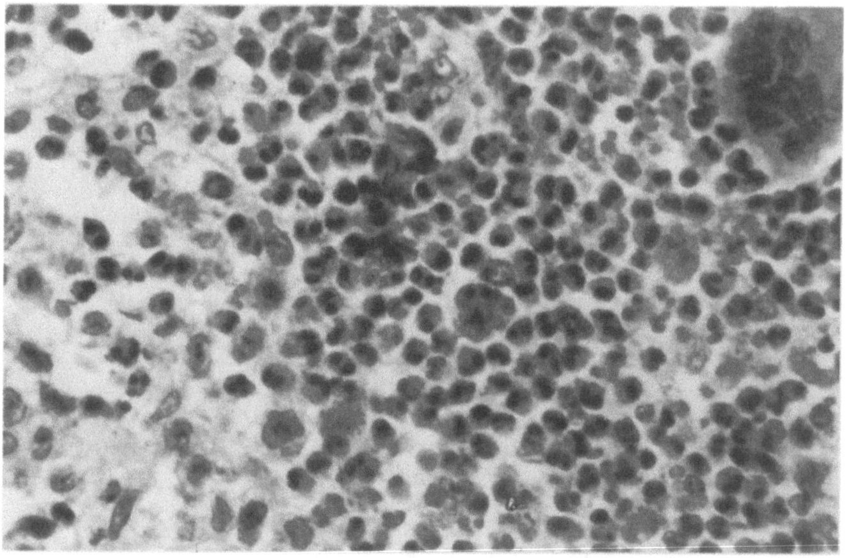

*Fig. 14. Histiocytosis X in bone with numerous eosinophils, some mononuclear cells and osteoclastic activity (H. & E. X625)*

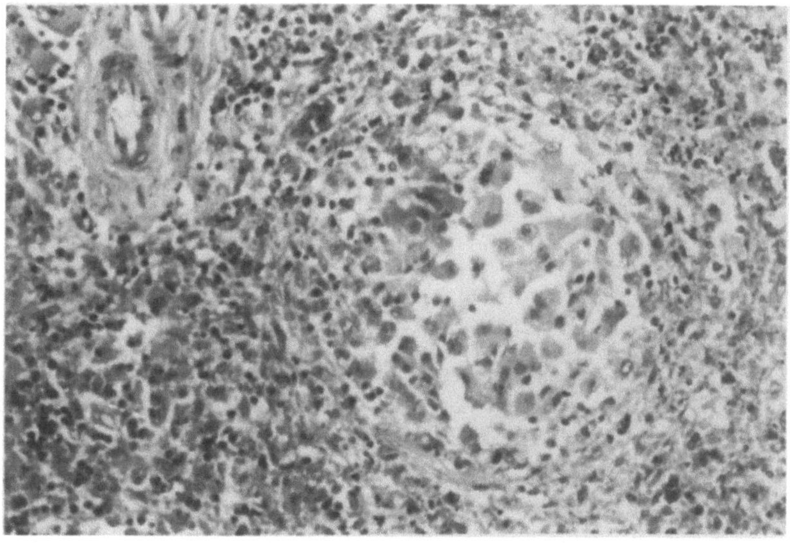

*Fig. 15. Spleen in histiocytosis X showing granuloma formation (H. & E. X250)*

diagnosis in the disease. Also it may be wrong to include the cases in a tumour register, as the neoplastic nature of the lesions is not absolutely certain. Nevertheless, histiocytosis X shows certain features compatible with it being a neoplasm of wandering reticuloendothelial cells, as it is radiosensitive and locally invasive, and, although there may be varying histological patterns, some cases show sheets of mononuclear cells without granuloma formation, resembling a reticulosarcoma. The problem has a certain similarity to that of the nature of Hodgkin's disease.

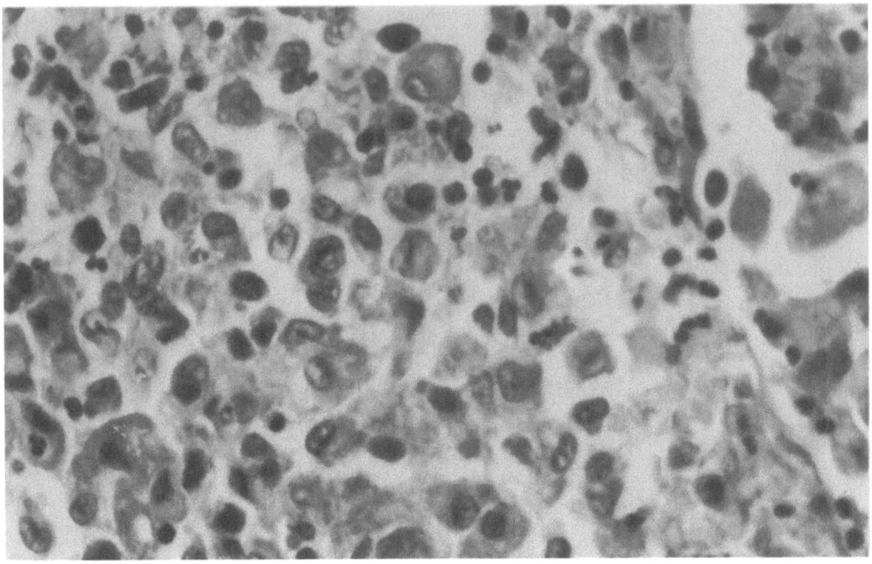

*Fig. 16. Diffuse mononuclear proliferation in histiocytosis X with some pleomorphism (H. & E. X625)*

Age and Sex. Histiocytosis X is seen mainly in early childhood - 38 of the 45 cases occurred before the age of 5 years (Table 2). There was no significant sex difference (Table 4).

Manifestation of the Disease. Since more than half of the children survive and autopsies were rarely performed on those who died, it is not possible to arrive at a completely accurate conclusion from the present series about the relative frequency of organ involvement. However, an attempt is made in Table 12 to indicate the sites of the lesions based largely on the clinical findings.

Diagnosis. The bone lesions of histiocytosis X are characteristically sharply defined osteolytic areas with minimal new bone formation. Although it is undesirable to make a diagnosis of this disease without a biopsy, the clinician may be justified in doing so if the typical punched-out areas are confined to inaccessible parts of the body (e.g. the base of the skull). When the disease is suspected, it is essential to do a skeletal survey before doing a biopsy so that the surgeons can select the most accessible rather than the presenting lesion.

Prognosis. Histiocytosis X has a better prognosis than other reticulo-endothelial tumours - 27 out of the 45 children in the Manchester series are still alive. Since all the deaths occurred within 2 years of diagnosis and the remaining children have been followed up for at least 3 years, it is hoped that none of the 27 survivors has active disease. However, histiocytosis X in certain sites (see below) can leave sequelae so that mere survival rates do not give the whole prognostic picture.

Fourteen out of the 25 boys and 13 out of the 20 girls in the Manchester series survived. Therefore sex did not appear to affect the prognosis. The three factors which were of major prognostic significance were the age of the patient, the extent of the disease, and the involvement of certain special sites.

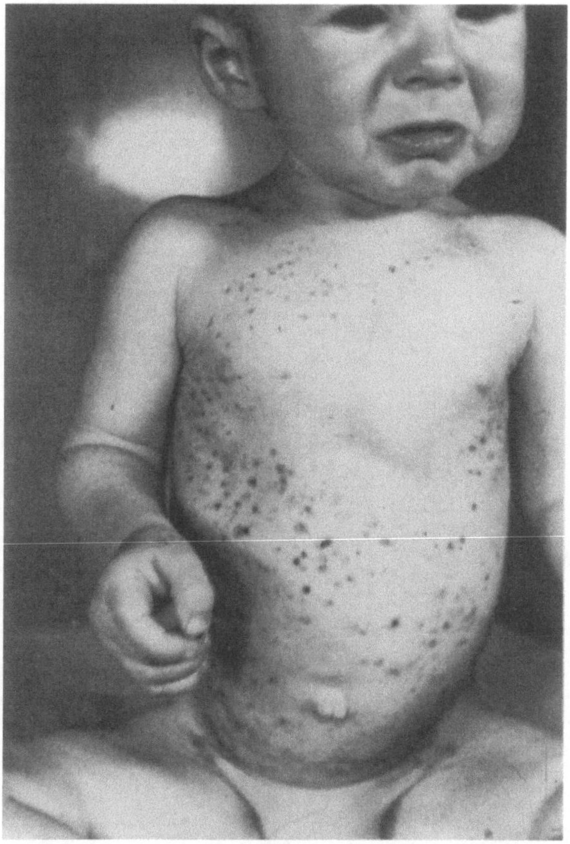

*Fig. 17. Characteristic eruption of histiocytosis X, almost entirely limited to trunk and consisting of small desquamating brownish-red papules interspersed with petechial lesions*

Table 12. Histiocytosis X. Relation between organ involvement and mortality

| | Affected Total | Affected Dead | Not affected Total | Not affected Dead |
|---|---|---|---|---|
| Skeleton | 27 | 9 | 18 | 9 |
| Skin | 20 | 12 | 25 | 6 |
| Lungs | 23 | 15 | 22 | 3 |
| Liver | 8 | 4 | 37 | 14 |
| Spleen | 13 | 10 | 32 | 8 |
| Anaemia &/or WBC >20,000 | 2 | 1 | 43 | 17 |
| Platelets down | 6 | 5 | 39 | 13 |
| Diabetes insipidus | 4 | 1 | 41 | 17 |
| Nodes | 8 | 6 | 37 | 12 |
| Ears | 8 | 4 | 37 | 14 |
| Gums | 3 | 1 | 42 | 17 |
| Parotids | 1 | 1 | 44 | 17 |
| Kidneys | 1 | 1 | 44 | 17 |
| Thymus | 2 | 2 | 43 | 16 |
| Gut | 2 | 2 | 43 | 16 |

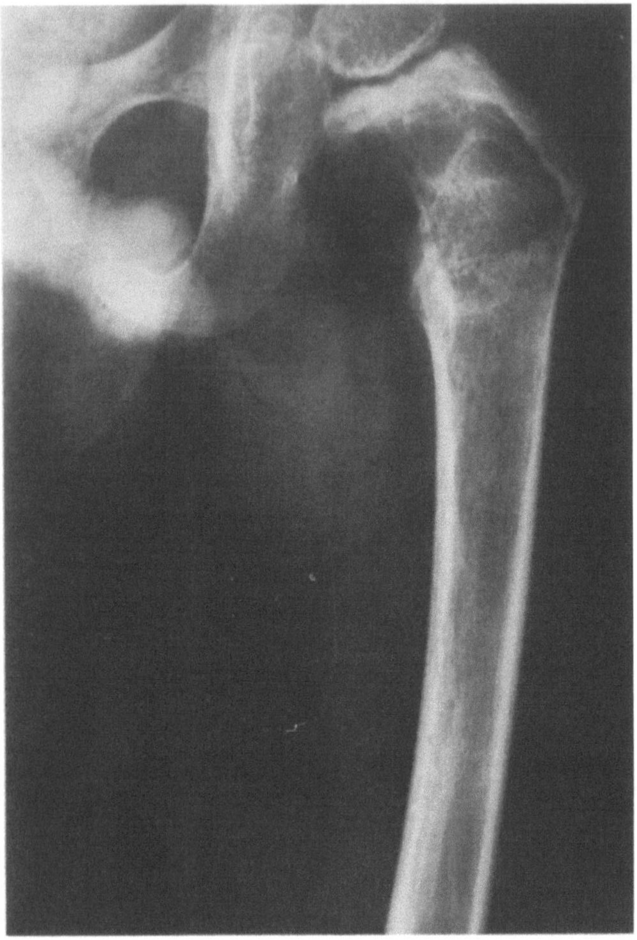

*Fig. 18. Punched-out osteolytic lesion in femoral neck due to histiocytosis X*

Age of Patient. Children who developed the disease in infancy did badly, whereas 10 of the 11 children who presented over the age of 3 years survived (Table 13).

Extent of the Disease. LAHEY (1962) in an analysis of 69 cases suggested a method of expressing the extent of the disease by giving a score of 1 to each organ system involved. He showed that all the children in his series with a score of 1 - 2 survived, whereas all with a score of 8 died. LAHEY specifically excluded from his analysis those patients with only one bone lesion (eosinophilic granuloma). His method was applied to the Manchester series with the modification that single bone lesions were included and given a score of one and multiple bone lesions were given a score of two. The relationship between the extent of the disease and the mortality rate is shown in Figure 19 which confirms LAHEY's findings.

Involvement of Special Sites. The relationship between the sites of the lesions and the mortality is shown in Table 12. There are four manifestations of histiocytosis X which may by themselves be dangerous or cause disability in those who survive.

Table 13. Histiocytosis X

| Age (years) at first consultation | -1 | -2 | -3 | -4 | -5 | -6 | -7 | -8 | -9 | -10 | -11 | -12 | -13 | -14 | -15 |
|---|---|---|---|---|---|---|---|---|---|---|---|---|---|---|---|
| Alive | 6 | 7 | 4 | 2 | 1 | 0 | 2 | 2 | 1 | 1 | 0 | 0 | 0 | 1 | 0 |
| Dead | 10 | 4 | 3 | 0 | 1 | 0 | 0 | 0 | 0 | 0 | 0 | 0 | 0 | 0 | 0 |

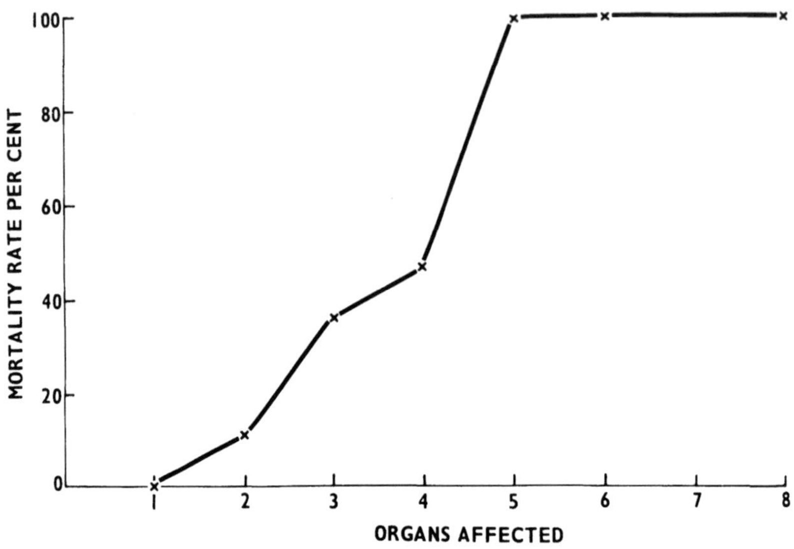


*Fig. 19. Histiocytosis X. Relationship between number of organs involved and mortality rate in the Manchester cases*

1) Diabetes Insipidus. Four of the Manchester children developed this condition - in one case the patient died soon after the onset of the diabetes insipidus, possibly due to electrolyte imbalance. In those who survived, the condition persisted although it could be satisfactorily controlled. Involvement of the pituitary sometimes also resulted in stunting of growth. BRAUNSTEIN and KOHLER (1972) carried out an examination of the pituitary function in 13 patients with histiocytosis X and found that growth stunting was usually found when diabetes insipidus was present. They concluded that the stunting was due to quantitative deficiency of the pituitary growth hormone apparently due to lack of release of this hormone secondary to infiltration of the hypothalamus.

2) Thrombocytopenia. Six of the children had thrombocytopenia and 5 of these died. Two appeared to die of haemorrhage presumably due to the low platelets.

3) Deafness. This occurred in 4 survivors in the Manchester series and appeared to be due to local involvement of the middle ear or a lesion of the temporal bone.

4) Lung Involvement is the most important and serious of the complications of histiocytosis X. In 15 of the 18 children who died there was evidence of pulmonary infiltration (Table 12) and in 8 of these, death was directly due to the lung involvement. LAHEY (1962) reported that 35 of the 69 children in his series had pulmonary involvement and 20 of the 25 deaths occurred in this group. LEWIS (1964) was able to find 75 reports in the literature of pulmonary involvement and described a further 12 adult patients personally studied by him. He pointed out that if the patient survives, this condition can result in considerable disability; the fibrosis resulting in emphysema and recurrent spontaneous pneumothoraces. This is illustrated by one of the cases in the Manchester series.

CTR.35/57. Boy, aged 1 year, attended hospital on 14/1/57 with rapid breathing and a slight cough. X-rays of the chest showed reticulation throughout both lungs. He became very dyspnoeic and cyanosed and was

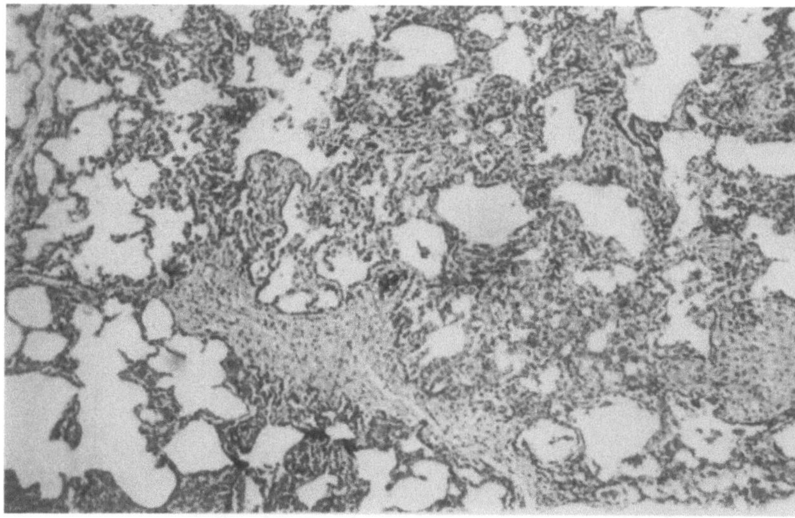

*Fig. 20. Lung in histiocytosis X showing interstitial mononuclear infiltration and emphysema (H. & E. X60)*

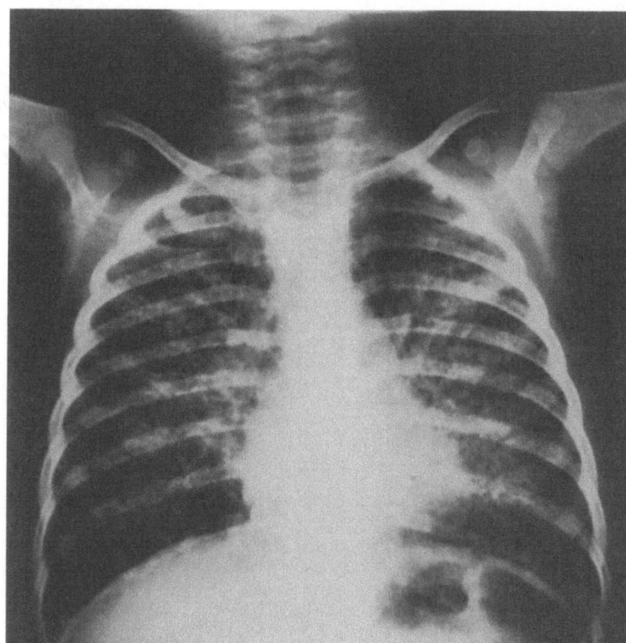

*Fig. 21 a, b & c. Reticulation of lung in case of histiocytosis X.*
*a) 16.1.57. Patient extremely dyspnoeic and cyanosed but symptoms disappeared following steroid therapy*

treated with oxygen and cortisone 50 mg 6 - hourly. On 1/2/57 a small pneumothorax was noted and a little later a skin rash appeared. The dyspnoea continued until April 1957 and the steroids were given up to December 1957. Although by then he was symptom-free, the lung reticulation remained. On 25/10/61 he developed a spontaneous pneumothorax,

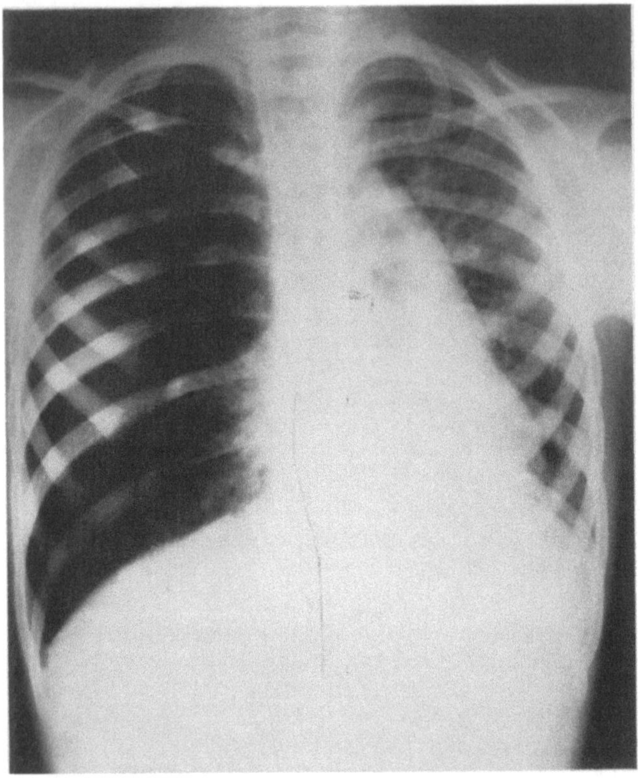

*b) 28.10.61. Development of spontaneous pneumothorax when patient had been symptom-free for over three years*

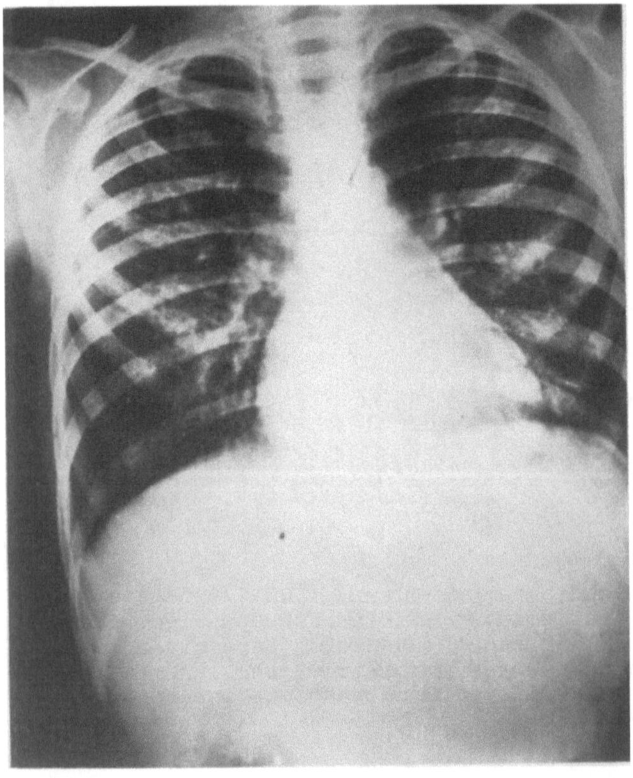

*c) 4.12.61. Persistence of reticulation without symptoms*

which recurred in July 1962. Although after this he was symptom-free, the lung reticulation remained.

## Clinical Management

In planning the treatment of children with histiocytosis X it is essential to determine as far as possible the extent of the disease so that it can be decided whether local or general treatment is required. In addition, it is necessary to determine whether the disease involves the lungs, pituitary or ears so that, if possible, the sequelae resulting from such involvement may be minimised.

Thus, in taking the history, care should be taken to enquire specifically into a history of polyuria, polydipsia, ear discharge, dyspnoeic episodes or "chest infection". The following investigations are necessary:

1. Chest X-ray
2. Full skeletal survey
3. Full blood count and platelets
4. Bone marrow aspiration
5. Urinary specific gravity

In cases where pituitary involvement is suspected, sophisticated investigations of pituitary function should be carried out, including urinary concentration and dilution tests, serum and urinary osmolality, response of urine osmolality to antidiuretic hormone and investigations of growth hormone.

In children who have evidence of lung involvement but who are not acutely ill, assessment of the lung function at the outset and sequential serial studies indicate whether permanent impairment of lung function is occurring.

Clinical assessment in association with these investigations will allow patients to be placed in the subclassification of OBERMAN (1961) and to score them according to LAHEY (1962).

Treatment. Single bone lesions are best treated by radiotherapy which results in immediate relief of pain and permanent destruction of the lesions.

For small lesions a single field to cover them with a margin of normal bone is used, and normally, treatment is restricted to a single dose of 600 rads using 4 MeV X-rays. If lesions are larger, or the deposits are near the pituitary or ears, a short fractionated course is given. For the pituitary a parallel pair of fields and a dose in the mid-plane of 1000 rads in 4 exposures is used and for the ear and some bone lesions 1200 rads is given in a single field in 4 exposures. These doses can be repeated, but this is rarely necessary provided care is taken that no part of the lesion is missed. Check films should always be taken. Apart from lesions in the gums, there seems to be no indication for X-ray therapy to other soft tissue involvement such as the lungs, although localised skin involvement will respond to superficial X-ray therapy in a dose of 450 rads in a single exposure. As the prognosis is often very good, radiation doses used should be as low as possible, so that any long-term effects are minimised.

When multiple lesions occur in sequential fashion and are not appearing rapidly, radiotherapy is also the treatment of choice. If the lesions occur with great frequency, the addition of chemotherapy is indicated.

In general, any involvement of organs or soft tissues requires chemotherapy. The only real exceptions to this are those cases with bone lesions and a sparse rash only. There is evidence that steroids and cytotoxic drugs reduce mortality. However, it is very difficult to assess accurately the relative efficiency of the various drugs, due to the variable behaviour of the disease. Histiocytosis differs from most tumours in that, even in the absence of specific treatment, it may regress spontaneously. This happened in three of the Manchester cases.

When the LAHEY score is 3 - 5, we have tended to use high doses of steroids - prednisolone 40-60 $mg/m^2$ daily for an initial period of three weeks and if the response has been obvious a lower maintenance dose of 20 $mg/m^2$ over a prolonged period of time. Usually these children have had combinations of bone, skin and lymph node lesions with lung, pituitary and haematological manifestations in some instances. In cases with more widespread disease, especially initial hepatosplenomegaly, we have combined steroids in the above dosage with either vincristine sulphate 1.5 $mg/m^2$ weekly or vinblastine sulphate 10 $mg/m^2$ weekly or 6-mercaptopurine 50 $mg/m^2$ daily or chlorambucil 1-2 mg daily; all given initially for 4 - 6 weeks. Vincristine has been the first line drug and if there is a failure of response or progression of disease, cyclophosphamide or methotrexate has also been used, but without success in our hands.

Histiocytosis X has a natural tendency to burn itself out, even when it has been widespread, and therefore treatment strategy does not necessarily consist of the attempted destruction of all the disease. The child may only need supportive measures and enough chemotherapy to keep the disease in check for a while. In the acute, severe forms blood and platelet transfusions may be indicated. Oxygen and humidification are necessary during periods of dyspnoea, and in those with diabetes insipidus adequate hydration is essential until the disease is brought under control. Fluid loss may also result from fever and rapid respiration.

Exophthalmos caused by histiocytosis X may stretch the optic nerve and cause impairment of vision. There should be no delay in carrying out orbital decompression in any case where radiation or chemotherapy fails to cause quick regression of the exophthalmos.

There are an appreciable number of survivors who have evidence of growth hormone defect . These children should be appropriately investigated and given replacement therapy if they are to achieve optimum growth.

## ERYTHRAEMIC MYELOSIS (di Guglielmo's Disease)

There have been 3 children with this disease.
CTR.123/56. A girl, aged 2 years. Attended on 5/3/56 with pallor, bruising, and petechiae; Hb. 52%, R.B.C. 2,46 million. Nucleated cells 12,600 (Polys. 12%, Lymphs 77%, Monos 1%, late normoblasts 10%), platelets 18,000. Subsequent peripheral blood counts showed atypical erythroid cells, with bizarre nuclear forms and mitoses and the proportion of reticulum cells varied between 6 and 30%. In the marrow the myeloid: erythroid ratio was 1 : 2. No megakaryocytes were seen and the red cell precursors showed mitotic forms. Coombs test negative. No increase in excretion of urobilinogen or urobilin. At varying periods during her illness the girl was given folic acid 100 mg /daily, cortisone 200 mg /

daily, and prednisolone 40 mg /daily, but there was no noticeable improvement attributable to these drugs. Splenectomy was of no avail. From 1/7/56 to 7/7/56, 6-mercaptopurine 25 mg /daily was given, but was stopped after one week as the total nucleated count had fallen to 1800 per c.mm. However, it was noted that for the following two weeks the proportion of abnormal cells was greatly reduced. By the beginning of August 1956 the nucleated cell count had risen to 22,800 per c.mm. She continued with a low platelet count and a large number of reticulum and erythroid cells in her peripheral blood and she needed repeat transfusions. She died on 19/11/56. At autopsy there was widespread invasion by erythroid and undifferentiated cells, particularly in the liver, spleen and kidneys.

CTR.61/60. Boy, aged 10 years, attended hospital in February 1960 with a six weeks' history of vomiting, loss of appetite and pallor. Hb. 49%, nucleated blood cells, 2,800, Polys. 37%, Lymphs. 19%, Monos. 10%, Eos. 3%, late normoblasts 21%, reticulocytes 1%, platelets 48,000. Indirect Coombs test negative. The marrow was cellular; the megakaryocytes were very small and did not show platelet formation and there was a great increase of erythroid elements. The boy was given prednisolone 40 mg daily for 5 weeks, with no improvement. On 5/5/60, 6-mercaptopurine 100 mg/daily was started. By 3/6/60 the platelets had risen to 83,000 and the normoblasts had almost disappeared from the peripheral blood. However, the W.B.C. was only 2600 and the 6-mercaptopurine was stopped. Ten days later the platelets had fallen to 31,000 and the nucleated blood cells were 2,400 with 14% normoblasts. 6-mercaptopurine 150 mg daily was then started and a transfusion given. Twelve days later Hb. 52%, W.B.C. 3,600, Polys. 66%, Lymphs. 31%, Monos. 3%, platelets 350,000. No normoblasts in the peripheral blood. The 6-mercaptopurine was reduced to 100 mg/daily and by 22/7/60 the count was completely normal. On 30/9/60 the 6-mercaptopurine was reduced to 50 mg/daily and it was stopped on 30/8/62. The blood count has remained normal ever since and the patient remains well 16 years after the disease started.

CTR.68/62. Girl, aged 9 years. In March 1962 she became tired, pale, and had abdominal pain and vomiting. In April 1962 the patient was found to have marked hepatosplenomegaly. Hb. 6 g /100 ml , P.V.C. 18%, M.C.H.C. 33%, W.B.C. 5,100, Polys. 34%, Lymphs. 59%, Monos 7%, nucleated red cells 11 per 100 white cells. Direct Coombs test negative. She was transfused and given prednisolone 50 mg without improvement. In August 1962 6-mercaptopurine 150 mg daily as well as prednisolone was given for 2 weeks. From 26 September to 19 October, 6-mercaptopurine in doses between 50 and 100 mg daily was given, but the blood count never returned to normal. The prednisolone was continued in a dose of 30 mg daily and ascorbic acid 100 mg/daily was added on the 27th October. 22/11/62 the blood picture was normal. However, at the end of January the blood picture changed to stem cell leukaemia and she died on 15/3/63.

## Conclusion

The fact that in case 2 (CTR.61/60) the giving of 6-mercaptopurine in large doses resulted in the control of the disease and probably the cure of the patient, and in case 1 (CTR.123/56) it appeared to have caused a temporary improvement, suggests that this drug is useful in erythraemic myelosis.

## MICROGLIOMATOSIS

The one child with this disease was a boy (CTR.8/57), aged 14 years, who became ataxic in September 1956. In November 1956 he developed right facial palsy and soon afterwards palatal palsy. In September 1956 it was realised that he had right nerve deafness. The C.S.F. showed no abnormality. Air ventriculograms and blood counts normal. He had no headaches.

He died on 19/1/57. At autopsy there were soft grey areas about 1 cm in diameter in the middle cerebellar peduncle, the centrum semiovale, the cornu and the medullo-pontine angle. Sections showed these areas to consist of aggregations of cells, some of which looked like lymphocytes and some had vacuolated cytoplasm. The other organs were normal.

Theoretically this child might have been cured by irradiation of the whole central nervous system as is used for the treatment of medulloblastoma. However, it is difficult to see how the diagnosis could have been made during life.

## MYCOSIS FUNGOIDES

The one child with this condition was a boy (CTR.107/68), aged 8 years, who was admitted to hospital on 30/10/68 with a 2 weeks' history of enlarged axillary and cervical nodes, shivering and sweating. Blood count normal. Marrow hypercellular due to neutrophil increase with a few blast cells present. On 11/11/68 a purple maculopapular rash appeared. In spite of antibiotics the child was very ill and pyrexial and died on 21/12/68. At autopsy there were purple areas about 10 cm in diameter of wrinkled, indurated skin in each axilla. They were infiltrated with tumour cells. Apart from this the only naked eye lesion was a mass of glands 6 cms in diameter near the pancreas. However, microscopically only small groups of tumour cells were seen in these nodes and also in the thymus.

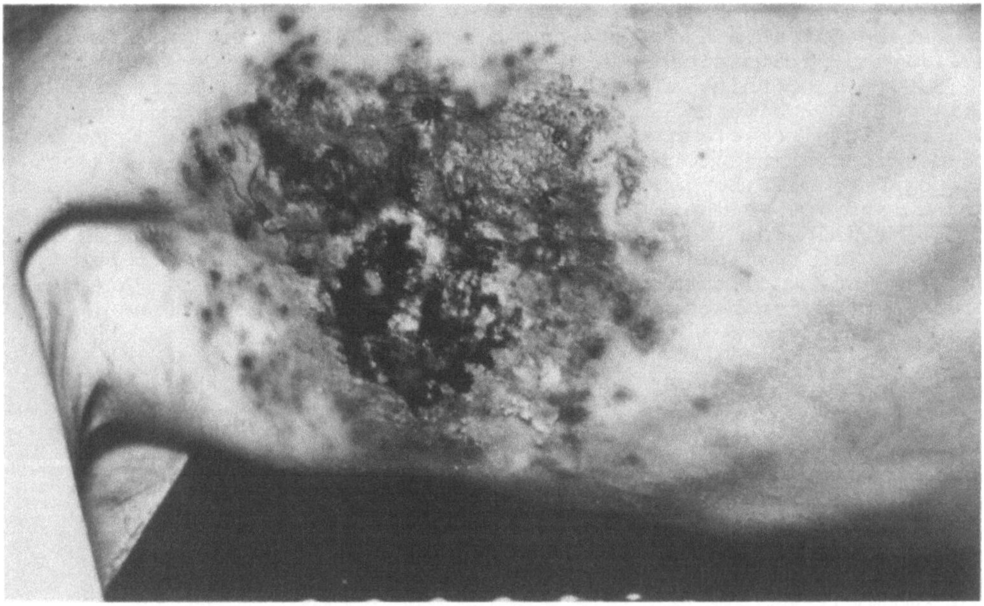

*Fig. 22 a & b. Mycosis fungoides (a) Purple ulcerating papular rash over right side of chest. (b) Skin with heavy infiltration by hyperchromatic pleomorphic tumour cells mainly in upper dermis (H.&E. X125)*

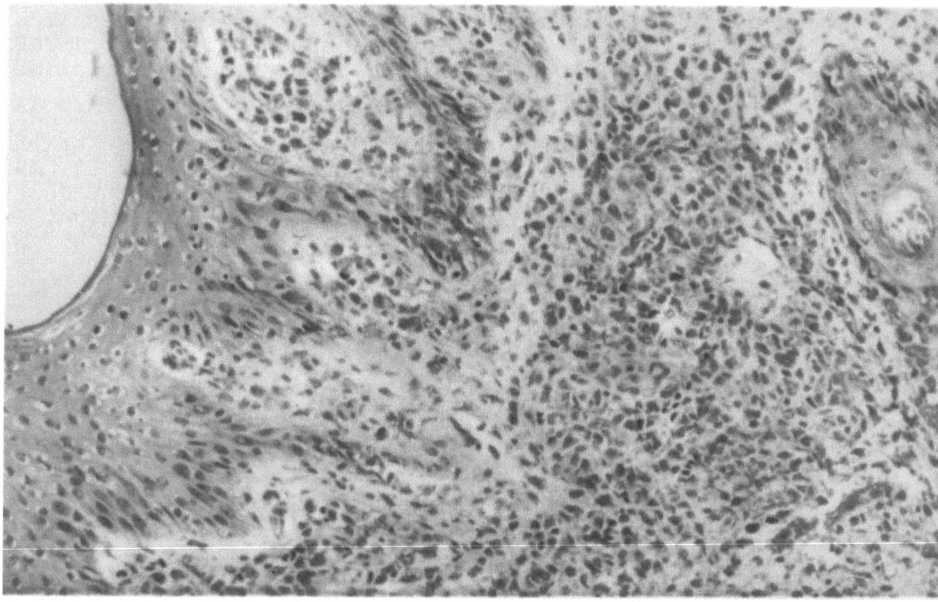

MYELOSARCOMA (CHLOROMA)

There is one example of this tumour in the Manchester series before 1968. CTR.19/65, girl, aged 6 years, developed a flaccid paraplegia in December 1964. Thoracic laminectomy on 16/2/65 revealed a fleshy extradural tumour which, when placed in hydrosulphite, became green.

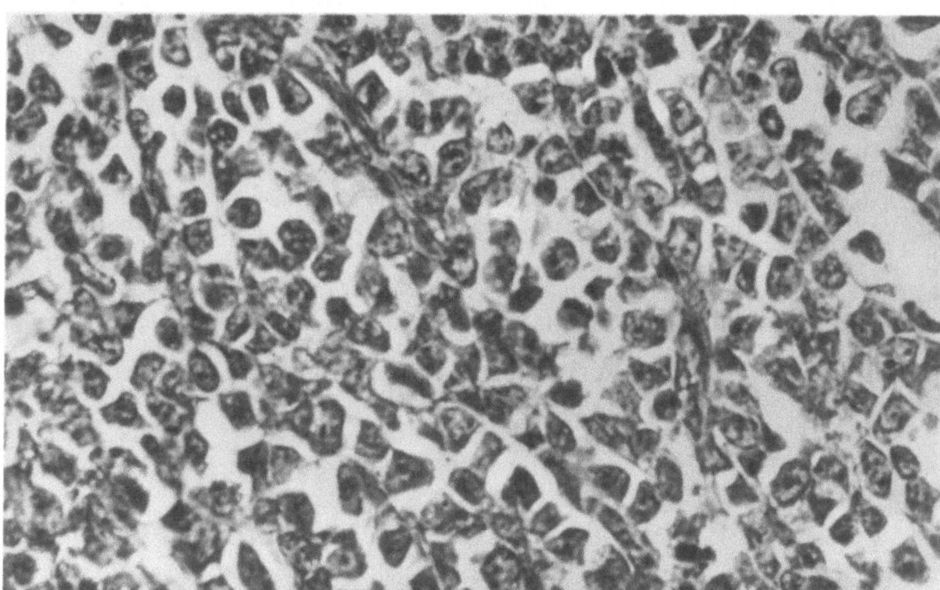

*Fig. 23. Myelosarcoma. Diffuse proliferation of myeloid cells (H. & E. X625)*

After partial removal of the tumour the dorso-lumbar spine was irradiated (3,520 rads in 20 days). The child remained well up to 16/12/65, when she developed acute myeloid leukaemia. She went into remission on prednisolone and 6-mercaptopurine. She died on 16/1/67.

There has been one more case of myelosarcoma in the Register, which occurred since 1968. The patient was a Jamaican girl (CTR.14/72) who died after a short illness. At autopsy there were green tumour deposits in the orbits, retrosternal glands, kidneys, femur and heart.

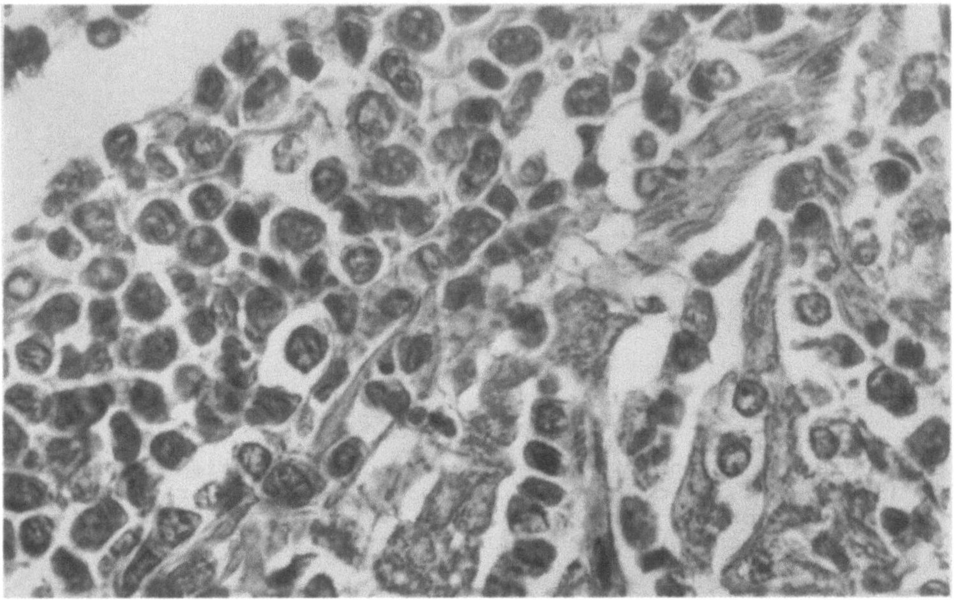

*Fig. 24. Chloroma. Invasion of cardiac muscle by cells of myeloid type (H. & E. X625)*

Histologically, the myelosarcoma can be distinguished from the lymphosarcoma by the fact that the cells have more irregular nuclei with a variable amount of cytoplasm. Histochemical demonstration of naphthol-ASD-chloracetate esterase activity may be helpful in the detection of cells of the myeloid series (LEDER, 1964).

In the first child (CTR.19/65) the interval between clinical onset and the development of leukaemia was 1 year, which is much longer than occurred in any of the Manchester patients with leucosarcoma. In the second child (CTR.14/72) death occurred within 1 week of clinical onset and the bone marrow, although abnormal, was not definitely leukaemic.

## HISTIOCYTOSIS AND RETICULOENDOTHELIOSIS

There are a number of syndromes, some of which are familial, in which histiocytic proliferation is a prominent feature. In familial haemophagocytic reticulosis (FARQUAHAR et al., 1958) there is marked erythrophagocytosis and nucleated cells are engulfed to a lesser degree. OMENN (1965) described 12 infants in 6 sibships dying with disease of the reticuloendothelial system associated with eosinophilia. Hepatosplenomegaly, skin involvement, lymphadenopathy and infiltration of the meninges by lymphocytes and histiocytes were features. Generalized lymphohistiocytic infiltration in members of the same family was reported by NELSON et al. (1961). In these cases proliferation of reticulum cells and histiocytes with erythrophagocytosis was seen in the sinuses of the lymph nodes and there was meningeal infiltration. The thymus showed depletion with absence of Hassall's corpuscles in some cases.

Thymic dysplasia was a feature of the cases described by CEDERBAUM et al. (1974) under the title of "combined immunodeficiency presenting as the Letterer-Siwe syndrome", in which a rash and eosinophilia were clinical features and sinusoidal, endothelial and histiocytic cells with erythrophagocytosis and some degree of nuclear phagocytosis were found on lymph node microscopy. Thymic involvement was reported in histiocytosis X by LEIKIN et al. (1973) in a discussion on the immunologic parameters of this disease. The thymic lesions described in 3 infants with the Letterer-Siwe syndrome by these authors were considered to be due to immunosuppressive therapy.

In the Chédiak-Higashi syndrome, a familial disease with constitutional stigmata and inclusions in the leucocytes, DONOHUE and BAIN (1957) reported dense infiltration by histiocytes, reticular cells, lymphocytes, and cells with a myelocytic appearance in a number of organs.

ROSAI and DORFMAN (1972) described sinus histiocytosis with massive lymphadenopathy as a pseudolymphomatous benign disorder. In an analysis of 34 cases collected from various parts of the world these authors showed that cervical node involvement was the principal feature with sinus histiocytosis on microscopy. Lymphocytes and to a lesser degree erythrocytes and plasma cells were engulfed by the histiocytes. The general condition of the patients was good, but evidence of more disseminated lesions including other nodes, eye, skin, spleen and bone involvement was apparent in a minority of cases. In the two cases who died thymic dysplasia with absence of Hassall's corpuscles was noted. Defects of cellular immune function were thought to be important in the pathogenesis of this condition following the studies of BECROFT et al. (1973) on a 16-month-old boy from New Zealand who had been included in ROSAI and DORFMAN's survey.

CTR.39/75. A Caucasian female child having spontaneous hyphaema at the age of 5 1/2 months. Small nodules were noted over the scalp and left hypochondrium and firm lymph nodes were palpable in the groins and occipital region. She was a first child, the parents being healthy. A maternal aunt had bronchial carcinoma at the age of 24 years. Biopsy of a skin nodule showed heavy infiltration of the dermis and subcutaneous fat by pale mononuclear cells. The blood count was normal and also the immunoglobulins. A diffuse nodular rash became apparent. Bone marrow examination showed numerous mononuclear and undifferentiated cells. There was persistent fever and cellulitis of the orbital and perineal regions developed. Anti-leukaemic therapy was given but there was steady deterioration and the child died after one month. At autopsy there was moderate hepatosplenomegaly with generalized enlargement of lymph nodes which were purple in colour and up to 2 cm in diameter. The thymus was 6 g in weight, pale, and hard in consistency. Microscopically the lymph node sinuses were distended by histiocytes which contained numerous lymphocytes in some areas and erythrocytes and large mononuclear cells in others (Figs. 25 and 26). All three cell types were engulfed in some cells. The bone marrow showed patchy replacement by histiocytes and there was subperiosteal extension in places. Lymphophagocytosis was seen in the marrow. The spleen was replaced by sheets of similar cells and there was perisplenitis. Histiocytes were confined

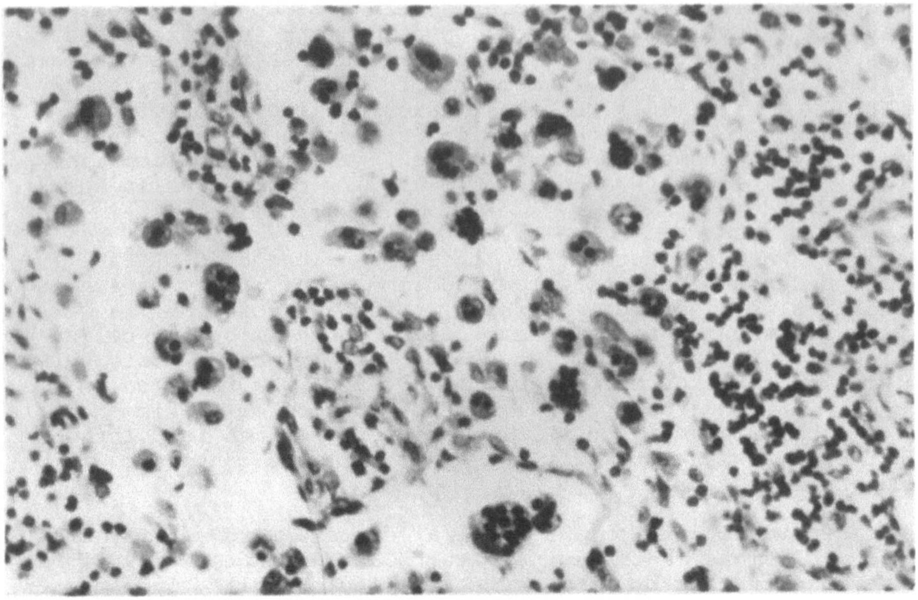

*Fig. 25. Sinus histiocytosis. Intracellular lymphocytes are a prominent feature (H. & E. X 250)*

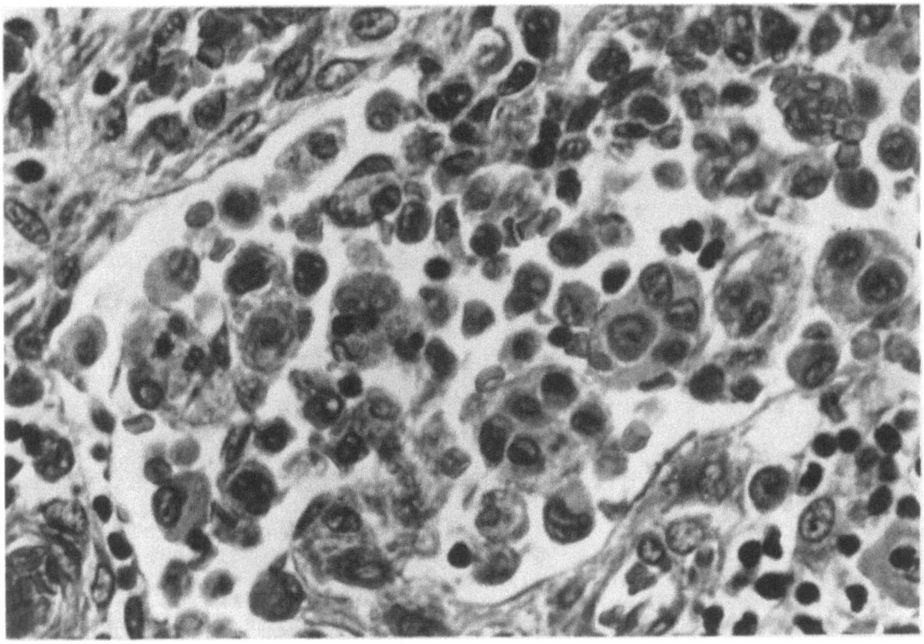

*Fig. 26. Sinus histiocytosis. Intracellular monocytes and erythrocytes predominate in this field (H. & E. X750)*

to the sinusoids in the liver. Heavy infiltration by mononuclear cells was seen in the epicardial fat and there were similar cells and lymphocytes in the meninges. The thymus showed scanty lymphocytes, large numbers of histiocytes and occasional degenerate Hassall's corpuscles.

The findings in this patient show a number of the features seen in the reported cases. The histiological appearances, namely sinus histiocytosis with engulfed nucleated cells principally lymphocytes, are similar to those described by ROSAI and DORFMAN (1972). However, larger mononuclear cells are also seen inside the histiocytes and erythrophagocytosis is a more prominent feature. The clinical features are different and the disseminated lesions are more in keeping with generalized lymphohistiocytic infiltration. The thymus is abnormal, a finding which is reported in sinus histiocytosis, combined immuno-deficiency with eosinophilia, generalized lymphohistiocytic infiltration and some cases of the Letterer-Siwe syndrome. It is clear that further immunological studies are needed in this unusual and important group of diseases.

## REFERENCES


ATWOOD, W. A., MILLER, R. C., NELSON, C. T.: Arch. Derm. 94, 144 (1966)

AUR, R. J. A., HUSTU, H. O., SIMONS, J. V., PINKEL, D.: Cancer 27, 1328 (1971)

BECROFT, D. M. O., DIX, M. R., GILLMAN, J. C., MacGREGOR, B. J. L., SHAW, R. L.: J. Clin. Path. 26, 463 (1973)

BERARD, C. W., THOMAS, L. B., AXTELL, L. M., KRUSE, M., NEWELL, G., KAGAN, R.: Canc. Res. 31, 1776 (1971)

BRAUNSTEIN, G. D., KOHLER, F. O.: New Eng. J. Med. 286, 1225 (1972)

BURN, C., DAVIES, J. N. P., DODGE, O. G., NIAS, B. C.: J. Nat. Canc. Inst. 46, 37 (1971)

CARBONE, P. P., KAPLAN, H. S., MUSSHOFF, K., SMITHERS, D. W., TUBIANA, M.: Canc. Res. 31, 1860 (1971)

CARBONE, P. P.: Cancer 30, 1511 (1972)

CEDERBAUM, S. D., NIWAYAMA, G., STIEHM, E. R., NEERHOUT, R. C., AMMANN, A. J., BERMAN, W. Jr.: J. Ped. 85, 466 (1974)

COOKE, J. V.: J. Amer. Med. Ass. 119, 547 (1942)

CORREA, P., O'CONOR, C. T.: Int. J. Cancer 8, 192 (1971)

DE VITA, V. T., CANELLOS, G. P., MOXLEY, J. H.: Cancer 30, 1495 (1972)

DIAMANDOPOULOS, C. T., SMITH, E. B.: Cancer 17, 329 (1964)

DONOHUE, W. L., BAIN, H. W.: Pediat. 20, 416 (1957)

DORFMAN, R. F.: Cancer 18, 418 (1965)

DORFMAN, R. F.: Canc. Res. 31, 1786 (1971)

EASSON, E. C., RUSSELL, M. H.: Brit. Med. J. 1, 1704 (1963)

FARQUHAR, J. W., MacGREGOR, A. R., RICHMOND, J.: Brit. Med. J. 2, 1561 (1958)

GOLDFARB, B., COHEN, S. S.: J. A. M. A. 211, 1525 (1970)

GRESHAM, C. A., ACKERLEY, A. G.: J. Clin. Path. 11, 244 (1958)

GROSSMAN, H., WINCHESTER, P. H., BRAGG, D. G., TAN, C., MURPHY, M. L.: Am. J. Roentgenol. 108, 354 (1970)

HAYES, D. M., HIPPLE, R. C., ISAACS, H., KARON, H.: J. Ped. Surg. 7, 517 (1972)

JACKSON, H., PARKER, F.: Hodgkin's disease and allied disorders. New York: Oxford Univ. Press (1947)

JENKIN, R. D. F., PETERS, M. V., DARTE, J. M. M.: Am. J. Roentgenol. 100, 222 (1967)

JONES, B., KLINGBERG, W. C.: J. Ped. 63, 11 (1963)

LAHEY, M. E.: J. Ped. 60, 664 (1962)

LEDER, L. D.: Klin. Wschr. 42, 553 (1964)

LEIKIN, S., PURUGANAN, G., FRANKEL, A., STEERMAN, R., CHANDRA, R.: Cancer 32, 796 (1973)

LEWIS, J. G.: Quart. J. Med. 33, 337 (1964)

LOWENSTEIN, S., RAMSEY, H., SUTHERLAND, J., SERPICK, A. A.: Am. J. Med. 50, 49 (1971)

LUKES, R. J., BUTLER, J. J., HICKS, E. B.: Cancer 19, 317 (1966)

MARSH, J. C., DELONTI, R. C., HUBBARD, S. P.: Canc. Chemotherapy Rep. 55, 599 (1971)

NELSON, P., SANTAMARIA, A., OLSON, R. L., NAYAK, N. C.: Pediat. 27, 931 (1961)

NEWELL, C. R., COLE, S. R., MITTINEN, O. S., MacMAHON, B.: J. Nat. Canc. Inst. 45, 311 (1970)

OBERMAN, H.: Pediat. 28, 307 (1961)

OMENN, G. S.: New Eng. J. Med. 273, 427 (1965)

PETERS, M. V.: Canc. Res. 31, 1713 (1971)

ROSAI, J., DORFMAN, R. F.: Cancer 30, 1174 (1972)

ROSENBERG, S. A.: Canc. Res. 26, 1310 (1966)

SALZMAN, J., KAPLAN, H. S.: Cancer 27, 471 (1971)

STOKER, T. A. M.: Proc. Roy. Soc. Med. 64, 661 (1971)

STRUM, S. B., RAPPAPORT, H.: Pediat. 46, 748 (1970)

SULLIVAN, M.: Pediat. 29, 589 (1962)

TEILLET, F., BOIRON, M., BERNARD, J.: Canc. Res. 31, 1723 (1971)

WANTANABE, S. A., KAPLAN, H. S.: California Medicine 113, 23 (1970)

# Chapter 6
# Intracranial and Spinal Tumours

The central nervous system is the second commonest site of tumour formation in children. In contrast with lethal neoplasms elsewhere, those in the central nervous system very rarely spread to other organs but are dangerous because they invade and destroy adjoining vital centres. Thus the prognosis depends as much on site as on histological type. The fact that in children these tumours often arise close to the midline structures at the base of the brain, limits the extent of local treatment which can be given safely.

A basic requirement of tumour diagnosis is either histological or biochemical proof. However, neoplasms of the central nervous system present a special problem in this respect. It is very seldom justifiable to biopsy lesions in the brain stem or third ventricle and pathological material from tumours in these areas is generally only obtained if an autopsy is performed. In order to obtain a proper picture of the therapeutic problem it is necessary therefore to include those cases in which the clinical evidence points very strongly towards a diagnosis of neoplasm even though pathological proof is lacking.

Three hundred and thirty-three children with proven or presumed primary intracranial or spinal tumours were included between 1954 and 1968. In 291 cases histological material was available but in 42 cases the diagnosis was based on clinical and radiological evidence alone.

## Types of Tumour

The present study is limited as regards classification, not only because pathological material was completely absent from some cases, but also because if only a small biopsy is taken it is not possible to obtain the true picture of a glioma which may vary from one part to another. In addition, problems of definition and nomenclature bedevil the study of these tumours and make comparative statistics difficult or even impossible. Many large series are not specially concerned with the problems as seen in young people; others, such as HARE and WOLF (1934); BAILEY et al. (1939); WALKER and HOPPLE (1949); CRAIG et al. (1949); BODIAN and LAWSON (1953) and MATSON (1969 a) who report surveys of tumours occurring specifically in childhood, may show selective bias because the occurrence rates are not truly population-based.

The practical value of any histological classification depends on whether it can be correlated with the behaviour of the tumour. In the past, once the neurosurgeon had operated on a glioma, all he needed to know was whether the tumour was likely to recur and, if so, whether further excision or radiotherapy might be beneficial. With the advent of adjuvant chemotherapy, more precise information is required. Since many anti-tumour agents act mainly during a limited period of the cell cycle, a chemotherapy regime needs to be planned with some knowledge of the speed of growth of the tumour. Although there is little experimental evidence on the growth kinetics of gliomas, a certain amount can be deduced from their clinical behaviour. For instance, the fact that medulloblastomas sometimes recur many years after initial treatment indicates that this tumour may contain clones which either have a very long cell cycle or which may be in a resting phase for a very long time. Thus a drug like vincristine which acts mainly during mitosis would need to be given over a long period to kill all the cells in such a tumour.

In an attempt to provide clinical guidance KERNOHAN et al. (1949) applied Broder's system for grading epithelial tumours to the gliomas. This involved the recognition of four stages of cytological anaplasia for each tumour type and implied a corresponding clinical progress. However, the effect on the patient of a tumour in the central nervous system is so dependent on the site that any correlation with histological appearance is often blurred, and this applies particularly to the midline gliomas in children which may be fatal, not because of their rapid growth, but because they invade vital structures or obstruct the flow of C.S.F.
The classification which is used here is basically that which originated with BAILEY and CUSHING (1926), BAILEY (1931) and PENFIELD (1931) and resembles that used by ZÜLCH (1965 a), RUSSELL and RUBINSTEIN (1971 a),

Table 1. Manchester Children's Tumour Registry Primary intracranial and spinal tumours 1954 - 1968 (assessed 1972)

| | Alive | Dead | Total |
|---|---|---|---|
| Astrocytomas | 58 | 72 | 130 |
| Medulloblastomas | 14 | 61 | 75 |
| Ependymomas | 8 | 32 | 40 |
| Oligodendrogliomas | 1 | 3 | 4 |
| Gliomas (uncertain origin) | 0 | 5 | 5 |
| Cerebellar, brain stem and cord gliomas (clinical diagnosis only) | 8 | 23 | 31 |
| Craniopharyngiomas | 9 | 8 | 17 |
| Third ventricular (clinical diagnosis only) | 5 | 4 | 9 |
| Pinealomas | 0 | 7 | 7 |
| Teratomas | 1 | 4 | 5 |
| Connective tissue | 4 | 1 | 5 |
| Pituitary adenomas | 1 | 1 | 2 |
| Microglioma | 0 | 1 | 1 |
| Meningeal melanoma | 0 | 1 | 1 |
| Acoustic neuroma | 1 | 0 | 1 |
| | 110 | 223 | 333 |

and KOOS and MILLER (1971 a). In Table 1 the frequency and prognosis of the various tumour types in the Manchester series are shown. It will be seen that over 70% of these patients had tumours of three main types - medulloblastomas, astrocytomas, or ependymomas, thereby differing from the situation in adults in whom meningiomas, neurinomas, and metastatic carcinomas are common.

Table 2. The sites of the main groups of central nervous system tumours

| | Astro-cytoma | Medullo-blastoma | Ependymoma | Oligoden-droglioma | Glioma (uncertain type) | Pine-aloma | Cranio-pharyn-gioma | Clinical diagnosis only | Total |
|---|---|---|---|---|---|---|---|---|---|
| Cerebellum | 45 | 68 | 16 | 1 | 0 | 0 | 0 | 4 | 134 |
| Brain stem and 3rd ventricle | 36 | 5 | 11 | 1 | 2 | 7 | 17 | 33 | 112 |
| Cerebrum | 31 | 1 | 9 | 2 | 3 | 0 | 0 | 0 | 46 |
| Optic nerve | 12 | 0 | 0 | 0 | 0 | 0 | 0 | 1 | 13 |
| Cord | 6 | 1 | 3 | 0 | 0 | 0 | 0 | 2 | 12 |
| Separate from brain | 0 | 0 | 1 | 0 | 0 | 0 | 0 | 0 | 1 |
| Total | 130 | 75 | 40 | 4 | 5 | 7 | 17 | 40 | 318 |

## Sites of Tumours

Many authors have commented on the fact that most intracranial tumours in children are subtentorial and in this respect they differ from neoplasms in adults (CRITCHLEY, 1925; CUSHING, 1927; WALKER and HOPPLE, 1949). Seventy percent of the gliomas in the Manchester series were below the tentorium.

In Table 2 the sites of the main groups of central nervous system tumours are shown. It will be seen that the commonest type of tumour in the cerebrum, brain stem, and cord was the astrocytoma. In the cerebellum there were considerably more medulloblastomas than astrocytomas. Ependymomas were much rarer in the Manchester series and were most commonly cerebellar. Tumours in the third ventricle were frequently not biopsied but many of those whose histology was known were astrocytomas with craniopharyngiomas, ependymomas, and pinealomas being less common.

Table 3. Sites of intracranial gliomas

| | Cerebellum | Brain stem, third ventricle, optic nerve | Cerebrum |
|---|---|---|---|
| Manchester (272 cases) | 49% | 34% | 17% |
| Chicago (76 cases) | 51% | 42% | 7% |
| London (115 cases) | 60% | 25% | 15% |

In Table 3 the sites of the gliomas in the Manchester series are compared with those in two other series of children's gliomas - one reported from Chicago by BAILEY et al. (1939) and the other from the Hospital for Sick Children, London, by BODIAN and LAWSON (1953).

In comparing these figures it must be realised that the Chicago and London series consisted entirely of histologically proven cases, and that the Chicago study was carried out at a time when patients with intracranial tumours had exploratory operations which would not be considered justifiable at the present time. Such operations increased the opportunity for histological examination. Even though these three studies were carried out under different conditions they gave similar results. From the point of view of practical therapy it is fortunate that the cerebellum is the commonest site but the fact that so many tumours arise in the brain stem, cord and diencephalon inevitably limits the efforts of the surgeon and radiotherapist and contributes to the high overall mortality.

The distribution of tumours in the central nervous system of children must be a reflection of those factors which give rise to them. In a child aged 3 years the combined weight of the vermis and brain stem is approximately 40 g. Although these structures comprise only 3% of the total mass of the central nervous system, over half of the gliomas arose in them. The reasons why this small area of the central nervous system, situated at the cephalic end of the primitive neural tube, is so liable to be the site of tumour formation in children, are unknown. Perhaps it is because it contains cells capable of tremendous growth during early embryonic development and these cells may go through a phase when they are sensitive to some carcinogenic agent which would not affect more mature tissues. This might suggest that the cause of children's gliomas should be sought in early foetal life.

MEDULLOBLASTOMA. This tumour shows a markedly greater incidence in boys than girls - in the Manchester series 55 boys were affected compared with 20 girls (see Table 4, Chapter 1). It is considered to be a primitive tumour which may have the potential for neuronal or glial differentiation although its exact nature is not certain. It usually arises in the midcerebellar region. Fifty-two of the 75 Manchester medulloblastomas involved the cerebellar vermis. In 12 of the remaining 23 cases the tumours were in the cerebellum, but there was no note of whether they were midline, and in 3 cases the tumours arose in the cerebellar hemisphere. Only 8 children had medulloblastomas arising outside the cerebellum (Table 4) and these figures are in agreement with the observations of RINGERTZ and TOLA (1950) who found 86% of medulloblastomas to be midcerebellar.

Table 4. Sites of Medulloblastomas

| | | |
|---|---|---|
| | ( vermis | 52 |
| Cerebellum | ( exact site unknown | 12 |
| | ( hemisphere | 3 |
| Brain stem | | 6 |
| Spinal cord | | 1 |
| Cerebrum | | 1 |
| | | 75 |

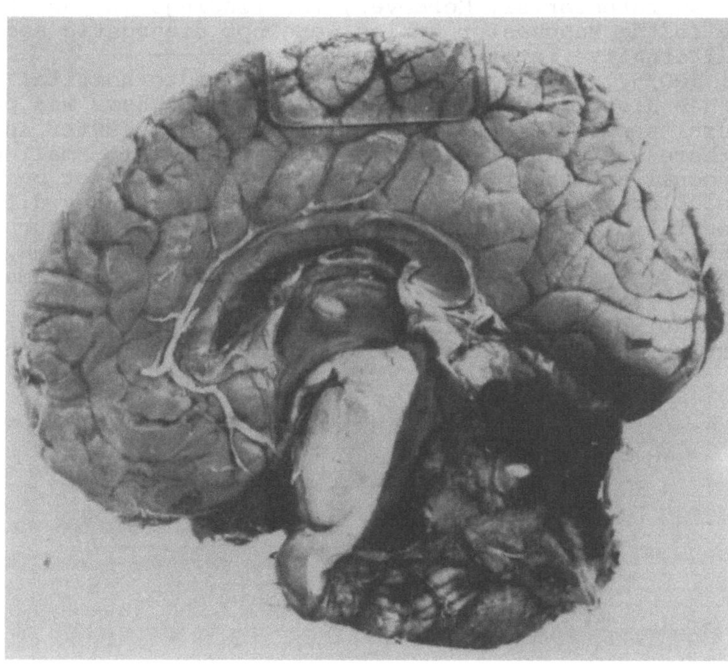

*Fig. 1. Medulloblastoma in roof of 4th ventricle. Tumour had not invaded floor of ventricle*

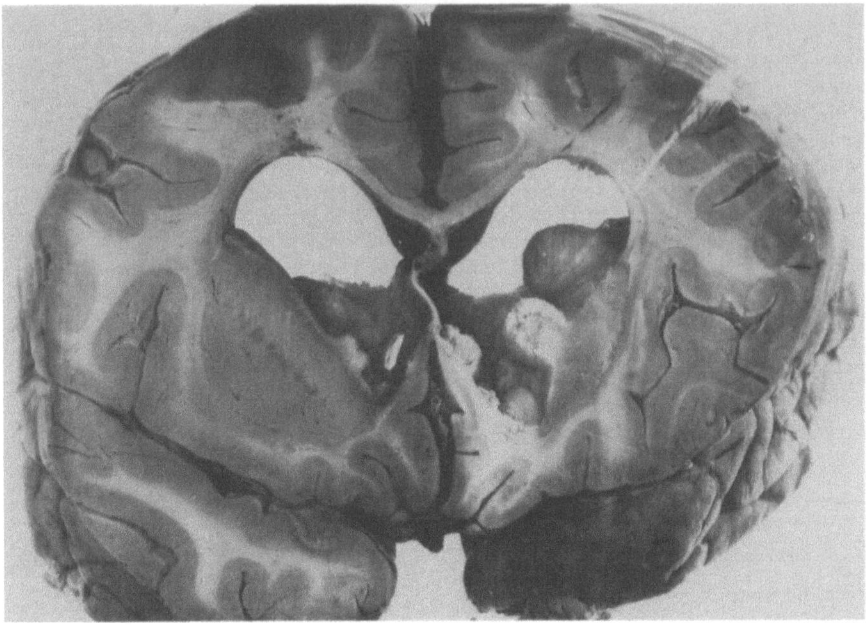

*Fig. 2. Deposits in lateral ventricles from cerebellar medulloblastoma which has caused hydrocephalus from obstruction of 4th ventricle*

The medulloblastomas in the Manchester series were, with one exception, subtentorial, whereas 15 out of the 51 cases of BODIAN and LAWSON (1953) were supratentorial. Moreover, the findings in the one supratentorial case in the Manchester series were not diagnostic and could be open to an alternative interpretation.
CTR. 100/57. Boy, aged 5 years. Admitted to hospital on 21/9/57 with a month's history of headache and vomiting. There was papilloedema and sutural separation and the child died 4 days after admission. At autopsy there was a large necrotic and haemorrhagic small-celled tumour with polygonal and short spindle cells which could not be distinguished from a medulloblastoma, although in the absence of any differentiating features the diagnosis must remain unproven. The tumour involved the entire right cerebral hemisphere and had remained localised, a feature which might be regarded as evidence against medulloblastoma.

The medulloblastoma spreads from its primary site throughout the ventricular system causing blockage of C.S.F. flow and hydrocephalus and

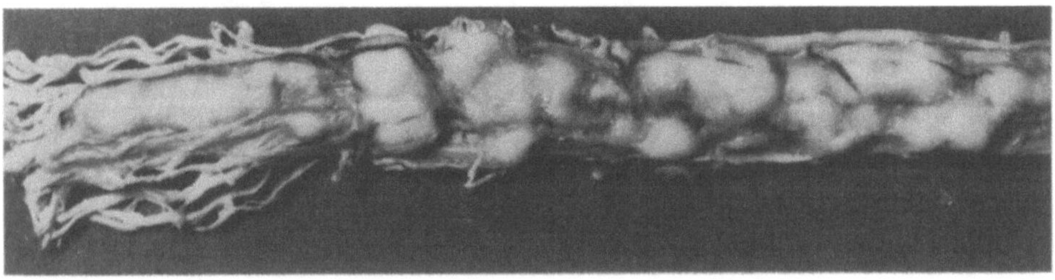

*Fig. 3. Deposits from medulloblastoma surrounding and invading spinal cord*

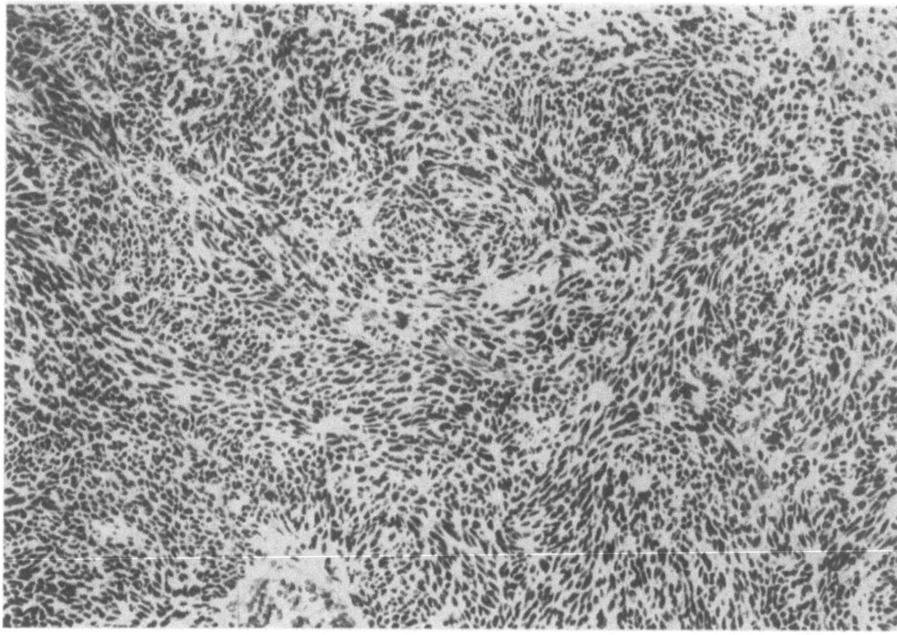

*Fig. 4. Medulloblastoma. Streams and interweaving bundles of spindle- and carrot-shaped cells forming random patterns (H. & E. X 100)*

it also spreads to the subarachnoid space. Following therapy, extensive spinal deposits may be found at autopsy without any recurrence at the primary site. Invasion of the arachnoid occurs early, and it is probable that, by the time of diagnosis, metastases are present through much of the nervous system. At the sites of invasion of meninges there is considerable stromal reaction; nevertheless there is little to support the suggestion that many of these tumours are really meningeal sarcomas. Very rarely the medulloblastoma may metastasise to other organs (PATERSON, 1961). Five patients in the Manchester series developed metastases outside the central nervous system (Table 5).

There were no common clinical or histological features of these 5 cases indicating the reason for the metastatic spread. It might be thought that the haematogenous dissemination could have occurred during the original biopsy of the primary tumour. However, in one case (CTR.33/67) no tumour was seen when the posterior fossa was explored at the beginning of the child's illness and a purely clinical diagnosis was made which was eventually confirmed at autopsy. All 5 children were given a full course of craniospinal irradiation.

Histologically the Manchester medulloblastomas were undifferentiated tumours made up of short spindle- or carrot-shaped cells with more spheroidal and polygonal forms arranged in a hardly recognisable pattern. Mitoses were prominent in a minority of cases although this did not appear to be correlated with the rate of growth. Nevertheless, it was noticed that mitoses were not a feature in the tumours of any of the survivors. The proportion of spindle to polygonal cells varied in individual tumours and one or other type showed considerable predominance in some cases.

A mosaic distribution of areas dense with tumour cells alternating with paler areas in which the nuclei were separated by greater amounts

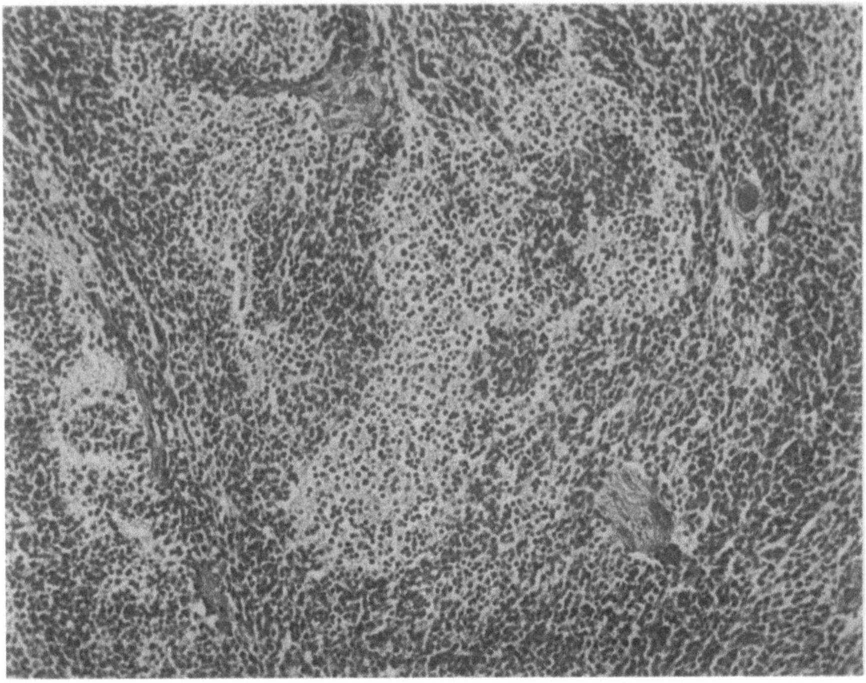

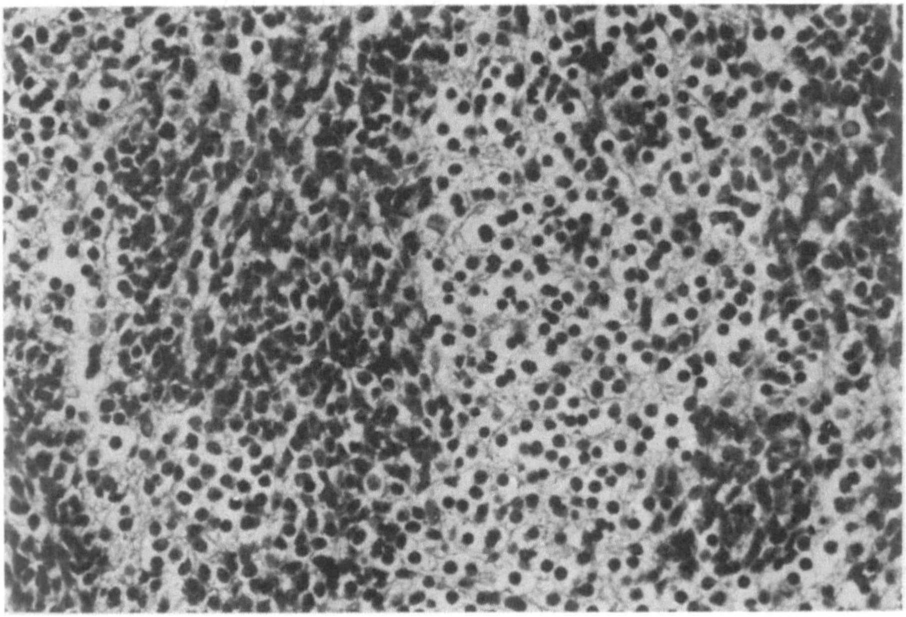

*Figs. 5a and b. Medulloblastoma. Mosaic pattern of tumour cells, the paler areas closely resembling swollen oligodendroglia (a) (H. & E. X 100) (b) (H. &. E. X 250)*

Table 5. Medulloblastomas metastasising outside the C.N.S.

| C.T.R. Number | Sex | Age at clinical onset | Interval from clinical onset to treatment of primary | Primary site | Interval from primary treatment to signs of metastases | Interval from signs of metastases to death | Sites of metastases | Signs of recurrence in C.N.S. | Comments |
|---|---|---|---|---|---|---|---|---|---|
| 95/55 | M | 3 years | 5 months | Vermis | 9 months | 1 month | Bones | No | |
| 87/63 | M | 2 1/2 years | 1 month | Vermis | 3 years 8 months | 3 months | Bones | Yes | |
| 139/63 | F | 10 years 11 months | 1 month | Vermis | 8 months | 3 weeks | Bones and lung | No | |
| 33/67 | M | 9 years 3 months | 3 months | Cerebellum | 3 years 5 months | 2 years 3 months | Bones | Yes | Primary not biopsied |
| 17/68 | F | 4 years | 3 months | Vermis | 5 months | 6 months | Bones | No | |

of cytoplasmic and fibrillary processes was a distinctive feature of rather less than a quarter of the tumours. Astrocytes were seen in a similar number, and as reported by BAILEY (1971), they appeared to be mature and surrounded by undifferentiated cells or in small spaces having a rosette appearance. True rosettes and neurones were exceptional and were more irregular and less densely packed than the typical neuroblastoma rosette.

Giant cells were seen in 8 of the tumours and in one of these, strap forms and bizarre eosinophilic giant cells suggested a diagnosis of medullomyoblastoma (RUSSELL and RUBINSTEIN, 1971b). However, clearly defined cross striations were not seen in the haematoxylin and eosin sections and no other material was available for further study. Giant cells in irradiated medulloblastomas have been described by OPPENHEIMER (1969) but no such treatment had been given to the Manchester cases prior to biopsy. Areas of necrosis were noted in about a quarter of the cases and calcification was seen in 8 tumours. Foam cells were a feature in a similar number and although they may have been phagocytic, large vacuolated cells isolated in cellular areas of healthy tumour tissue were sometimes noted.

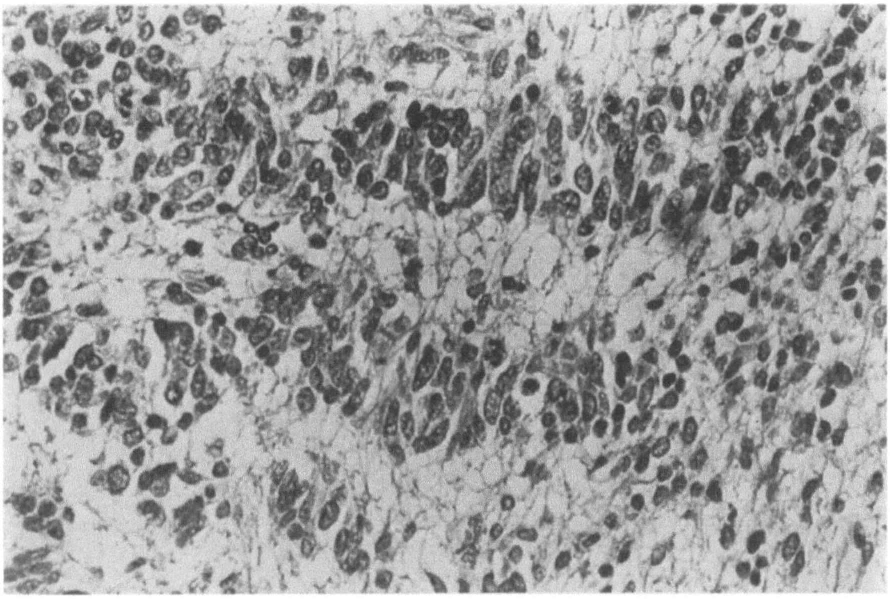

*Fig. 6. Medulloblastoma. Regimented columns or palisades of tumour cells (H. & E. X 300)*

BODIAN and LAWSON used the term 'differentiating medulloblastoma' and regarded oligodendroglial and astrocytic differentiation as a feature of the tumour. Although the cases in the Manchester series have been classified simply as 'medulloblastoma', it is appreciated that considerable variation can be encountered not only in the histological features but also in the naked eye appearance and consistency of these tumours. The paler, relatively hypocellular islands with glial fibre formation show cells having a resemblance to astrocytes and oligodendroglia. Oligodendroglial areas may sometimes be seen in astrocytic tumours and transitional forms between these cell types may be found in oligodendrogliomas (BAILEY and BUCY, 1929; RUSSELL and RUBINSTEIN,

1971 c). However, as stated by ZÜLCH (1965 b), it may be difficult to distinguish areas of degeneration in an astrocytoma from oligodendroglial cells. Additional difficulties are produced by the presence of invaded cerebellar tissue which may account for the differentiated glial and neuronal cells within the tumour, and by the limits of histological techniques regarding the nature of small groups of cells showing little differentiation. The medulloblastoma can be regarded, therefore, as sometimes showing evidence of glial differentiation but the direction of that differentiation may not be certain. Maturation towards the neurone was not encountered in the Manchester material.

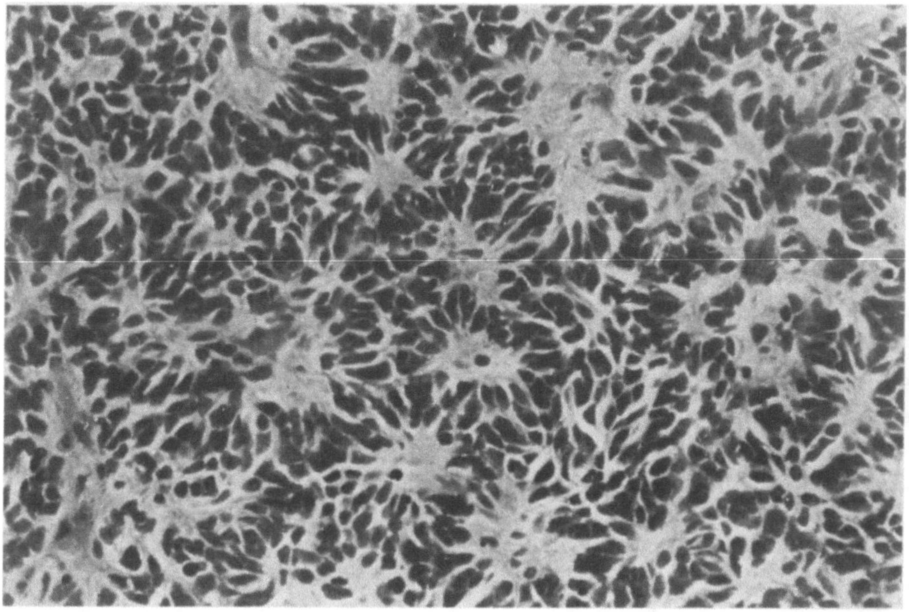

*Fig. 7. Medulloblastoma. Carrot-shaped, unipolar tumour cells forming rosettes. Fibres from cells run to centre of rosettes where large, presumably non-neoplastic, astrocytes can be seen (H. & E. X 250)*

The medulloblastoma was thought by STEVENSON and ECHLIN (1934) to have arisen from remnants of Obersteiner's external foetal granular layer. This layer covers the folia of the lateral lobes as well as the vermis, and it is difficult on this theory to account for the very great predominance of midline tumours.

In the present series there were no clearly defined histological features which could be related to prognosis. However, in the small number of survivors there was no tumour with numerous mitoses, and large differentiated glial islands in the tumours of survivors appeared to be more frequent than in the series as a whole.

## Tissue Culture

Three main outgrowths from medulloblastomas in tissue culture have been reported. KREDEL (1928 and 1929) and NAGAI et al. (1967) observed the presence of small cells with short processes. KERSTING (1961) described small bipolar cells similar to those seen in his retinoblastoma cultures. LUMSDEN (1971) strongly contends that medulloblastomas in vitro produce a thick radial outgrowth of neurite-like processes. Eleven medulloblastomas have been studied in tissue culture by us, and all three types of growth described in the literature were observed. However, unlike LUMSDEN's cases, the Manchester tumours produced only a limited number of neurites. The changes in nuclear morphology with growth described by KERSTING were also seen in the Manchester cases. These studies suggest that the medulloblastoma is made up of a number of cell types, some of which resemble neural and others glial elements. Different cultures of the same tumour varied in the proportion of the different cell types. The tissue culture of children's tumours is discussed in Chapter 14.

## ASTROCYTOMA

Astrocytomas constituted more than half of the gliomas in the Manchester series. Their sites are shown in Table 6. Histologically they could be

Table 6. Sites of Astrocytomas

| | Alive | Dead | Total |
|---|---|---|---|
| Cerebellum | 33 | 12 | 45 |
| Cerebrum | 7 | 24 | 31 |
| Brain stem | 6 | 17 | 23 |
| Third ventricle | 4 | 9 | 13 |
| Optic nerve | 7 | 5 | 12 |
| Cord | 1 | 5 | 6 |
| | 58 | 72 | 130 |

separated into five types - juvenile, adult, mixed, giant-cell, and gemistocytic. The relative frequency of these tumours is shown in Table 7. It will be seen that the great majority fall into either the juvenile or adult groups and that the smallness of the mixed group indicates that there is little overlap between them.

### Juvenile Astrocytoma

This term has been adapted from RUSSELL and RUBINSTEIN (1971 d) to mean a very slowly growing tumour seen mainly in children, made up of small piloid or protoplasmic astrocytes or a combination of these. ZÜLCH (1965 c) regards these tumours as spongioblastomas and gives an age range of 8 months to 60 years with a peak incidence between 8 months and 15 years. However, in paediatric oncology the suffix "-blastoma" implies a rapidly growing cellular embryonic tumour whereas the most characteristic feature of the juvenile astrocytoma is its extremely slow growth even if its cells might look like primitive glia. In addition large, well-formed typical astrocytes can be seen in a number of cases.

The characteristic histological features of the juvenile astrocytoma are:

1. Areas of piloid astrocytic bundles made up of small fusiform cells with bipolar glial processes.

Table 7. Types and sites of astrocytomas

| | Juvenile | Adult | Mixed juvenile and adult | Gemistocytic | Giant cell (tuberous sclerosis) | Total |
|---|---|---|---|---|---|---|
| Cerebellum | 40 | 5 | 0 | 0 | 0 | 45 |
| Cerebrum | 8 | 17 | 1 | 1 | 4 | 31 |
| Brain stem | 8 | 13 | 2 | 0 | 0 | 23 |
| Third ventricle and optic nerve | 21 | 4 | 0 | 0 | 0 | 25 |
| Cord | 4 | 0 | 2 | 0 | 0 | 6 |
| | 81 | 39 | 5 | 1 | 4 | 130 |

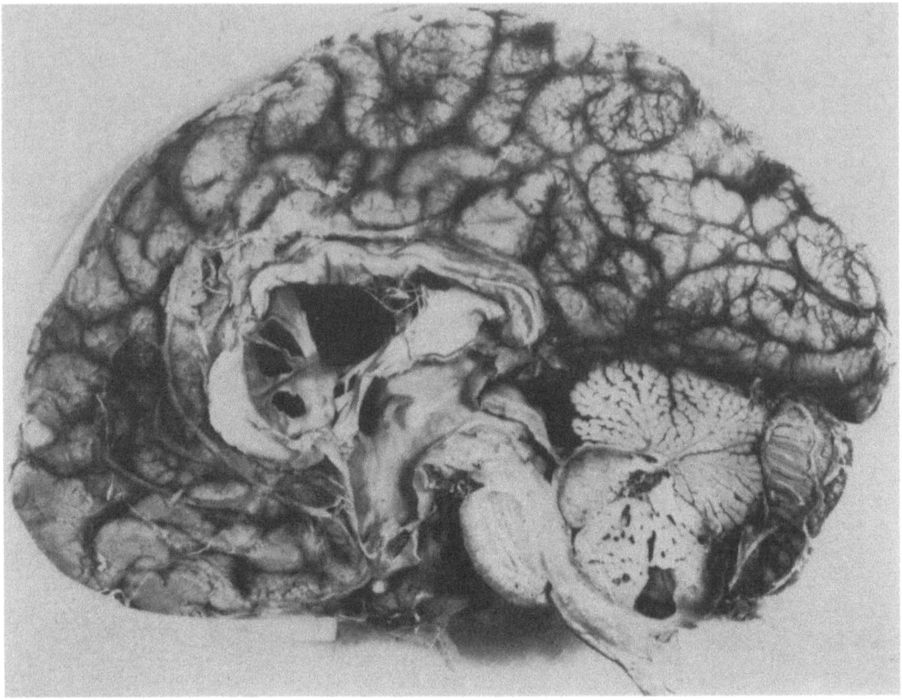

*Fig. 8. Cystic cerebellar juvenile astrocytoma causing hydrocephalus*

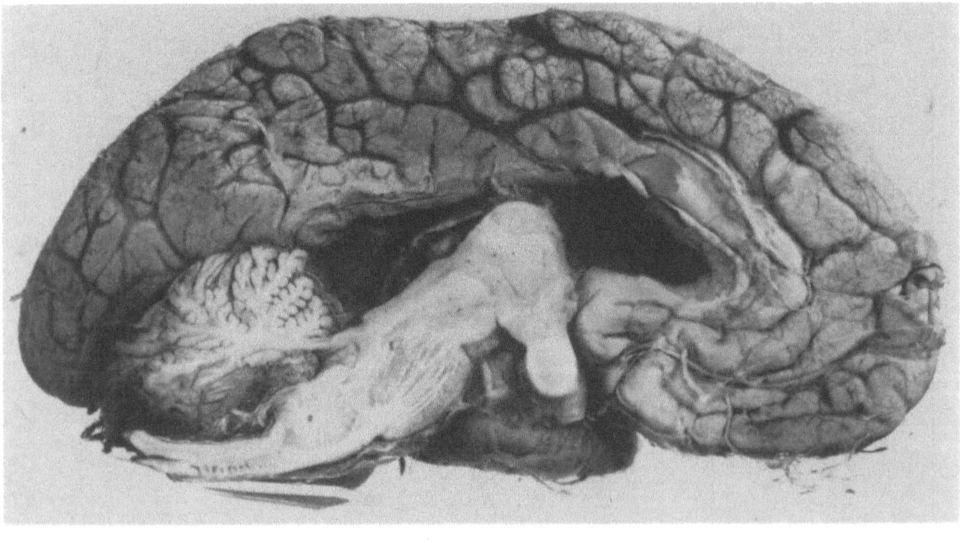

*Fig. 9. Juvenile astrocytoma of optic nerve which caused obstruction of left foramen of Monro*

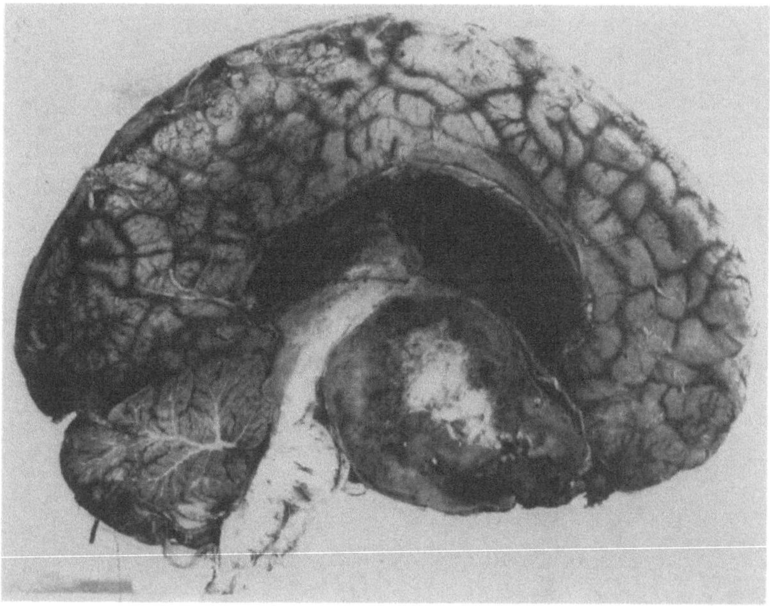

*Fig. 10. Hypothalamic piloid glioma of infundibuloma type (WOLMAN, 1959)*

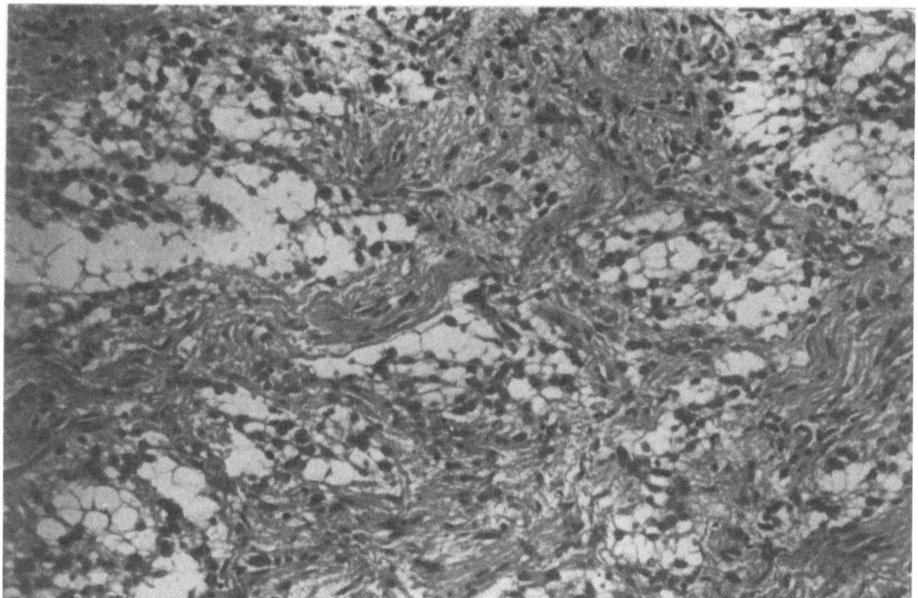

*Fig. 11. Juvenile astrocytoma of cerebellum showing arrangement of tumour cells and bundles of fibres (H. & E. X 100)*

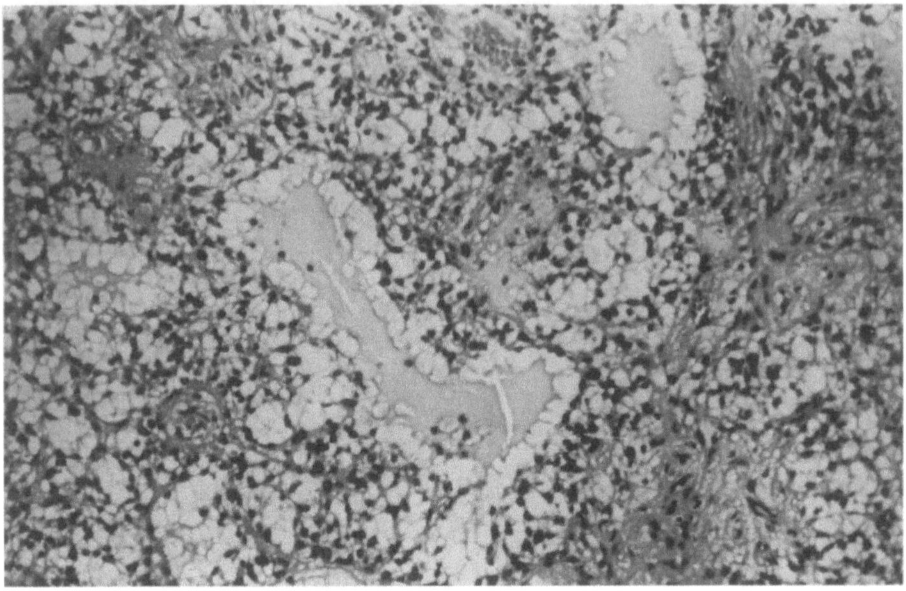

Fig. 12. Juvenile astrocytoma of cerebellum to show microcyst formation amongst loosely arranged stellate tumour cells (H. & E. X 100)

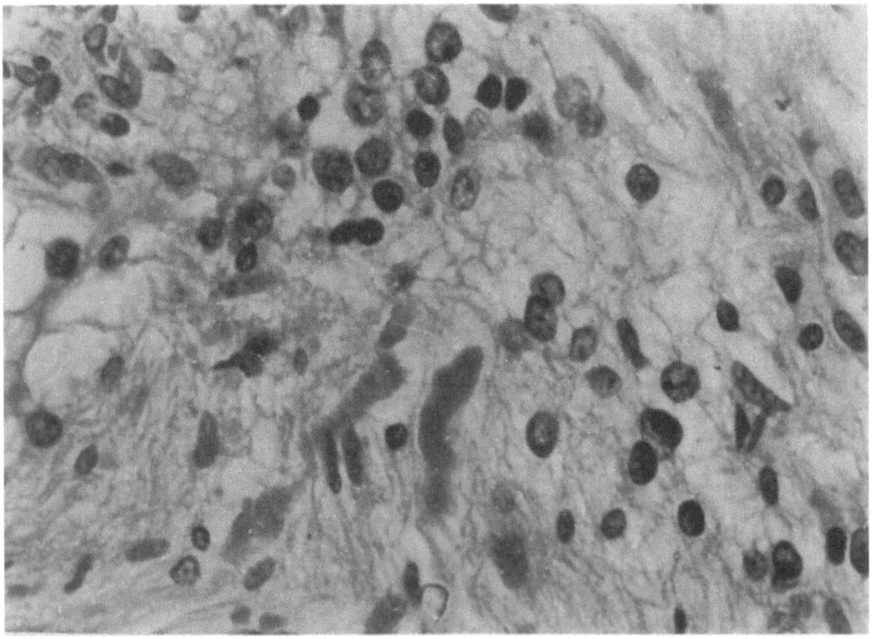

Fig. 13. Juvenile astrocytoma. Elongated, tadpole-shaped Rosenthal bodies in fibrillary area of tumour (H. & E. X 400)

2. Groups of small stellate protoplasmic astrocytes giving a "spider's web" appearance, the fibres being separated by fluid. Larger astrocytes may also be seen.

3. Microcyst formation due to coalescence of liquefactive areas, a feature particularly seen in cerebellar astrocytomas.

4. Broad, refractile, and acidophilic structures (Rosenthal fibres) are found particularly in the piloid areas (GRCEVIC and YATES, 1957) and are of considerable diagnostic help when present. Such fibres were seen in rather more than one-third of the Manchester juvenile astrocytomas.

5. Capillary proliferation, sometimes with non-canalised cords or cells was a feature of about 20% of the cases.

6. Calcification was noted in about 10% of cases.

7. Mitotic figures are absent.

## Adult Astrocytoma

Whereas most astrocytomas in children belong to the characteristic juvenile group, a considerable minority has the varied histological appearance and malignancy of astrocytomas which occur in patients of all ages, and are therefore termed adult astrocytomas. Histologically, these tumours are of varying cellularity with pleomorphic stellate and spindle astrocytes and sometimes bizarre giant cells in the more active tumours. Mitotic figures may be present. There are no piloid bundles or microcysts. Necrotic areas and calcification may occur in a small number of cases. All grades between relatively hypocellular forms with considerable uniformity and highly cellular pleomorphic tumours may be seen. This is in accordance with the classification of SCHERER (1940) in which adult astrocytomas, anaplastic tumours, and

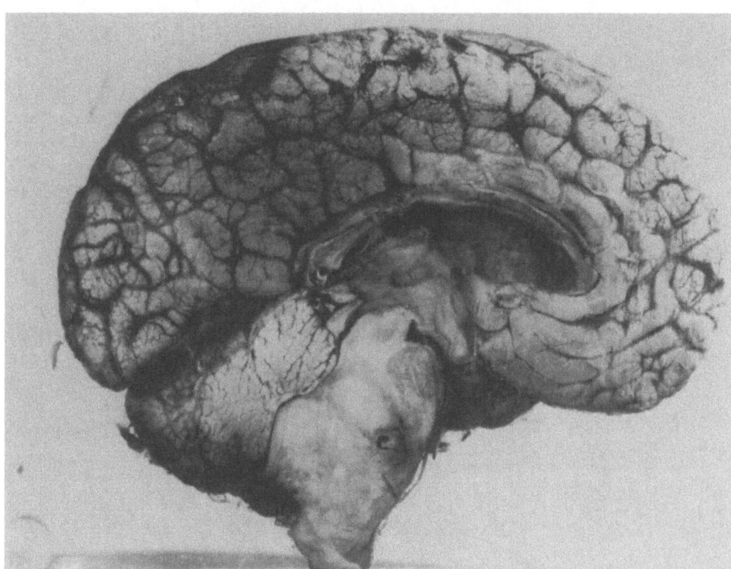

*Fig. 14. Diffuse pontine astrocytoma ("Macrogliosis of pons")*

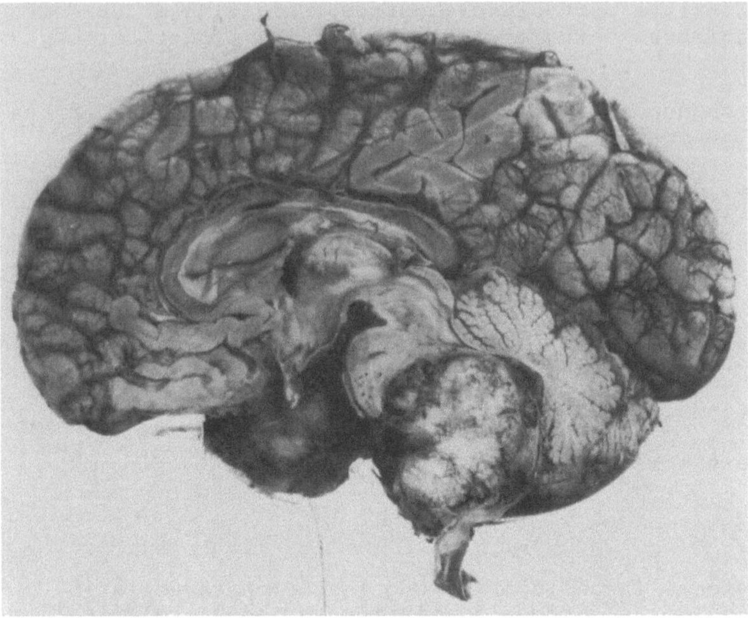

*Fig. 15. Localised ponto-medullary astrocytoma causing blockage of 4th ventricle*

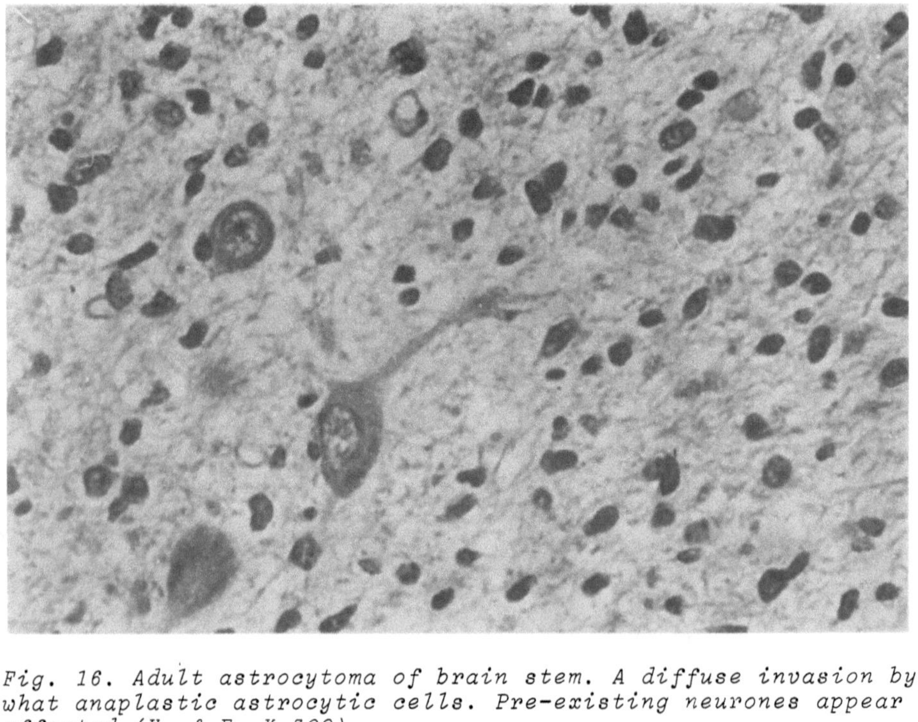

*Fig. 16. Adult astrocytoma of brain stem. A diffuse invasion by somewhat anaplastic astrocytic cells. Pre-existing neurones appear little affected (H. & E. X 300)*

glioblastomas are regarded as aspects of a single disease process. It has similarities to the classification of KERNOHAN et al. (1949).

It should be stressed that the separation of astrocytomas into juvenile and adult types is based on histological evidence and does not indicate that they present in children of different ages. In the Manchester series the average age of the children with juvenile astrocytomas was 6 years 2 months and in those with adult astrocytomas it was 6 years 9 months.

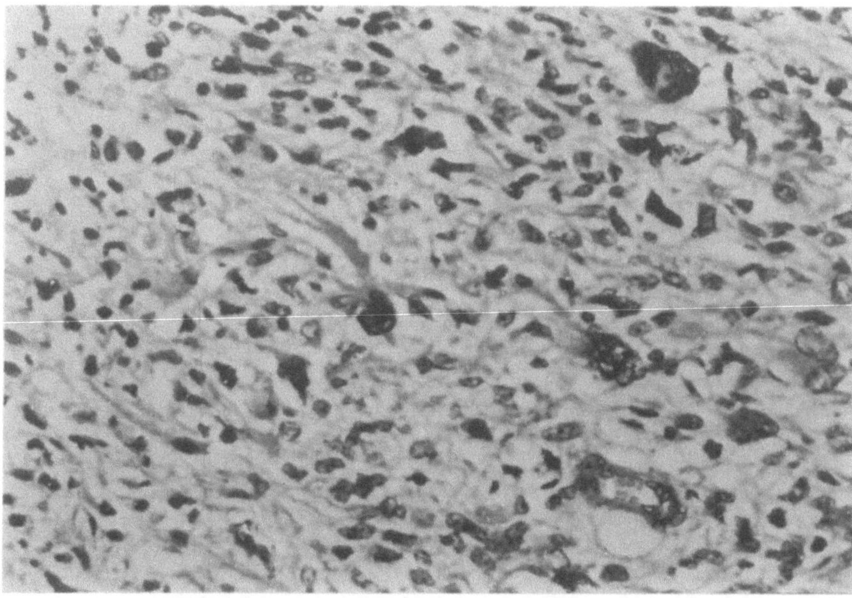

*Fig. 17. Adult astrocytoma of cerebrum. Pleomorphism of tumour cells. Mitotic figures were common (H. & E. X 100)*

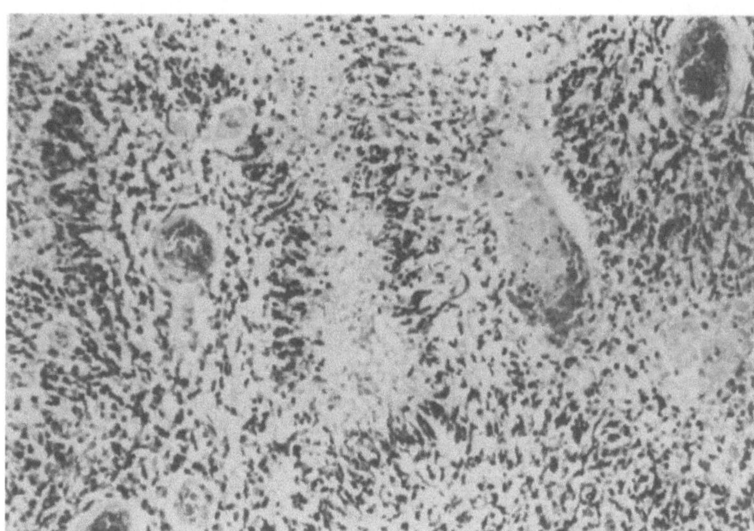

*Fig. 18. Adult astrocytoma. Palisaded arrangement of anaplastic tumour cells around ribbons of necrosis. This is characteristic of astrocytic glioblastoma (H. & E. X 100)*

## Giant Cell Astrocytoma

Four of the Manchester tumours were giant cell astrocytomas. Two of the patients had the stigmata of tuberous sclerosis and another had a sister who had died of this disease. Although the fourth patient showed no clinical or familial evidence of tuberous sclerosis, the histological appearance of her tumour was essentially the same as that seen in the other three. It consisted of large polygonal, eosinophilic cells, superficially resembling neurones and having a predominantly

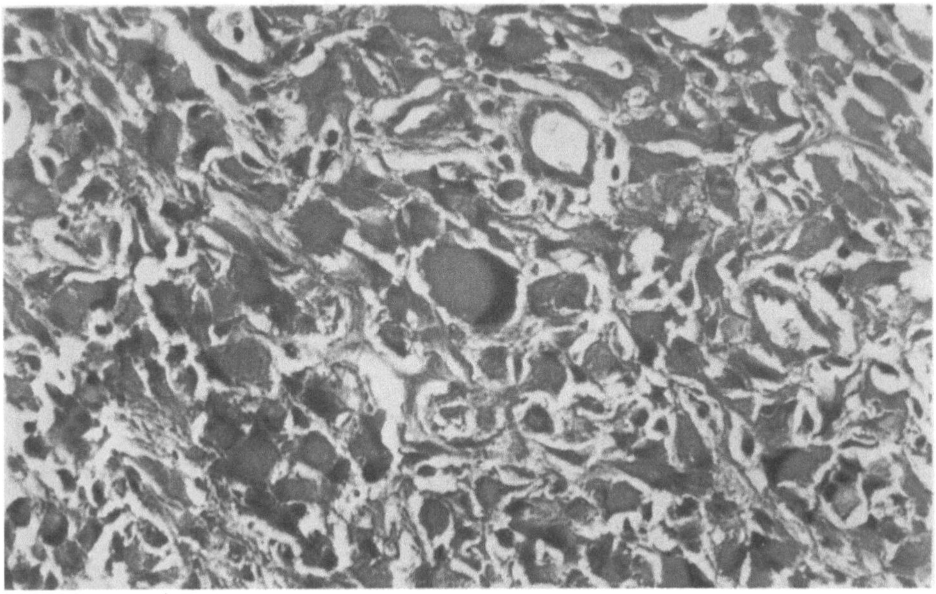

*Fig. 19. Giant cell astrocytoma in a 12-year-old girl with tuberous sclerosis (H. & E. X 300)*

perivascular arrangement. This type of tumour has been called an astroblastoma but the cells do not show any features suggesting lack of differentiation. In the three cases associated with tuberous sclerosis similar cells were encountered together with large spindle cells, pleomorphism, and giant cells.

RUSSELL and RUBINSTEIN (1971 e) have shown that although giant cells are a typical feature of astrocytomas associated with tuberous sclerosis, they are not always present.

## Gemistocytic Astrocytoma

One case showed the swollen cells which are usually described as gemistocytes. The histological appearance is entirely different from the giant-cell astrocytoma.

## Relationship of the Histological Classification of Astrocytomas to Their Sites and Prognoses

### Site

The frequency of the various types of tumour in different parts of the brain is shown in Table 7. It will be seen that juvenile astrocytomas are predominantly tumours of the cerebellum and third ventricle, while the adult variety occurs mainly in the cerebral hemispheres and brain stem.

## Prognosis

The main practical value of the division into juvenile and adult types is in prognosis (see section on Survival Times on pages 185 to 187 and Figures 41 and 42). Whereas all of the Manchester children with adult astrocytomas died within 3 years of diagnosis, those with juvenile astrocytomas usually lived for many years provided they survived the initial postoperative period and this long-term survival may occur even if the only treatment given has been partial surgical excision of the tumour.

The recognition of giant cell astrocytomas as a separate group is important because these tumours grow much more slowly than their pleomorphic histological appearance would suggest (RUSSELL and RUBINSTEIN, 1971 e; KOOS and MILLER, 1971). Two of the 4 Manchester children with this tumour are still alive 16 and 12 years after diagnosis and another survived for 2 years 10 months. However, the 2 surviving children are mentally subnormal due to tuberous sclerosis.

## EPENDYMOMAS

Ependymomas make up the remaining major group of glial tumours. Although SCHEINKER (1945) and CHASON (1956) showed that astrocytes may be present in these tumours, the term "ependymoma" is better than "subependymoma" or "subependymal glioma" (BODIAN and LAWSON, 1953) to describe the group as a whole, the term "subependymoma" being reserved for a subgroup. Ependymomas occur in all parts of the central nervous system, but in the Manchester cases they were mainly subtentorial (Table 8).

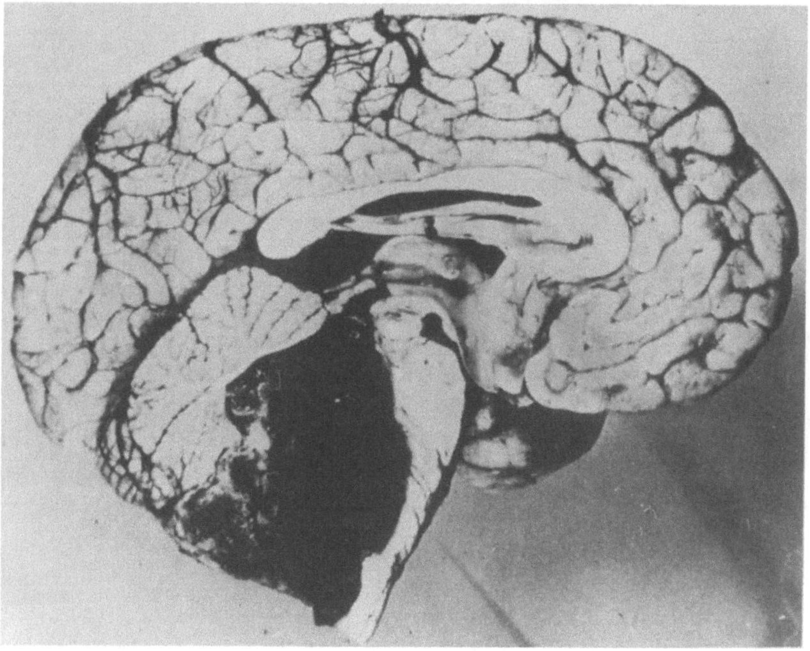

*Fig. 20. Ependymoma growing into 4th ventricle and invading brain stem*

Table 8. Sites of ependymomas

| | Alive | Dead | Total |
|---|---|---|---|
| Brain stem | 1 | 9 | 10 |
| Cerebellum | 3 | 6 | 9 |
| Cerebello-pontine angle | 0 | 7 | 7 |
| Cerebrum | 3 | 6 | 9 |
| Third ventricle | 0 | 1 | 1 |
| Cord | 0 | 2 | 2 |
| Filum terminale | 1 | 0 | 1 |
| Separate from brain | 0 | 1 | 1 |
| | 8 | 32 | 40 |

Five histological subgroups can be recognised:

1. Choroid plexus tumour
2. Myxopapillary ependymoma
3. Subependymal glioma (subependymoma)
4. Epithelial ependymoma
5. Malignant epithelial ependymoma

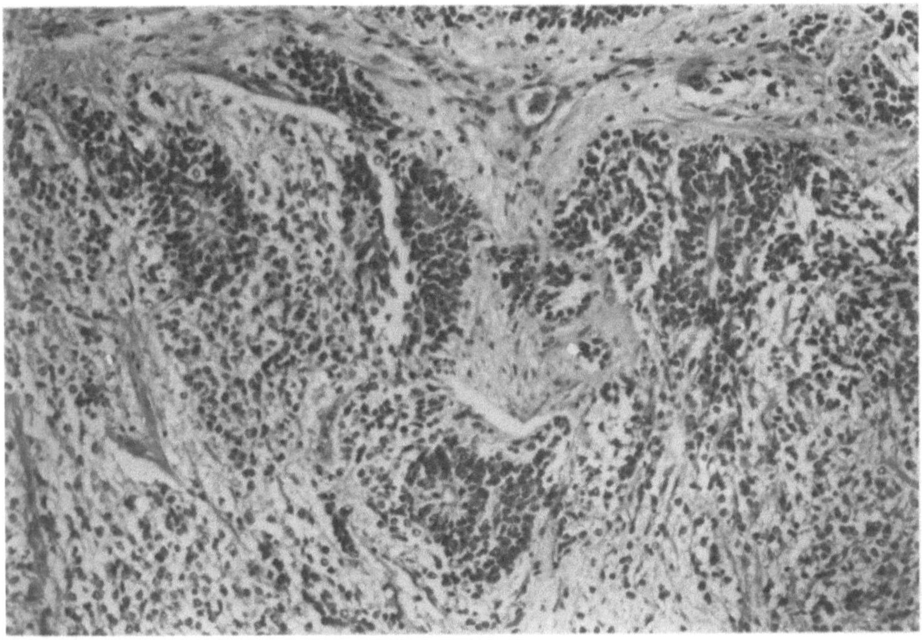

*Fig. 21. Ependymoma. Condensations of tumour cells within which develop epithelial cavities (H. & E. X 100)*

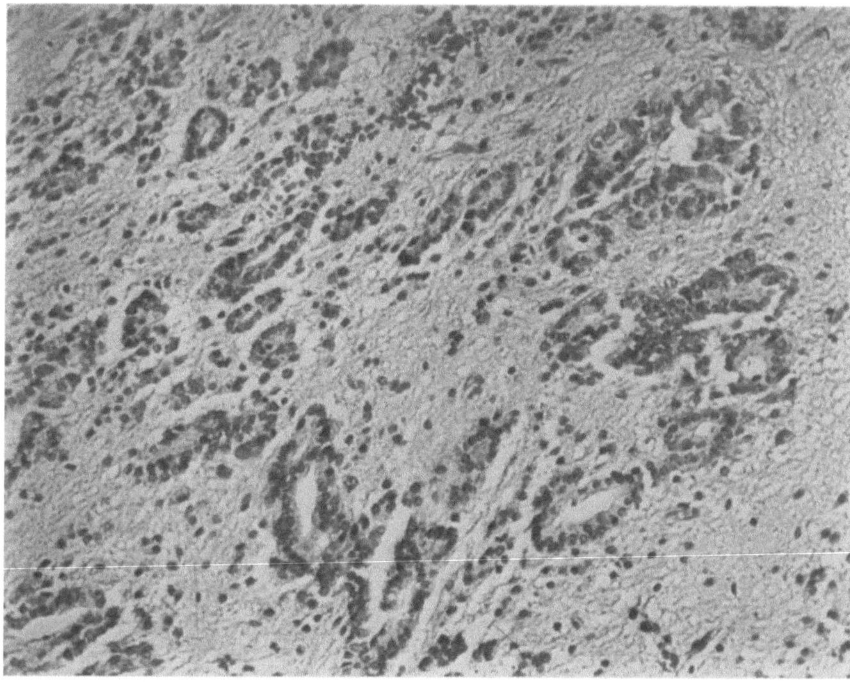

*Fig. 22. Ependymoma. Epithelial-lined cavities (H. & E. X 100)*

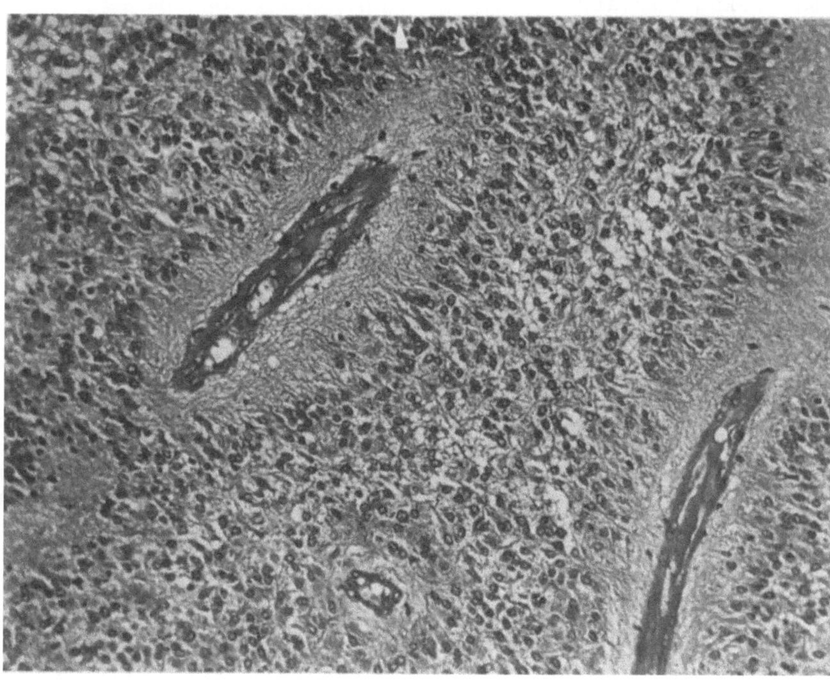

*Fig. 23. Ependymoma. Perivascular orientation of tumour cells to form "glio-vascular systems" (H. & E. X 100)*

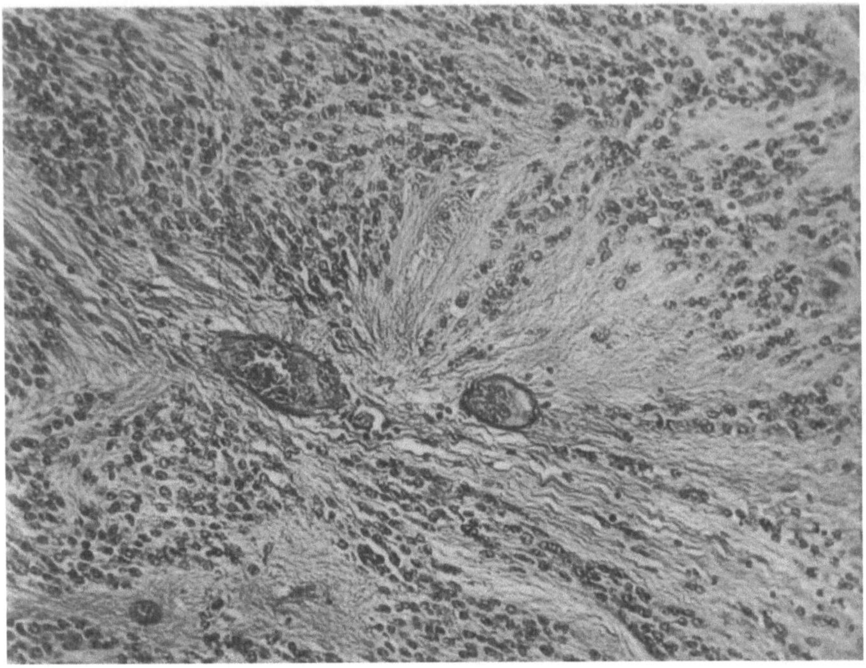

*Fig. 24. Ependymoma. Islands of tumour cells from which stream fibrous processes toward blood vessels. The so-called subependymoma (H.&E.X100)*

Choroid Plexus Tumours

According to ZÜLCH (1965 d) these tumours occur most frequently in childhood and are usually in the fourth or lateral ventricles. The two tumours in the Manchester series were both in the lateral ventricles. One arose in the right lateral ventricle of a 6-weeks-old boy and the other in the left lateral ventricle of a girl aged 2 years 11 months. The girl died postoperatively. The boy's tumour could be completely excised but he remains severely mentally handicapped. Both tumours closely resembled mature choroid plexus, but in one Manchester case seen recently, the tumour was not so mature. Some choroid plexus tumours may be clearly malignant and spread via the cerebrospinal fluid.

The myxopapillary ependymoma is essentially a slowly growing tumour of the filum terminale, having an epithelial papillary structure with mucoid or myxoid changes in the supporting connective tissue.

The subependymal glioma (subependymoma) shows a focal or diffuse arrangement of uniform cell bodies, with a tendency of the glial fibres to form collections round blood vessels, often known as gliovascular systems. The cellularity of these tumours varies and true ependymal canals may be present but they are relatively scarce.

Epithelial ependymomas merge with subependymomas but the cells in them are more cuboidal or polygonal and true ependymal canals are frequent.

Malignant ependymal tumours are very cellular with hyperchromatic cells and some pleomorphism. In one of the three Manchester cases, giant cells were present. Meningeal spread may occur. In all three cases true ependymal canals were present. The prognosis was uniformly poor with a rapidly fatal outcome.

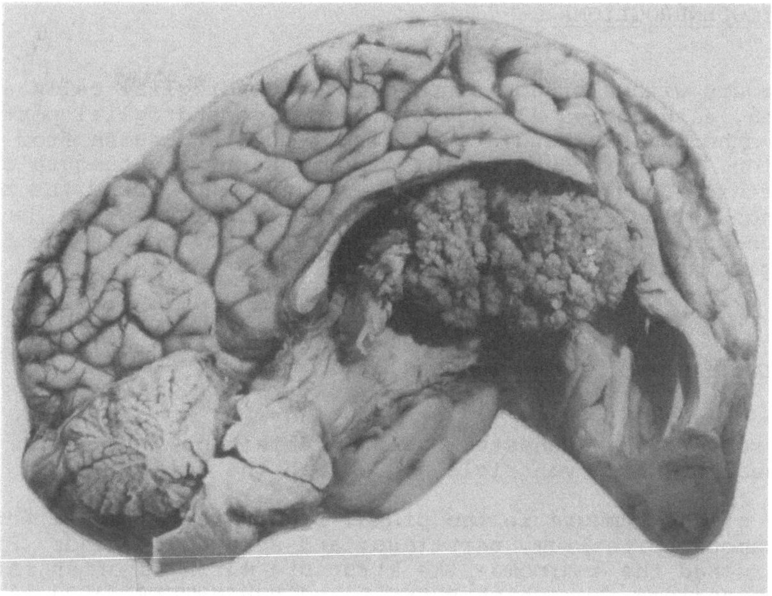

*Fig. 25. Papilloma of choroid plexus*

Ependymomas may contain necrotic areas. There was calcification in 12 and thrombosis of blood vessels in 7 tumours. Cartilage was present in one tumour (CTR.114/63), which was hypocellular with ependymal canals and calcification. RUSSELL and RUBINSTEIN (1971 b) and SEQUEIRA and BUCY (1966) describe a chondroma arising in a mixed glioma of astrocytic and ependymal type.

Blepharoplasts, which are small intracytoplasmic bodies related to the ciliary mechanism, may occur in tumours with well differentiated epithelial features. They are difficult to identify in other ependymomas.

Mitoses are not a prominent feature of ependymomas except in the malignant epithelial forms.

The frequency and prognosis of the types of ependymomas are shown in Table 9.

Table 9. The frequency and prognosis of the types of ependymoma

| | Alive | Dead | Total |
|---|---|---|---|
| Choroid plexus papilloma | 1 | 1 | 2 |
| Myxopapillary | 1 | 0 | 1 |
| Subependymal | 3 | 21 | 24 |
| Epithelial | 3 | 7 | 10 |
| Malignant epithelial | 0 | 3 | 3 |
| | 8 | 32 | 40 |

## OLIGODENDROGLIOMA

Tumours with a predominance of oligodendroglial cells are rare in children, although as already stated, oligodendroglial portions may be seen in other gliomas and are difficult to distinguish from areas of degeneration. The oligodendrogliomas are essentially tumours of the cerebral cortex of adults, and EARNEST et al. (1950) found the highest incidence in the fourth and fifth decades. There were 4 Manchester children with this tumour - 2 in the cerebrum, one in the third ventricular region and one in the medulla.

## TERATOMAS AND PINEAL TUMOURS

There were 12 Manchester cases in this group, 11 in the region of the pineal or third ventricle and one in the spinal cord.

One of the tumours in the pineal region was a mature teratoma with squamous epithelium, cartilage, and sebaceous glands. Five pineal tumours had the seminoma-like structure which is often referred to simply as pinealoma, but which RUSSELL and RUBINSTEIN (1971 g) interpret as a teratoid tumour akin to the seminoma of the testis or dysgerminoma of the ovary. They showed the well-known mosaic appearance of large spheroidal cells and stroma infiltrated with lymphocyte-like cells. One tumour had a granulomatous reaction of sarcoid-type which has been described previously in these tumours (RUSSELL and RUBINSTEIN, 1971 g). Similar giant-cell reactions are seen in dysgerminomas. Another showed cysts lined by squamous epithelium together with the seminomatous tis-

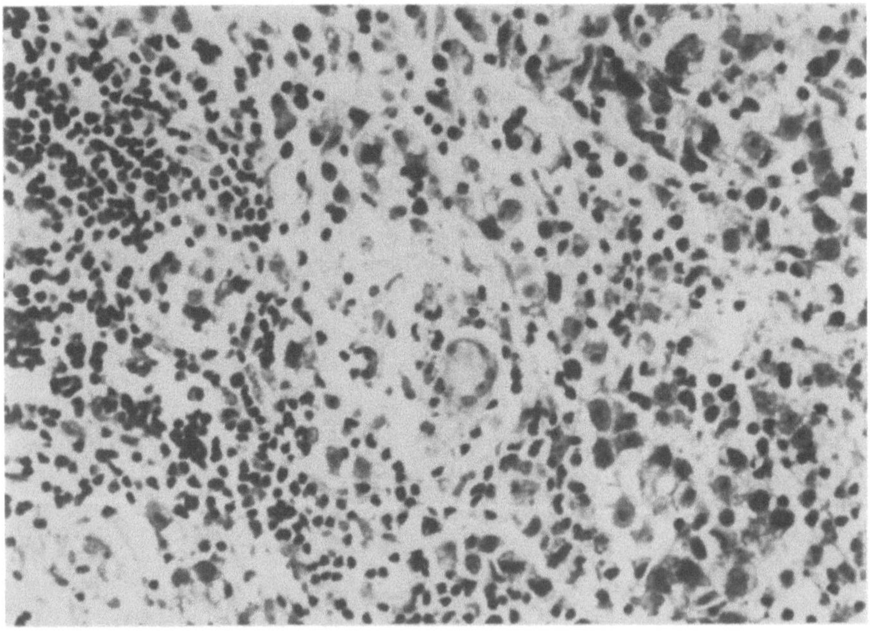

*Fig. 26. Pinealoma (seminoma-type) showing spheroidal cells infiltrated by smaller lymphocyte-like cells and containing giant cell granuloma (H. & E. X 250)*

sue. The other three pineal tumours had a more uniform appearance, being called pineoblastomas when the cells were small and pineocytomas when the cells were larger. In one of these less differentiated tumours some of the cells were spindle-shaped, having the appearance of small piloid astrocytes. The undifferentiated pineal tumours were all in young children, none of whom survived for more than 6 months. Those with the seminoma-teratomatous structure occurred in older children one of whom survived for 4 years.

Seven of the 9 pineal tumours were in boys, none of whom showed precocious puberty. However, recently in Manchester, a 9-year-old boy with a pinealoma of seminoma type presented with marked evidence of precocious puberty and a high gonadotrophin excretion level. The association between precocious puberty and pineal tumours is obscure. Only boys appear to be affected and DI GEORGE (1964) states that as many as one-third of boys with this tumour have these changes. The pineal has been shown to secrete melatonin, a derivative of 5-hydroxy-tryptamine, which, according to WURTMAN et al. (1964) has an inhibitory effect on sexual development. Pinealectomy in young rats leads to enlargement of the reproductive organ and the early onset of puberty. However, the tuber cinereum is thought to have a similar effect (MATSON, 1969 b) and involvement of this region or the presence of associated hydrocephalus may be contributory factors. In the recent Manchester case there was no hydrocephalus and the lesion appeared at operation to be confined to the pineal although hypothalamic involvement cannot be excluded.

The prognosis of the teratomas in the central nervous system seemed to be related largely to site rather than to type. Only the one child who had the spinal tumour is still alive, having survived for 18 years. One of the hypothalamic tumours was histologically malignant with seminoma-like areas. Three months after the primary was removed, a metastasis appeared in the cervical subdural space.

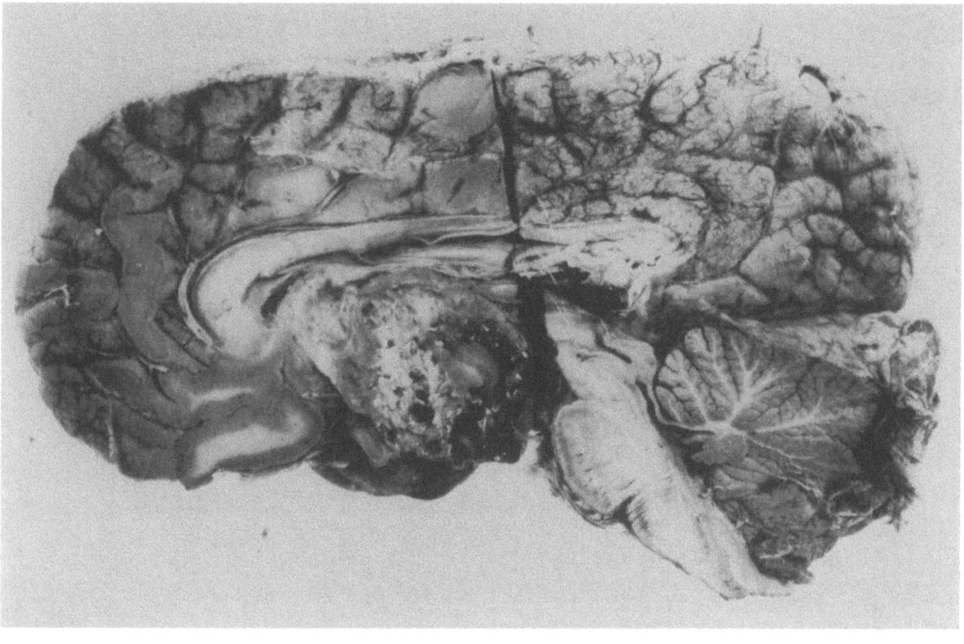

*Fig. 27. Craniopharyngioma with cyst formation and calcification*

CRANIOPHARYNGIOMA

These tumours consist of epithelial islands or trabeculae growing slowly in the floor of the third ventricle and hypothalamus which they may replace almost completely. The epithelium commonly has an outer columnar layer which may show swollen, vacuolated and degenerate cells and an inner reticular zone containing keratinizing nodules. Areas of prickle cell formation may be seen. Microcysts lined by dark epithelium are present and larger cysts lined by more mature squamous epithelium

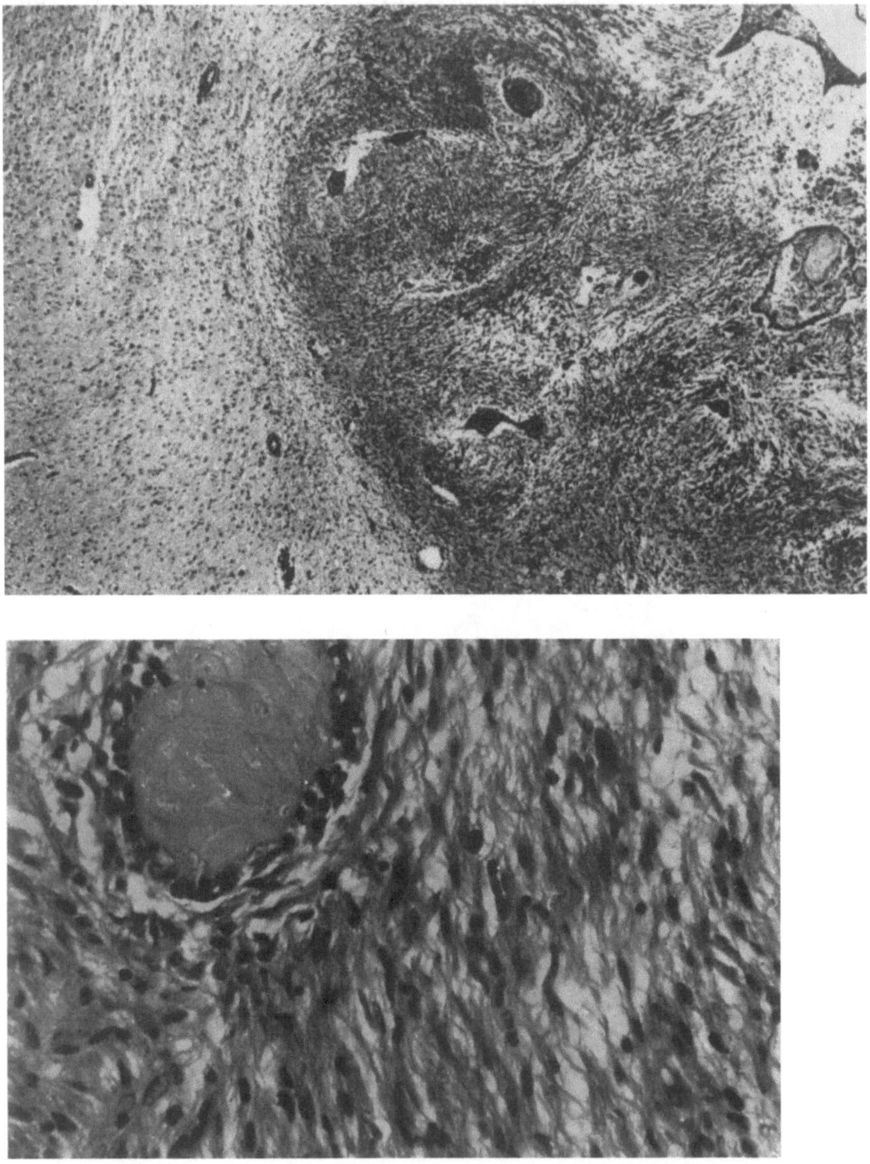

*Fig. 28a and b. Craniopharyngioma showing epithelium surrounded by dense glia (H. & E. X 35 a); X 250 b) )*

may be prominent. Eosinophilic degenerate squamous masses, calcification, lymphocytic infiltration, cholesterol clefts, foreign body giant cells, haemosiderosis, macrophages, and bone formation are all features which may be encountered.

The supporting connective tissue may be loose in structure or consist of more mature collagen, occasionally with glial proliferation which appears to be part of the tumour itself and separated from the adjacent brain tissue. The latter shows softening and astrocytic reaction sometimes with Rosenthal fibres and the glial proliferation within the tumours may show many Rosenthal fibres which may be even more prominent than in piloid juvenile astrocytoma (GRCEVIC and YATES, 1957).

## MENINGEAL TUMOURS

Meningeal tumours are rare in childhood and only four examples were seen in the Manchester series. A similar number was recorded by MATSON (1969 c) in a series of 750 intracranial tumours in children.

The first Manchester case was a 10-year-old girl (CTR.39/58) with a fibroblastic meningioma in the lower thoracic region.

The second was a 1-week-old boy (CTR.21/59) with a large tumour (10 x 2.5 cm ) in the right parietal region. It was a fibroblastic meningioma with groups of arachnoidal cells. The patient's father and grandfather had extracranial nodules considered to be fibromata.

The third tumour (CTR.113/61) was of similar size and was removed from the left temporal region of a 3-year-old girl. It was of typical meningiothelial type.

The fourth patient (CTR.93/62) was a 1-year-old girl who had a tumour which was in the medulla and left cerebellar peduncle and surrounded the vertebral artery. The medulla itself was involved and isolated neurones appeared in the tumour. Histologically it contained meningothelial and fibroblastic elements.

The only fatality in this group was the third child (CTR.113/61) who died during the operation to remove the tumour. The other 3 children survived, but one (CTR.21/59) was mentally retarded.

## PITUITARY TUMOURS

There have been 2 children with tumours of the anterior pituitary. One was a 12-year-old girl (CTR.92/57) with a year's history of headaches. She was 5 feet 8 inches in height with very large hands and feet. At operation the pituitary tumour, which had burst through the capsule, was removed piecemeal and proved to be a pituitary adenoma. She was given postoperative irradiation to the pituitary. She continued to grow and was 7 feet high when she was 17 years old. After removal of parts of her tibiae and femora her height was reduced to 6 feet and she has remained well since. The other pituitary adenoma occurred in a 3-month-old boy (CTR.90/59) who presented with Cushing's syndrome of obesity with hair on the chin and pubis and hypertension. He died 3 weeks later and at autopsy there was a well-defined pituitary adenoma measuring 3.5 cm in diameter.

MICROGLIOMA

This tumour of the macrophage cells of the central nervous system has been the subject of considerable debate. Some deny its existence, suggesting that reported cases are examples of inflammation or of a generalised reticulosis. RUSSELL et al. (1948) described 7 such cases in

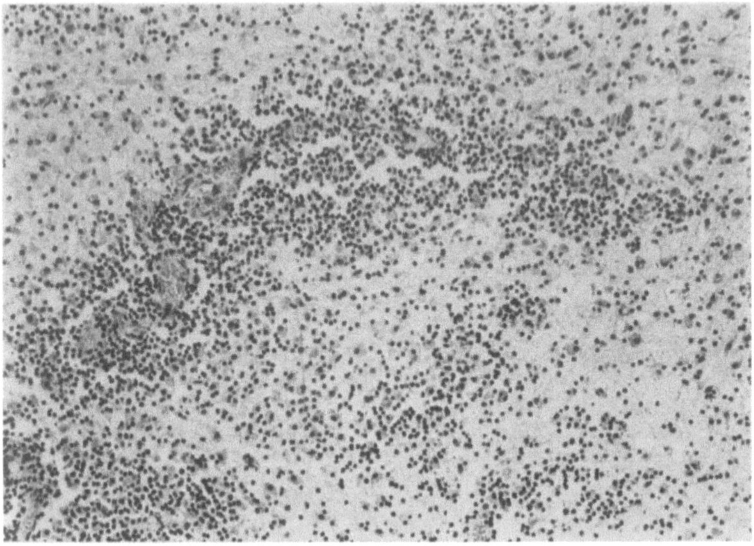

*Fig. 29. Microglioma. Infiltration of brain by perivascular growth of small round cells (H. & E. X 100)*

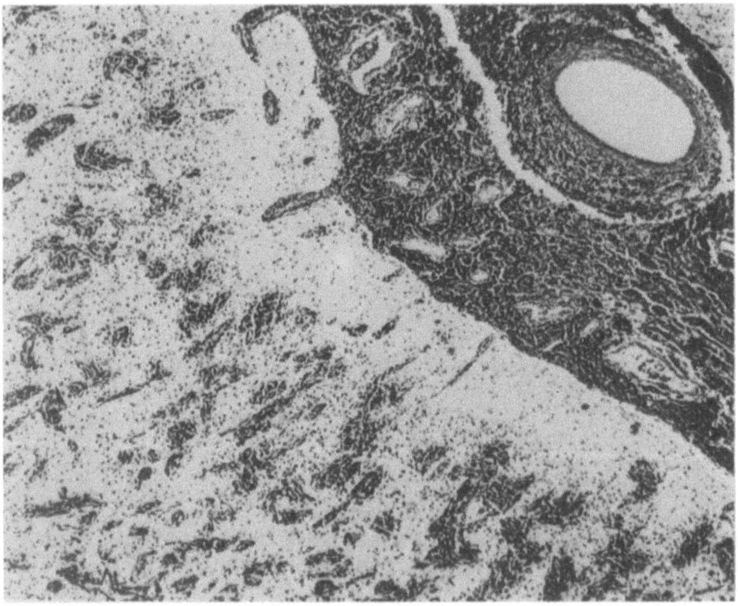

*Fig. 30. Meningeal melanoma showing infiltration of underlying cortex (H. & E. X 25)*

4 of which the lesions were confined to the brain. One child in the Manchester series (CTR.8/57) died within 6 months and had a tumour which fitted in with this diagnosis (see also Chapter 5). The characteristic feature is infiltration of brain tissue around the blood vessels. The cells which are argyrophil and have irregular nuclei containing a coarse chromatin net, sometimes resemble reticulum cells. Lymphocyte-like cells may also be present. Mitotic figures are common. There is a tendency for the condition to be multifocal as in the Manchester case, spreading perhaps in the subarachnoid space.

## MELANOMA

The pia mater normally contains melanin-bearing cells which are usually found on the surface of the medulla. Occasionally these give rise to a malignant melanoma which spreads widely on the surface of the nervous system, invading the brain and cord along perivascular spaces. One such case (CTR.67/60) which occurred in the present series has been reported more fully elsewhere (FOX et al., 1964). These cases often show pigmented naevi of the skin.

## ACOUSTIC NEUROMA

The only child in the Manchester series with this tumour was a 13-year-old boy (CTR.95/65) who started with headaches and clumsiness in 1964. A year later he attended a neurosurgical clinic and was found to have bilateral papilloedema and left-sided deafness. At operation a large neurilemmoma in the left cerebello-pontine angle was removed. The patient was alive and well in December 1974. A similar tumour is reported in the right cerebello-pontine angle in a 13-year-old boy by ANDERSON and BENTINCK (1972). These authors refer to 7 acoustic tumours in children, the youngest patient being 8 1/2 years old.

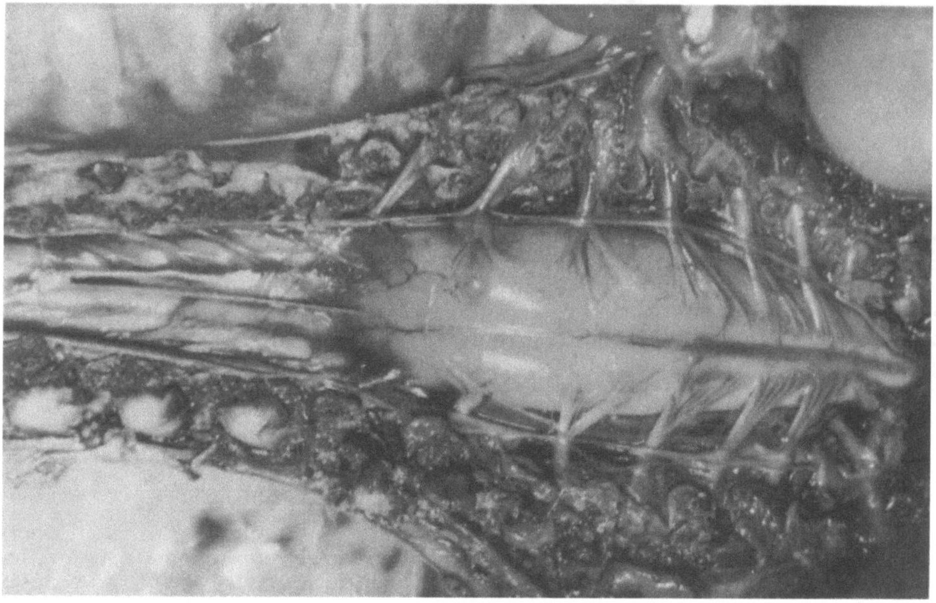

*Fig. 31. Spinal astrocytoma*

## SPINAL TUMOURS

Thirty-seven children (17 boys and 20 girls) presented with primary tumours in the vertebral canal. Their ages were evenly distributed throughout childhood. The tumours could be divided into three groups (Table 10).

Table 10. Types of spinal tumours

| | |
|---|---|
| Intramedullary gliomas | 12 |
| Extradural tumours | 22 |
| Intradural tumours | 3 |
| | 37 |

### Intramedullary Gliomas

The types of spinal gliomas are shown in Table 11.

Table 11. Types and prognosis of spinal gliomas (assessed 1972)

| | Alive | Dead | Total |
|---|---|---|---|
| Astrocytomas | 1 | 5 | 6 |
| Ependymomas | 1 | 2 | 3 |
| Medulloblastomas | 0 | 1 | 1 |
| Clinical diagnosis only | 0 | 2 | 2 |
| | 2 | 10 | 12 |

Seven of these tumours were in the cervical region, four in the thoracic, and one in the lumbosacral region. The frequency of cervical gliomas may be a reflection of the same factors which cause the preponderance of brain stem gliomas.

Eight of the 12 children with gliomas died within 3 years of diagnosis, one child with a subependymoma died after 8 years and a child with a mixed astrocytoma died 3 years after diagnosis. One of the survivors is well 16 years after a myxopapillary ependymoma was removed, but the other survivor has been paraplegic ever since he had a juvenile astrocytoma of the cervical cord removed in 1966.

### Extradural Tumours

The 22 extradural tumours fell into three categories shown in Table 12.

Sympathetic tumours comprised the largest single group in the Manchester series and it may well be that this group should be even larger since most of the tumours which were called "malignant unclassified" occurred before the diagnostic importance of the level of catecholamine excretion had been discovered.

Table 12. Types and prognosis of extradural spinal tumours (assessed 1972)

| | Alive | Dead | Total |
|---|---|---|---|
| Neuroblastomas | 1 | 6 | 7 |
| Ganglioneuromas | 1 | 0 | 1 |
| Embryonic sarcomas | 0 | 2 | 2 |
| Neurofibromas | 3 | 0 | 3 |
| Lymphosarcomas | 0 | 2 | 2 |
| Myelosarcomas | 0 | 1 | 1 |
| Malignant unclassified | 2 | 4 | 6 |
| | 7 | 15 | 22 |

In contrast with the preponderance of intramedullary gliomas in the cervical cord, extradural tumours tended to occur lower down in the vertebral canal; only three were cervical, 11 were thoracic, and 8 were in the lumbosacral region. Fifteen of the tumours were continuous with paravertebral masses through the intervertebral foramina.

Fourteen of the 22 children died within 3 years of diagnosis. One child with a neuroblastoma died of pneumonia after more than three years and at autopsy there was no residual tumour. Seven children with extradural tumours are still alive, one with a neuroblastoma, one with a ganglioneuroma, three with neurofibromas, and two with malignant unclassified tumours.

### Intradural Tumours

There were 3 children with intradural tumours. Two are still alive - a girl who presented at the age of 11 years with a lumbar teratoma and a boy who had a lower thoracic meningioma removed when he was 10 years old. The only fatality was a 6-year-old boy with a family history of von Recklinghausen's disease, who died from a neurofibrosarcoma of the cauda equina.

## SECONDARY TUMOURS IN THE CENTRAL NERVOUS SYSTEM

Secondary tumours in the central nervous system are much less common in children than in adults. Nevertheless, in two children's tumours - leukaemia and retinoblastoma - spread to the brain is a well-recognised and important complication.

In the Manchester series the central nervous system was affected in the following cases:

1. Leukaemia. Infiltration of the brain and spinal cord by leukaemic tissue has become much more common in recent years, presumably because anti-leukaemic drugs are able to cause haematological remissions but do not penetrate the blood-brain barrier. Often, nervous system involvement occurs in a patient who is haematologically under control and it usually presents either as a diffuse lesion causing raised intracranial

pressure or by obesity due to neuroendocrine disturbance. Rarely neurological symptoms may occur in a patient in whom the diagnosis of leukaemia had not been suspected (GRAHAM POLE, 1973). Leukaemic infiltration of the central nervous system is discussed in Chapter 4.

2. Retinoblastoma. Growth along the optic nerve to the brain is the commonest method of extraocular spread of the retinoblastoma and when it has occurred the prognosis is poor. For this reason the optic nerve

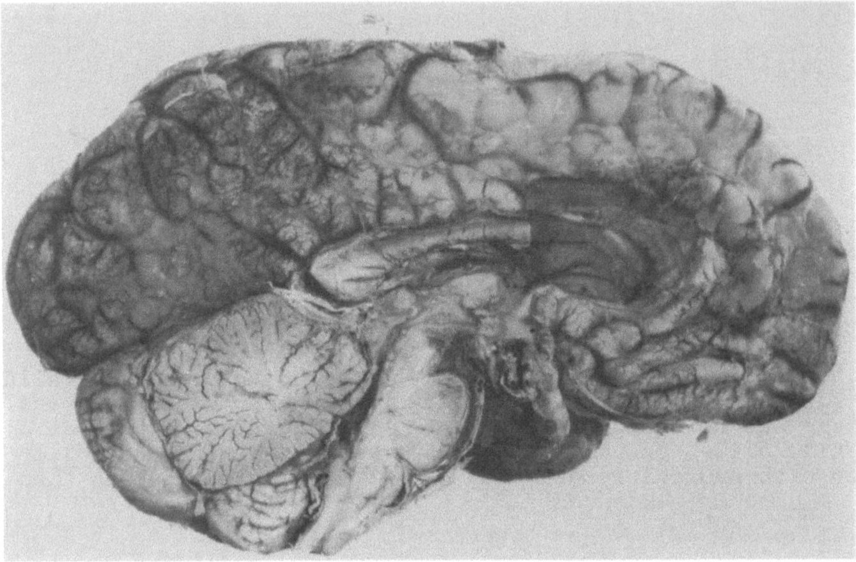

*Fig. 32. Retinoblastoma extending along optic nerve into ventricles and spreading over surface of brain*

must be cut as far back as possible when enucleating an eye for retinoblastoma. By comparison haematogenous spread to bones and viscera is rare.

3. Embryonic sarcoma of the middle ear or neck may spread directly into the brain.

4. Fibrosarcoma of the base of the skull may invade the brain.

5. Carcinoma of the nasopharynx (lymphoepithelioma) may spread through the base of the skull.

6. Malignant presacral teratoma may grow into the vertebral canal causing paraplegia.

7. Chordoma. One 8-year-old Manchester boy (CTR.136/68) presented with cranial nerve palsies and was found to have a chordoma pressing on the brain stem.

8. Malignant melanoma. One child in the Registry who died from a malignant melanoma of the skin had evidence of intracranial metastases.

## CLINICAL MANIFESTATIONS

Since so many children's tumours arise in the central axis of the brain, they frequently cause obstruction to the flow of cerebrospinal fluid. Consequently a child with an intracranial tumour is much more often brought to hospital because of the general signs due to raised intracranial tension than because of any local signs caused by the tumour. One hundred and ninety-four (68%) of the 285 children with gliomas had raised tension at the time of diagnosis. Medulloblastomas, since they encroach on the fourth ventricle, are particularly liable to obstruct the cerebrospinal fluid - 90% of the Manchester children with this tumour had raised tension on hospital admission.

### General Symptoms and Signs

The main symptoms of increased tension are headache, vomiting, and diplopia due to sixth nerve palsy but the presentation is somewhat different from that in adults. In children vomiting may occur without any apparent headache. Both vomiting and headache quite often occur at any time and not necessarily first thing in the morning. The headaches may not be well localised especially in younger children. Often they are frontal but sometimes with posterior fossa tumours they are occipital and may be accompanied by neck pain, stiffness and retraction. Bilateral sixth nerve palsy, due to stretching of these nerves in their long intracranial course, is usually due to raised pressure and is of no localising significance.

Raised tension not only causes papilloedema but also, in children, separation of the sutures of the cranial bones. This is seen mainly in younger patients but may happen even in later childhood; one Manchester child who had this sign was aged 10 years. Sometimes this separation is so marked that the enlargement of the head is clinically obvious. Raised pressure may cause absorption of the inner table of the skull vault. Sometimes distension of the third ventricle results in erosion of the sella turcica with destruction of the posterior clinoid processes.

### Localising Signs

The clinical effects of an intracranial tumour depend both on the site and the rate of destruction of adjacent nervous tissue - a rapidly growing neoplasm causes more disturbance than a slowly growing one.

### Cerebellar Tumours

A lesion involving the vermis causes ataxia of gait which is sometimes present before incoordination of voluntary limb movements is evident. Thus a child with a vermis tumour may have great difficulty in walking and yet be able to perform the finger-nose and heel-knee tests well while lying in bed. This vermis ataxia, which is the commonest localising sign of a medulloblastoma, may be very disabling and in its more advanced form the child may not even be able to sit up. By contrast with the ataxia caused by the rapidly growing medulloblastoma, the cerebellar dysfunction due to an astrocytoma is usually much less disabling and it is often not mentioned by the parents although incoordination of limb movements may be obvious on clinical examination. Nystagmus may accompany the ataxia and its presence is evidence in favour of a tumour being cerebellar.

## Brain Stem Tumours

The gliomas of the pons may by their growth upset or destroy the function of the nuclei or origins of the third, fourth, fifth, sixth, or seventh nerves. Facial and external ocular palsies are thus relatively common localising features of pontine tumours. Medullary involvement may cause dysarthria and dysphagia. Coincident involvement of the motor and sensory tracts is frequent and cerebellar function may also be affected. In pontine tumours backward bowing of the aqueduct of the mid-brain is usual because the dorsum of the sphenoid and occipital bones prevents much forward growth of the tumour which therefore has to expand backwards. So characteristic is the appearance of this bowing that ventriculography is the most usual method of clinching the diagnosis. Thus, radiology offers a relatively safe method of diagnosis and since it is never possible to excise this tumour, surgical exploration is not justifiable.

## Tumours of the Hypophysis, Hypothalamus, and Optic Chiasma

Lesions in this area present some of our most difficult surgical problems. Because this region contains many delicate and important structures, function may be disturbed long before massive invasion of the third ventricle causes blockage to the flow of cerebrospinal fluid.

Invasion or compression of the optic nerves or chiasma result in unilateral or bilateral optic atrophy or the various hemianopic field defects. Blindness may come on rapidly or be so insidious that a young child may be blind by the time medical help is sought. Endocrine dysfunction due to damage to the hypothalamus or hypophysis may cause stunting in growth, precocious puberty, obesity, diabetes insipidus, or hypopituitarism with a pale skin rather like Simmond's disease in an adult. Drowsiness, apathy, and mental confusion can occur and reduce the child to a pitiable state. Appetite changes, either anorexia or voracious eating, may be a feature of tumours in this region.

## Cerebral Tumours

Cerebral tumours in children seldom cause symptoms until they are very large and then they usually present with evidence of raised intracranial pressure rather than with focal symptoms and signs. In 19 of the 46 Manchester children with cerebral tumours there were no symptoms or signs apart from those due to raised tension. Fifteen patients presented with hemiparesis and there was a history of epilepsy in 7 children (Table 13).

BAILEY et al. (1939) state that 7 of their children with cerebral tumours had histories of convulsions. They note, however, that epilepsy in children is very rarely caused by intracranial neoplasms.

## Spinal Tumours

The mode of presentation of spinal tumours did not depend on whether the lesions were intramedullary, extradural or intradural. Twenty-five of the 37 children complained of nerve root pain which was sometimes severe and could be associated with rigidity of the spine. In 26 children there was weakness or paralysis which was sometimes confined to one limb but paraplegia or even tetraplegia could occur. This could be associated with bladder paralysis, a patulous anus and, in a cervical tumour, with dyspnoea.

Table 13. Children with cerebral gliomas preceded by epilepsy

| C.T.R. Number | Sex | Age (years) | | Site of tumour | Type of tumour | Outcome (in 1973) | Comment |
|---|---|---|---|---|---|---|---|
| | | At onset of epilepsy | At diagnosis of tumour | | | | |
| 17/56 | M | 9 | 10 | left frontal | Adult astro. | Died after 7 months | |
| 26/60 | F | 5 | 12 | Left temporal | Giant cell astro. | Alive | Tuberous sclerosis |
| 124/63 | M | 3 | 14 | Left parietal | Giant cell astro. | Alive | Tuberous sclerosis |
| 69/64 | M | 5 | 12 | Left frontal | Giant cell astro. | Died post-op. | |
| 133/66 | F | 6 | 12 | Right parietal | Oligodendrogl. | Alive | |
| 59/67 | M | 4 | 5 | Right parietal | Adult astro. | Died after 1 year | |
| 148/68 | M | < 1 | 5 | Left temporal | Ependymoma | Alive | |

Differential Diagnosis

In Manchester, the following diagnostic difficulties were encountered:

1. The ataxia due to a cerebellar tumour may be confused with the clinical picture of chorea, hysteria, or the encephalitides. The latter, which may be associated with the common infectious fevers such as

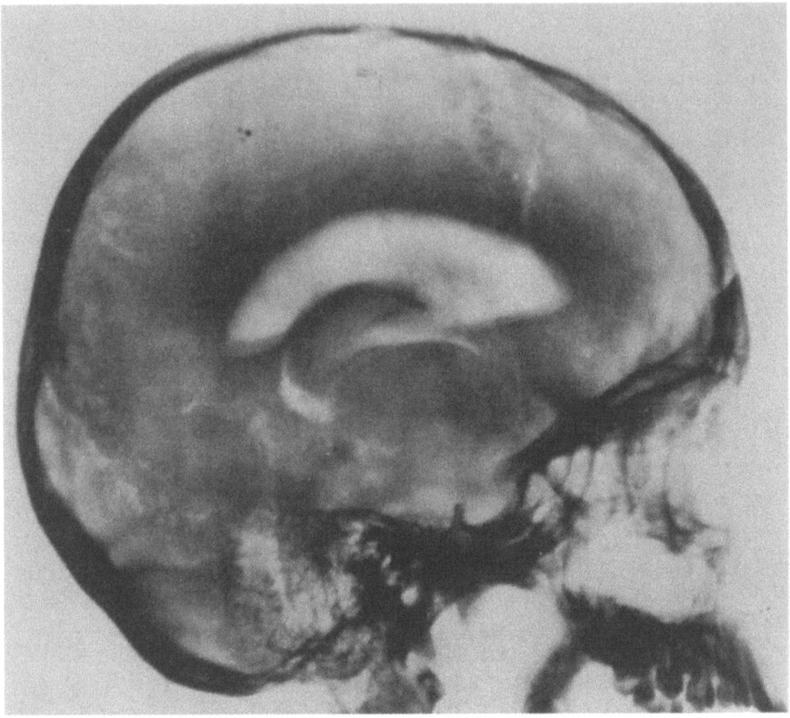

*Fig. 33. Craniopharyngioma. Air ventriculogram. Floor of third ventricle is displaced and posterior clinoid is eroded*

measles or mumps, present with unsteadiness and perhaps palsy of one of the cranial nerves. Usually children with post-infective encephalitis recover completely.

2. Non-neoplastic space-occupying lesions such as congenital anomalies (dermoids or arachnoid cysts) or chronic inflammatory conditions (abscesses, tuberculomas, or gummas) may present like tumours.

3. The raised intracranial tension encountered in lead encephalopathy may be confused with that due to a tumour, especially when the lead poisoning causes difficulty in walking due to foot drop. Examination for punctate basophilia, glycosuria, coproporphyrinuria, lead lines in the bones, and abnormal levels of lead in the blood and urine should enable the correct diagnosis to be made.

4. The combination of headache, vomiting, and neck stiffness due to a posterior fossa tumour may cause the clinician to suspect meningitis, particularly tuberculous.

5. Head enlargement in an infant is much more likely to be due to congenital hydrocephalus than a tumour. However, when papilloedema is associated with infantile hydrocephalus a tumour is almost certain to be present.

6. The proptosis due to an intra-orbital optic glioma may be confused with infantile glaucoma (buphthalmos), particularly as both conditions may be manifestations of von Recklinghausen's disease

7. The fact that a brain tumour in a child may cause vomiting without headache may lead to the patient being investigated for some metabolic defect.

## Diagnostic Delay in Tumours of the C.N.S.

It was pointed out in Chapter 1 that the speed with which children's tumours were diagnosed depended on the mode of presentation. This is summarised in Table 14.

It will be seen that there was considerable delay in referring children with brain tumours to hospital, but once they were there the diagnosis was usually made quickly. Those with spinal tumours were referred to hospital more rapidly, but there was sometimes some delay in making a diagnosis thereafter. It is extremely likely that diagnostic delay has a significant bearing on the survival rate of children with intracranial tumours and also on the brain damage which is sometimes seen in the survivors.

There are two reasons for the delay in referring these children to hospital:

1. The early manifestations of these tumours may be intermittent - a child may have headaches and vomiting for a few days and then be well for some weeks or even months.

2. The absolute incidence of intracranial and spinal tumours in children is low. In the Manchester Region there are 1600 general practitioners and 20 children develop intracranial tumours each year. Thus, on an average a general practitioner would see only one child with a glioma every 80 years.

Under these circumstances it is difficult to see how any programme, aimed to make lay people or general practitioners more aware of the problem, could be expected to result in earlier diagnosis.

## Special Investigations

It cannot be stressed too strongly that a lumbar puncture should never be done on a child suspected of having an intracranial tumour. Any draining of fluid from below may result in the cerebellar tonsils being forced down through the foramen magnum with compression of the medulla, causing respiratory paralysis and decerebrate rigidity which can only be relieved by immediate surgical decompression in the foramen magnum region. Although every medical student knows this, the temptation to do a lumbar puncture before referring the child to a neurosurgeon is not always resisted by paediatricians. Admittedly, coning only occurs in a minority of cases but in Britain, where neurosurgical services are readily available, it is absolutely unjustifiable to subject a child with a dangerous disease to any unnecessary hazard.

Table 14. Diagnostic delay in C.N.S. tumours compared with other children's tumours (summarised from Tables 9 and 10 of Chapter 1)

| Mode of presentation | Clinical onset to hospital consultation | | Hospital consultation to diagnosis | |
|---|---|---|---|---|
| | Median interval (weeks) | % cases with over 3 months delay | Median interval (weeks) | % cases with over 3 months delay |
| Brain | 8.1 | 40 | 1.1 | 16 |
| Spinal | 4.9 | 25 | 2.5 | 11 |
| All children's tumours | 5.4 | 24 | 0.5 | 11 |

## Plain X-rays

Convolutional impression of the inner table of the skull vault ("beaten silver" effect) is a very common feature produced by raised intracranial tension in children and in those up to the age of ten years it occurs in all except the most acute cases. Stretching of the cranial sutures is the most important radiological sign of raised pressure in children and is most often seen in posterior fossa tumours. Erosion and decalcification of the dorsum sphenoid or posterior clinoid processes due to a distended third ventricle occur less often in children than adults in whom the pressure cannot be relieved by separation of the sutures.

Plain X-rays of the skull sometimes give localising signs. The occipital bone over a cerebellar astrocytoma may be thinned out. Sharpening and erosion of the anterior clinoid processes by local pressure or the finding of speckled calcification in the suprasellar region may clearly demonstrate the presence of a craniopharyngioma. A very characteristic mottled calcification occasionally occurs in certain of the cerebellar astrocytomas and is also seen in oligodendrogliomas. Enlargement of the optic foramen may be caused by an optic glioma.

## Angiography and Ventriculography

Since the posterior fossa is the commonest site for children's tumours, ventriculography was, up to a few years ago, more frequently used than

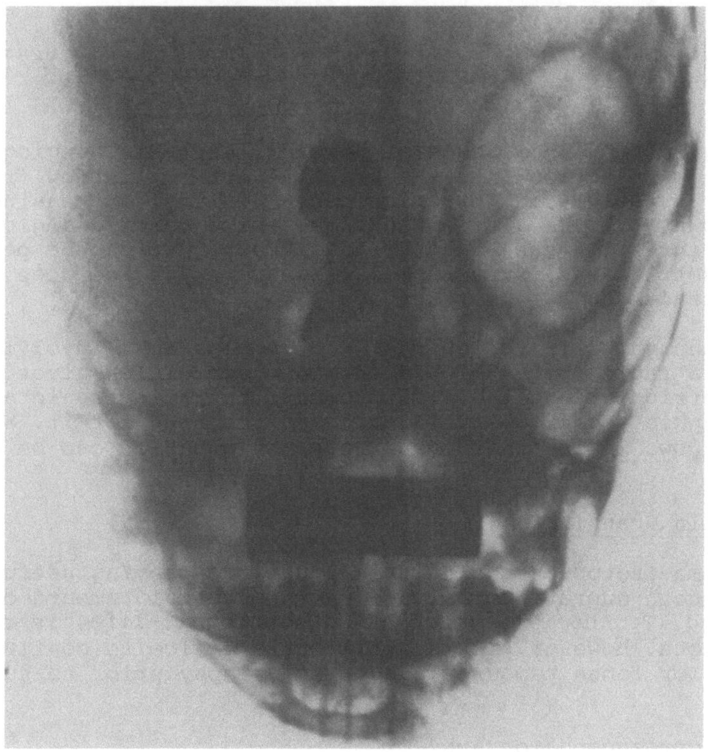

*Fig. 34. Cerebellar medulloblastoma. Antero-posterior myodil ventriculogram. There is a filling defect of 4th ventricle*

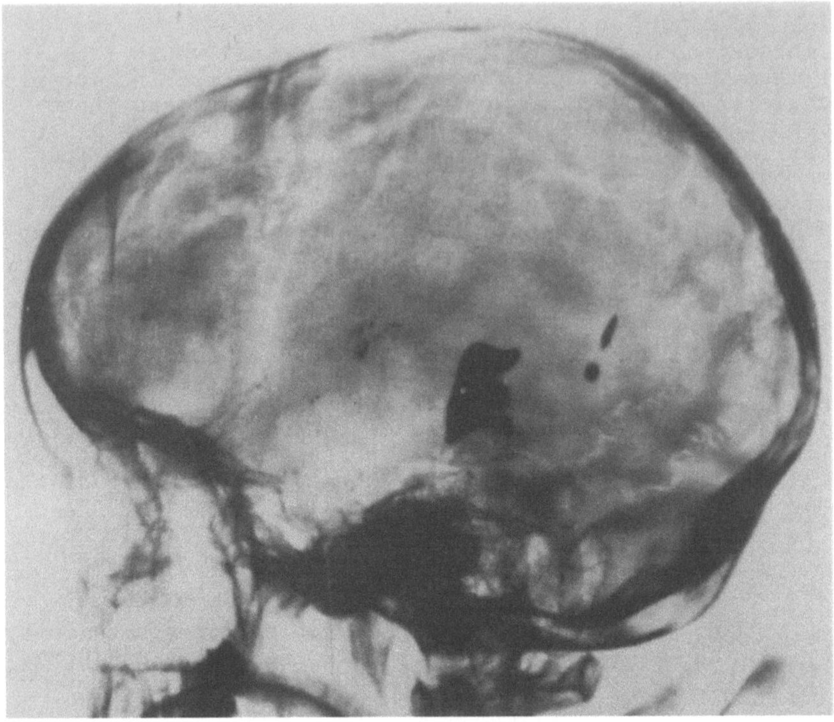

*Fig. 35. Mid-brain astrocytoma. Lateral myodil ventriculogram. The aqueduct is occluded*

angiography in diagnosis. However, vertebral angiography, using retrograde injection into the brachial artery, is now frequently employed in investigating posterior fossa lesions. Increasing experience has shown it to be a safe technique. Like carotid angiography which is used to investigate supratentorial tumours, it can be performed without upsetting the intracranial pressure state and does not require the attendance of a neurosurgeon.

Although positive contrast ventriculography involving the injection of a radio-opaque liquid into the ventricles gives a sharp and clear ventricular outline, improvements in radiographic apparatus and tomographic techniques have decreased the need for it. With tomography, air shadows in the third ventricle and aqueduct can be clearly seen.

## Brain Scanning

Gamma-isotope scanning techniques are proving useful in the diagnosis of both supratentorial and infratentorial tumours of infancy and childhood. Technetium, which has a short half-life, is reliable and not hazardous. However, it is still our practice to confirm a suspected posterior fossa tumour by ventriculography prior to surgical intervention.

## Electroencephalography

Electroencephalography has a very limited place in the diagnosis of intracranial tumours in children. Occasionally a record showing a

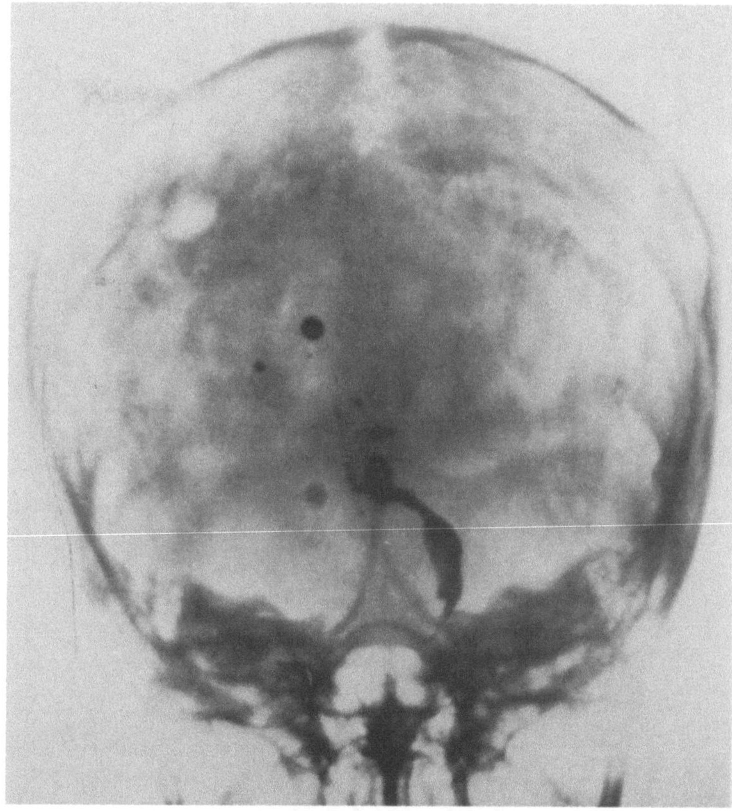

*Fig. 36. Cerebellar astrocytoma. Antero-posterior myodil ventriculogram. There is a filling defect of 4th ventricle*

serious upset of electrical activity and excessive amount of slow waves may alert the clinician to the need for more specific investigations.

## Computerised Transverse Axial Tomography

Tumours may be visualised by this method using the E.M.I. scanner and the results may be enhanced by intravenous contrast material. It is suggested by O'CONNOR (1974) that this technique may revolutionise neuroradiological diagnosis.

## TREATMENT

The treatment of children with intracranial tumours requires the co-operation of even more disciplines than are needed with other children's neoplasms. Children with such lesions as cerebellar astrocytomas may sometimes be completely cured by surgical excision and subsequently lead useful and happy lives. However, it is now realised that the outcome is often much less satisfactory, since, in a significant number of cases, survival following a brain tumour is accompanied by a variety of

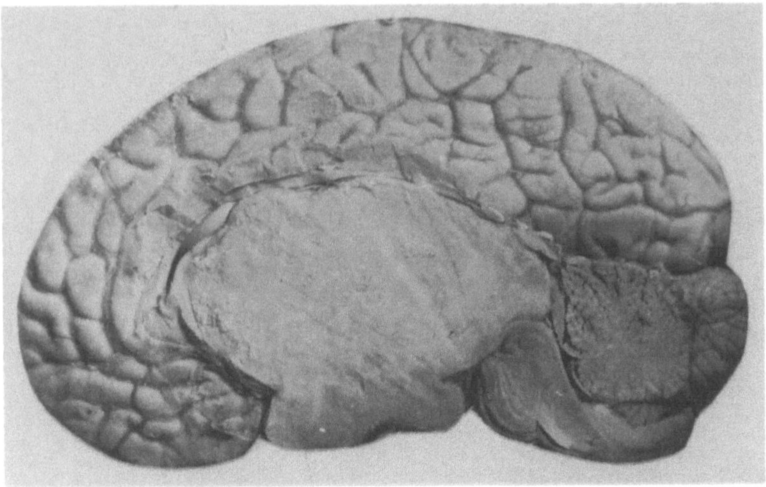

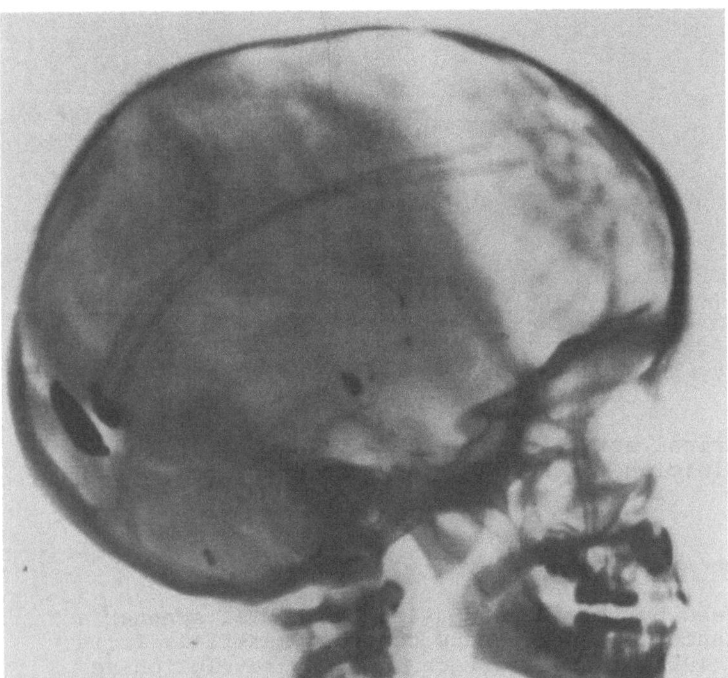

*Figs. 37. Astrocytoma filling 3rd ventricle. The ventriculocisteronostomy tube can be seen both in (a) gross specimen and in (b) lateral myodil ventriculogram*

sensory, motor or intellectual defects, some of which, such as optic atrophy, have developed before the start of treatment. Thus, therapeutic success must be judged not merely by whether the child lives or dies, but also by the quality of survival, and it is very important to assess any neurological change in the patient following treatment. To do this, a detailed history should be obtained from the parents of the presenting symptoms, length of history, previous status of the child and any deterioration in general behaviour, achievements, vision or hearing.

Particular attention should be paid to birth history, convulsions and personality changes. In children of school age a report should be obtained from teachers and the results of any I.Q. test which may have been carried out. Sometimes it may be possible to do an I.Q. test as part of the pre-operative neurological examination. In the absence of a proper assessment of the initial status of the child any retrospective attempt to analyse the aetiology of subsequent neurological defects is difficult or impossible.

## Surgery

The surgeon has the following aims:

1. Complete removal of the tumour may be possible with astrocytomas of the cerebellum or optic nerves. Meningiomas, cerebellar haemangioblastomas and acoustic neuromas may also be excised completely but are exceedingly rare in children.

2. Posterior fossa exploration is necessary with medulloblastomas, not only to establish the diagnosis but to relieve the obstruction which is almost always present. The surgeon is usually able to diagnose this tumour at operation when he sees a purple or reddish mass extending from the vermis, spreading out into the cerebellar hemispheres and bulging

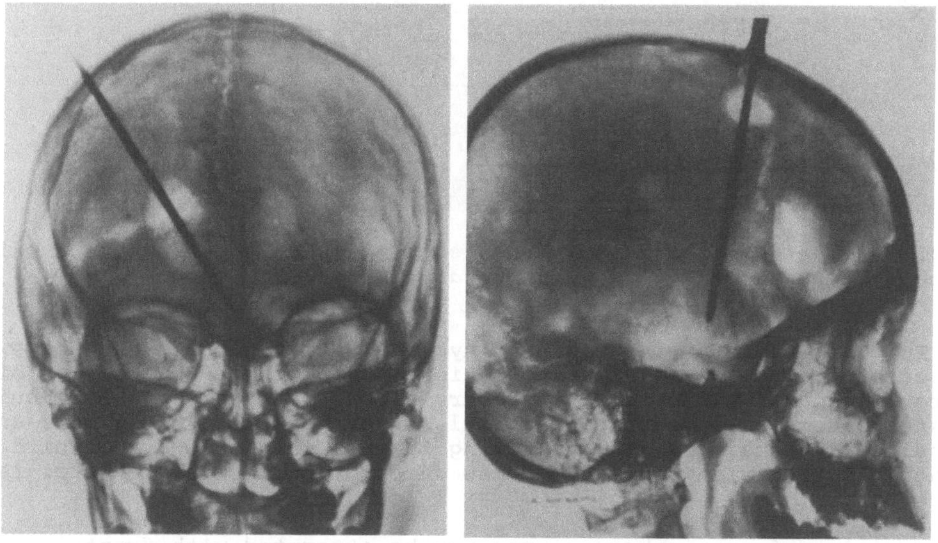

*Fig. 38. Craniopharyngioma showing cannula inserted to drain cyst in tumour*

in the fourth ventricle with sometimes a tongue-like extension up the iter. However, as stated in the pathology section, there is considerable variation in the naked eye appearance of this tumour. Many fragile vessels enter the tumour and haemorrhage is difficult to control. The proximity of the vital centres on the floor of the fourth ventricle makes this operation difficult and any attempt to remove nodules of tumour which have seeded there may result in dangerous disturbance of circulation and respiration which may require tracheostomy. By contrast, it is quite easy to excise or suck away those parts which have invaded the hemispheres so long as the dentate nuclear regions are not disturbed. Sometimes the bulk of the tumour can be removed.

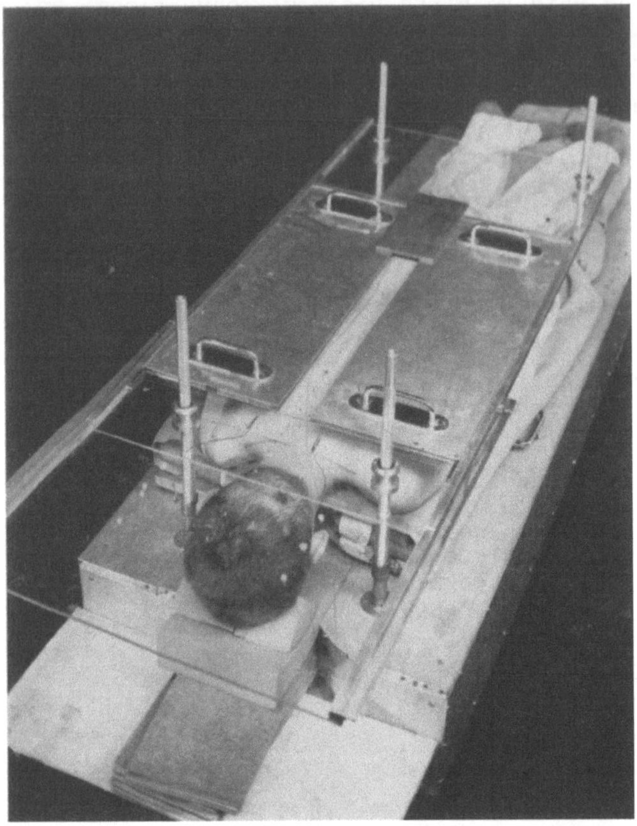

*Fig. 39. The medulloblastoma table showing lead shielding which only allows X-rays to reach spine and head*

3. Tumours involving the pons and hypothalamic regions cannot be excised but it may be possible to relieve the blockage to the flow of cerebrospinal fluid by a diversionary procedure such as a ventriculo-cisternostomy or a ventriculo-atrial shunt. This is usually more successful with the more slowly growing tumours which block the third ventricle than with pontine gliomas which often show evidence of rapid growth.

4. Excision of craniopharyngiomas may be attempted with frontal or temporal craniotomies and the possibilites of safer surgery under hypothermia are being explored. Subsequent endocrine replacement therapy may be required. The masses of glia surrounding the epithelial elements in the craniopharyngioma may make excision impossible and in some centres the direct craniotomy approach has been abandoned in favour of relieving the block to the C.S.F. flow by diversionary procedures. Tapping of the cyst in a craniopharyngioma under X-ray control and the injection of corrosive fluid has been tried with partial success in some centres.

## Radiotherapy

The dramatic relief of the ataxia of a child with a medulloblastoma following X-ray therapy indicates clearly that this tumour is radiosensitive. Early experience showed that, if only the primary was treated, the metastases soon showed in the spinal cord and, even if these were subsequently treated, cure was impossible. It was therefore decided that the whole central nervous system should be irradiated at the outset and this was originally done using a separate field to the head and several contiguous fields down the spine. Even with this treatment success was rare, and it was disappointing to see recurrences at the junctions of the fields. This led to the present widely used technique being developed, where the whole of the head and spinal column is subtended by a single posterior field, the radiation dose in the anterior half of the skull being raised to the desired dose by additional lateral or anterior head fields (PATERSON and FARR, 1953). The single posterior field is achieved by using 250 - 300 KV X-rays and a 20 x 5 cm applicator with an F.S.D. of 40 cm . This field size is increased to the necessary length by increasing the F.S.D. This also gives sufficient width to subtend the whole head, and lead shielding over the trunk reduces the width of the spinal field to 5 cm . The field subtends from the top of the head to a level 2 1/2 cm, below the second sacral vertebra. 4 MeV X-rays are now used for the head fields with a special wedge which gives little radiation to the back of the head and enough to the anterior half of the head to bring up the dose here to the required level. A minimum tumour dose of 2700 rads is given at approximately 4 cm deep in the spine and to the whole of the head. This rises to a skin dose of the order of 3800 - 4000 rads depending on the size of the child.

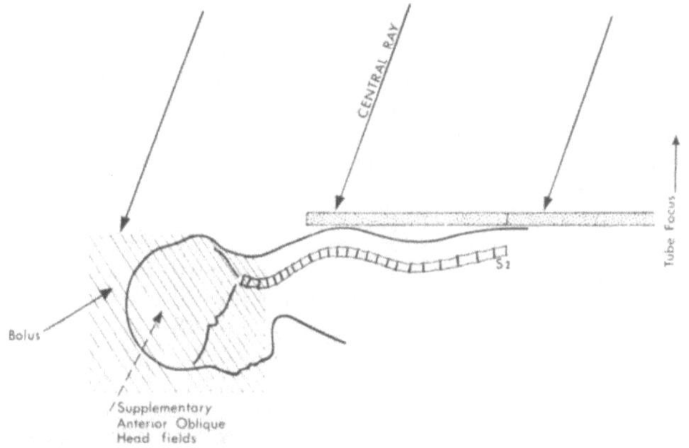


*Fig. 40. Diagram showing dominant posterior field reinforced by anterior head fields used in treatment of medulloblastoma*

In treating other central nervous system tumours with radiation the policy at the Christie hospital has been to use larger rather than smaller fields, and to take the volume of brain irradiated to tolerance levels (TODD, 1963). In the case of cerebellar astrocytomas, this consists in treating the whole of the posterior fossa. This can be achieved in a child with a volume of approximately 7 x 7 x 7 cubic centimetres, using two wedged megavoltage fields, roughly at right angles and delivering a dose of 4250 rads in 3 weeks. The midbrain is treated by parallel opposed megavoltage fields - in children 7 x 5 x 6 cubic cm is adequate to cover this region and again a dose of 4250 rads in 3 weeks is used. Tumours in the cerebrum and spinal cord are treated with fields which give a wide margin to all clinically recognisable tumour. Cerebral tumours will usually require at least half the brain to be treated and occasionally the whole of both hemispheres. The dose given may vary from 3000 rads to 4000 rads in 3 weeks depending on the volume. It is usually possible with spinal cord tumours to deliver 4000 rads in 3 weeks using a single megavoltage field.

The place of irradiation in the treatment of children with central nervous system tumours is discussed in the section on prognosis.

### Chemotherapy

For some time evidence has been accumulating of the efficacy of cytotoxic chemotherapy in bringing about symptomatic remissions in recurrent brain tumours (LASSMAN et al., 1965; LAMPKIN et al., 1967; BRAHAM et al., 1969). In Manchester we have treated approximately 15 children with recurrent medulloblastomas, ependymomas, and malignant gliomas and have been encouraged by the response which, in some cases, has been complete for periods up to 9 months. Most commonly we have used vincristine in a dose of 1.5 - 2.0 mg/$m^2$ weekly for 3 weeks. If this initial course is associated with clinical evidence of improvement, similar courses have been given every 12 weeks - i. e. 3 weeks on and 9 weeks off therapy for 12 months. More recently we have also used B.C.N.U. (1,3-Bis (2-Chloroethyl) -1-Nitrosourea), but as yet our experience is too limited to comment on its usefulness in recurrent tumours. Other authors have reported on B.C.N.U. (WALKER et al., 1970; WILSON et al., 1970; WALKER, 1973) and C.C.N.U. (1-(2-Chloroethyl)-3-Cyclohexyl-1-Nitrosourea) (WALKER et al., 1971) intrathecal methotrexate (WILSON et al., 1969) and mithramycin (KENNEDY et al., 1965) have also been used.

Because of our own experience and that of others with the chemotherapy of recurrent intracranial tumours, we began in 1970 to give vincristine sulphate 2 mg / $m^2$ weekly for 3 weeks immediately after the confirmation of tumour at operation. The first effect of this therapy was a less stormy postoperative period and hence the children could be referred earlier for radiotherapy, usually 10 - 12 days postoperatively. The courses of vincristine were repeated every 12 weeks for 1 year. It is far too early to say whether there will be an improvement in survival but at the present time the 3-year survival rate for medulloblastomas treated in this way is 68% compared with 36% for those having no chemotherapy. The similar rates for astrocytomas are 85% and 72%.

During the past 2 years we have been conducting a randomised study giving all newly diagnosed cases vincristine sulphate paraoperatively as above and then B.C.N.U. 100 mg /$m^2$ and vincristine sulphate 2.0 mg/ $m^2$ 6 weeks after the completion of radiation and repeating the course every 6 weeks for 2 years. The first cases in this study are just reaching the end of chemotherapy. We have not encountered any severe toxic effects other than vomiting on the day of administration of B.C.N.U. and this has been controlled with oral chlorpromazine 12.5 mg - 25 mg half an hour before the injection. In this study there has been so far not a single tumour recurrence. Possibly we are merely delaying the onset of recurrence but at present these results are very encouraging.

## PROGNOSIS

It was mentioned at the beginning of the section on treatment that children who survive intracranial tumours may be left with varying degrees of brain damage. Therefore, in discussing prognosis, not only survival rates but also the quality of survival must be considered.

## Survival Rates in Manchester Children Treated during 1954 - 1968

### Astrocytomas

The survival curves for children with astrocytomas of the brain during the 3 years after diagnosis is shown in Figures 41 and 42. It will be seen that there is a great difference between the behaviour of juvenile and adult astrocytomas. Children with juvenile astrocytomas in any part of the brain rarely died provided they survived the immediate postoperative period. This meant that 3 years after diagnosis 55 out of 77 (71%) of these patients were still alive and the 3-year survival rate of those with cerebellar juvenile astrocytomas was 33 out of 40 (82%). None of the children with juvenile astrocytomas confined to the cerebellum, cerebrum, third ventricle or optic nerves has died more than 3 years after diagnosis but three with this tumour in the brain stem have done so.

1. CTR.80/57. Boy, who attended hospital in June 1957 when 14 years old, with a 10 months' history of headaches. Found to have bilateral papilloedema, nystagmus, and 6th nerve palsy. Myodil ventriculograms showed

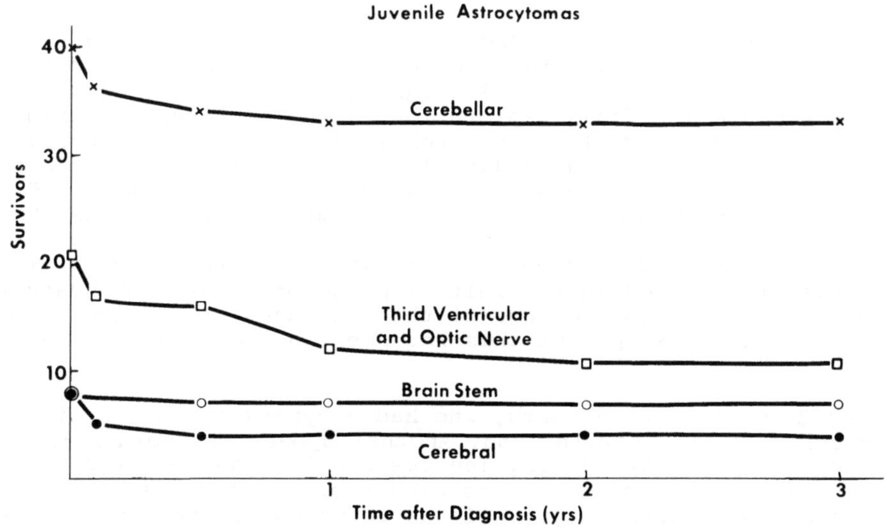


*Fig. 41. Survival curve of children with juvenile astrocytomas*

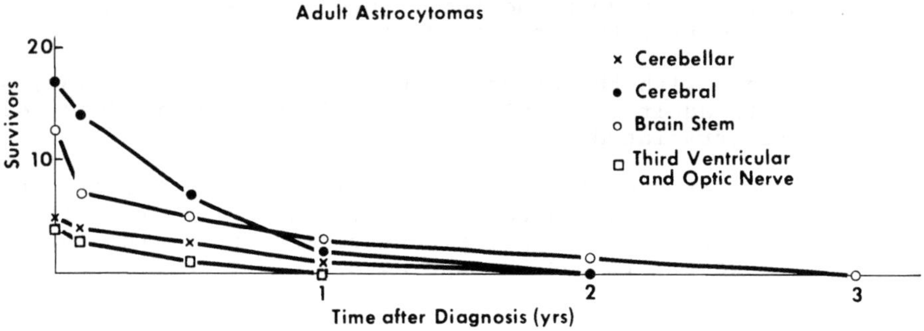


*Fig. 42. Survival curve of children with adult astrocytomas*

obstruction of the iter. Posterior fossa exploration failed to reveal any definite tumour and a Torkildsen's bypass operation was performed. The patient lost all signs of raised intracranial tension but his manner was effeminate and eventually he became an established transsexual. Apart from this he remained well up to August 1971, when he suddenly died. At autopsy he had bilateral gynaecomastia and a low grade astrocytoma with Rosenthal fibres involving the cerebellum, third and fourth ventricles.

2. CTR.86/58. Girl, who presented with right hemiparesis in April 1958 at the age of 6 years. There was no sign of raised intracranial pressure. Air encephalography showed slight enlargement of the ventricles without any shift. The films suggested a brain stem lesion and the child was treated with X.R.T. Afterwards she did not use her right arm fully and was mentally backward, but apart from this she remained well up to November 1967, when she gradually became blind in her left eye, her right hemiplegia got worse and she had headaches. Insertion of a Holter valve caused an improvement but she eventually died in January 1973. Autopsy revealed a diffuse tumour extending from the midcerebellar region to both cerebral peduncles, filling the fourth ventricle and distorting the third ventricle. Histologically it was a hypocellular astrocytoma with liquefaction, Rosenthal fibres, and thrombosis.

3. CTR.146/66. Girl, who attended hospital in December 1966 at the age of 10 years with visual deterioration and headaches. Obstruction of the iter was found and a Holter valve inserted. She was re-admitted in April 1967 when posterior fossa exploration failed to reveal a tumour. She remained reasonably well up to March 1973 when following a fall she became unconscious and died in June 1973. At autopsy the iter was replaced by honeycomb tissue containing cysts up to 5 mm in diameter. Histologically the lesion was a juvenile astrocytoma containing Rosenthal fibres.

Thus, in all the fatal juvenile astrocytomas in the Manchester series death either occurred in the initial phase or after many years when it appeared to be due to blockage of the iter due to invasion of the brain stem. A striking example of this was seen in the following Manchester case:

CTR.26/53. Girl, aged 3 years, who had a bypass operation for an obstruction of the iter in 1953. Another bypass was needed in 1957 but no other treatment was given. The obstruction was relieved until the patient was 20 years old when she died shortly after having been admitted to hospital. At autopsy a juvenile astrocytoma of the midbrain was found. Although 25 of the children with juvenile astrocytomas who survived were treated with irradiation, it is very doubtful whether this was of any real benefit in view of the fact that patients with untreated juvenile astrocytomas of the brain stem can live for so many years. Five of the Manchester survivors had their juvenile astrocytomas only partially excised and no radiotherapy was given.

In sharp contrast with the prognosis of juvenile astrocytomas, all the 39 children with adult astrocytomas died within 3 years (Fig. 42), even though 25 were irradiated.

Thus the Manchester experience makes it difficult to believe that radiotherapy by itself has any value either with juvenile or adult astrocytomas - in the former it appears unnecessary and in the latter it is ineffective. However, it may perhaps have a place in conjunction with chemotherapy.

The situation with giant cell astrocytomas is not clear although the chances of survival here appear much better than with adult astrocytomas with which they may be confused histologically. Two Manchester children with giant cell astrocytomas are alive 12 and 16 years after treatment which included irradiation but they require institutional care for their tuberous sclerosis.

Medulloblastomas

In spite of the radiosensitivity of the medulloblastoma and the fact that, for many years, Manchester children with this tumour have been treated with irradiation to the whole neuraxis, the overall survival rate is low - only 14 (19%) out of the 75 patients were alive in 1972 (Fig. 43). This is lower than the 41% 5-year survival rate at the

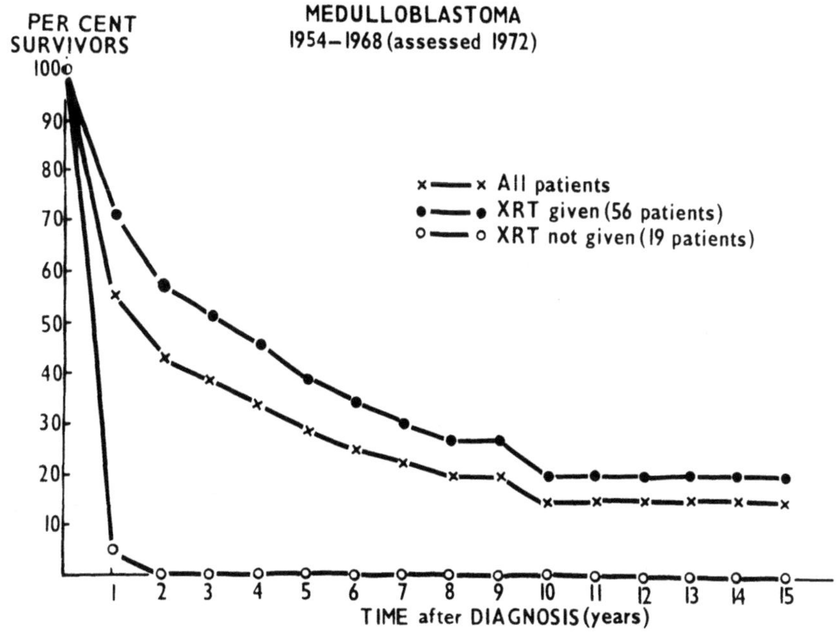


*Fig. 43. Survival curve (calculated by life table methods) of children with medulloblastomas*

Christie Hospital reported by PATERSON (1958). However, the difference becomes less striking when it is realised that 20 children in the Register died before a full course of X-rays could be given, one child was not irradiated because the tumour was misdiagnosed and another was so paralysed that it was decided that irradiation would only prolong an intolerable existence. Thus 14 (26%) of the 53 children who had a

Table 15. Manchester Children's Tumour Registry 1954 - 1968 (assessed 1972)

Time from diagnosis to death in fatal cases of medulloblastoma

| Diagnosis to death (years) | - 1/12 | - 1/2 | - 1 | - 2 | - 3 | - 4 | - 5 | - 6 | - 7 | - 8 | - 9 | - 10 |
|---|---|---|---|---|---|---|---|---|---|---|---|---|
| Number of cases | 18 | 7 | 9 | 8 | 4 | 4 | 3 | 3 | 2 | 1 | 1 | 1 |

full course of X-ray treatment before the end of 1968 were still alive in 1972. Another reason for the discrepancy between the earlier Christie reports and the Registry figures is the fact that this tumour may recur several years after treatment. Eight children in the Manchester series died from medulloblastomas more than 5 years after diagnosis (Table 15).

Death is nearly always due to recurrence within the central nervous system - metastatic spread to other sites only occurred in 5 children (see Table 5) and therefore had little effect on the overall survival rate.

## Ependymomas

The length of survival of the 40 children with ependymomas during the first three years after diagnosis is shown in Fig. 44. Three children died from the tumour after this period had elapsed, two with tumours in the cerebellum after 4 and 6 years and one in the cord after 8 years.

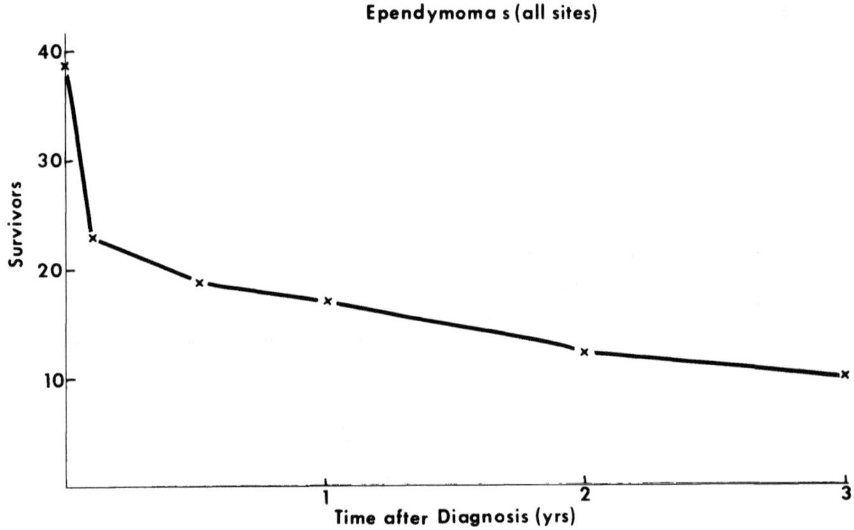


*Fig. 44. Survival curve of children with ependymomas*

Amongst the survivors, three of the tumours were cerebellar, three cerebral, one in the fourth ventricle and one in the filum terminale. Seven of the 8 survivors had been treated with irradiation.

In the description of the histology of the ependymoma in the Manchester series it was mentioned that there was some variation in the malignancy of these tumours as judged by their histological appearance. There did not appear to be any difference in survival time between those children with tumours having a "subependymal" structure and those with an "epithelial" one, but the three children with "malignant epithelial" tumours fared badly, dying 3 days, 10 days, and 4 months after diagnosis.

## Oligodendrogliomas

Three of the 4 children with oligodendrogliomas have died after intervals varying between 2 days and 19 months from diagnosis. The history

of the one survivor is as follows:
CTR.13/66. Girl, who started with focal epilepsy at the age of 6 years. At that time skull X-rays showed a small calcified area in the right parietal region. However, she was not investigated further until she was 12 years old when the calcified area had increased in size. Exploration revealed a calcified oligodendroglioma measuring 3 x 2 cm in the right parietal lobe. The tumour was excised and the child remains well 6 years later.

## Pinealomas

All the children with pinealomas have died. The 5 children who had no treatment all died within 6 months of diagnosis. However, 2 patients with seminoma-like tumours treated with radiotherapy lived for much longer. One survived for 2 years 9 months, while in the other who lived for 4 years, there was no sign of residual tumour found at autopsy.

## Craniopharyngiomas

Nine of the children with craniopharyngiomas are still alive and 8 have died. The survivors have lived for between 4 and 14 years after diagnosis and have received a variety of treatments. No treatment was given in one case, the tumour was partially removed in another, partial removal was followed by irradiation in 5 cases and the tumours were excised completely in two children. In those who died, the interval between diagnosis and death varied between 14 months and 4 years 9 months.

## Tumours of the Brain Stem and Third Ventricle, Diagnosed on Clinical and Radiological Evidence Only

Although histological examination of every tumour is desirable before the diagnosis can be considered to be certain, biopsies of tumours of the brain stem or third ventricle are often impossible to carry out without endangering the patient's life. In order to get a true picture of the therapeutic problem it is therefore necessary to include those cases in which a diagnosis of tumours in these regions appears very probable on clinical and radiological grounds alone. Such tumours in the brain stem are very likely to be gliomas while those in the third ventricle could be gliomas (mainly juvenile astrocytomas), craniopharyngiomas, pinealomas or teratomas. It has been seen that juvenile astrocytomas and craniopharyngiomas grow so slowly that children suffering from them may survive for many years even though the treatment given could not have destroyed the tumour.

In the Manchester series the 3-year survival of those children with brain stem, third ventricular, and optic nerve tumours diagnosed on clinical and radiological evidence only, is shown in Figure 45. Two of these children died from their original tumours more than three years after diagnosis - one in the brain stem after 4 years and one in the third ventricle after 12 years. Another child who had a brain stem tumour died from an abdominal sarcoma 9 years after his brain tumour was diagnosed (see discussion of second primary tumours in Chapter 1, page 4).

## Quality of Survival

A recent detailed analysis of 30 Manchester children who had intracranial tumours 5 - 24 years ago has shown the frequency of neuro-

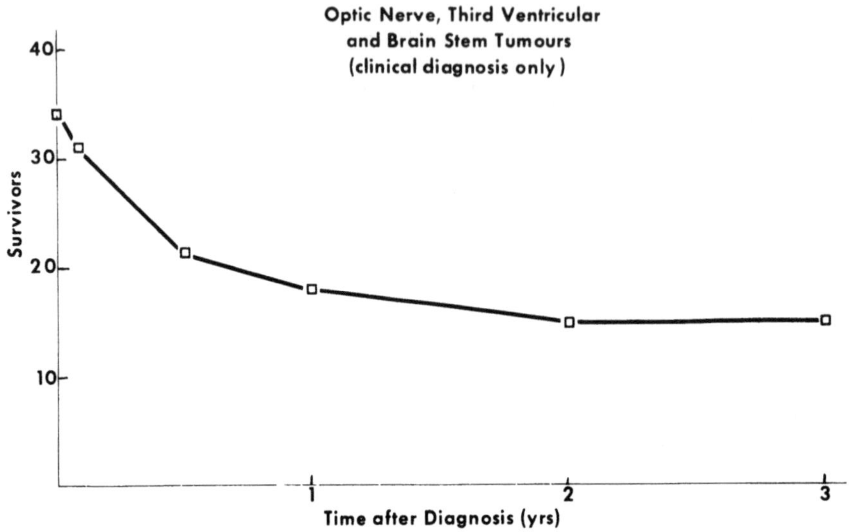


*Fig. 45. Survival curve of children with optic nerve, third ventricular or brain stem tumours (clinical diagnosis only)*

logical defects in these survivors. These patients had a variety of lesions - medulloblastomas, astrocytomas, brain stem gliomas, angiomas or craniopharyngiomas. Thirteen are mentally handicapped and 4 others are of low average intelligence. Three are blind and 3 partially-sighted while 11 have correctable visual defects. One child is deaf. All those treated before the age of 11 years are of short stature, falling on or below the 25th centile. This fact applies whether or not they initially had cranial or craniospinal irradiation. All those already over the age of 18 years are below the 3rd centile and the growth velocity of the younger children is below normal, suggesting that they too will fall below the norm. Preliminary studies suggest that a specific growth hormone deficit may be the cause of the failure to grow in these cases.

## FOLLOW-UP OF CHILDREN WITH C.N.S. TUMOURS

The histories of the Manchester cases demonstrate the need for close and prolonged follow-up of all children with C.N.S. tumours. Those who have suffered brain damage need to be helped to lead as useful and happy lives as their abilities will allow. Medulloblastomas may recur many years after diagnosis and the development of new forms of therapy may enable these recurrent tumours to be treated satisfactorily. Children with juvenile astrocytomas of the brain stem must be under neurosurgical supervision for the rest of their lives since the flow of C.S.F. may become obstructed at any time.

The history of one Manchester patient showed that clinical deterioration of a child who has had a glioma is not necessarily due to recurrence of the tumour.
CTR.80/69. A boy, aged 6 years, who had a cerebellar juvenile astrocytoma in June 1969. Most of the tumour was removed but some was left behind and postoperative irradiation (4000 rads in 21 days) was given. The child remained well up to September 1972 when he started to have headaches and vomiting and was found to have bilateral papilloedema.

Because of parental objection to blood transfusion on religious grounds, it was decided not to re-explore the posterior fossa, but a bypass operation was performed. He was then given treatment with B.C.N.U. and vincristine. However, his condition deteriorated and he died on the 9th September 1973. At autopsy the pons and medulla were flattened by a large cyst of the fourth ventricle with adhesions at the foramina. The cyst measured 4 cm in diameter and contained yellow fluid. There was extensive thrombosis of recent origin. Only fragments of the juvenile astrocytoma remained.

## REFERENCES


ANDERSON, M. S., BENTINCK, B. R.: Cancer 29, 231 (1972)

BAILEY, O. T.: In: Pathology of the Nervous System. MINCKLER, J. (ed.). New York: McGraw-Hill Co., 1971, Vol. II, p. 2075

BAILEY, P.: Cellular types in primary tumors of the brain. In: Penfield's cytology and cellular pathology of the Nervous System. New York: Hoeber, 1931, Vol. III

BAILEY, P., BUCHANAN, D. N., BUCY, P. C.: Intracranial tumors of infancy and childhood. Chicago: Univ. Chicago Press, 1939

BAILEY, P., BUCY, P. C.: J. Pathol. 32, 735 (1929)

BAILEY, P., CUSHING, H.: Tumors of the glioma group. Philadelphia: Lippincott, 1926

BODIAN, M., LAWSON, D.: Brit. J. Surg. 40, 368 (1953)

BRAHAM, J., SAROVA-PIHAS, I., GOLDHAMMER, Y.: Neurochirurgia 12, 195 (1969)

CHASON, J. L.: J. Neuropath. exp. Neurol. 15, 461 (1956)

CRAIG, W. McK., KEITH, H. M., KERNOHAN, J. W.: Acta psychiat. neurol. 24, 375 (1949)

CRITCHLEY, M.: Brit. J. Child. Dis. 22, 251 (1925)

CUSHING, H.: Amer. J. Dis. Child. 33, 551 (1927)

DI GEORGE, A. M.: In: Textbook of Pediatrics. NELSON, W. E. (ed.) 8th ed. Philadelphia: W. B. Saunders Company, 1964, p. 1263

EARNEST, F., KERNOHAN, J. W., CRAIG, W. McK.: Arch. Neurol. Psychiat. 63, 964 (1950)

FOX, H., EMERY, J. L., GOODBODY, R. A., YATES, P. O.: Arch. Dis. Child. 39, 508 (1964)

GRAHAM POLE, J.: Arch. Dis. Child 48, 867 (1973)

GRCEVIC, N., YATES, P. O.: J. Path. Bact. 73, 467 (1957)

HARE, C. C., WOLF, A.: Arch. Neurol. Psychiat. 32, 1230 (1934)

KENNEDY, B. J., BROWN, J. W., YARBRO, J. W.: Cancer Chemotherapy Reports 48, 59 (1965)

KERNOHAN, J. W., SVIEN, H. J., MABON, R. F., ADSON, A. W.: Proc. Mayo Clin. 24, 53 (1949)

KERSTING, G.: Die Gewebszüchtung menschlicher Hirngeschwulste. Berlin: Springer 1961, p. 14

KOOS, W. Th., MILLER, M. H.: Intracranial Tumours of Infants and Children. St. Louis: C. V. Mosby Co. 1971 a, Chap. 1

KOOS, W. Th., MILLER, M. H.: Intracranial Tumours of Infants and Children. St. Louis: C. V. Mosby Co., 1971 b, p. 141

KREDEL, F. E.: Amer. J. Path. 4, 337 (1928)

KREDEL, F. E.: Arch. Surg. 18, 2008 (1929)

LAMPKIN, B. C., MAUER, A. M., McBRIDE, B. H.: Pediatr. 39, 761 (1967)

LASSMAN, L. P., PEARCE, G. W., GANG, J.: Lancet 1, 296 (1965)

LUMSDEN, C. E.: In: Pathology of tumours of the Nervous System, 3rd ed., RUSSELL, D. S., RUBINSTEIN, L. J. (eds.). London: Edward Arnold, 1971, p. 375

MATSON, D. D.: Neurosurgery of Infancy and Childhood, 2nd ed., Springfield: Thomas 1969 a, p. 406

MATSON, D. D.: Neurosurgery of Infancy and Childhood, 2nd ed., Springfield: Thomas 1969 b, p. 540

MATSON, D. D.: Neurosurgery of Infancy and Childhood, 2nd ed., Springfield: Thomas 1969 c, p. 624

NAGAI, M., HOSHINO, T., TSUCHIDA, T., SATO, F., SANO, K.: Brain Nerve (Tokyo) 19, 1055 (1967)

O'CONNOR, J. F.: Ped. Clin. North America 21, 323 (1974)

OPPENHEIMER, D. R.: J. Neurol. Neurosurg. and Psychiat. 32, 94 (1969)

PATERSON, E.: J. Fac. Radiol. 9, 170 (1958)

PATERSON, E.: Brain, 84, 301 (1961)

PATERSON, E., FARR, R. F.: Acta Radiol. Stockh. 39, 323 (1953)

PENFIELD, W.: Brit. Med. J. 1, 337 (1931)

RINGERTZ, N., TOLA, J. H.: J. Neuropath. 9, 354 (1950)

RUSSELL, D. S., MARSHALL, A. H. E., SMITH, F. B.: Brain 71, 1 (1948)

RUSSELL, D. S., RUBINSTEIN, L. J.: Pathology of tumours of the Nervous System. 3rd ed. London: Arnold, 1971 a, Chap. 6

RUSSELL, D. S., RUBINSTEIN, L. J.: Pathology of Tumours of the Nervous System, 3rd ed. London: Arnold 1971 b, p. 15

RUSSELL, D. S., RUBINSTEIN, L. J.: Pathology of Tumours of the Nervous System, 3rd ed. London: Arnold 1971 c, p. 151

RUSSELL, D. S., RUBINSTEIN, L. J.: Pathology of Tumours of the Nervous System, 3rd ed. London: Arnold 1971 d, p. 121

RUSSELL, D. S., RUBINSTEIN, L. J.: Pathology of Tumours of the Nervous System, 3rd ed. London: Arnold 1971 e, p. 124

RUSSELL, D. S., RUBINSTEIN, L. J.: Pathology of Tumours of the Nervous System, 3rd ed. London: Arnold 1971 f, p. 16

RUSSELL, D. S., RUBINSTEIN, L. J.: Pathology of Tumours of the Nervous System, 3rd ed. London: Arnold 1971 g, Chap. 7

SCHEINKER, I. M.: J. Neurosurg. 2, 232 (1945)

SCHERER, H. J.: Am. J. Cancer 40, 159 (1940)

SEQUEIRA, E. B., BUCY, P. C.: J. Neuropath. and exp. neurol. 25, 667 (1966)

STEVENSON, L., ECHLIN, F.: Arch. Neurol. Psychiat. Chicago 31, 93 (1934)

TODD, I. D. H.: Brit. J. Radiol. 36, 645 (1963)

WALKER, A. E., HOPPLE, T. L.: J. Pediatr. 35, 671 (1949)

WALKER, M. D.: Cancer Chemotherapy Reports, Part 3, Vol. 4, No. 3, p. 21, 1973

WALKER, M. D., HURWITZ, B. S.: Cancer Chemotherapy Reports, Part 1, Vol. 54, No. 4, p. 263, 1970

WALKER, M. D., ROSENBLUM, M. L., SMITH, K. A., REYNOLDS Jr., A. F.: Proc. Am. Ass. Canc. Res. 12, 51 (1971)

WILSON, C. B., BOLDREY, E. B., ENOT, K. J.: Cancer Chemotherapy Reports, Part 1, Vol. 54, No. 4, p. 273, 1970

WILSON, C. B., NORRELL, H. A.: Cancer 23, 1038 (1969)

WOLMAN, L.: J. Path. Bact. 77, 283 (1959)

WURTMAN, R. J., AXELROD, J., TOCH, R.: Nature 204, 1323 (1964)

ZÜLCH, K. J.: Brain Tumours, their Biology and Pathology. London: Heinemann Medical Books Ltd., 1965 a, Chap. 2

ZÜLCH, K. J.: Brain Tumours, their Biology and Pathology. London: Heinemann Medical Books Ltd., 1965 b, p. 159

ZÜLCH, K. J.: Brain Tumours, their Biology and Pathology. London: Heinemann Medical Books Ltd., 1965 c, p. 152

ZÜLCH, K. J.: Brain Tumours, their Biology and Pathology. London: Heinemann Medical Books Ltd., 1965 d, p. 186

# Chapter 7
# Tumours of the Sympathetic System

The sympathetic nervous system is the fourth commonest site of tumour formation. Since this system consists of cells which are scattered over a wide area, sympathetic tumours could theoretically start almost anywhere, but in practice they usually arise where there are concentrations of sympathetic cells in or beside the vertebral column or near the kidneys.

## CLASSIFICATION

It is usual to divide sympathetic tumours into neuroblastomas, ganglioneuromas or phaechromocytomas depending on the degree and direction of cell maturation. In examining the 114 cases in the Manchester series it was apparent that this classification would fit only if it was recognised that a neuroblastoma might contain areas showing different degrees of maturation, including fully mature ganglion cells. On this basis the frequency of the three groups is as shown in Table 1.

Table 1. Sympathetic tumours 1954 - 1968 (assessed 1972)

| | Alive | Dead | Total |
|---|---|---|---|
| Neuroblastomas | 13 | 88 | 101 |
| Ganglioneuromas | 10 | 0 | 10 |
| Phaeochromocytomas | 2 | 1 | 3 |
| | 25 | 89 | 114 |

### Site of Origin

Six of the ganglioneuromas arose in the thorax, three were in the abdomen and one in the neck. All 3 phaechromocytomas were abdominal, 2 arising in the adrenals and 1 being extra-adrenal. The exact sites of origin of the neuroblastoma primaries were sometimes difficult to determine for the following reasons:

1. During recent years the fact that these tumours can be diagnosed biochemically has eliminated the need for surgical exploration in some cases.

2. At autopsy the disease was often very widespread.

3. There might be multiple tumours arising in the normal sites of sympathetic tissue.

4. Children with solid tumours often die at home and in any series many patients do not have autopsies.

Although it is impossible to be certain in every case, the frequency of the primary sites of the neuroblastomas in the Manchester series appeared to be as shown in Table 2.

Table 2. Primary sites of neuroblastomas

| | Alive | Dead |
|---|---|---|
| Abdomen | 7 (4 near kidneys) | 71 (62 near kidneys) |
| Thorax | 2 | 14 |
| Neck | 4 | 1 |
| Abdomen and thorax (mutliple primaries) | 0 | 1 |
| Not known | 0 | 1 |

## Adrenal and Extra-Adrenal Primaries

When an adrenal is replaced by neuroblastoma it is often assumed to be the site of the primary tumour and various authors give the proportion of tumours arising in the adrenal in their series (STOWENS, 1957 - 39%; BLACKLOCK, 1934 - 16 out of 18 cases). It may, however, be difficult to exclude the possibility that a neuroblastoma in the adrenal is a metastasis. If there is no other tumour at the normal sites of sympathetic tissue it is reasonable to assume that the adrenal was the primary site. However, the problem becomes more complicated if, as sometimes happens, the tumours in the adrenals are very small in comparison with masses elsewhere. In 27 of the 81 Manchester neuroblastomas it was known that there was tumour tissue in the adrenals while in a further 28 cases there was clinical evidence that the primaries were near the kidneys and might have been in the adrenals. Thus, the adrenal appeared to be the primary site in approximately half of all the Manchester neuroblastomas.

## Multiple Primaries

There are reports (e. g. POTTER and PARRISH, 1942) in which there is convincing evidence of a multifocal origin of neuroblastoma. In some cases (e. g. CTR.125/56) in which there were tumours in both adrenals and the mediastinum) one may suspect a multifocal origin, but proof is impossible. However, in one 14-year-old boy in the Manchester series, there were multiple tumours along the sympathetic chains on both sides of the vertebral column in the abdomen and thorax and it was very likely that there were multiple primaries.

# HISTOLOGICAL CHARACTERISTICS

## a) Neuroblastoma

1. The most frequent finding was the presence of eosinophilic fibrillary material which was detected in 80% of the specimens examined. These fibrils could be traced to the neuroblasts from which they appeared to

be processes. Sometimes the fibrils were replaced by amorphous eosinophilic substance.

2. A very definite lobular appearance was present in the majority of tumours with thin connective tissue septa between individual groups of cells which were sometimes clustered along the edge of the lobule.

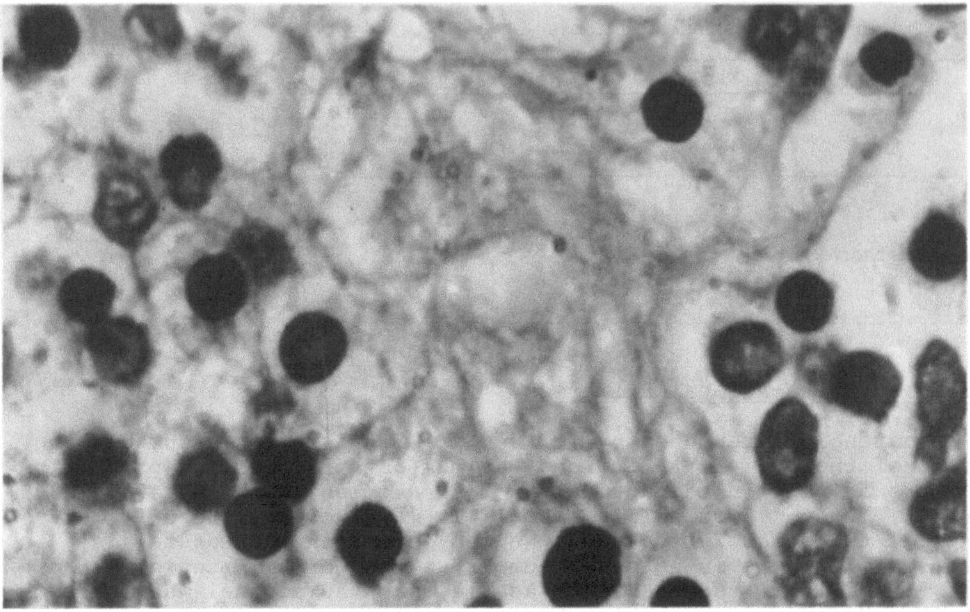

*Fig. 1. Neuroblastoma showing eosinophilic fibrillary material (H. & E. X 1250)*

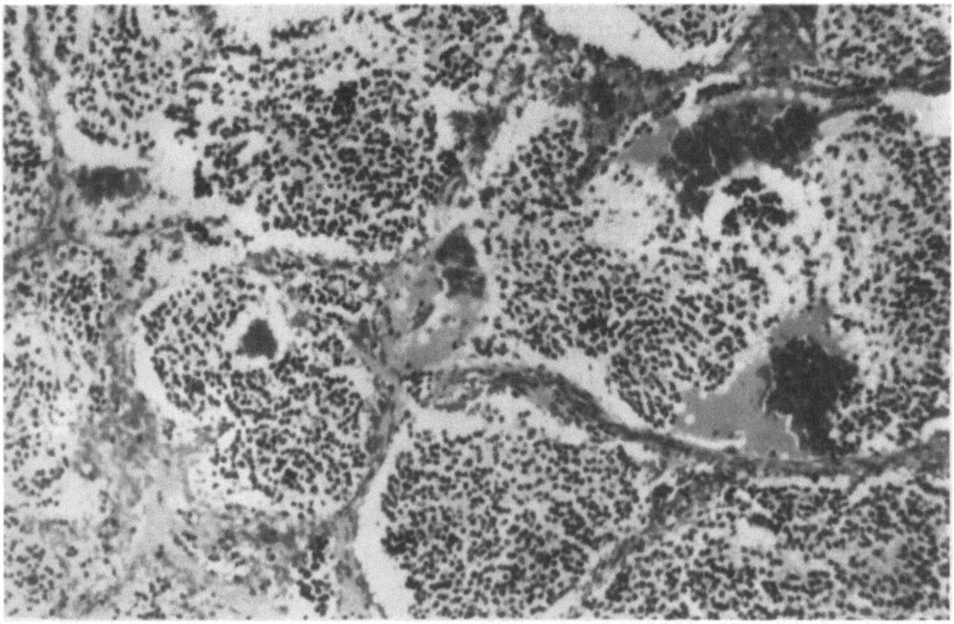

*Fig. 2. Lobular arrangement in neuroblastoma (H. & E. X 125)*

3. Evidence of maturation towards ganglion cells was detected in about half of the specimens and even tumours which were largely undifferentiated showed occasional cells with large nuclei, prominent nucleoli and an increase in the amount of cytoplasm.

4. Calcification was the next commonest feature and typically consisted of small granules no larger than individual cells.

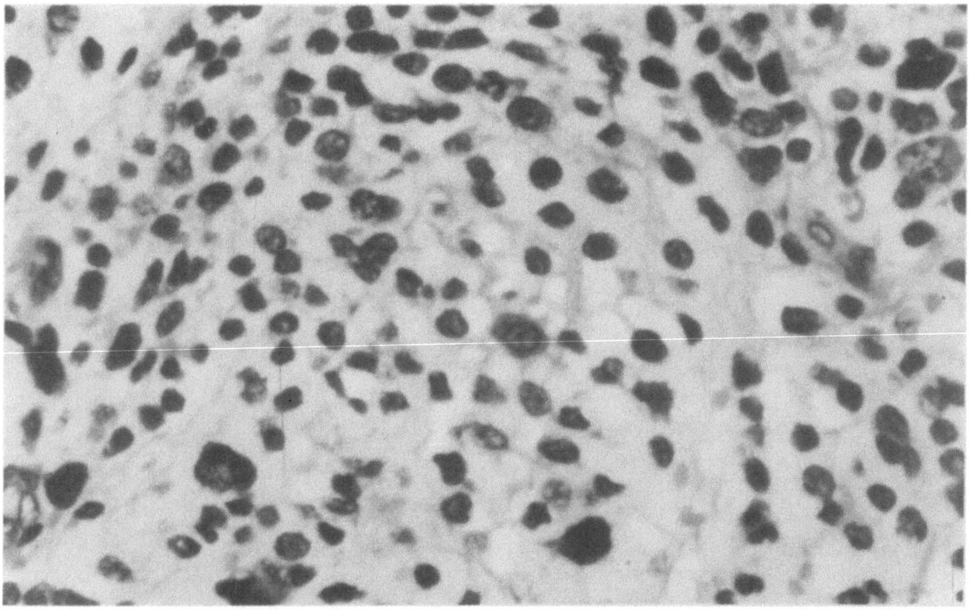

*Fig. 3. Maturation towards ganglion cell in neuroblastoma (H.&E.X500)*

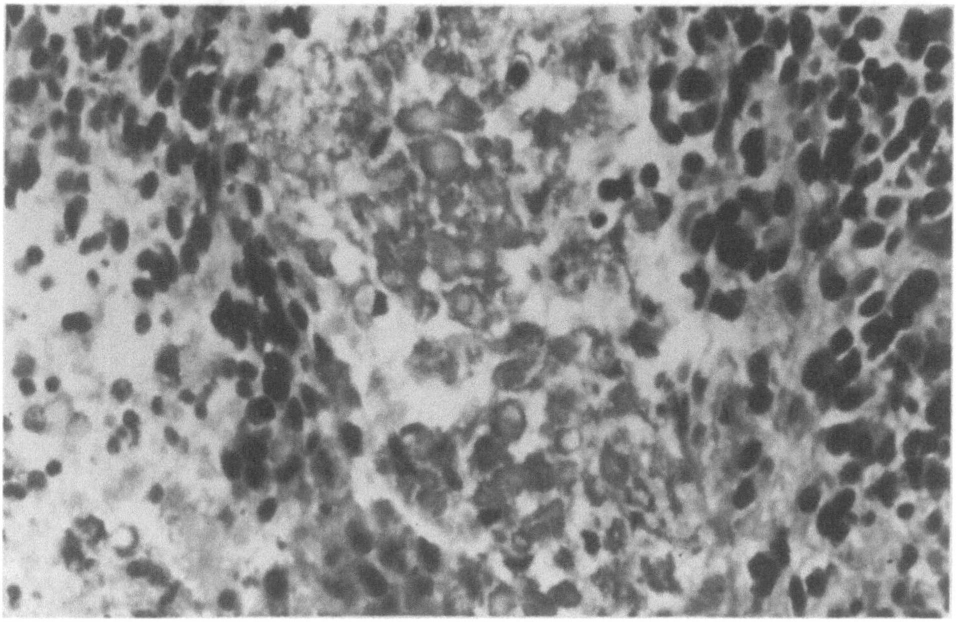

*Fig. 4. Calcification in neuroblastoma (H. & E. X 500)*

5. Rosettes were only seen in about one-third of cases.

6. Giant cells with pleomorphic nuclei were occasionally seen.

7. Unequivocal glycogen has been seen in a few Manchester cases by light and electron microscopy. PRICE (1973) gives a figure of 18% compared with 59% in Ewing's tumours.

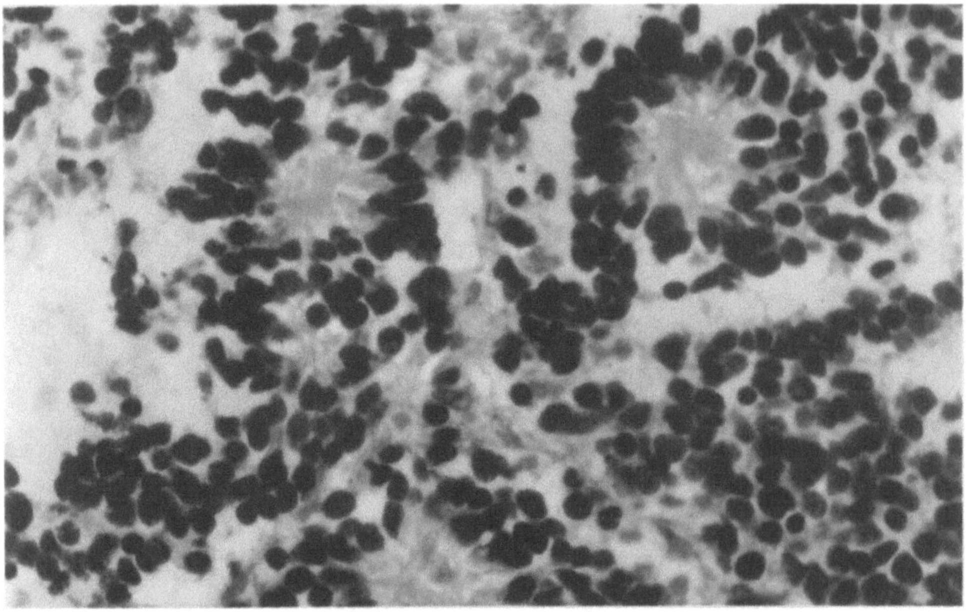

*Fig. 5. Neuroblastoma with rosettes (H. & E. X 500)*

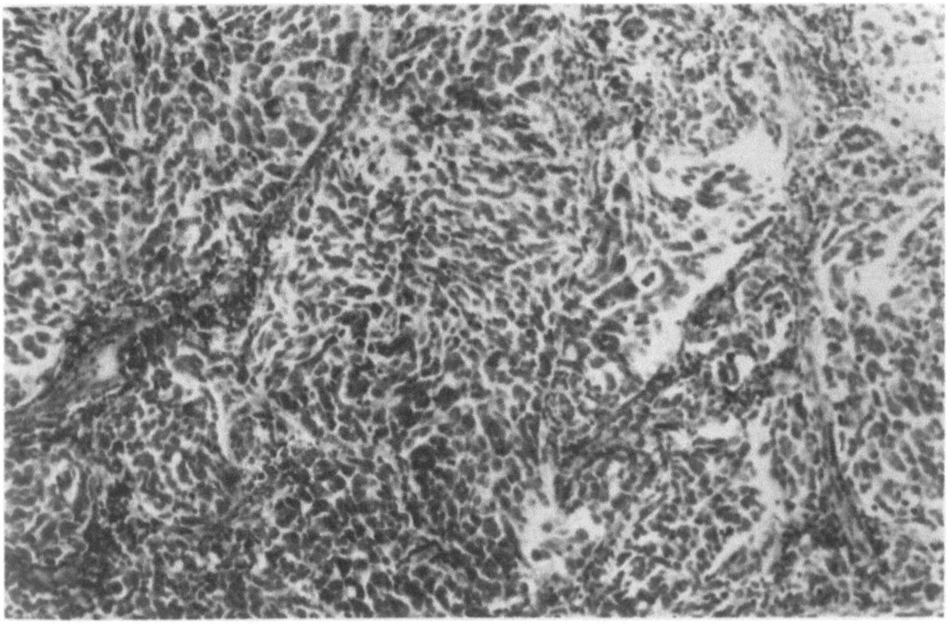

*Fig. 6. Giant cells in neuroblastoma (H. & E. X 125)*

b) Ganglioneuroma

The tumours consisted of sympathetic ganglion cells with neurofibrillary and neural sheath tissue. The neurones varied considerably in number with scanty cells rather diffusely scattered in some tumours and numer-

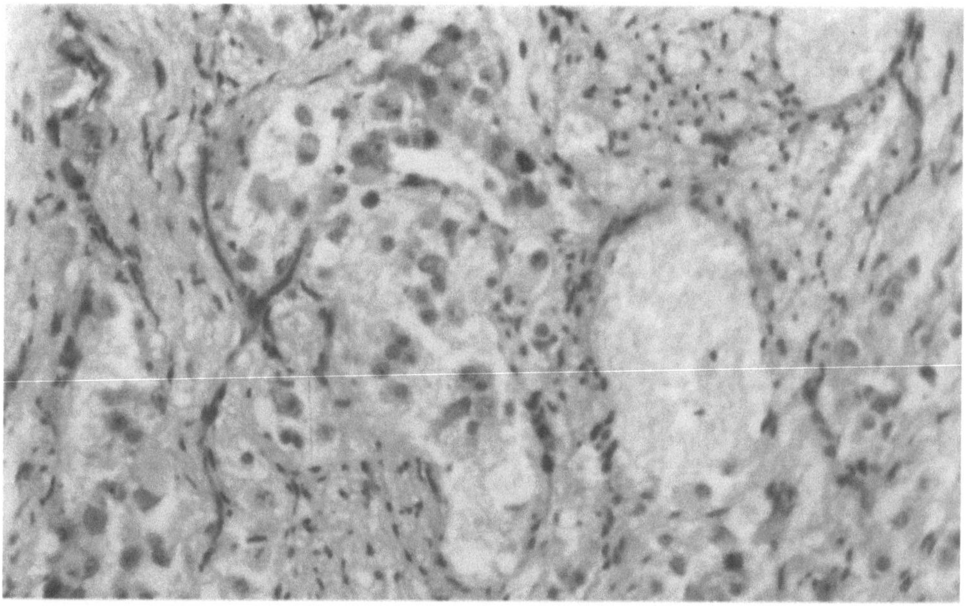

*Fig. 7. Ganglioneuroma showing neurones of varying size and lobular arrangement (H. & E. X 250)*

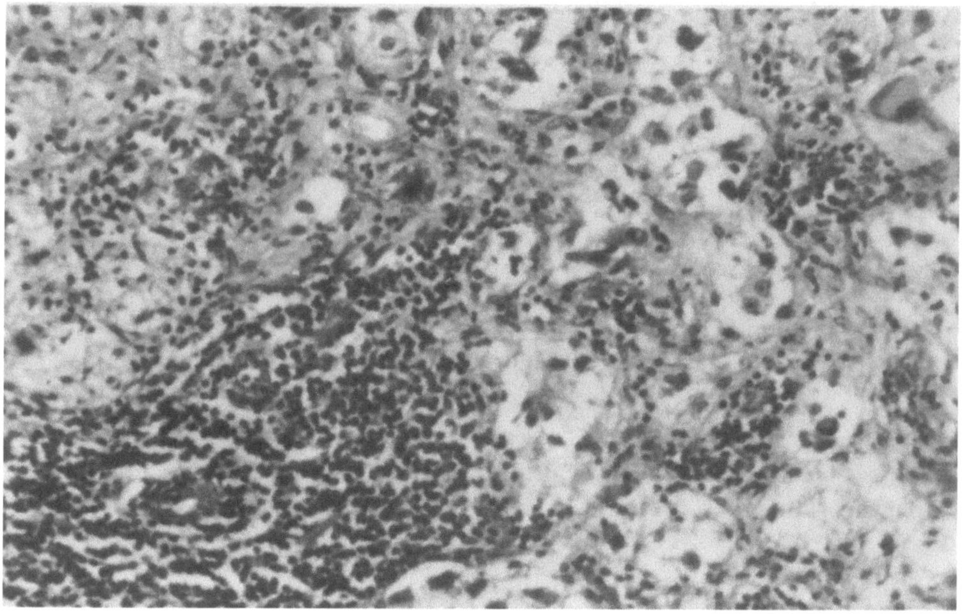

*Fig. 8. Lymphocytic infiltration in ganglioneuroma (H. & E. X 250)*

ous clustered cells having the lobular arrangement of the neuroblastoma in others. The ganglion cells showed variation in size with relatively normal cells and large multipolar and multinucleate forms. Swollen, degenerate, eosinophilic granular neurones were also seen. Lymphocytic infiltration was noted in several of the tumours and the resemblence to immature neuroblasts might cause confusion. Calcification was a feature in some cases. Islands of neurofibrillary material were seen and bundles of nerve fibres were sometimes embedded in the tumour tissue. A fibrous capsule was present in some parts but this was not a constant feature although the tumours were circumscribed and did not show invasive tendencies. Mature collagen and neurilemmal tissue were present in varying amounts and oedema with separation of fibres similar to that in nerve sheath tumours was encountered.

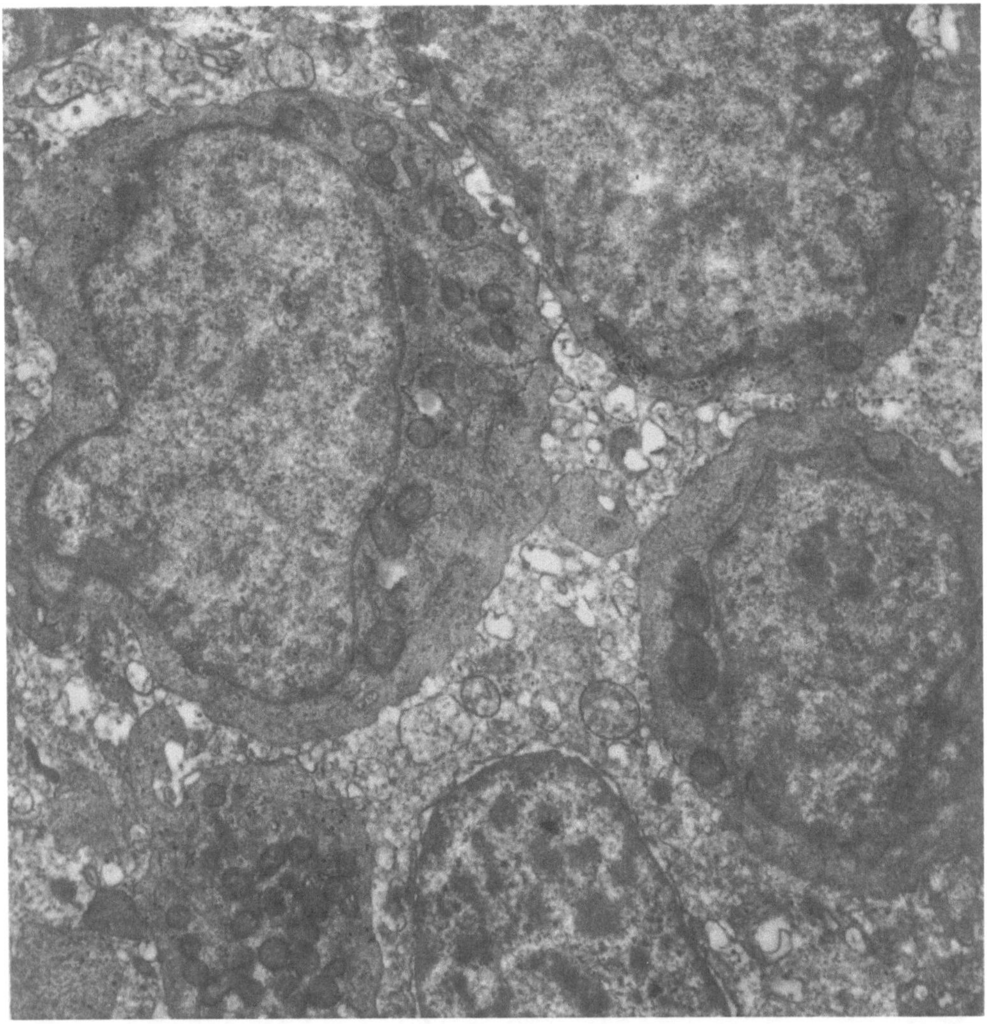

*Fig. 9. Undifferentiated neuroblastoma. Note the large nucleus and a sparcity of cytoplasmic organelles (X 7,500)*

## Electron Microscopy of Neuroblastoma and Ganglioneuroblastoma

In contrast to the many reports on the histological and biochemical characteristics of neuroblastomas very little has been written on the ultrastructural features of this tumour (MISUGI et al., 1968).

The variations in differentiation which are apparent by light microscopy can also be seen at the ultrastructural level. In undifferentiated neuroblastomas the tumour cells are rounded or ovoid and the rounded nucleus occupies most of the cell. Characteristically there is a sparsity of cytoplasmic organelles. Some cells contain a few mitochondria and occasional Golgi complexes (Fig. 9). The morphology of more differentiated tumours is very different. The cells have much more cytoplasm in which numerous mitochondria can be seen as well as an increase in the number of vesicles of rough-surfaced endoplasmic reticulum. Many differentiated cells contain membrane-bound homogeneous osmiophilic granules (Fig. 10) which resemble the catecholamine granules

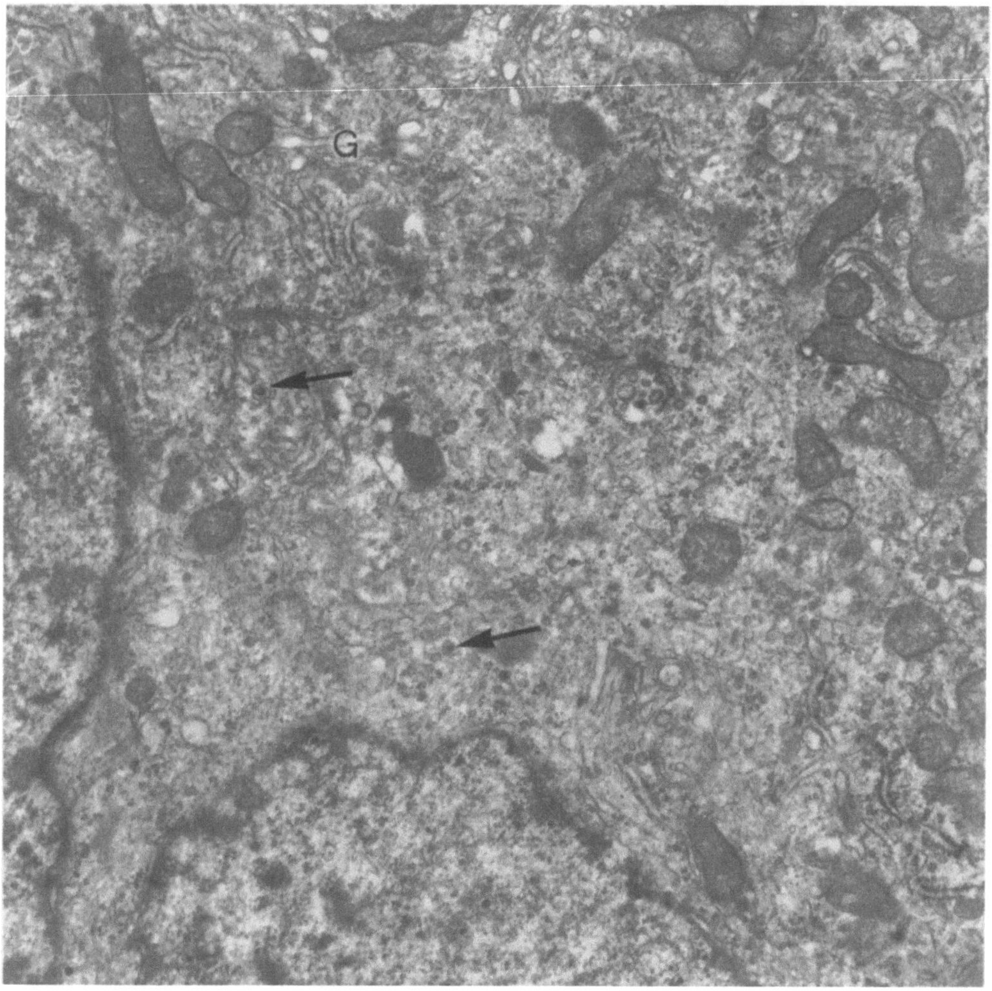


*Fig. 10. Differentiated neuroblastoma. Note numerous mitochondria, well-developed Golgi complex (G) and membrane-bound granules (arrow heads) (X 20,000)*

described in the adrenal medulla (DE ROBERTIS and FERREIRA, 1957). In the better differentiated neuroblastomas cell processes of varying length containing numerous fine filaments are present. The picture becomes more complex in tumours which can be described as "ganglio-neuroblastomas" in which the cytoplasm contains various organelles and inclusions and the intracellular spaces are filled with cell processes and neurites (Fig. 11).

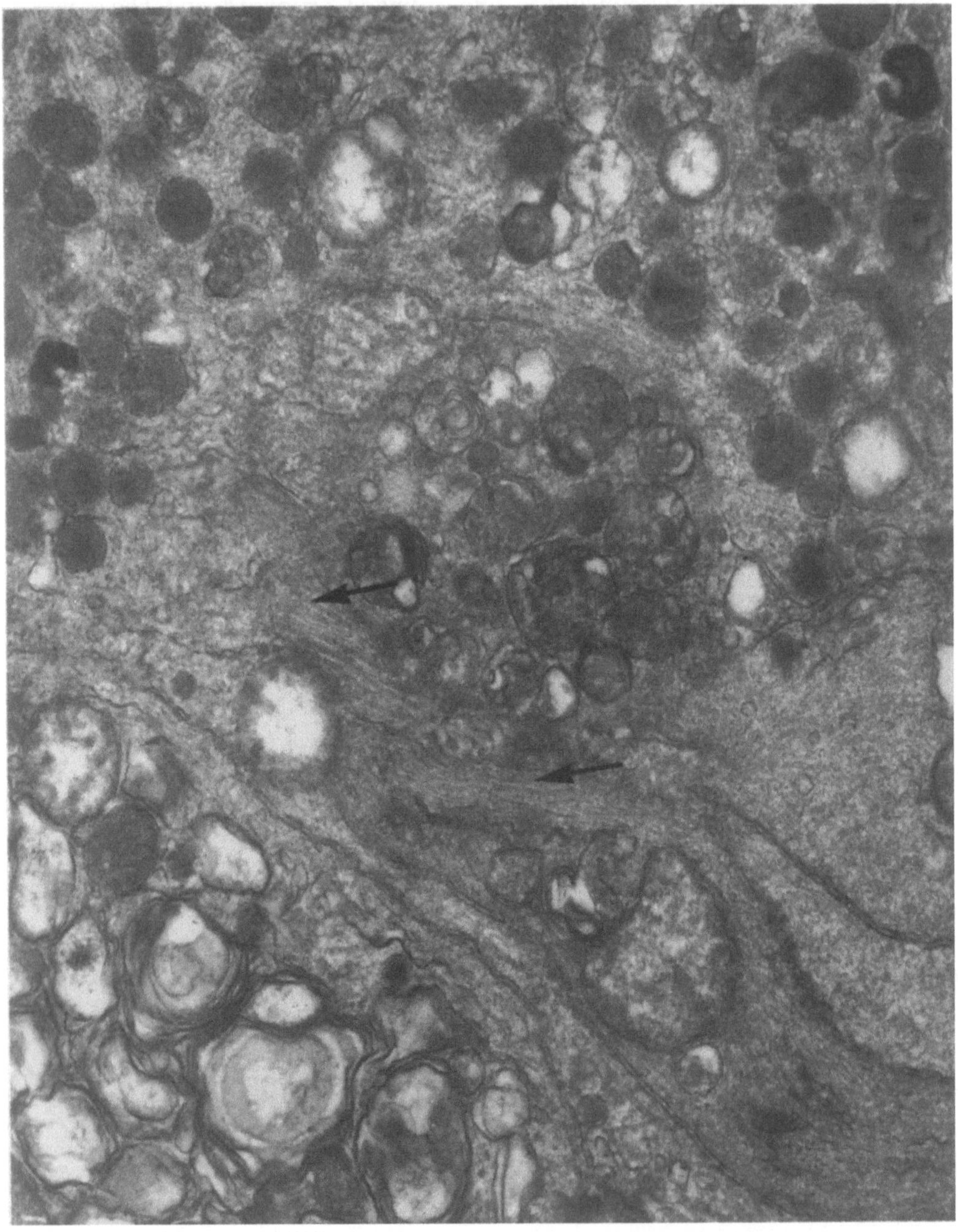

*Fig. 11. Ganglioneuroblastoma. Cytoplasm contains numerous inclusions. Note adjacent neurites (arrows) (X 25,000)*

c) Phaeochromocytoma

The three cases in the Register showed similar features with certain differences. A prominent capsule was noted in each case with compressed adrenal cortical cells adjacent to it. Lobular arrangement reminiscent

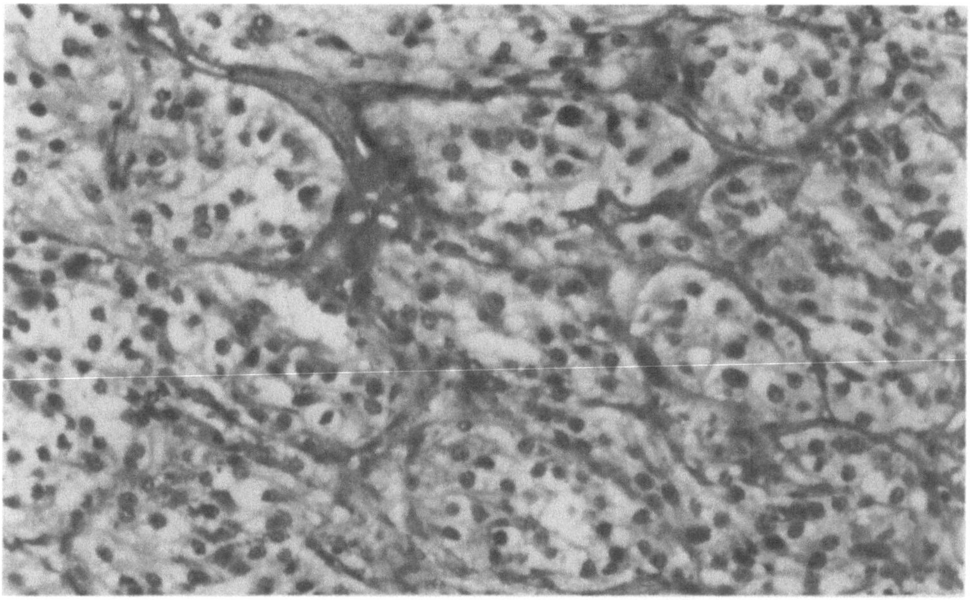

*Fig. 12a. Phaeochromocytoma with lobular arrangement of spheroidal and polygonal cells possessing granular cytoplasm (H. & E. X 250)*

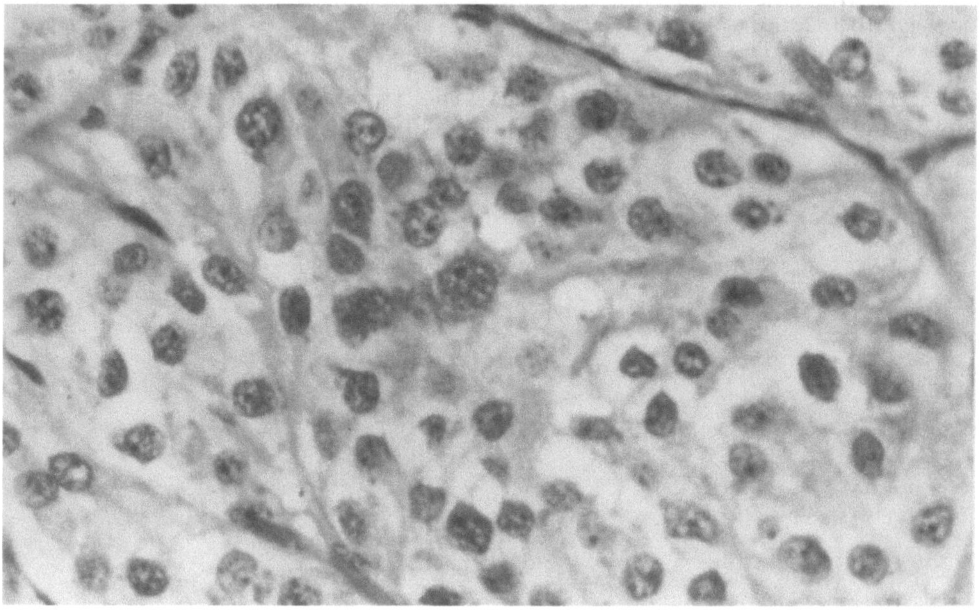

*Fig. 12b. Detail of Fig. 12a (H. & E. X 625)*

of the neuroblastoma was a feature in common although in one case the septa were rather thicker and less obvious than the delicate tracery seen throughout the tumour in another patient. Thin-walled vascular sinuses were prominent and areas of necrosis were noted. The cells in the lobules were rather large, spheroidal and polygonal, with some more spindle-shaped, and possessed abundant granular eosinophilic cytoplasm. In one case the cells were quite uniform while another showed pleomorphism with giant cells, nuclear vacuolation and inclusions. Brown pigment, mostly intracytoplasmic, independent of the chromaffin reaction, was sometimes present. Composite tumours consisting of phaeochromocytoma, neuroblastoma, and ganglioneuroma may be seen on occasion. In one of the tumours examined there were clusters of small cells which could have had a sympathetic neural origin and some of the larger forms had nuclear, nucleolar and cytoplasmic features consistent with developing neurones.

## THE CHEMICAL PATHOLOGY OF SYMPATHETIC TUMOURS

### Catecholamines

The three types of sympathetic tumours have one very important property in common - they are, in the main, active tumours secreting catecholamines and their metabolites. This generalisation has been questioned in the case of ganglioneuromas but, in our experience, even these tumours secrete although it is never possible to be absolutely certain that a ganglioneuroma does not contain neuroblastic foci. These compounds are usually excreted in the urine of affected subjects and there are quantitative and qualitative variations in the excretion patterns.

### Catecholamine Synthesis

The catecholamines (o-dihydric phenols with a side chain carrying an amino group) noradrenaline, adrenaline and dopamine are located in the adrenal medulla, the sympathetic nerves and the brain. Noradrenaline is present mainly in the central and sympathetic nervous system including the adrenal medulla. Adrenaline is mainly in the adrenal medulla. Dopamine is present in the central nervous system and has

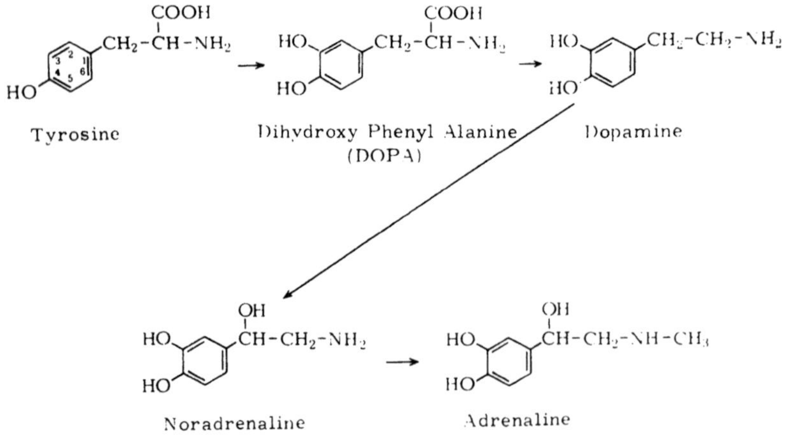


*Fig. 13. Catecholamine synthesis*

also been detected in the adrenal medulla among other tissues. It serves as a precursor of noradrenaline and is also thought to act as a neurotransmitter. The main pathway for the synthesis of noradrenaline and adrenaline from phenylalanine and tyrosine was suggested by BLASCHKO (1939) and this is still accepted as the major route (Fig. 13).

The enzymes concerned in catecholamine formation from phenylalanine have now all been demonstrated. Pathways have been studied in rats in which radioactive phenylalanine, tyrosine and dopa give rise to radioactive adrenaline in the adrenal medulla. Similarly pathways for the conversion of tyrosine to noradrenaline have been demonstrated in sympathetic nerves and ganglia, brain and heart. Adrenaline is not found in these tissues but appreciable amounts of dopamine may be present. The hydroxylation of phenylalanine to tyrosine requires two enzymes. Tyrosine hydroxylase converts L-tyrosine to L-dopa. This enzyme appears to be specific for L-tyrosine and is inhibited by catecholamines. L-dopa is converted to dopamine by the non-specific dopa decarboxylase.

Dopamine is converted in the storage granules to noradrenaline by the enzyme dopamine-β-hydroxylase. Noradrenaline is converted to adrenaline by the enzyme phenylethanolamine N-methyl transferase (PNMT), the methyl donor being S-adenosylmethionine and a second N-methyl group can be added to form N-methyladrenaline. This pathway goes to completion in the adrenal medulla but in sympathetic tissue noradrenaline is the final product. Most of the steps in the pathways occur in the cell cytoplasm, the conversion of dopamine to noradrenaline specifically in the chromaffin granules. The rate-limiting step seems to be the conversion of tyrosine to dopa. The lack of specificity of the enzymes makes other pathways theoretically possible giving rise to other metabolites e. g. octopamine, tyramine, etc. These alternative pathways are unimportant in normal metabolism.

## Metabolism of Catecholamines

In 1957 ARMSTRONG et al. demonstrated the presence of 4-hydroxy-3-methoxy mandelic acid (HMMA) in normal urine and showed it to be a major metabolite of noradrenaline. Other workers confirmed this finding and

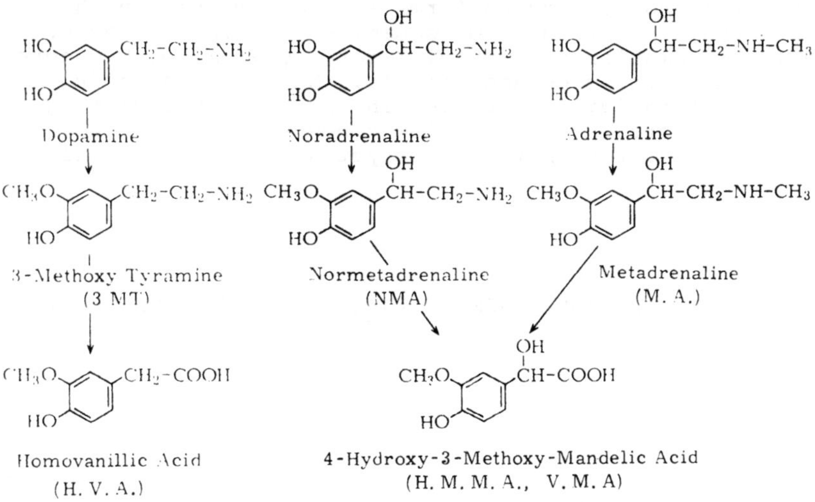


*Fig. 14. Catecholamine metabolism (showing major products of value in diagnosis of sympathetic tumours)*

showed that adrenaline is metabolised in essentially the same manner. Dopamine also has a similar degradation pathway, the major metabolite being 4-hydroxy-3-methoxyphenylacetic acid (homovanillic acid, HVA). As a result of these findings the pathway for the metabolism of catecholamines has been confirmed and a simplified version is shown in Figure 14. Two enzymes are mainly concerned in the catabolism and hence inactivation of adrenaline and noradrenaline. O-methylation in the liver has been shown to be a major pathway, the enzyme catechol-O-methyl transferase (COMT) catalysing the transfer of a methyl group from S-adenosylmethionine to the m-phenolic group of catecholamines. The enzyme may also act locally where noradrenaline is released. Noradrenaline and adrenaline are converted to normetadrenaline and metadrenaline which have little pressor effect and are excreted in normal urine both in the free state and as sulphates and glucuronides.

The second enzyme monoamine oxidase (MAO) is a widely distributed non-specific mitochondrial enzyme which can convert a number of monoamines to the corresponding aldehydes. The aldehyde is usually converted to the acid by a dehydrogenase but reduction to the alcohol may occur. Normetadrenaline and metadrenaline are both converted to HMMA by the action of MAO followed by oxidation. The aldehyde formed by MAO may be reduced to form the alcohol 4-hydroxy-3-methoxyphenylglycol (HMPG). Adrenaline and noradrenaline may also give rise to other compounds such as the 3, 4-dihydroxy acid and 3, 4-dihydroxyphenylglycol and these may occur in small amounts in the urine. The two enzymes (COMT and MAO) are also concerned in the formation of 3-methoxytyramine and 4-hydroxy-3-methoxyphenylacetic acid (HVA). There are also relatively small amounts of other derivatives of dopamine in the urine.

The catecholamines in the brain are synthesised in situ as those in the blood do not cross the blood-brain barrier. Products of brain metabolism found in the CSF include HMMA and HVA but the main product of noradrenaline in the brain appears to be HMPG.

HMMA is the main metabolite of adrenaline and noradrenaline and is excreted in the urine in the free state in normal subjects. Normetadrenaline and metadrenaline are also present in smaller amounts, chiefly in the conjugated form. Only small amounts of the unstable unchanged amines are found while small amounts of other compounds e. g. the dihydroxy acids in the free and conjugated forms and HMPG mainly in the conjugated form are present. The products of dopamine excreted in the urine are chiefly HVA with smaller amounts of 3-methoxytyramine. The determination of the output of these metabolites is, therefore, a useful means of assessing the catecholamine turnover in the body. Circulating catecholamines are normally present in very low concentration and their estimation is difficult, requiring methods not yet suitable for routine analysis.

## SYNTHESIS OF CATECHOLAMINES IN TUMOURS OF THE SYMPATHETIC NERVOUS SYSTEM

### 1. Phaeochromocytoma

The tumour tissue is able to synthesise noradrenaline and adrenaline from tyrosine and all the enzymes required have now been demonstrated. GOLDSTEIN et al. (1970) have shown that the activities of tyrosine hydroxylase in phaeochromocytoma and neuroblastoma tumour tissue are of the same order and are comparable with that found in bovine and rat adrenal glands.

Dopa decarboxylase has been found in levels comparable with or even higher than that found in normal human adrenal medulla. Dopamine-β-hydroxylase has also been studied by GOLDSTEIN (1966). The enzyme PNMT which catalyses the conversion of noradrenaline to adrenaline in the medulla has been shown to be dependent on, and require a high level of, corticosteroids in the adrenal blood and it has been considered that extra-adrenal tumours might contain little or no adrenaline because they are not exposed to a high concentration of corticosteroids. Occasionally, however, adrenaline is found in high concentrations in some extra-adrenal tumours and GOLDSTEIN et al. (1970) have shown that a non-inducible enzyme present in frog tissue has some properties in common with the enzyme present in tumour tissue. Many phaeochromocytomas are able to synthesise large amounts of catecholamines but tyrosine hydroxylase is said to be inhibited by these compounds. It has been suggested that tyrosine hydroxylase from tumour tissue might be less sensitive to inhibition by noradrenaline but GOLDSTEIN et al. (1970) have shown that the enzyme isolated from two tumours was sensitive to end-product inhibition. The enzymes responsible for inactivation have been detected in the tissue. COMT has been detected following the addition of S-adenosylmethionine to the in vitro system. MAO has been found, although the activity is relatively low compared with that found in liver, kidney or neuroblastoma tissue. The fact that the tumour is able to liberate catecholamines is shown by the presence of increased amounts of these compounds or their metabolites in the plasma and urine. In the majority of patients it would appear that the active catecholamine (chiefly noradrenaline), is released into the circulation.

## 2. Neuroblastoma

Fewer studies of the enzymes responsible for synthesis in neuroblastoma have been reported. GOLDSTEIN (1966) detected tyrosine hydroxylase in tumour tissue and the activity of this enzyme was found by other workers to be comparable with that present in the adrenal medulla, and it has

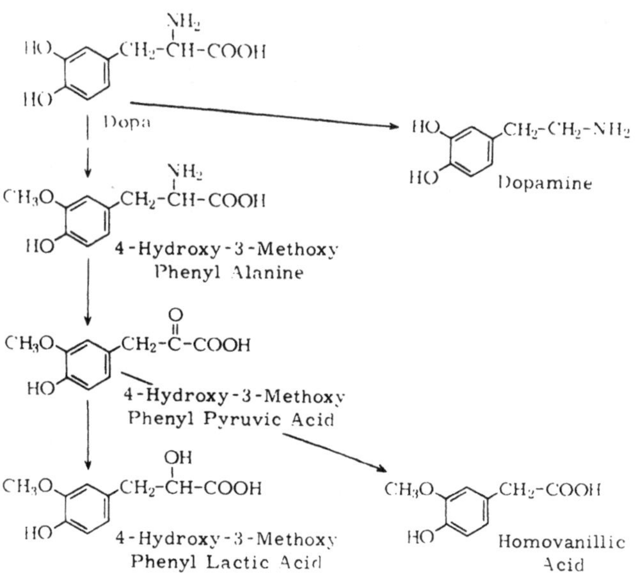


*Fig. 15. Alternative pathway of catecholamine metabolism encountered in certain cases of neuroblastoma*

been reported that the enzyme from neuroblastomas is inhibited by catecholamines. Dopamine-β-hydroxylase has been demonstrated by BOHUON and GUERINOT (1966) and GOLDSTEIN et al. (1970) have also shown it to be present in varying amounts in tumour tissue but the activity in neuroblastoma tissue is significantly lower than in phaeochromocytoma. PNMT activity has also been demonstrated in some neuroblastoma tissue by GOLDSTEIN et al. (1970), but again the activity is less than that in phaeochromocytoma.

COMT and MAO have been detected and the activities, although they varied between tumours, were comparable with the levels found in the liver. MAO activity in general was found to be higher than in phaeochromocytoma tissue. Most of the neuroblastomas do not liberate noradrenaline in an active form and it is possible that the presence of the enzymes responsible for inactivation results in the metabolism of a large part of the catecholamines within the tumour and the inactive metabolites are released. There is some evidence that a disturbance of metabolism may occur in some cases at a stage in the synthesis earlier than that of noradrenaline. Dopamine may be liberated and metabolised peripherally. Figure 15 illustrates an alternative pathway found in a few cases. Here dopa may be liberated and metabolised to 4-hydroxy-3-methoxyphenyllactic acid or HVA or it may be decarboxylated to form dopamine. GJESSING (1964) found an increase in the excretion of dopa metabolites in all of the 10 cases of neuroblastoma studied and 2 of these cases showed predominantly dopa metabolites.

## Determination of Catecholamines and Their Metabolites in Urine

In 1950 an increase in the urinary excretion of catecholamines by patients with phaeochromocytoma was shown by ENGEL and Von EULER and it was recognised that the estimation of these compounds could be of value in the diagnosis of this condition. Similarly, in 1957, MASON et al. reported an increase in the excretion of pressor amines in a child with neuroblastoma, and adrenaline and noradrenaline were detected in the tumour tissue. This was followed by numerous other reports. In 1960 VOORHESS and GARDNER published figures for the urinary excretion of noradrenaline and adrenaline and HMMA in 5 infants and children with a histological diagnosis of neuroblastoma. Interest was originally directed towards the estimation of noradrenaline and adrenaline in urine but the levels of these compounds present in the urine of normal infants and children are low and the increase may be small in some cases. It was later shown, however, that the precursors of noradrenaline namely dopa and dopamine may be increased together with their metabolites in the urine of some cases. BELL and STEWARD (1961) reported an increase in dopamine and HVA in several neuroblastoma patients and this finding was confirmed by other workers. Von STUDNITZ (1961) also reported an increase in HVA in 17 out of 25 cases with neuroblastoma and dopa was found to be increased in some of the cases.

### 1. Catecholamines

Both biological and chemical methods have been employed for the estimation of catecholamines in urine. Plasma levels have also been measured but the normal values are very low. The biological methods usually estimate the non-conjugated physiologically active substances.

Some of the chemical methods determine noradrenaline and adrenaline, others include dopamine. Catecholamines may be separated from urine using either alumina which adsorbs at the catechol group, or a suitable ion exchange resin to adsorb the amine group. Methods for evaluation following separation are usually fluorimetric. The "trihydroxyindole" methods involve oxidation of the catecholamines followed by conversion to fluorescent derivatives in alkaline medium, a stabilising agent being incorporated. The fluorescence obtained from dopamine is negligible since it does not possess the β-hydroxyl group and for routine purposes the error introduced is insignificant. Noradrenaline and adrenaline may be determined together at pH 6.0, but at 3.5 only adrenaline is oxidised and this method may, therefore, be used for the differential estimation of these compounds. With the "ethylenediamine" method all three catecholamines will form fluorescent derivatives after prior oxidation. A number of interfering substances will also fluoresce under these conditions. Methods are available for the estimation of dopamine but these are not always suitable for routine purposes. It seems reasonable, therefore, to use a method which will estimate all three catecholamines (BELL et al., 1958).

A number of drugs will fluoresce in alkaline solution, but the use of urine blanks will eliminate this interference. A volume of urine equivalent to 5-10 mg of creatinine output is used and the results are expressed in terms of dopamine. If a fluorimeter is not available a suitable source of UV light may be used. Kits are available for the estimation of catecholamines and these are usually based on the trihydroxyindole reaction and dopamine is not assayed. These kits may have a use in the investigation of suspected cases of phaeochromocytoma. Normal values are quoted in some procedures as being up to 100 μg per 24h expressed as noradrenaline, but this level is grossly in excess of normal values in young children. Similarly a screening test devised by HINGERTY (1957) to differentiate between normal excretion and levels in excess of 180 μg of noradrenaline and adrenaline per 24h is not generally suitable for use in childhood. WEIL-MALHERBE (1964) proposed that dopamine could be estimated by the difference between the value obtained for total catecholamines using condensation with ethylenediamine and that for noradrenaline and adrenaline with the trihydroxyindole method. Dopamine may also be estimated using other fluorimetric and colorimetric procedures.

## 2. Methylated Derivatives

The methylated amines are excreted largely as conjugates and they must be hydrolysed to the free base before assay. PISANO (1960) published a method for the estimation of metadrenaline and normetadrenaline, 3-methoxytyramine not being included. Chromatographic techniques may be used, but these methods are more time-consuming and, therefore, less suitable for routine use.

## 3. Phenolic Acid Metabolites

The chromatographic methods are based on those proposed by ARMSTRONG et al. (1956). Various modifications have been made but in general the acids are extracted from acidified urine with ethyl acetate. Two-dimensional chromatography is often used and standards are included. These methods involving visual comparison are usually only semiquantitative but it is possible to detect high excretion values of both HMMA and HVA if a suitable location reagent is used. Attempts to make the procedure more quantitative by eluting the developed spots with a suitable reagent have been made. Single phase chromatography has also been used for screening. High voltage electrophoresis may be used and simple electrophoresis has also been employed. Gas-liquid chromatography and isotope dilution methods are available but these techniques are less suited to routine use. SANDLER and RUTHVEN (1961) introduced a method for the estimation of HMMA which involved adsorption, elution, extraction, and conversion of HMMA to vanillin which was measured spectrophotometrically. In 1962 PISANO et al. published a method for the estimation of HMMA also based on the formation of vanillin. This procedure is less time-consuming than that proposed by SANDLER and is widely used. A urine blank should be used. No interference due to the ingestion of drugs, coffee, or vanilla products has been found. Other modifications involve the removal of interfering substances but this makes the procedure more complicated and time-consuming.

Various screening techniques for the detection of raised levels of HMMA have been proposed in an attempt to make the chemical detection of these conditions more readily available and to assist in early diagnosis. GITLOW et al. (1960) introduced a screening test for the detection of phaeochromatocytoma but it was not found to be sufficiently sensitive for this purpose; however, it is possible to use it as a screening test for neuroblastoma using the criteria suggested by BELL (1966). This test is based on the coupling of HMMA following extraction from acidified urine with diazotised p-nitroaniline. The coloured complex is extracted into amyl alcohol and the optical densities at 450 and 550 nm are determined and expressed as a ratio. This reaction is non-specific and there may be interference due to dietary pigments or drugs. Dietary restriction is necessary and medications should be withdrawn. A fasting morning specimen is recommended in the original procedure. Ratios greater than 1.3 are found in normal subjects. Values between 1.0 and 1.3 are of doubtful significance and below 1.0 is said to indicate increased excretion of HMMA. It is recommended that all negative results require further study. The test is usually quite satisfactory where the increase is large and ratios of 0.5 may be obtained but occasionally ratios of 1.3 or over have been found in cases where the excretion is known to be elevated. It is also not always possible to impose dietary restrictions and in this case it is more satisfactory to carry out a quantitative assay and, indeed, this may be true in most instances if the facilities are available. Modifications of this procedure have been made in an effort to overcome interference. YOUNG et al. (1963) introduced a semiquantitative technique based on the GITLOW test. Again dietary restrictions are essential and 24 hour collections are used. A much simplified spot test on filter paper was proposed and discussed by LA BROSSE (1968), which is said to be negative at levels less than 20 μg per mg creatinine, i. e. if interfering pigments are not present. This procedure has recently been reviewed by EVANS et al. (1971). GITLOW et al. (1970) proposed a further test which can be carried out at the bedside by non-skilled operators using drops of urine and this test is also likely to be positive at levels in excess of 20 μg/mg creatinine. LEONARD et al. (1972) introduced a test in which a HMMA dipstick is used and is said to be sensitive to a concentration of 20 μg/ml of HMMA or normetanephrine. In our experience not all the cases excrete these compounds at levels in excess of 20 μg/ml. It is suggested that such a stick might be used for mass screening at birth and at intervals during the first 6 or 7 years of life in an effort to detect neuroblastomas prior to the development of clinical symptoms.

These simple screening tests which have all been devised to make the diagnosis of the conditions by chemical means more readily available, are rapid and require no specialised equipment and may be carried out by those who are not familiar with laboratory procedures. It is recognised that early detection might lead to an improvement in prognosis and, therefore, mass screening using a simple test may be of value but it must be realised that while a strongly positive result is highly suggestive of a tumour of neural crest origin a negative result does not rule out the possibility of such a diagnosis, since not all the cases excrete increased amounts of HMMA, nor does an excess, if present, always exceed 20 μg/mg creatinine. Also these tests are often carried out on random specimens and it has been shown that there is sometimes a variation in the excretion throughout the day. A negative finding in the presence of strong clinical evidence should be followed by quantitative assay using a 24h collection.

Reagent kits have been introduced using thin layer chromatography and again it must be remembered that the levels quoted by the manufacturers are not always realistic when dealing with urine from small children and the procedure must be modified. An excess of HVA may be detected using chromatography and other techniques are available but they are not always suitable for routine purposes. GITLOW et al. (1970) claim that the quantitative assay of HMPG appears to offer the greatest reliability for biochemical diagnosis of neuroblastoma, 97% of the patients tested being found to excrete increased amounts. Methods are available for the estimation (RUTHVEN and SANDLER, 1965) and paper chromatography may be used.

The excretion pattern of catecholamines and their metabolites in neuroblastomas is very variable and since no one test can be relied upon to be diagnostic in all cases, a combination is recommended. The choice, in the main, will depend on the facilities available. BELL (1966) proposed a scheme using the estimation of total catecholamines and HMMA and he found it to give 100% reliability. There are few reports where a full range of determinations has been carried out; GJESSING (1963) stresses the importance of estimating as many metabolites as possible. WILLIAMS and GREER (1963) suggest that the estimation of HMMA and HVA would identify 95% of the cases whilst GITLOW (1970) claims HMMA to be raised in 95% and HMPG in 97%, HVA in 92%, and metanephrines in 87%.

## Catecholamine Excretion in Manchester Children

In the Manchester series total catecholamines were estimated by a modification of the method of BELL et al. (1958), increased volumes of urine being used depending on the creatinine output. Metadrenalines (NMA and MA) were determined by the method of PISANO (1960) and HMMA according to PISANO et al. (1962) and again increased amounts of urine were used for HMMA. The GITLOW screening test (1960) and two-phase paper chromatography have been used on occasions.

## Collection of Specimens

With three exceptions the estimations in the Manchester series have been carried out on 24h collections. Ten ml of 5N HCl was added as preservative in older children and 1 ml per year of age in infants and young children. Urine was stored at 4°C during collection and prior to estimation. No dietary restrictions were imposed. Originally, random samples were used but this was discontinued when it was realised that there is variation in the excretion over the 24h period. An increase in both HMMA and metadrenalines has been found in incomplete 24h specimens but the levels were well within normal limits when the full collection was analysed. This variation has been discussed by McKENDRICK and EDWARDS (1965) and VOORHESS (1968). It may not always be possible to obtain a full collection and a borderline result may be of doubtful significance.

The results have been expressed in terms of creatinine excretion and no difficulty has been encountered with dilute urines. The excretion has also been related to time, bodyweight or surface area, or even volume by other workers.

## Normal Values

The following values (Table 3) were found in children whose ages ranged from a few weeks to 11 years and who were in-patients in the Royal Manchester Children's Hospital. They were all subjects on whom the investigations were requested but in whom the diagnosis of tumour of the sympathetic system was later discounted.

Table 3. Normal values in children aged between a few weeks and 11 years

| | No. cases | Range (µg/mg creatinine) |
|---|---|---|
| Total catecholamines[a] | 70 | 0.2-1.5 (66 cases <1.0) |
| Total metadrenalines | 50 | <1.05 (49 cases <1.0) |
| HMMA | 55 | 1.3-10 (51 cases 1.3-8.0) |

[a]catecholamines are expressed as dopamine

In order to find the normal range for total catecholamines and HMMA in 24h specimens and to relate them to the patients' ages, 50 children aged between 3 days and 7 years were examined. They were all in-patients and were either due to leave hospital within the next 48h or the reason for admission was not thought likely to affect the catecholamines. They were as far as possible not receiving any drugs and dietary restrictions were not imposed (Table 4). These figures are in agreement with those published by VOORHESS (1967). When expressed in relation to creatinine excretion the levels decrease with age because of the increase in muscle mass in older children compared with the rate of catecholamine turnover. In the GITLOW test 85% had ratios greater than 1.3 with readings at 450 nm up to 0.475 and at 550 nm up to 0.32.

Elevated results have occasionally been found in other conditions besides sympathetic tumours e. g. a child with a terminal liver disease had total catecholamines 6 µg/mg creatinine, total metadrenalines 1.8 µg/mg creatinine and HMMA 22 µg per mg creatinine. Raised values have also occurred in intracranial haemorrhage. BARSON and HODGE (1971) reported an increase in HMMA output in infants with spina bifida and hydrocephalus and McKIBBEN et al. (1969) found an increase in one or other of several compounds in 96% of 55 cases with meningomyelocele. In familial dysautonomia the excretion of HMMA is reduced and HVA is increased (SMITH et al., 1963). The possibility of increased excretion in stress and postoperative conditions has not been confirmed by McKENDRICK and EDWARDS (1965). Some patients with carotid body tumours may have raised levels (ROBINSON, 1966) and the catecholamine content of these tumours may be increased (WINKLER and SMITH, 1972).

## CATECHOLAMINE EXCRETION IN CHILDREN WITH SYMPATHETIC TUMOURS

### Neuroblastomas and Ganglioneuromas

Since 1963, 44 children with neuroblastomas and 4 children with ganglioneuromas have been investigated at the Royal Manchester Children's Hospital. Twenty-four-hour collections were made in all except three cases. The upper limits of normal for children not suffering from sympathetic tumours were considered to be: total catecholamines 1.5 µg/mg

Table 4. Total catecholamines, HMMA and Gitlow test in normal children of various ages

| Age | No. cases | Total catecholamines[a] µg/mg creatinine Range | Mean | µg/24 hours Range | Mean | HMMA µg/mg creatinine Range | Mean | µg/24 hours Range | Mean | Gitlow Test OD 450/550 nm |
|---|---|---|---|---|---|---|---|---|---|---|
| 3 days - 1 year | 16 | 0.5-2.4 | 1.4 | 32-132 | 74 | 7-20 | 9.6 | 210-1600 | 590 | 1.1 - 2.0 |
| 1 - 3 years | 15 | 0.6-1.4 | 0.78 | 33-210 | 90 | 3.5-20 | 8.2 | 345-2400 | 1100 | 0.9 - 1.5 |
| 3 - 7 years | 19 | 0.4-1.2 | 0.78 | 60-420 | 185 | 3-11 | 4.5 | 500-3000 | 1230 | 0.9 - 1.3 |

[a]catecholamines are expressed as dopamine

Table 5. Excretion of catecholamines and their metabolites in 44 children with neuroblastomas and 4 with ganglioneuromas

| | No. cases | No. positive | % positive | No. of cases with excretion ratios[a] of 1-2 | -3 | -5 | -10 | -20 | -30 | -40 | -50 |
|---|---|---|---|---|---|---|---|---|---|---|---|
| Total Catecholamines | 47 | 43 | 92 | 14 | 3 | 9 | 3 | 5 | 6 | 0 | 3 |
| Total Metadrenalines | 43 | 40 | 93 | 11 | 7 | 4 | 10 | 5 | 2 | 0 | 1 |
| HMMA | 44 | 39 | 89 | 9 | 9 | 5 | 7 | 7 | 1 | 0 | 1 |

[a]The excretion ratio is the multiple of the upper limit of normal

creatinine, total metadrenalines 1.0 µg/mg creatinine, HMMA 10 µg/mg creatinine. Raised levels were sometimes expressed as excretion ratios, i. e. multiples of the upper limit of normal (see Table 5).

## Results

1. Total catecholamines. Forty-seven children were studied and the values were raised in 43. The levels ranged from 1.8 to 75 µg/mg creatinine and exceeded 10 times the upper limit of normal in 14 cases.

2. Total metadrenalines. Forty-three children were studied and the values were raised in 40. The levels ranged from 1.1 to 44 µg/mg creatinine and were over 10 times the upper limit of normal in 8 cases.

3. HMMA. Forty-four children were studied and the values were raised in 39. The levels ranged from 11.5 to 400 µg/mg creatinine and were over 10 times the upper limit of normal in 9 cases.

In 43 children all three investigations - total catecholamines, total metadrenalines and HMMA - were carried out and all were raised in 32 cases. The total catecholamines were normal in 4 cases, the total metadrenalines were normal in 3 cases, and the HMMA was normal in 5 cases.

The results are summarised in Table 5.

## GITLOW Screening Test

This was carried out on 48 children with neuroblastomas or ganglioneuromas and was positive in 31 (65%) compared with 89% positives using the quantitative assay for HMMA. There were 12 cases which could be regarded as borderline since the ratio ranged from 1.0 to 1.3

## Ganglioneuromas

VOORHESS (1968) considered that a pure ganglioneuroma without the diarrhoea syndrome does not show any abnormality in catecholamine excretion. Negative findings were also reported by KASER et al. (1964) but SMELLIE and SANDLER (1961) and BELL (1962) describe raised levels. All 4 Manchester children with ganglioneuromas had increased excretion of catecholamines. Two had all three components affected and one had an isolated twofold increase in catecholamines. The fourth child (CTR.81/71) presented at the age of 8 months with normal total catecholamines but the metadrenalines and HMMA were increased 15-20 times. The child was treated with chemotherapy and irradiation before the tumour was removed 9 months later and during this time the levels changed markedly. The total catecholamines rose, the metadrenalines fell to normal, and the HMMA decreased considerably, but did not become completely normal until the tumour was excised. Although the excision specimen consisted of completely differentiated tumour, its previous response to irradiation indicated that it had contained undifferentiated tissue (Table 6).

Table 6. Levels of catecholamines and metabolites in child CTR.81/71

| Date | Total catecholamines[a] (µg/mg creatinine) | Metadrenalines (µg/mg creatinine) | HMMA (µg/mg creatinine) |
|---|---|---|---|
| 17. 6.71 | 1.4 | 15.2 | 178 |
| 26. 8.71 | 6.8 | 2.2 | 43 |
| 6.12.71 | 8.2 | 0.5 | 11.2 |
| 14. 3.72 | 18 | 0.7 | 13 |
| | Excision of tumour | | |
| 28. 3.71 | 0.8 | 0.4 | 9.2 |

[a]catecholamines are expressed as dopamine

In all 4 children with ganglioneuromas the increase in excretion of total catecholamines at the time of operation was greater than that of HMMA (Table 7).

Table 7. Excretion ratios of total catecholamines and HMMA in children with ganglioneuromas

| | Excretion Ratio | | |
|---|---|---|---|
| | Total catecholamines | HMMA | HMMA / catecholamines |
| Case 1 | 4 | 1.1 | 0.275 |
| Case 2 | 1.4 | 1.2 | 0.86 |
| Case 3 | 1.6 | 0.93 | 0.58 |
| Case 4 | 12 | 1.3 | 0.11 |

It will be seen that there is a wide range in the excretion patterns in patients with neuroblastomas and ganglioneuromas and attempts have been made to relate these to the type of tumour (BELL, 1966). However, evidence on this is difficult to obtain because serial estimations on the same patient may show alterations in the relative levels of the various components. One Manchester child with a differentiating neuroblastoma had an initial increase in all three values but 3 days later, in a 24h specimen, the HMMA had increased to three times the previous reading, the metadrenalines were only marginally raised and the total catecholamines were normal.

The estimation of a single component is obviously inadequate in all cases for the diagnosis of neuroblastomas or ganglioneuromas but by using a suitable combination of estimations it was possible in the Manchester series to demonstrate abnormal levels in all histologically proven cases. Patients with sympathetic tumours have been reported with no catecholamine abnormality. VOORHESS et al. (1963) quoted 5 such cases with proven neuroblastoma, 3 of whom were in an older age group, and VOORHESS described 2 infants with cervical neuroblastoma with normal catecholamines and HMMA (VOORHESS, 1971).

Serial estimations may be used to indicate whether, following treatment, there is any residual tumour. After complete surgical excision the levels rapidly return to normal as was found in 6 cases in this series.

In the Manchester series irradiation has sometimes resulted in a slow decrease in the levels but has never caused them to become completely normal.

VOORHESS and GARDNER (1962) quote a case in which a persistently high level indicated the need for operative removal of residual tumour. In the Manchester series an infant of 2 weeks was found to have an abnormal catecholamine excretion but laparotomy failed to reveal a tumour. Two doses of cyclophosphamide were given but the catecholamines remained raised and at a second exploration a neuroblastoma was removed. Twelve days later the catecholamines had fallen to normal.

## Phaeochromocytoma

Only one patient, a boy aged 13 years, was investigated in the Manchester series. The total catecholamines and HMMA were only marginally raised being respectively 1.1 µg and 13.6 µg per mg creatinine. The greatest increase was in the metadrenalines which were 3.2 mg/24h (3.6 µg/mg creatinine). This finding is in agreement with other reports indicating that the levels are not as high as in neuroblastomas and that the metadrenalines are most significant in this tumour. CROUT and SJOERDSMA (1964) included 5 children in their series of 24 patients with phaeochromocytomas and the excretion patterns and tissue content were the same in adults and children. It has been suggested that a raised excretion of dopamine metabolites indicates a malignant phaeochromocytoma (ROBINSON, 1966) but GITLOW et al. (1972) demonstrated increased HVA levels in three children with benign phaeochromocytomas as well as marked increases in HMMA and metadrenalines. In the first edition of this book a case was quoted of a child with a benign phaeochromocytoma excreting 6 mg of dopamine per day. Another child with a benign ganglioneuroma had increased HVA. Although no histologist, however many sections he examines, can be sure that a particular tumour does not contain some malignant cells, it seems that for practical purposes a child with a benign sympathetic tumour can excrete increased amounts of dopamine and its metabolites.

Hypertension in patients with phaeochromocytoma is due to overproduction of pressor amines and it has been suggested that when the blood pressure is normal, dopa secreted by the tumour may prevent the action of the pressor amines. In neuroblastomas the hypertension is much less marked and this may also be due to the blocking action of dopa.

## TISSUE CATECHOLAMINES

### 1. Neuroblastoma

MASON et al. (1957) first reported the presence of catecholamines in neuroblastoma tumour tissue; an equivalent of 0.14 mg of pressor amines/g tumour being found. VOORHESS (1968) reported that the noradrenaline and adrenaline content was lower in neuroblastomas than in phaeochromocytoma tissue. It was found that in neuroblastomas the amount of HVA and HMMA was low and that there was little correlation between the tissue content of catecholamines and their excretion in the urine. However, such a correlation may exist in phaeochromocytomas. Neuroblastomas are not thought to have any storage mechanism for catecholamines and LA BROSSE (1968) suggests that the noradrenaline which is synthesised is rapidly metabolised to HMPG.

In the Manchester series three neuroblastomas have been found to have a catecholamine content of 4 µg, 7 µg, and 7.5 µg/g tissue. Total catecholamines were not detected in one ganglioneuroma but SMELLIE and SANDLER (1961) isolated noradrenaline, dopamine, and dopa from a ganglioneuroma. There was no evidence of a chromaffin reaction to bichromate in their tumour and this would accord with the finding of MARSDEN (1963) in neuroblastoma tissue although in the latter report a weak colour reaction for reducing substances of the catecholamines type was shown to be present.

### 2. Phaeochromocytoma

The presence of catecholamines in phaeochromocytoma tissue has been recognised for many years. Most tumours contain at least 1-10 mg/g tissue and some contain much more. The normal human adrenal medulla contains less than 1 mg/g tissue, mostly as adrenaline. In phaeochromocytomas noradrenaline usually predominates. In the first edition of this book two children's phaeochromocytomas were reported to contain noradrenaline in a concentration of 1-2 mg/g tissue with only a trace of adrenaline in one. VOORHESS (1968) quotes levels of 515 μg/g and 336 μg/g tissue for noradrenaline in two children aged 10 and 13 years and the corresponding adrenaline levels were 20 μg/g and nil. These levels were much lower than were found in phaeochromocytomas in adults but were still much higher than the levels in neuroblastomas. HVA and HMMA were virtually absent, suggesting that these metabolites do not occur within the phaeochromocytoma.

## OTHER COMPOUNDS OF INTEREST

GJESSING (1964) showed that cystathionine was present in tumour tissue in 6 cases of neuroblastoma but not in a ganglioneuroma or a benign phaeochromocytoma. It was suggested that the presence of cystathionine and β-amino-isobutyric acid in the urine might be of value in assessing the degree of malignancy of sympathetic tumours. Urinary cystathionine is attributed to increased production and decreased breakdown of this compound in the tumours as well as to leakage of the substance from it. However, cystathionine is present in other conditions, e. g. hepatoma and glycogen storage disease. SHAW et al. (1967) examined 3000 urine specimens from children by two-dimensional paper chromatography and found substantial quantities of cystathionine in the urine of many children with neuroblastomas and also other conditions. The increase in cystathionine may be due to a partial deficiency of pyridoxine in the liver and it has been suggested that there is an increase in methionine metabolism in neuroblastoma due to increased methylation of catecholamines. Vitamin B6 is supposedly inactivated by catecholamines and this will in turn result in the inhibition of cystathionase (GJESSING, 1963).

An increase in mucopolysaccharides in the blood of a patient with neuroblastoma has been reported by BROUGHTON et al. (1970) but no increase in urinary catecholamines or HMMA was found in this patient on three occasions nor were there any mucopolysaccharides in the urine. Mucopolysaccharides have also been reported in the blood and urine in Wilms' tumour and therefore their presence cannot be considered to be diagnostic of neuroblastoma.

Dopamine-β-hydroxylase has been estimated in the serum of 22 patients with neuroblastoma and in 27 controls (GOLDSTEIN et al., 1972). Ten of the patients had very high levels and they excreted large amounts of HMMA. There was no correlation between the enzyme levels and the excretion of dopamine and HVA. It is suggested that the assay of this enzyme may be of diagnostic value but it is doubtful whether this estimation could be performed routinely in most hospital laboratories.

Cushing's syndrome, a rare condition in childhood, has been reported in association with neuroblastoma and other tumours of neural origin, e. g. ganglioneuroblastoma (KENNY et al., 1967); KOGUT and DONNELL (1961) and more recently DAHMS et al. (1973). It is thought that the tumours might secrete material which stimulates the cortex to produce excessive amounts of corticosteroids. KENNY et al. (1967) report that the steroid levels in their patients fell after the removal of the neuroblastoma. No such association has been found with any of the cases in this present series, but MARSDEN (1963) reports the occurrence of adrenal hyperplasia and neuroblastoma in a Manchester child before the start of the Registry in 1953.

## Neuroblastomas and the Nerve Growth Factor

The remarkable effects of the Nerve Growth Factor (NGF) on sympathetic ganglia in vitro and in vivo (LEVI-MONTALCINI and ANGELETTI, 1968; ZAIMIS, 1972) led to the hope that this substance might have some effect on the growth of sympathetic tumours. NGF is found in the submaxillary glands of adult male mice and in snake venom and is detected by its effect on cultures of chick embryo ganglia which, in its presence, become surrounded by a dense halo of neurites. An antiserum against it can be produced which, when injected into newborn mice, destroys most of their sympathetic ganglia. BURDMAN and GOLDSTEIN (1964) found that sera from 7 children with neuroblastoma caused some neurite outgrowth from chick ganglia, but the effect was much weaker than that produced by NGF itself. Nil responses were observed in 20 controls. These results were taken to mean that sera from neuroblastoma patients have an abnormally high NGF activity. However, using much larger groups of controls, BILL et al. (1969) and WAGHE et al. (1970), showed that the serum of many normal individuals will stimulate neurite outgrowth and that children with neuroblastoma have no greater NGF activity than that seen in the normal population. Furthermore, KUMAR et al. (1970) showed that anti-NGF had no effect on neuroblastomas in culture and that the injection of purified NGF into 3 children with widespread neuroblastoma did not alter the course of the disease.

# CLINICAL MANIFESTATIONS

## Age of Onset

Ganglioneuromas and phaeochromocytomas may occur at practically any age (STOUT, 1947). Neuroblastomas are most common in early childhood (see Table 8).

In four children the tumours were discovered within a few days of birth, indicating that the disease must have started *in utero.* Three of these cases were described by EVANS (1965). Twenty-three children with neuroblastomas were included by WELLS (1940) in his review of congenital tumours.

# MODE OF PRESENTATION

## Ganglioneuroma

The modes of presentation of the 10 cases of ganglioneuroma in the Register are shown in Table 9.

It will be seen that in 2 of the abdominal tumours (CTR.35/54 and CTR. 73/64) the symptoms were probably attributable to the tumour, but in 4 other patients the ganglioneuromas were certainly symptomless and in another 4 there was possibly no connection between the symptoms and the tumour.

The ganglioneuroma is generally diagnosed by the radiologist reporting a paravertebral shadow in the mediastinum. It characteristically lies posteriorly - farther back than the usual situation of enlarged lymph nodes or a teratoma. STOUT (1947) reported ganglioneuroma presenting as lumps in a wide variety of situations.

Table 8. Sympathetic tumours

| Age (years) | Age at diagnosis <1 | 1 | 2 | 3 | 4 | 5 | 6 | 7 | 8 | 9 | 10 | 11 | 12 | 13 | 14 |
|---|---|---|---|---|---|---|---|---|---|---|---|---|---|---|---|
| Neuroblastomas | 29 | 21 | 11 | 15 | 9 | 2 | 2 | 5 | 2 | 1 | 0 | 1 | 2 | 0 | 1 |
| Ganglioneuromas | 0 | 0 | 1 | 1 | 1 | 3 | 1 | 1 | 0 | 0 | 0 | 1 | 0 | 1 | 0 |
| Phaeochromocytomas | 0 | 0 | 0 | 0 | 0 | 0 | 0 | 0 | 0 | 0 | 0 | 1 | 1 | 1 | 0 |

Table 9. Ganglioneuromas

| CTR. | Site | Clinical presentation |
|---|---|---|
| 35/54 | Abdomen | Pain |
| 102/55 | Chest | No symptoms - chance X-ray finding |
| 95/56 | Chest | Cough - X-ray finding |
| 115/58 | Chest | No symptoms - chance X-ray finding |
| 76/59 | Chest | Respiratory infection - X-ray finding |
| 13/60 | Chest | Respiratory infection - X-ray finding |
| 15/62 | Abdomen | Respiratory infection - chance finding |
| 116/63 | Neck | No symptoms - lumps felt |
| 73/64 | Abdomen | Pain and vomiting |
| 99/66 | Chest | Attacks of screaming and restlessness |

## The Neuroblastoma Primary

The mode of presentation of primary neuroblastoma depends on its situation. If the tumour is in the abdomen it may cause pain, which, because of the youth of the patients, is not accurately localised or described. Often the pain is accompanied by vomiting or anorexia, and in the majority of cases a mass can be felt. X-rays may show a characteristic mottled calcification in the tumour. A pyelogram may reveal renal displacement which is usually outwards and/or downwards because

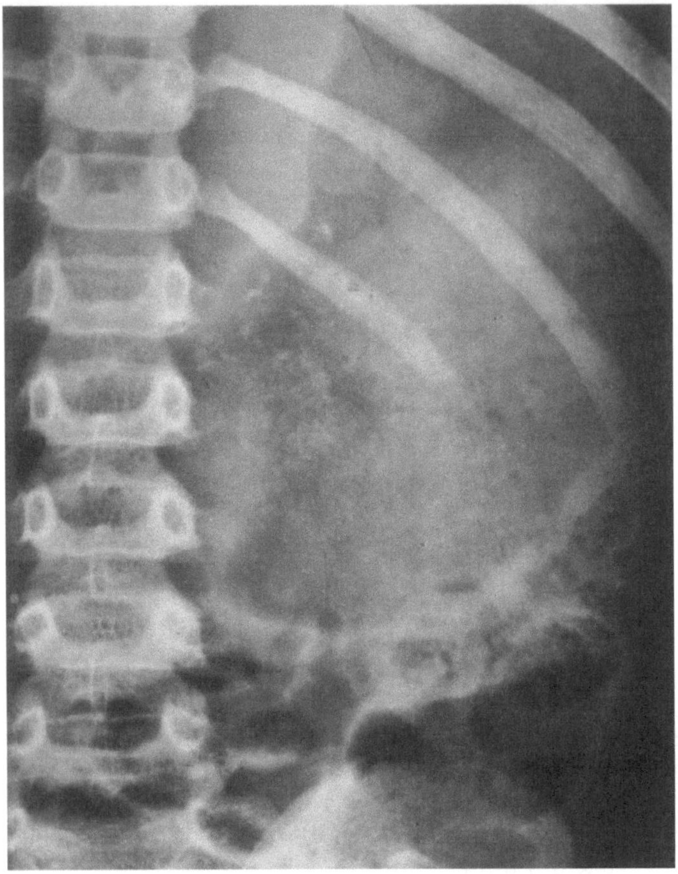

*Fig. 16. Mottled calcification in abdominal neuroblastoma*

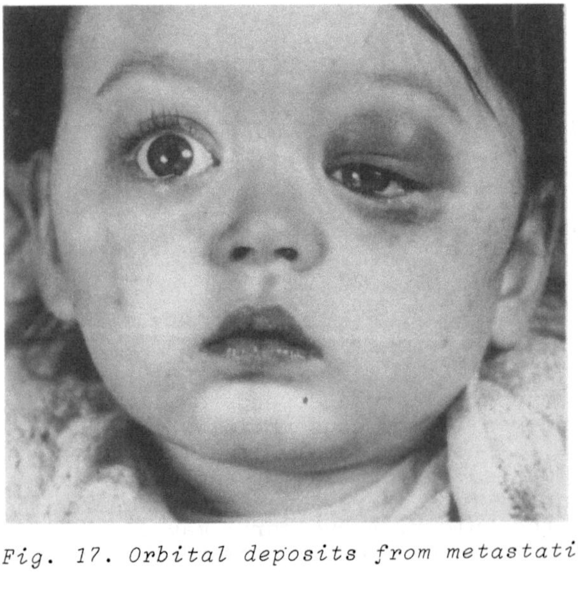

*Fig. 17. Orbital deposits from metastatic neuroblastoma*

the tumours generally arise either in the adrenal or in sympathetic tissue medial to the kidneys. The majority of abdominal neuroblastoma primaries can be detected either clinically or radiologically but very occasionally a case is encountered in which there are widespread secondaries and a primary which is so small that it can only be detected at operation or autopsy. Sometimes an abdominal neuroblastoma may press on the bile duct causing obstructive jaundice. An extradural primary manifests itself as a paralysis which may affect one or two or four limbs and usually causes a patulous anus. Root pain and sensory loss may occur. In a child the commonest primary extradural tumour is a neuroblastoma (see Chapter 6, Table 13). Primary neuroblastomas in the chest nearly always arise in the posterior mediastinum and by spreading

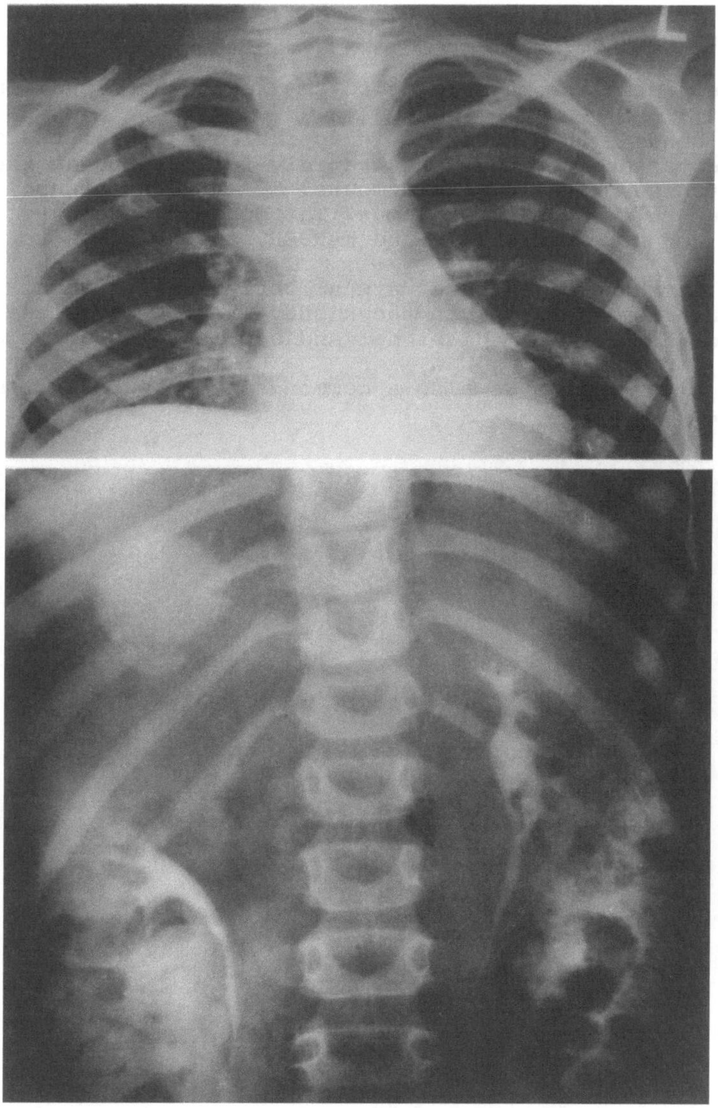

*Fig. 18. Upper and lower. Spread to mediastinum from calcified neuroblastoma above right kidney*

forwards may cause cough, dyspnoea, recurrent respiratory infections, and superior vena caval obstruction. They may be associated with extradural tumours.

In most of the Manchester children with neuroblastoma there was no record of the blood pressures having been taken. However, in nine children some evidence of hypertension was noted. In general this was not severe, the highest recorded pressure being 160/120 in a 7-year-old child.

Diarrhoea has been reported together with abnormal catecholamine excretion but this must be a rare manifestation. It was only noted in 4 children in the Manchester series.

## Secondary Neuroblastoma

The neuroblastoma spreads to the following situations:

1. Bones - this occurred in approximately half the Manchester cases. One osseous secondary was rapidly followed by another until the skeleton was riddled with tumours. Often these became evident first in the skull and neck of femur. The bones of the hands and feet are usually not affected (WYATT and FARBER, 1941).

2. Lymph nodes - these were slightly less frequent than in bones. Neuroblastomas arising in the kidney region may spread to the para-aortic and then to the mediastinal and supraclavicular nodes.

3. Liver - this is also a common site of spread from abdominal neuroblastoma.

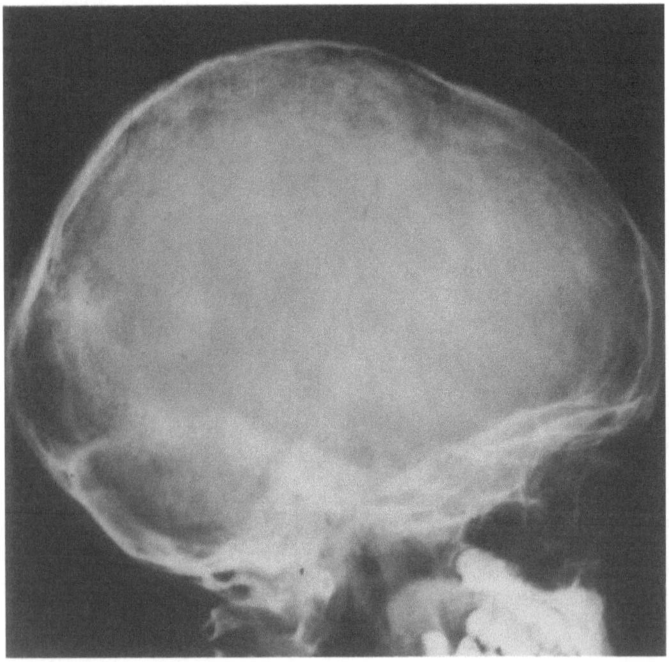

*Fig. 19. Skull in case of neuroblastoma showing multiple small deposits in vault*

4. Lung - the infrequency of pulmonary metastases is one of the most striking features of neuroblastoma. In the Manchester series 8 children developed tumour in the lung. In 3 cases this was due to direct spread from the mediastinum or through the diaphragm. Six children had multiple pulmonary deposits which were confined to the subpleural region in 4 cases. Only 2 children had multiple metastases throughout the lung parenchyma.

5. Skin - this is a rare site of secondaries. It occurred in only 2 Manchester children, one aged 3 months and the other aged 11 months. Possibly the neuroblastoma resembles leukaemia in metastising to skin in infancy rather than in later childhood.

The commonest symptom of bone involvement is pain accompanied by an unwillingness to move the affected limbs and a toddler may stop walking. Subperiosteal tumours may cause palpable lumps, usually in the scalp. Radiologically, osteolytic lesions are seen, but at clinical diagnosis

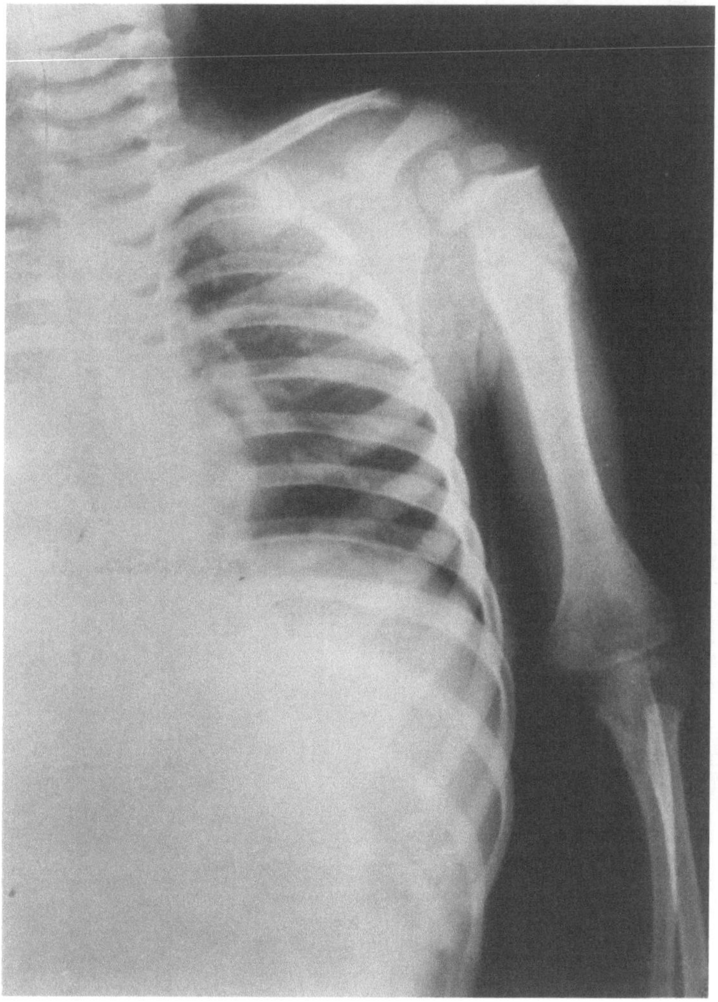

*Fig. 20. Metastatic neuroblastoma deposit in humerus*

they are often so small that the bone changes are minimal. The common sign of subperiosteal invasion is a thin covering layer of reactive bone. More rarely a "sun-ray" appearance is seen. Since skeletal involvement makes a patient ill and restricts his activities, pathological fractures are rare. Bone secondaries are often accompanied by a considerable degree of anaemia. Less commonly, they may be preceded

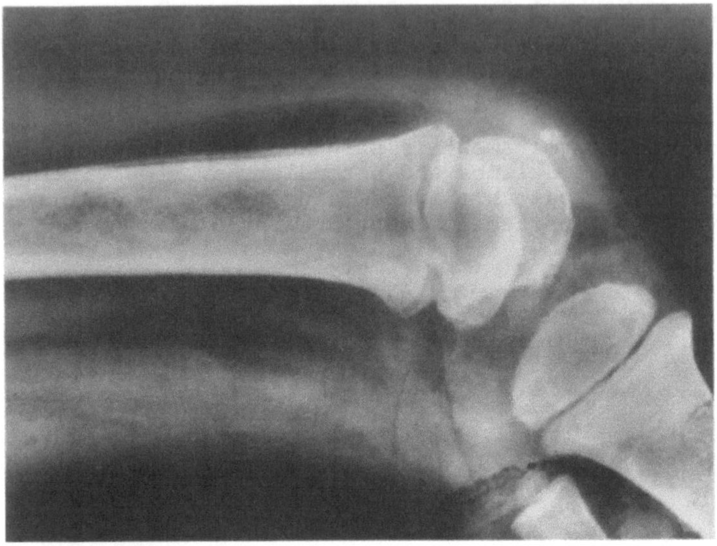

*Fig. 21. Femur showing subperiosteal invasion by metastatic neuroblastoma with elevation of periosteum*

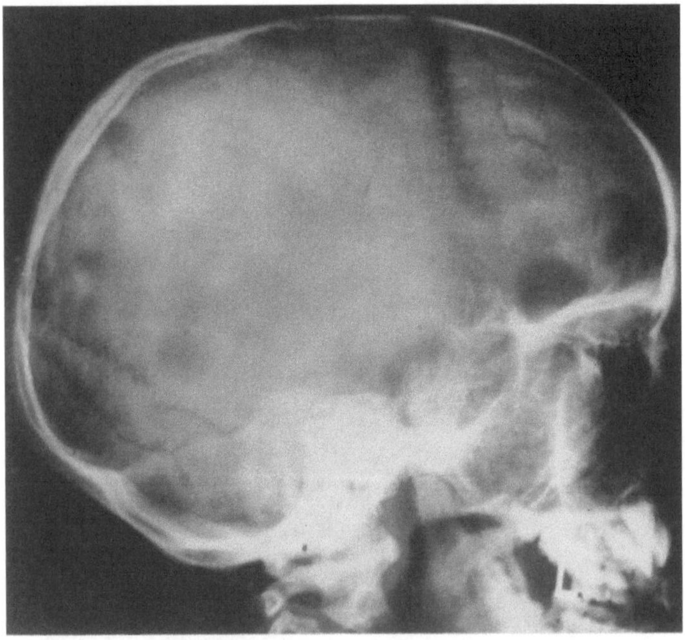

*Fig. 22. Metastatic neuroblastoma in base of the skull with radiating spicules of bone*

by a period of joint stiffness, which may be mistaken for Still's disease. Skeletal involvement is often associated with orbital deposits. Typically such deposits cause proptosis accompanied by local subcutaneous bruising, but sometimes the bruising may precede the proptosis by several weeks.

Hepatic metastases are usually symptomless. Occasionally they grow so rapidly that the liver enlargement may be obvious from day to day (a phenomenon seen also in lymphosarcoma). Lymph node involvement in the abdomen is also usually symptomless, but in the mediastinum it may cause respiratory and venous obstruction. The progressive spread from a primary near the kidneys to the para-aortic nodes, up through the diaphragm to the mediastinum and then to the cervical nodes, is quite typical of neuroblastoma.

When a neuroblastoma presents with anaemia and lymphadenopathy the clinical picture may at first suggest that the child is suffering from some disorder of the reticuloendothelial system. Examination of the marrow in such a case may reveal cells resembling reticulum cells and

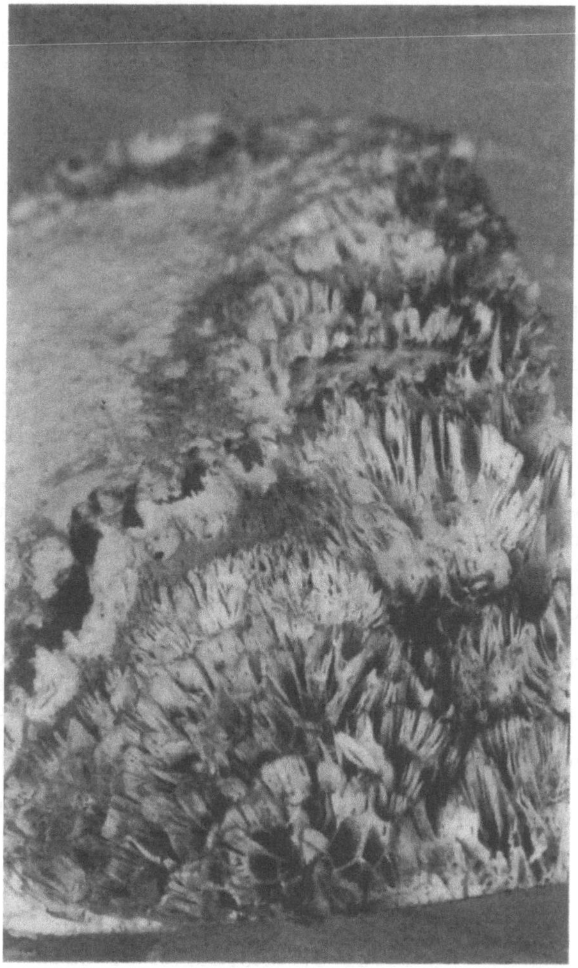

*Fig. 23. Calvarium from case of metastatic neuroblastoma showing bone spicules*

the diagnosis of "an unusual form of reticulosis" be made (PINEY et al., 1950). A mass in the left loin may be interpreted as splenomegaly. This syndrome is really due to widespread bone invasion by neuroblastoma; the loin mass being the primary tumour. In any child presenting with a widely metastasising tumour, examination of the catecholamine excretion should be carried out to exclude the possibility of a neuroblastoma.

Although anaemia in a child with neuroblastoma almost always indicates a bad prognosis, one Manchester case was an exception.
CTR.61/55. A girl aged 7 months, admitted to hospital with a month's history of pallor. Her haemoglobin was 5.4 gms/100 ml, RBC 1.9 million, WBC normal. The marrow was not examined. A localised neuroblastoma behind her right kidney was removed and she was given X-ray treatment to her abdomen. She remains alive and well 18 years later.

One case of neuroblastoma with myoclonic encephalopathy (the "Dancing Eyes syndrome") has been seen in Manchester. The patient is a 4-year-old girl with a highly differentiated thoracic tumour in whom symptoms had been present for one year prior to histological diagnosis. BRANDT et al. (1974) found 3 out of 42 cases of neuroblastoma with this syndrome and WILLIAMS et al. (1972) report a figure of 2%. During the period in which this one case was encountered in Manchester, 150 sympathetic tumours have been included in the Register.

The excretion of catecholamines and their metabolites appears to be less frequently elevated in tumours with cerebellar symptoms, and of 57 cases in Manchester in whom total catecholamines, noradrenaline, metadrenaline and HMMA were estimated, the case with the myoclonic encephalopathy was the only one where no increase was detected on repeated occasions.

## Differential Diagnosis of Neuroblastoma

The primitive neuroblast is an undistinguished-looking cell consisting merely of a nucleus surrounded by a thin layer of cytoplasm. Since most sympathetic tumours arise in those concentrations of sympathetic tissue beside the vertebral column and near the kidneys, the primary tumour may be confused with a Wilms' tumour or a lymphosarcoma. Radiologically, a distinguishing feature of a neuroblastoma is the presence of finely mottled calcification. Once the neuroblastoma has metastasised, its manifestations are protean. It may mimic other diseases causing enlarged liver, mediastinum or lymph nodes and may be confused with bone tumours or osteomyelitis or reticuloendothelial involvement of bone marrow.

Every pathologist encounters anaplastic tumours whose site of origin is uncertain and if these occur in children he may be tempted to diagnose neuroblastoma on very little evidence. This tendency is to be deplored; a tumour of the sympathetic system can be diagnosed only if there is evidence that some at least of the cells show definite neural differentiation. Before it was realised that sympathetic tumours secreted catecholamines, this evidence had to be purely histological and was sometimes difficult to obtain since there was no reliable staining method by means of which an immature neurite could be distinguished from an immature connective tissue fibre.

However, the demonstration that almost all neuroblastomas can be diagnosed by the level of excretion of catecholamines and related compounds has greatly simplified the position. Nowadays, if a child with neuroblastoma is properly investigated, it is practically always possible to make the diagnosis from the clinical, radiological and biochemical data. Thus, it is hardly ever justified to perform an operation merely to take a diagnostic biopsy in this disease. Such a procedure may be very dangerous in the case of a large mediastinal tumour and any child with metastatic neuroblastoma has enough to suffer without being subjected to an unnecessary operation.

Phaeochromocytoma

The clinical manifestations of the phaeochromocytoma are due not to pressure effects but to the secretory activity of the tumour which results in hypertension, hypermetabolism and hyperglycaemia. This secretory activity may vary from time to time in the same patient and appears to be stimulated by surgical procedures. Hypertension is the most dangerous effect and may be intermittent or sustained. Sweating may be a marked feature. Glycosuria, an abnormal glucose tolerance curve and polyuria may be caused by the disturbance in carbohydrate metabolism. For a more detailed account of the pathological and clinical features of the phaeochromocytoma in patients of all ages, the reader is referred to EVANS (1963). TEVETOGLU and LEE (1956) and CONE et al. (1957) review the literature of this tumour as it occurs in children.

The three children with phaeochromocytoma in the Registry all presented with severe hypertension associated with headache.
CTR.6/59. Boy, aged 12 years, who in November 1958 started with severe nocturnal headache and nausea. He also complained of excessive sweating. He had left papilloedema, but no localising neurological signs. Ventriculograms normal. BP - systolic 230 to 140, diastolic 195 to 120. Two months later he developed a left homonymous hemianopia. In February 1957 a phaeochromocytoma of the right adrenal, measuring 5 cm in diameter, was removed and the patient has remained well with a normal blood pressure ever since. The family history is significant. The patient's sister and his father's nephew and cousin had phaeochromocytomas. The patient's father and sister had Von Hippel-Lindau's disease.
CTR.17/59. Boy, aged 11 years. In December 1958 he started with severe nocturnal headaches accompanied by profuse sweating. Towards the end of January 1959 he started vomiting every day. He was admitted to hospital where he was found to have bilateral papilloedema. BP - systolic 200 to 130, diastolic 150 to 90. On March 1st he collapsed and he died soon after a ventriculogram (which was normal) had been performed. At autopsy phaeochromocytomas of both adrenals were found (left 41 gm, right 22 gm). There was no family history of phaeochromocytoma.
CTR.58/68. Boy, aged 13 years. He started in April 1968 with headaches which usually occurred in the morning. The systolic blood pressure varied between 170 and 190 and the diastolic between 100 and 125. In June 1968 laparotomy showed that the adrenals were normal but there was a phaeochromocytoma 3 x 4 cm in diameter adherent to the aorta and inferior vena cava at the level of L2. It was removed. The patient has remained well with a normal blood pressure ever since.

Usually the phaeochromocytoma is histologically benign, although it may be multifocal. However, acceptable cases of malignant phaeochromocytoma have been described, the most frequent modes of spread being to liver, lung, skeleton, abdominal and mediastinal lymph nodes (EVANS, 1963).

The hypertensive headaches and papilloedema due to this tumour may cause the diagnosis of an intracranial tumour or hypertension to be considered. In those cases in which there is profuse sweating the clinical picture may resemble thyrotoxicosis.

COURSE OF DISEASE

Since the phaeochromocytoma manifests itself by its secretory activity which bears little relationship to tumour size, it is impossible to measure its growth rate from the clinical course of the disease. However, some idea of the speed at which ganglioneuromas and neuroblastomas grow can be inferred from the clinical histories of the patients and the histological appearance of the tumours.

A mature ganglioneuroma shows no histological evidence of mitotic activity. However, it is possible that a tumour might enlarge due to an increase in the amount of nerve fibres or connective tissue or it might swell due to oedema. Only two of the 10 ganglioneuromas showed evidence of enlargement. One was in a 2-year-old boy (CTR.116/63) who was first noticed to have a cervical swelling in July 1963. This was not excised until January 1964, when it was found to measure 6 x 4 x 3 cm. The other was in a 5-year-old girl, who had always walked with a slight limp. A week prior to admission she developed paraparesis with loss of bladder control. At operation a dumb-bell ganglioneuroma extending from T12 - S3 was removed. Sections of the tumour showed no evidence of active growth. One child with a thoracic ganglioneuroma was kept under observation for 6 months before operation and during that time the tumour did not alter in size. In another case, the surgeon considered that he had only partially removed a thoracic ganglioneuroma but it has not recurred during 10 years postoperative surveillance.

In contrast with ganglioneuroma, the neuroblastoma grows rapidly. Histologically it contains mitotic figures. The time from diagnosis to death of the children with fatal neuroblastoma in the Register is shown in Table 11. It will be seen that only 2 of these survived for longer than 1 year.

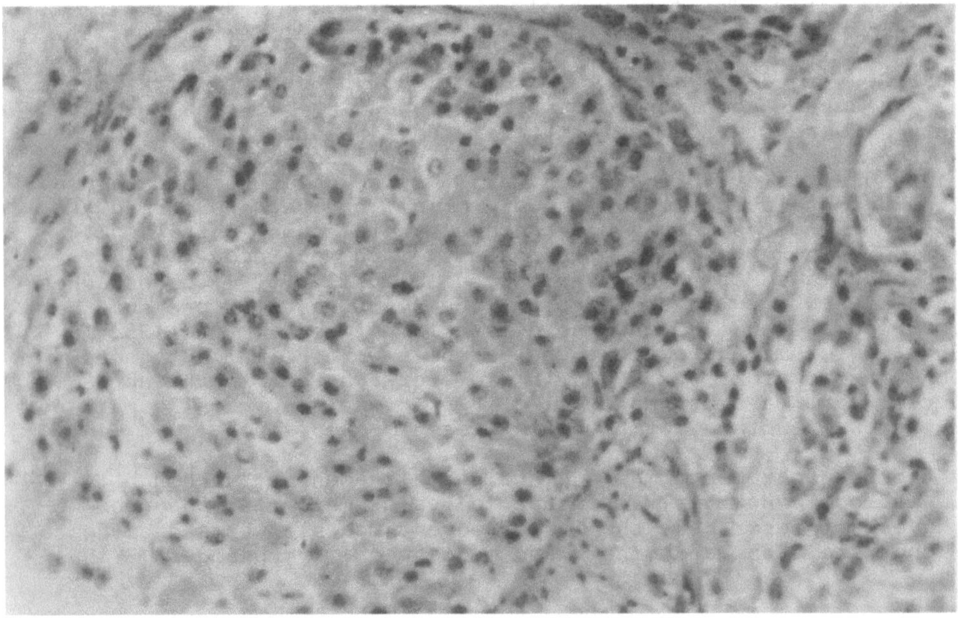

*Fig. 24. Cellular ganglioneuroma, possibly ganglioneuroblastoma (CTR.116/63) with poorly developed neurones, which showed some evidence of active growth (H. & E. X 250)*

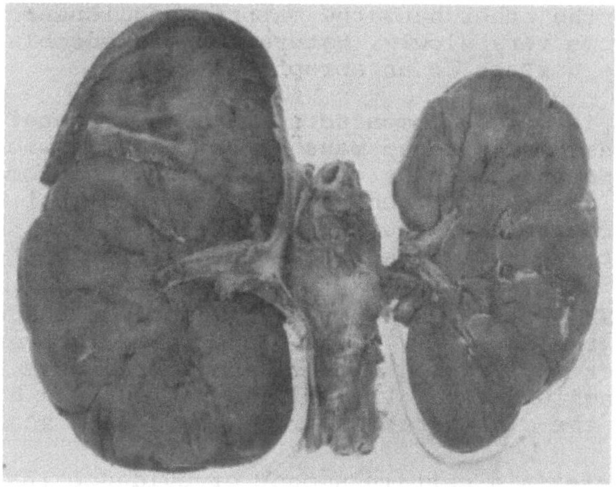

*Fig. 25a. Ganglioneuroma in the suprarenal gland found at autopsy. The child died with widespread neuroblastomatous deposits*

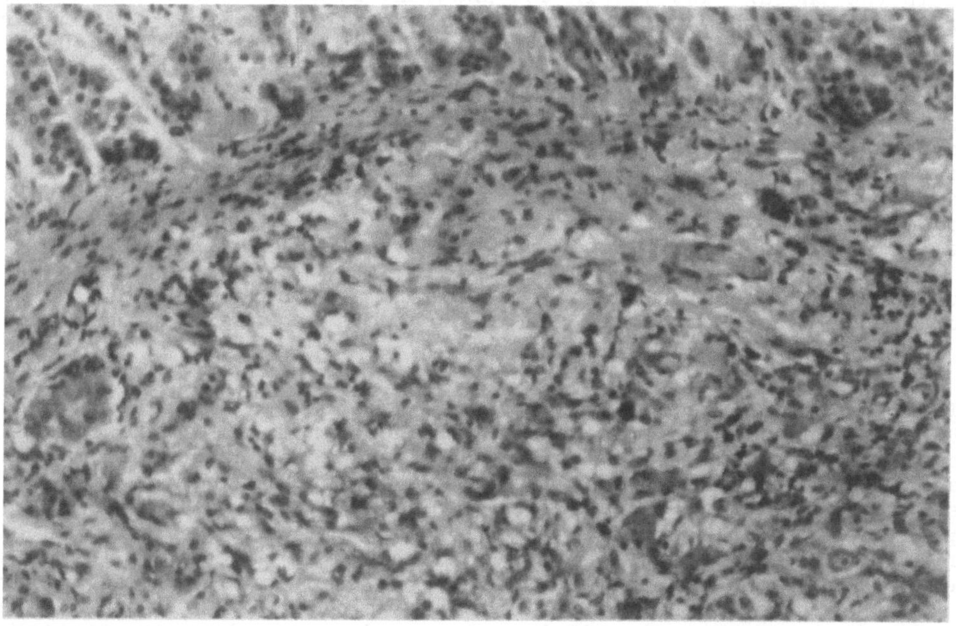

*Fig. 25b. Photomicrograph of suprarenal of same case showing medullary ganglioneuroma with intact cortex (H. & E. X 250)*

The most rapidly growing neuroblastoma was in a girl (CTR.69/59). At birth her abdomen was somewhat enlarged, but at the age of 1 month it had become so distended by the tumour that laparotomy was impossible.

## Maturation and Spontaneous Regression of Neuroblastoma

The striking feature of the growth rate of sympathetic tumours is that, on the one hand, the neuroblastoma grows and metastasizes rapidly while on the other hand the mature ganglioneuroma does not grow at all or grows very slowly. Maturation of neuroblasts to ganglion cells brings the disease to an abrupt halt.

It is quite common to see groups of ganglion cells in sections of neuroblastomas. In two Manchester children who died of widespread neuroblastoma the adrenals contained ganglioneuromas - presumably these were the primaries. In these cases it seemed that maturation and growth of the tumours were occurring at the same time, but unfortunately the maturation was not widespread enough to halt the disease.

CUSHING and WOLBACH (1927) described the case of a boy who, in 1911, at the age of 1, had a biopsy of a paravertebral neuroblastoma. A further exploration in 1921 showed that the tumour had changed into a ganglioneuroma. In 1957 the patient was again examined and a biopsy of the old operation site showed only scar tissue (FOX et al., 1959).

There is a certain amount of evidence that the site of the tumour may influence its tendency towards maturation. Six out of the 10 ganglioneuromas in the Register occurred in the chest and one was in the neck, whereas 78 out of the 101 neuroblastomas arose in the abdomen. STOUT (1947) reviewed 243 ganglioneuromas and found that 24 were in the neck, 62 in the thorax and 134 in the abdomen. STOWENS (1957), in an analysis of material in the Armed Forced Institute, reported that 38% of ganglioneuromas occurred in the chest compared with only 12% of neuroblastomas. The relative frequency of ganglioneuromas in the thorax may, of course, be an artefact since most of them are discovered by chance when the patient's chest is X-rayed, and they are more liable to be missed in the abdomen. However, it may be that sympathetic tumours above the diaphragm do have a greater tendency to mature. Sympathetic cells in the chest only have to migrate to the sympathetic chain, while in the abdomen many of them migrate further afield. When these two groups of cells become neoplastic, they may well behave differently.

Spontaneous regression of the neuroblastoma is not always due to maturation. In one Manchester case spontaneous regression probably played a part in the survival of one patient.

CTR.41/62. A girl, aged 11 months, was admitted to hospital in April 1962 with an abdominal mass and subcutaneous nodules in the chest and abdomen. The nodules were excised and found to be neuroblastoma metastases. Laparotomy revealed a left suprarenal neuroblastoma with liver metastases. Abdominal X-rays were given (2000 rads MV in 31 days). In April 1963 a nodule appeared on the scalp, but this was not treated. In August 1963 X-rays of the sphenoid showed an osteolytic lesion with new bone formation. A few weeks later the child's vision deteriorated rapidly and the sphenoidal lesion was irradiated (1900 rads in 3 days). At the same time Vitamin B12 2 mg i. m. alternate days was started and continued until early 1966. After 1963 the retro-orbital lesion gradually increased in size but there has been little change in the X-ray appearance since March 1965. However, proptosis has developed and the child is blind. Her general condition is excellent.

EVERSON and COLE (1966) from a review of the literature describe twenty-nine cases of spontaneously regressed neuroblastoma - in 5 of these there was maturation of the tumours. The most striking feature of these cases was that they all occurred in very young patients - 21 out of the 29 children were under 6 months old and none of them was over 2 years old. It seems likely that this tendency towards spontaneous regression of neuroblastomas in infants is in some way connected with the better prognosis of this disease in children under 2 years old.

## The Frequency of Spontaneous Regression of Neuroblastoma

Before 1963 it was considered that spontaneous regression of neuroblastoma was a very rare phenomenon. However, in that year BECKWITH and PERRIN (1963) reported that amongst 1571 autopsies done on infants under the age of three months at the Los Angeles and Cincinnati Children's Hospitals there were seven instances of in situ neuroblastoma. If it is assumed that this is representative of the incidence of neuroblastoma during the first three months of life, it means that approximately one in every 250 infants in this age group have the tumour, but only one in 10,000 manifest the disease later. In other words, 39 out of every 40 neuroblastomas present at birth regress spontaneously.

Table 10. Children with neuroblastoma metastatic to bone

| | Age at diagnosis | | | | | | | | | | | | | | |
|---|---|---|---|---|---|---|---|---|---|---|---|---|---|---|---|
| Age (years) | <1 | 1 | 2 | 3 | 4 | 5 | 6 | 7 | 8 | 9 | 10 | 11 | 12 | 13 | 14 |
| No. Cases | 5 | 13 | 5 | 12 | 6 | 1 | 2 | 3 | 2 | 0 | 0 | 0 | 0 | 0 | 1 |

## The Hutchison and Pepper Syndromes

The liver and bones are two of the common sites of metastases of neuroblastoma. PEPPER (1901) described six cases in which spread to the liver was a marked feature, while HUTCHISON (1907) reported 10 in which there were osseous metastases. Although the clinical manifestations of neuroblastoma must not be too sharply divided into these two syndromes, some authors (WILBERDINK, 1957; SOFFER et al., 1961) have pointed out that the PEPPER syndrome occurs more frequently in infancy, whereas the

Table 11. Neuroblastomas

| | Time from diagnosis to death | | | | | | | | | | | | | | |
|---|---|---|---|---|---|---|---|---|---|---|---|---|---|---|---|
| Time (months) | <1 | 1 | 2 | 3 | 4 | 5 | 6 | 7 | 8 | 9 | 10 | 11 | 12 | 13-22 | 23 |
| All neuroblastomas | 25 | 12 | 8 | 10 | 7 | 6 | 3 | 6 | 1 | 1 | 0 | 0 | 1 | 0 | 1 |
| Neuroblastomas with bone metastases | 9 | 10 | 6 | 6 | 5 | 4 | 2 | 4 | 1 | 1 | 0 | 0 | 0 | 0 | 1 |

HUTCHISON type occurs in older children. In the Manchester series there were only six children who presented with massive liver involvement without bone metastases and all of them were less than 4 months old. The age of the 50 Manchester children with the HUTCHISON syndrome is given in Table 10. Thus it seems that massive liver involvement is much rarer than spread to bones and tends to occur at a younger age.

If bone metastases are going to develop they are usually apparent early in the clinical course of the disease. In 41 of the 50 children skeletal involvement was present at clinical onset while in nine it developed later on. All except one of the children with skeletal metastases in the Register have died - 98% within 1 year of the first sign of a bone lesion (see Table 11).

The history of the 1 child who died nearly 2 years after the first sign of skeletal invasion is as follows:
CTR.62/61. Boy, aged 6 years. Admitted to hospital in May 1961 with a 6 months' history of abdominal pain. Laparotomy revealed a large inoperable retroperitoneal tumour. A biopsy showed this to be a neuroblastoma and this diagnosis was confirmed by a high catecholamine excretion. Postoperative irradiation caused the mass to disappear. At the end of June 1961 there were X-ray changes in both femora suggestive of metastases, but these did not alter up to April 1962 when suddenly there was an increase in the size and number of the bone lesions. Palliative irradiation was given but by December 1962 the child was very ill and had the typical picture of the HUTCHISON'S syndrome. In spite of vincristine, the catecholamines rose and the child died in April 1963.

The fact that the femoral lesions remained unchanged for 9 months suggests that the long survival of the child was due either to the nature of the tumour or some host resistance rather than to the treatment given.

## PROGNOSIS OF SYMPATHETIC TUMOURS IN MANCHESTER CHILDREN 1954 - 1968

### Ganglioneuromas

All the 10 children with ganglioneuromas were treated satisfactorily by surgical excision of their tumours and remain alive and well.

### Phaeochromocytomas

Two of the 3 children with phaeochromocytomas remain well, having been treated by surgery alone. The other child died while being investigated and before any treatment was given.

### Neuroblastomas

Thirteen of the children with neuroblastomas are alive and 88 have died. In 7 cases the tumours were small incidental autopsy findings in infants who had died from non-neoplastic causes. In one child death was due to bronchopneumonia 3 years after the neuroblastoma was treated and no residual tumour was found at autopsy.

The treatment given to these patients is shown in Table 12. It will be seen that in the period under review reliance was placed much more on local treatment than on chemotherapy.

Table 12. Treatment[a] given to Manchester children with neuroblastoma 1954 - 1968

| | Alive | Dead | Total |
|---|---|---|---|
| Surgery alone | 2 | 6 | 8 |
| Surgery and XRT | 10 | 5 | 15 |
| XRT alone | 0 | 33 | 33 |
| Surgery or XRT with vincristine or cyclophosphamide | 1 | 10 | 11 |
| Surgery or XRT with actinomycin D | 0 | 2 | 2 |
| Vincristine, cyclophosphamide, or actinomycin D only | 0 | 4 | 4 |
| No treatment | 0 | 21 | 21 |
| | 13 | 81 | 94 |

[a]Treatment with Vitamin B12 has been ignored

All those with fatal neuroblastomas died within 2 years of diagnosis (see Table 11) and this agrees with the findings in other centres (GROSS et al., 1959; EVANS et al., 1971). The overall 2-year survival rate in the Manchester cases was 14/94 (15%).

The following factors influenced the prognosis:

1. The age of the patient
2. The extent of the disease, particularly the presence of bone metastases
3. The histological appearance of the tumour
4. The site of the primary

In analysing the effect of these factors and their relationship to each other, 83 cases in which the tumour was examined histologically are considered. The remaining 18 cases (7 in which the tumours were incidental autopsy findings and 11 diagnosed purely on clinical or biochemical evidence) are excluded.

## 1. Age of Patient

The prognosis was better in younger children (Table 13). Children aged 6 months to 1 year seem to have the best survival rate. Only 3 children

Table 13. Neuroblastoma: Relationship between patient's age and survival rate

| Age | No. in group | Number alive at: 1 year | 3 years |
|---|---|---|---|
| 0 < 6 months | 10 | 2 | 2 |
| 6 months < 1 year | 11 | 6 | 6 |
| 1 < 2 years | 17 | 3 | 3 |
| 2 < 3 years | 8 | 2 | 2 |
| 3 < 4 years | 13 | 1 | 1 |
| 4 years + | 24 | 3 | 0 |

who were over 2 years old at diagnosis have survived and all three had tumours showing a considerable evidence of maturation (ganglioneuroblastomas). The 3-year survival rate in children aged less than two years was 28.9% and the difference between this and the survival rate in those over 4 years old (0%) is statistically highly significant ($\underline{P}$ = 0.004). However, the number of children aged between 2 and 4 years is too small for statistical comparison with the survival rates in the younger and older age groups.

## 2. Extent of the Disease

The striking effect of the presence of bone metastases on prognosis has already been noted. Only one of the 50 children who had X-ray evidence of bone involvement still survives. In this case the bone metastases appeared some time after the neuroblastoma was originally diagnosed.

EVANS et al. (1971) proposed the following system of clinical staging of neuroblastoma, which has prognostic significance and may be used for comparing the results of treatment.

Stage 1. Tumour confined to the organ or structure of origin.

Stage 2. Tumour extending in continuity beyond the organ or structure of origin but not crossing the midline. Regional lymph nodes on the same side may be involved. For tumours arising in midline structures penetration beyond the capsule and involvement of lymph nodes on the same side shall be considered Stage 2.

Stage 3. Tumour extending in continuity beyond the midline. Regional lymph nodes may be involved bilaterally. For tumours arising in midline structures bilateral extension of any sort shall be considered Stage 3.

Stage 4. Remote disease involving skeleton, organs, soft tissues or distant lymph node groups, etc. (see Stage 4 S).

Stage 4 S. Patients who would otherwise be Stages 1 or 2, but who have remote disease confined only to one or more of the following sites: liver, skin, or bone marrow (without radiographic evidence of bone metastases on complete skeletal survey).

To apply this system of clinical staging to any series, it is necessary that surgical exploration with lymph node biopsies and bone marrow examination should be carried out on all children except those in obvious Stage 4. Although this was done in only a few of the Manchester cases prior to 1969, it was possible to assign with reasonable certainty a clinical stage at diagnosis to 78 of the 83 cases (Table 14).

Table 14. Neuroblastomas: Relation between clinical stage at diagnosis and survival

| Clinical stage | No. in group | Crude survival rate at: 1 year | 3 years |
|---|---|---|---|
| 1 | 7 | 7/7 | 7/7 |
| 2 | 5 | 3/5 | 2/5 |
| 3 | 18 | 6/18 | 4/18 |
| 4 | 43 | 0% | 0% |
| 4 S | 5 | 1/5 | 1/5 |
| Not known | 5 | 0/5 | 0/5 |

It is quite obvious from this Table that survival depends on the extent of the disease as measured by clinical stage. The following differences in crude survival rates between adjacent stages are statistically significant: stage 1 vs stage 2 ($P < 0.05$) and stage 3 vs stage 4 ($P \approx 0.001$).

The survival rates of the Manchester cases were not as good as those reported by EVANS et al. (1971) in the Children's Cancer Study Group A. In particular these authors reported that 12 out of 16 children with stage 4 S disease survived compared with only 1 out of 5 in the Manchester series. Patients with stage 4 S neuroblastoma are usually under 1 year old and the fact so few of the Manchester children in this group survived might have been due to the unnecessarily pessimistic attitude which has sometimes been taken by paediatricians to the treatment of infants with cancer.

## 3. The Histological Appearance of the Tumour

MARTIN and BECKWITH (1968) and MÄKINEN (1972) reported that the prognosis of neuroblastoma is related to the maturation of the tumour cells. LAUDER and AHERNE (1972) suggested that a more important factor was the degree of lymphocyte infiltration of the tumour. The 83 Manchester cases were divided into the following histological grades:

Grade 1. Tumours showing a mixed pattern of undifferentiated cells and mature ganglion cells.

Grade 2. Tumours showing a mixed pattern of undifferentiated cells and some cells showing partial differentiation towards ganglion cells as evidenced by any of the following:
a) Vesicular nuclei
b) The presence of nucleoli
c) Increase in cytoplasmic-nuclear ratio
d) Formation of cytoplasmic processes

Grade 3. Completely undifferentiated tumours.

Table 15 shows there is an obvious difference between the survival rates for grade 1 and grades 2 and 3 combined. This difference is statistically highly significant, $P \ll 0.001$. Although (Table 16) histological grade was highly correlated with clinical stage (correlation

Table 15. Neuroblastomas: Effect of histological grade on survival

| Histological grade | No. in group | Crude survival rate at: 1 year | 3 years |
|---|---|---|---|
| 1 | 13 | 9/13 | 9/13 |
| 2 | 22 | 13.6% | 9.1% |
| 3 | 48 | 10.4% | 6.2% |

Table 16. Neuroblastomas: Relationship between histological grading and clinical stage at diagnosis

| Histological grade | Clinical stage at diagnosis: 1 | 2 | 3 | 4 | 4 S | not known |
|---|---|---|---|---|---|---|
| 1 | 4 | 2 | 3 | 2 | 2 | 0 |
| 2 | 2 | 1 | 7 | 10 | 1 | 1 |
| 3 | 1 | 2 | 8 | 31 | 2 | 4 |

coefficient r = 0.47, P << 0.001), an analysis of covariance showed that, even after eliminating the effect of stage on survival, the effect of histological grading was still statistically significant ($P < 0.05$).

The tumours were also placed in three groups according to the degree of lymphocyte infiltration (Table 17). None of the differences between

Table 17. Neuroblastomas: Relationship between lymphocyte infiltration and survival rate

| Lymphocyte infiltration grading | No. in group | Crude survival rate at: 6 months | 1 year | 2 years | 3 years |
|---|---|---|---|---|---|
| 0 | 35 | 20.0% | 14.3% | 14.3% | 14.3% |
| + | 38 | 44.7% | 28.9% | 21.1% | 21.1% |
| ++ | 10 | 2/10 | 2/10 | 2/10 | 2/10 |
| Total | 83 | 31.3% | 21.7% | 18.1% | 18.1% |

the groups is statistically significant: lymphocytic infiltration grading does not seem to affect survival.

## 4. Site of the Tumour

Most children (63/83 or 76%) had disease in the abdomen (Table 18). The numbers of children with disease in sites other than abdomen were

Table 18. Neuroblastomas: Relationship between site and survival

| Site | No. in Group | Crude survival rate at: 1 year | 3 years |
|---|---|---|---|
| Abdomen[a] | 63 | 14.3% | 12.7% |
| Chest | 13 | 3/13 | 2/13 |
| Neck | 5 | 4/5 | 4/5 |
| Not stated | 2 | 1/2 | 0/2 |

[a]including one child with abdomen and chest primaries

too small to enable a strict comparison of survival to be made between the different sites. However, the fact that 4 of the 5 children with tumours in the neck have survived, suggests that neuroblastomas in this site have a better prognosis.

## Other Factors

No correlations were found between age and stage, histological grading and age, and histological grading and site.

The above findings are discussed by HUGHES et al. (1974) and Tables 14-18 are from this article.

## CLINICAL MANAGEMENT

### Ganglioneuroma

All the Manchester children with ganglioneuromas were treated satisfactorily by surgical excision of the tumours.

### Neuroblastoma

Unlike most other solid tumours of childhood the prognosis for neuroblastoma has altered very little in the last decade. This is clearly due to the fact that about two-thirds of all cases were widely disseminated at the time of diagnosis (EVANS et al., 1971), and while many neuroblastomas are sensitive to chemotherapy there is no evidence to suggest that it is effective in eradicating disease as has been shown to be the case in Wilms' tumours and embryonic sarcomas (SUTOW, 1973; GHAVIMI et al., 1973). At present it is only possible to prolong life in disseminated cases by combinations of surgery, radiotherapy and chemotherapy but new chemotherapeutic regimes are under study in many centres and may be more effective. The studies on the immunological aspects of neuroblastomas hold out some hope that immunotherapy may prove useful in the future (BILL, 1969; HELLSTRÖM et al., 1970).

The use of Vitamin B12 was reported by BODIAN (1963) as showing a 50% response rate, but his results have not been upheld either in British or American studies (LANGMAN, 1970; SAWITSKY and DESPOSITO, 1965). The initial good results reported by BODIAN were probably due to the large number of young children in his series.

There are many reports of the use of single agents and combinations of various cytotoxic drugs. In most of these studies there are objective regressions of the order of 30% - 80%, but these are long-lasting or curative in very few instances (FARBER et al., 1951; PINKEL, 1961; PINKEL, 1962; JAMES and GEORGE, 1964; JAMES et al., 1965; EVANS et al., 1969).

The method of management of a child with neuroblastoma depends largely on the extent of disease at the time of diagnosis and also to a lesser degree on the age of the child. A programme of investigation similar to that outlined in the chapter on renal tumours is necessary to establish the diagnosis and extent of disease so that accurate staging can be achieved. As it is most unusual for either catecholamines or their metabolites not to be raised in cases of neuroblastoma, diagnosis should rarely be difficult or delayed, and except where pressure symptoms on the spinal cord call for urgent operative intervention, time should be spent in the ascertainment of the extent of disease. IVP, complete skeletal surveys and bone marrow aspiration are essential investigations. Radiologically obvious bone metastases indicate a very poor prognosis. Bone marrow involvement, if extensive, is also a bad prognostic finding, but can be eradicated by chemotherapy in some instances, and may also be a feature of Stage 4 S cases. The invasive nature of the primary tumour tends to make the neuroblastoma a much more difficult tumour to resect than a Wilms' tumour or embryonic sarcoma. Nevertheless, in patients with Stage 1, 2 and 3 disease every effort should be made to remove as much of the primary tumour as is possible. Incomplete removal has been shown to be associated with regression of remaining tumour (KOOP et al., 1955; KOOP and JOHNSON, 1971). In certain instances where preoperative radiological studies suggest that resection will not be possible, chemotherapy and/or radiotherapy can be given prior to surgery and in these cases the tumour may well become more easily removable.

Even in Stage 4 disease some people feel that removal of the primary tumour is indicated and certainly in Manchester this procedure has been associated with diminution in size of bone metastases and reduction in the pain in these lesions, although this has always been temporary. Radiotherapy has considerable effect on painful bones and gland masses.

## Surgery

When a neuroblastoma has an extension through an intervertebral foramen into the vertebral canal and causes cord compression, the spinal component must be dealt with first as a matter of urgency.

The operative treatment of abdominal neuroblastoma is made difficult by the variable site of origin and the tendency to spread retroperitoneally, especially towards the midline in front of the aorta, with encroachment on the large arteries. The relation of the tumour to other structures should be evaluated preoperatively as far as possible by X-rays and aortagrams. The anaesthetist must be prepared to deal with problems due to the hypertension which occurs occasionally. The operative approach should be transperitoneal since this gives the best opportunity to evaluate fully the extent of the tumour. It also provides the best chance of satisfactory removal with, in some cases, primary division of the venous drainage. A transverse or vertical incision is chosen, depending on the shape of the tumour, and the approach is similar to that for a Wilms' tumour. With right-sided tumours, an incision is made into the peritoneum posteriorly so that the colon and duodenum can be displaced medially and downwards. If possible the venous drainage should be divided first and if there is danger of serious bleeding the inferior vena cava must be isolated and controlled below and above the area. The kidney may or may not be removed with the tumour.

The colon is also mobilised if the tumour is left-sided, but in addition the spleen and body of the pancreas may have to be lifted forwards. A reasonable attempt must be made to remove the tumour but the danger to major vessels must be kept in mind, because the position of these vessels is often altered. Where the mass is not removable, incision into the capsule will allow much of the tumour to be removed piecemeal with the help of the sucker. The tissue is often friable, necrotic and haemorrhagic and comes away fairly easily.

With thoracic neuroblastomas the surgical approach depends on the exact site and on which side of the chest it projects. A curved incision over the upper sternum is useful. Its vertical limb runs down the midline and at the upper and lower ends it curves laterally to one or other side. A flap of skin and muscle is cleared to the side and the thorax is entered by incising a number of costal cartilages in a vertical line. This gives a good approach to the upper mediastinum. The tumours in this area are often encapsulated and not too vascular and can be removed despite the proximity of important structures.

## Radiotherapy

The irradiation should be on a regional basis - the area and volume treated being decided mainly on the site and, to a lesser extent, on the size of the primary. The dose delivered is of the order of 2500-3000 rads in 3-5 weeks. In the neck parallel opposed fields up to 15 cm long are used, giving a midline dose of 2500 rads at 300 KV or 3000 rads at 4 MV in three weeks, the trachea being shielded from the front field.

If the primary is in the chest or abdomen, the whole chest or whole abdomen should be irradiated to a dosage of 2500 rads at 300 KV or 3000 rads at 4 MV in 5 weeks. This treatment should be given even if there is invasion of the liver or vertebral canal. In abdominal cases the opposite kidney should be shielded after 2000 rads and hips shielded for the whole of the treatment. While it is possible, particularly with megavoltage, to treat in one volume a neuroblastoma which is in both the abdomen and the chest, the time needed to get in 2500 or 3000 rads would have to be extended to 7-8 weeks.

Although the neuroblastoma is usually sensitive to these doses, in some of the Manchester children the tumours have recurred in the irradiated areas. Rarely a primary may be completely radioresistant as is seen in the following case:
CTR.80/60. Boy, aged 8 years. Admitted to hospital on 21/6/60 with a large abdominal neuroblastoma. X-ray treatment was started on 4/7/60, but it was stopped after 3 days as the mass appeared to fluctuate in size. On 13/7/60 laparotomy was performed, but the tumour could not be removed. Irradiation was started again on 25/7/60 and completed on 3/9/60 when 2500 rads had been given. The abdominal mass never disappeared and fungated through the laparotomy wound. On 22/11/60 bone metastases began to appear and the child died on 14/1/61. At autopsy the abdominal tumour weighed 2240 g and sections showed that it consisted of actively growing neuroblastoma.

In addition to its curative role, irradiation is extremely valuable as a palliative treatment, particularly when the neuroblastoma has spread to the bones or orbits.

## Chemotherapy

Most experience has been gained with the use of cyclophosphamide and vincristine. The reported series show that survival time can be increased but none demonstrate any improvement in cure rate in the age group over 2 years at presentation. The cure rate in those under this age may be improved but because of the frequency of spontaneous cure, regression and maturation known to occur in this age group, it is difficult to assess accurately the effects of chemotherapy in small series (PINKEL et al., 1968; SUTOW et al., 1970; HELSON, 1972).

Even though accurate staging of the disease is simple, it is not possible to delineate a definitive plan of treatment stage by stage because of the great variation in the resectability of the tumours. In general terms, therefore, it is considered best to attempt as major a removal as possible as a primary procedure except in Stage 4 disease, and to follow this by chemotherapy and radiation. In Stage 1 cases where removal is complete no further therapy is indicated. In Manchester, vincristine and cyclophosphamide in the following regimen have been used in Stage 3 and 4 cases and in Stage 1 and 2 disease not completely resected.

| | | |
|---|---|---|
| Vincristine | 1.5 mg/m$^2$ IV | weekly for 6 weeks. |
| Cyclophosphamide | 600 mg/m$^2$ (IV or PO) | weekly for 6 weeks. |

The drugs are then alternated at weekly intervals for as long as the disease is controlled or for 6 months if there is no evidence of spread. The time interval between doses is then increased to 14 day intervals for a further six months.

More recently we have used adriamycin in conjunction with vincristine and cyclophosphamide initially, giving 20 $mg/m^2$ at weekly intervals for 6 weeks. In a small number of cases where there has been very satisfactory regression of disease we have continued the 3 drugs over 4 to 6 weeks increasing the dosage of adriamycin to 60 $mg/m^2$ on this regime. There is, however, a moderate degree of toxicity, manifest with vomiting, alopecia, and bone marrow depression.

Standardised trials of treatment are difficult to organise for neuroblastoma because of the multiple modes of presentation and the individual response. Progress in the future would seem to lie in the use of well tried and new drugs in ways which will increase the pool of actively dividing cells and allow for greater cell kill. These methods coupled with efforts to enhance the immune response may brighten the picture in this tumour.

## PHAEOCHROMOCYTOMA

This tumour is so rare in childhood that it is not possible to discuss its management in any detail. Its association with certain inherited disorders has already been discussed in Chapter 2. The presentation of phaeochromocytoma in childhood does not usually vary from the classic manifestations in adults and confirmation of diagnosis can be made by the presence of raised catecholamines and their metabolites.

The treatment should consist of removal of the primary tumour and if this is achieved in its entirety the hypertension settles and the prognosis appears good. It should be remembered, however, that the tumour may be multicentric in origin. Truly malignant phaeochromocytomas are only considered to be diagnosable when there is evidence of metastatic spread to other organs. Information regarding the effects of radiotherapy and chemotherapy in these cases is rare but it seems reasonable to suppose that a response could be expected.

## REFERENCES


ARMSTRONG, M. D., McMILLAN, A., SHAW, K. N. F.: Biochim. Biophys. Acta 25, 422 (1957)

ARMSTRONG, M. D., SHAW, K. N. F., WALL, P. E.: J. Biol. Chem. 218, 293 (1956)

BARSON, A. J., HODGE, J. S.: Develop. Med. Child Neurol. 13, Supp. 25 19 (1971)

BECKWITH, J. B., PERRIN, E. V.: Am. J. Path. 43, 1089 (1963)

BELL, M.: The Clinical Chemistry of the Monoamines (West-European Symposium on Clin. Chem. 1962). VARLEY, H., GOWENLOCK, A. H. (eds.), London: Elsevier, 1962, p. 82

BELL, M.: Neuroblastomas - Biochemical Studies. Recent Results in Cancer Research, BOHUON, C. (Ed.). Berlin: Springer 1966, Vol. II, p. 42

BELL, M., HORROCKS, R. H., VARLEY, H.: Practical Clinical Biochemistry 2nd ed., VARLEY, H. (ed.) 1958, p. 528, Heinemann (London)

BELL, M., STEWARD, J. K.: Lancet I, 1061 (1961)

BILL, A. H.: Surgery 66, 415 (1969)

BILL, A. H., BECKWITH, J. B., HARTMANN, J. R.: J. Nat. Canc. Inst. 43, 1221 (1969)

BLACKLOCK, J. W. S.: J. Path. Bact. 39, 27 (1934)

BLASCHKO, H.: J. Physiol. 96, 50 (1939)

BODIAN, M.: Arch. Dis. Child. 38, 606 (1963)

BOHUON, C., GUERINOT, F.: Clin. Chim. Acta 14, 414 (1966)

BRANDT, S., CARLSEN, N., GLENTING, P., HELWEG-CARLSEN, J.: Develop. Med. Child. Neurol. 16, 286 (1974)

BRAY, P. F., ZITER, F. A., LAHEY, M. E., MYERS, G. G.: J. Pediatr. 75, 983 (1969)

BROUGHTON, P. M. G., DYKES, J. R. W., HOLT, S., RIDLEY, J. W., STEEL, A. E.: J. Clin. Path. 23, 246 (1970)

BURDMAN, J. A., GOLDSTEIN, M. N.: J. Nat. Cancer Inst. 33, 123 (1964)

CONE, T. E., ALLEN, M. S., PEARSON, H. A.: Ped. 19, 44 (1957)

CROUT, J. R., SJOERDSMA, A.: J. Clin. Invest. 43, 94 (1964)

CUSHING, H., WOLBACH, S. B.: Amer. J. Path. 3, 203 (1927)

DAHMS, W. T., GRAY, G., VRANA, M., NEW, M. I.: Am. J. of Dis. Child. 125, 608 (1973)

DE ROBERTIS, E., FERREIRA, A. V.: Exp. Cell Res. 12, 568 (1957)

ENGEL, A., VON EULER, U. S.: Lancet 2, 387 (1950)

EVANS, A. E., BLORE, J., HADLEY, R., TANINDI, S.: Pediatrics 47, 913 (1971)

EVANS, A. E., D'ANGIO, G. J., RANDOLPH, J. A.: Cancer 27, 374 (1971)

EVANS, A. E., HEYN, R. M., NEWTON, W. A., LEIKIN, S. L.: JAMA 207, 1325 (1969)

EVANS, A. R.: J. Clin. Path. 18, 54 (1965)

EVANS, R. W.: In: The Clinical Chemistry of the Monoamines. VARLEY, H., GOWENLOCK, A. H. (eds.). London: Elsevier, 1963, p. 48

EVERSON, T. C., COLE, W. H.: In: Spontaneous Regression of Cancer. Philadelphia: W. B. Saunders Co., 1966, Chap. 3

FARBER, S.: Am. J. Dis. Child. 82, 239 (1951)

FOX, F., DAVIDSON, J., THOMAS, L. B.: Cancer 12, 108 (1959)

GHAVIMI, F., EXELBY, P. R., D'ANGIO, G. J., WHITMORE, W. F., LIEBERMAN, P. H., LEWIS Jr., J. L., MIKÉ, V., MURPHY, M. L.: Cancer 32, 1178 (1973)

GITLOW, S. E., BERTANI, L. M., GREENWOOD, S. M., WONG, B. L., DZIEDZIC, S. W.: J. Ped. 81, 1112 (1972)

GITLOW, S. E., BERTANI, L. M., RAUSEN, A., GRIBETZ, D., DZIEDZIC, S.W.: Cancer 25, 1377 (1970)

GITLOW, S. E., ORNSTEIN, L., MENDLOWITZ, M., KHASSIS, S., KRUK, E.: Amer. J. Med. 28, 921 (1960)

GJESSING, L. R.: Lancet 2, 1281 (1963)

GJESSING, L. R.: Scand. J. Clin. Lab. Invest. 15, 463 (1963)

GJESSING, L. R.: Scand. J. Clin. Lab. Invest. 16, 661 (1964)

GOLDSTEIN, M., FREEDMAN, L. S., BOHUON, A. C., GUERINOT, F.: New Eng. J. Med. 286, 1123 (1972)

GOLDSTEIN, M., JOH, T. H., GANG, H.: In: 7th Int. Congr. Clin. Chem. Geneva/Evian 1969, Basle: Karger 1970, Vol. III, p. 78

GOLDSTEIN, M.: Recent Results in Cancer Research. BOHUON, C. (ed.), Berlin: Springer, 1966, Vol. II, p. 66

GROSS, R. E., FARBER, S., MARTIN, L. W.: Pediatrics 23, 1179 (1959)

HELLSTRÖM, I., HELLSTRÖM, K. E., BILL, A. H., PIERCE, G., YANG, J.P.S.: Inter. J. Cancer 6, 172 (1970)

HELSON, L.: Cancer Chemotherapy Reports 56, 499 (1972)

HINGERTY, D.: Lancet 1, 766 (1957)

HUGHES, M., MARSDEN, H. B., PALMER, M. K.: Cancer 34, 1706-1711 (1974)

HUTCHISON, R.: Quart. J. Med. 1, 33 (1907)

JAMES, D. H., GEORGE, P.: J. Ped. 64, 534 (1964)

JAMES, D. H., HUSTU, O., WRENN, E. L., PINKEL, D.: JAMA 194, 103 (1965)

KÄSER, H., BETTEX, M., VON STUDNITZ, W.: Arch. Dis. Child. 39, 168 (1964)

KENNY, F. M., STAVRIDES, A., VOORHESS, M. L., KLEIN, R.: Am. J. Dis. Child. 113, 611 (1967)

KOGUT, M. D., DONNELL, G. N.: Pediatrics 28, 566 (1961)

KOOP, C. E., JOHNSON, D. J.: J. Ped. Surg. 6, 595 (1971)

KOOP, C. E., KIESEWETTER, W. B., HORN, R. C.: Pediatrics 16, 652 (1955)

KUMAR, S., STEWARD, J. K., WAGHE, M., PEARSON, D., EDWARDS, D. C., FENTON, R. L., GRIFFITH, A. H.: J. Ped. Surg. 5, 18 (1970)

LA BROSSE, E. H.: J. Ped. Surg. 3, 148 (1968)

LANGMAN, H. J. S.: Arch. Dis. Child. 45, 385 (1970)

LAUDER, I., AHERNE, W.: Brit. J. Cancer 26, 321 (1972)

LEONARD, A. S., ROBACK, S. A., NESBIT, M. E., FRIER, E.: J. Ped. Surg. 7, 528 (1972)

LEVI-MONTALCINI, R., ANGELETTI, P. U.: Physiol. Rev. 48, 534 (1968)

McKENDRICK, T., EDWARDS, R.W.H.: Arch. Dis. Child. 40, 418 (1965)

McKIBBEN, B., O'GORMAN, L., DUCKWORTH, T.: J. Clin. Path. 22, 687 (1969)

MÄKINEN, J.: Cancer 29, 1637 (1972)

MARSDEN, H. B.: In: Clinical Chemistry of the Monoamines. VARLEY, H., GOWENLOCK A. (eds.), London: Elsevier, 1963, p. 71

MARTIN, R. F., BECKWITH, J. B.: J. Ped. Surg. 3, 161 (1968)

MASON, G. A., HART-MERCER, J., MILLAR, E. J., STRANG, L. B., WYNNE, N. A.: Lancet 2, 322 (1957)

MISUGI, K., MISUGI, N., NEWTON, A. W.: Arch. Pathol. 86, 160 (1968)

PEPPER, W.: Am. J. med. Sci. 121, 287 (1901)

PINEY, A., MALLARMÉ, J., ROSS, M. S.: J. Clin. Path. 3, 230 (1950)

PINKEL, D.: Cancer 14, 36 (1961)

PINKEL, D.: Cancer 15, 42 (1962)

PINKEL, D., PRATT, C., HOLTON, C., JAMES, D., WRENN, E., HUSTU, O.: J. Ped. 73, 928 (1968)

PISANO, J. J.: Clin. Chim. Acta 5, 406 (1960)

PISANO, J. J., GROUT, J. R., ABRAHAM, D.: Clin. Chim. Acta 7, 285(1962)

POTTER, E. C., PARRISH, J. M.: Am. J. Path. 18, 141 (1942)

PRICE, C. H. G.: In: Colston Papers No. 24. Bone - Certain Aspects of Neoplasia. PRICE, C. H. G., ROSS, F. G. M. (eds.). London: Butterworth, 1973, p. 177

ROBINSON, R.: Recent Results in Cancer Research, BOHUON, C. (ed.), Berlin: Springer 1966, Vol. II, p. 37

RUTHVEN, C. R. J., SANDLER, M.: Clin. Chim. Acta 12, 318 (1965)

SANDLER, M., RUTHVEN, C. R. J.: Biochem. Journal 80, 78 (1961)

SAWITSKY, A., DESPOSITO, F.: J. Ped. 67, 99-103 (1965)

SHAW, K. N. F., LIEBERMAN, E., KOCH, R., DONNELL, G. N.: Am. J. Dis. Child. 113, 119 (1967)

SMELLIE, J. M., SANDLER, M.: Proc. Roy. Soc. Med. 54, 327 (1961)

SMITH, A. A., TAYLOR, T., WORTIS, S. B.: New Eng. J. Med. 268, 705 (1963)

SOFFER, L. J., DORFMAN, R. I., GABRILOVE, J. L.: The Human Adrenal Gland. London: Kimpton, 1961, Chap.14

STOUT, A. P.: Surg. Gyn. Obst. 84, 101 (1947)

STOWENS, D.: Arch. Path. 63, 451 (1957)

STUDNITZ, W. Von: Lancet 2, 215 (1961)

SUTOW, W. W.: Cancer 32, 1150 (1973)

SUTOW, W. W., FERNBACH, D. J., THURMAN, W. G., HOLTON, C. P., WATKINS, W. L.: Cancer Chemotherapy Reports 54, 283 (1970)

TEVETOGLU, F., LEE, C.: Am. J. Dis. Child. 91, 365 (1956)

VOORHESS, M. L.: J. Ped. 78, 680 (1971)

VOORHESS, M. L.: J. Ped. Surg. 3, 147 (1968)

VOORHESS, M. L.: J. Ped. Surg. 3, 152 (1968)

VOORHESS, M. L.: Pediatrics 39, 252 (1967)

VOORHESS, M. L., GARDNER, L. I.: Lancet 2, 651 (1960)

VOORHESS, M. L., GARDNER, L. I.: Pediatrics 30, 241 (1962)

VOORHESS, M. L., PICKETT, L. K., GARDNER, L. I.: Am.J. Surg. 106, 33 (1963)

WAGHE, M., KUMAR, S., STEWARD, J. K.: J. Ped. Surg. 5, 14 (1970)

WEIL-MALHERBE, H.: Z. Klin. Chem/2 Jahrg Heft 6, 161 (1964)

WELLS, H. G.: Arch. Path, 30, 535 (1940)

WILBERDINK, I.: Brit. J. Cancer 11, 378 (1957)

WILLIAMS, C. M., GREER, M.: J.A.M.A. 183, 836 (1963)

WILLIAMS, T. H., HOUSE, R. F., BURGERT, E. O., LYNN, H. B.: Cancer 29, 475 (1972)

WINKLER, H., SMITH, A. D.: In: Catecholamines. BLASCHKO and MUSCHOLL (eds.). Hdb exp. Pharmakol. Berlin: Springer, 1972, Vol. XXXIII,p.922

WYATT, G. M., FARBER, S.: Am. J. Roent. 56, 1485 (1941)

YOUNG, R. B., STEIKER, D. D., BONGIOVANNI, A. M., KOOP, C. E., EBERLEIN, W. R.: J. Ped. 62, 844 (1963)

ZAIMIS, E.: Nerve Growth Factor and its Antiserum. London: Athlone Press, 1972

# Chapter 8
# Retinoblastomas

J. L. S. SMITH and M. A. BEDFORD

## NATURE OF RETINOBLASTOMA

The investigation of the nature of this retinal cancer provides a fascinating story in itself, the unfolding of which has been mirrored in changes in nomenclature; to no other tumour has such a wealth of names been applied. Apart from one or two earlier observations, knowledge of this eye disease was first founded in the early 19th century, notably by WARDROP (1809) who must be credited with the first proper, clinical description of the "Fungus haematodes" of the eye, based on 17 cases; the actual tumours had a soft or "medullary" form with a resemblance to nervous tissue. In the succeeding quarter of a century these tumours were frequently reported as Fungus haematodes and/or medullaris, as by LANGENBECK (1822) and by MIDDLEMORE (1830). Somewhat later and in the middle decades of the 19th century this use of physical characteristics was continued, reflecting in particular the resemblance to cerebral matter, as "encephaloid tumour", "encephaloid degeneration of the retina" or even "encephaloma retinae" (CARTER, 1863) and perhaps prophetically "De l'encephaloide et du pseudo-encephaloide de la retine et du nerf optique" (SICHEL, 1859).

The "naked-eye" terminology now became boosted by the results of histological examination and the diversity of views expressed in relation thereto. VIRCHOW (1864) introduced the term "glioma retinae" and his authority was such that it persisted in general usage for many years, well into the present century. VIRCHOW derived these retinal tumours from the neuroglia which he had discovered in the central nervous system and its appendages and suggested in the more aggressive forms a transition to sarcoma, based on the finding of large, richly cytoplasmic cells in addition to the abundant small cells with scanty cytoplasm i. e. to gliosarcoma. Identification with the cerebral gliomata was inevitable (VETSCH, 1882, 1883; STRAUB, 1886) and, as many authors regarded the latter as sarcomata, this label with descriptive embellishments e. g. glioangiosarcoma or tubular gliosarcoma was accepted by many investigators, DA GAMA PINTO (1886) having emphasized the structural dependence of the tumour on the vessels but, as STRAUB pointed out, one could not logically continue to regard neuroglia as the mother tissue as its ectodermal origin had been demonstrated. In 1896 TREACHER COLLINS had pointed out the resemblance of the neoplastic tissue to the developing retina in the third and fourth month of foetal life, both consisting of rounded cells with scanty cytoplasm, some showing small projecting spicules. The histogenetic role of embryonic, neuroepithelial cells was supported by a number of authors, notably by VERHOEFF (1922) who derived these neoplasms from "retinoblasts" and on whose recommendation the American Ophthalmological Society in 1926 officially adopted the term "retinoblastoma".

However, the form of differentiation in particular continued to cause controversy. FAVALORO's claim (1937) to identify six categories of glial cells was expressed in his lavishly descriptive "ependymospongiofibrilloglioblastoma", accepting the bipotential nature of the retinoblasts but fighting shy of recognizing neuroblastic differentiation, as have GRINKER (1931) and PARKHILL and BENEDICT (1941). These last authors too have been at pains to emphasize the glial content and in company with DUKE-ELDER (1940) have favoured subdivision on basically similar lines, separating the highly undifferentiated retinoblastoma with, at most, a limited content of "spongioblastic cells" from the differentiated "neuroepithelioma retinae" with rosettes. Rosettes (Fig. 1) are found in

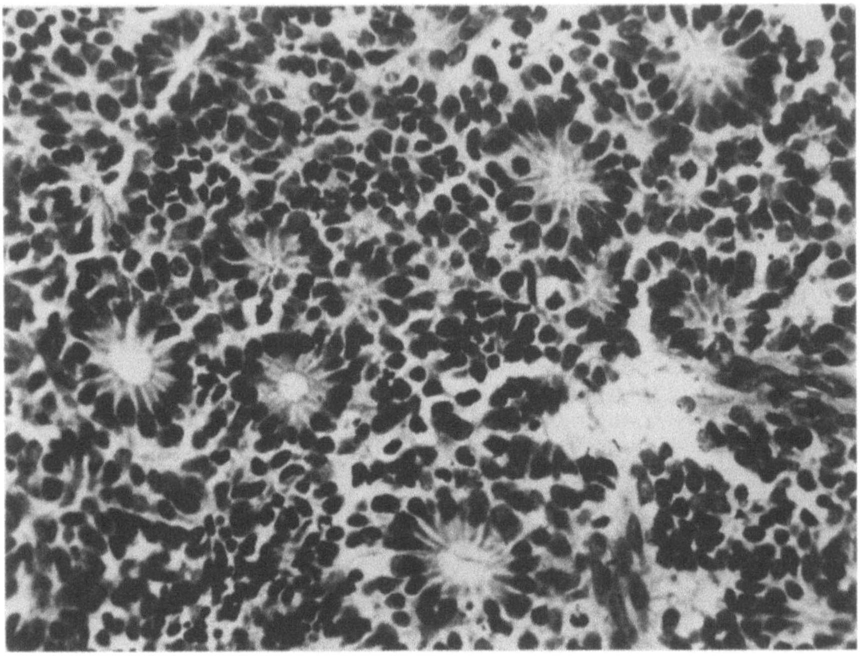

*Fig. 1. Neuroepithelial rosettes, one showing a mitotic figure (X450)*

a quarter to one-third of these tumours, usually appear circular in section but may be of more irregular shape, and frequently incomplete with or without some inward herniation of neighbouring cells. The lumen varies in size, usually being in the 5-20μ range and bordered by a limiting membrane through which project small bud-like structures belonging to the immediate lining cells which are of columnar type and which at their opposing end may reveal a fine, fibrillary process which becomes lost in the surrounding cells. This was noted by FLEXNER (1891) who gave the first proper description of the rosettes and within which he recognised the rudiments of rods and cones. FLEXNER therefore proposed "neuroepithelioma retinae" as appropriate and this was adopted by WINTERSTEINER (1897) as the title for his exhaustive, classical monograph on the subject. Identifying the rosettes as clusters of visual cells received general approval, as by WOLFF (1944) but there have been dissenters. Much of the argument as to the origin and quality of the constituent cells in these tumours has hinged on the nature of the rosettes and their bordering epithelium. They have been interpreted as an attempted formation of neural tubes (MARCHESANI, 1930) or optic vesicles (WOLTER, 1961) or, more specifically, as lined by primitive or ependymal spongioblasts as by GRINKER and FAVOLORO. Mitotic figures are not infrequent within the columnar cells - a feature which must have swayed opinion against accepting them as highly differentiated, visual elements. GINSBERG (1899) regarded them as embryonic cells not as yet differentiated into spongioblasts and neuroblasts. WINTERSTEINER even hypothecated an origin for these tumours from such misplaced visual cells in line with the "Cohnheim Theory" as rosettes are frequently to be found within a neoplastic inner nuclear layer which has been the one most favoured as the starting point i. e. on the basis of continuity in the border zone. In some tumours the rosettes may be confined to one or more areas but in others are almost universal and present in such numbers as to leave no doubt that they are structures which have differentiated. Furthermore, with intraocular spread they develop at remote sites, as on the iris, and are occasionally seen in distant metastases.

TS'O et al. (1969) studied five retinoblastomas, including two by electron microscopy. They selected these particular tumours as they contained pale staining regions of reduced cellularity where it was possible to demonstrate small bundles of cells showing photoreceptor differentiation and for which the name of "fleurette" was adopted, as the component cells had pear-shaped processes which fanned out as they projected in clusters through a common fenestrated membrane. This preliminary report was elaborated in two further communications (TS'O et al., 1970a, b), the main points of similarity with the normal visual cells being: 1. zonula-adherens-like attachments identical with the terminal bars of the normal external limiting membrane. 2. Cell processes filled by mitochondria resembling inner segments and lamellated membranes resembling outer segments of normal photoreceptors. 3. Cilia with 9 peripheral filaments but no central one. These findings were taken as clear indications that the cells of fleurettes are neurones modified for photoreception and almost identical in structure with the visual cells of normal retina though unaccompanied by glial (MÜLLER) cells and, beyond this, that retinoblastomas are "neuronal" neoplasms. These authors (1969) also demonstrated in a similar manner photoreceptor elements in the rosettes though exhibiting, as a rule, less advanced differentiation than those of the fleurettes and they comment upon the greater hyperchromatism of the nuclei. The recognition of fleurettes has contributed to our knowledge but experienced microscopists will be familiar with the occasional small fields showing differentiated cell groups arranged in crescentic or even horseshoe fashion and provided with a shared limiting membrane and projecting processes resembling rods and cones. Formations of this kind do not strike the eye, as any central lumen tends to be compressed to the point of absence (Fig. 2). Their structure is of course that of a fleurette and they are found in the paler areas where cell concentration is reduced; the darker and more actively growing tumour usually contains rosettes and one meets transitions. They were recognised by PARKHILL and BENEDICT (1941) as a variation of rosette structure and described as "irregular circles or segments of circles of cells surrounding a clear region containing fibrillary material".

The close resemblance of retinoblastoma cells to those of the nuclear layers has led many writers to consider either or both of the latter as sites of origin. The punctate chromatin pattern must be viewed as a pointer to the neuronal nature of the tumour cells, the density and coarseness varying somewhat within individual tumours but frequently so alike as to make it difficult to distinguish between neoplastic and normal cells: there is a contrast with the more vesicular appearance and greater variability in size shown by glial nuclei. As long ago as 1904 VERHOEFF identified bipolar cells with slender processes and WILLIS (1948) was able to demonstrate such with ordinary stains in "fibrillated" tumour tissue considering them, like VERHOEFF, to be neurones comparable with those of the inner nuclear layer. Even so, FISCHER's contention (1918) of an essential similarity with sym-

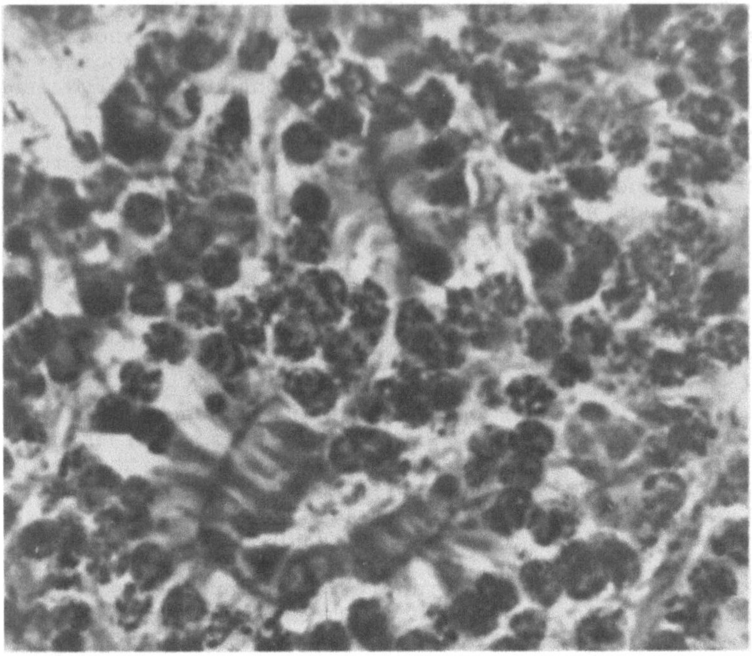

*Fig. 2. Two groups of differentiated visual cells complete with limiting membrane (X 800)*

pathetic neuroblastoma and his advocacy of "neuroblastoma retinae" evoked criticism by WILLIS as such a title did not take into account the obvious rod and cone cell differentiation shown by rosettes. BROWN (1966b) examined the urine in 12 children under treatment for retinoblastoma for the metabolites of catecholamines. In three patients the excretion of vanilmandelic and homovanillic acids would seem abnormally high, the most significant being a level of 46.2 microgrammes per milligramme of creatinine which fell to half this level following enucleation. A limited number of investigations along these lines in Manchester have proved negative, as would seem to apply elsewhere, but FREZOTTI et al. (1967) reported two cases of retinoblastoma with significantly increased levels of urinary vanilmandelic acid, though the amounts of dopamine, norepinephrine, and epinephrine were normal. In an electron microscopic study of 50 retinoblastomas by ALBERT (1974) in conjunction with LAHAV et al. one tumour, both in vivo and in tissue culture, showed numerous secretory granules consistent with those previously described in cells of sympathetic innervation (GEFFEN and LIVETT, 1971), predictable perhaps as the amacrine cells in a variety of vertebrate retinas have been shown to be catecholamine-containing (LATIES and JACOBOWITZ, 1966). Retinoblastoma has been reported in animals but, at least in the main, such examples have been medulloepitheliomas arising in the ciliary region and exhibiting tubular patterns or even rosettes, as occurs in man. Recently, KOBAYASHI and MUKAI (1974) have succeeded in inducing retinal tumours showing indifferent rosettes in rats using adenovirus type 12.

In essence, this retinal cancer must be regarded as a neuroblastoma of retinal origin, having at best only a small content of supporting glial cells, and likely to show an affinity with other neuroblastomata. Attempts at histological subdivision should be deprecated as retinoblastoma forms a signally specific and unitary group in which the results of statistical analysis will be valid.

## CLINICAL COURSE AND MORBID ANATOMY

Retinoblastoma presents as solitary or multiple lesions and if the latter applies, tends to be bilateral, especially if several independent foci have developed. The tumours lie more frequently in the lower half of the retina, as noted by HIRSCHBERG (1969). WINTERSTEINER was able to position the tumours in only 63 cases; excluding those in the centre-caecal region, 16 lay to the sides, 21 below and 4 above. DOLLFUS and AUVERT (1953) were able to position 47 solitary tumours; seven lay in the immediate region of the papilla, 15 in the upper, and 25 in the lower part of the globe. They comment upon the preference shown for the posterior pole but the vertical imbalance would appear the more striking. Multiple lesions vary in their stage of development and STALLARD (1968) has charted their delayed appearance other than at the original site in 23 children; he found mostly two or four additional islands after intervals of 3 - 18 months but a few at longer periods.

Clinically, retinoblastoma can be mimicked by several ocular diseases to which WINTERSTEINER also paid particular attention, setting them up in contrast under the name of "pseudoglioma". The conditions which can be confused with retinoblastoma have been succinctly stated by HOWARD and ELLSWORTH (1965) in the examination of 265 children and there seems to have been an increasing number of "battered baby" syndromes as reported by KIFFNEY (1964). Even today for an oculist the basic diagnostic problem remains one "of tumour or of pseudoglioma", and opinions may vary. To minimise mistakes, apart from a sound knowledge of alternative conditions, it is essential to appreciate the changing symptomatology as the disease evolves. WARDROP and others divided the clinical course into two main sections, the first covering the period up to perforation of the globe wall and the second that of extraocular spread and metastasis. Since the time of KNAPP (1968) it has been customary to recognise four stages in the progress of the disease, namely: 1. Intraocular growth, 2. Secondary glaucoma, 3. Extraocular spread, and 4. Distant metastasis, though most authors have combined the third and fourth stages, as once the tumour has extended beyond the retina and the chambers of the eye, extraglobal dissemination tends to be rapid. To some extent spread of the neoplasm is independent of the degree of global disorganization and, rarely, may be extraocular prior to the development of a frank second stage. From the ophthalmic angle the recognition of the second stage is particularly important for it is here nowadays that misdiagnoses are prone to occur, especially where it seems to be the start of the disease, the first stage having been overlooked. DOLLFUS and AUVERT rightly discuss modes of onset in some detail, notably in regard to local complications such as haemorrhage into the anterior chamber, cataract, pseudo-inflammatory phenomena and pseudo-iridocyclitis.

### 1. Stage of Visual Failure (Amaurotic Cat's Eye)

Impaired retinal function may be indicated by (a) visual defect (b) strabismus (c) nystagmus.

With few exceptions the tender age of most of these children effectively rules out any direct complaint of deteriorating vision. For the most part one is dependent on the parent's noting a difference between the two eyes in their response to visual stimuli, as in ability to fix or appreciate movement. Walking children may bump into objects on the one side. Suspected blindness may then be tested, as by covering the other eye.

In young children any interference with visual ability will favour squint. In developing retinoblastoma ocular deviation is attributable to retinal damage, especially at the macula resulting from the tumour and/or associated detachment, though later on opacification of the media may be contributory. The squint may be convergent or divergent, the latter being especially significant as there is a much higher relative incidence than applies in childhood strabismus in general, reflecting in part the tendency of blind eyes to deviate outwards. In the Manchester series during the last 50 years the ratio of convergent to divergent strabismus has been at the low figure of less than 2 : 1. In clinical practice one would accept such squints as secondary in nature but in some patients they can be incidental or even antedate the appearance of the tumour. Experience suggests that strabismus has a greater prevalence within the families of these patients than one would expect by chance. FALLS and NEEL (1951) examined 94 parents, finding five examples of divergent strabismus, well in excess of the expected number.

Rarely, nystagmus draws attention to the disease and one would equate this manifestation with macular lesions, in particular. In his total collection of 497 cases WINTERSTEINER was able to quote only three examples, only one being bilateral. One of the unilateral cases, that of LINCKE (1834), differed in being of late onset and having an associated microcornea in both eyes. Again in this context, as with strabismus, it seems that the relationship is not a simple one. In the entire Manchester series, 5 survivors of unilateral retinoblastoma show a coarse ocular nystagmus in the fellow eye.

As is well known, the major and often sole presenting symptom is expressed in the classical term "amaurotic cat's eye", in general use since the time of BEER (1817) though more recent, and especially Ameri-

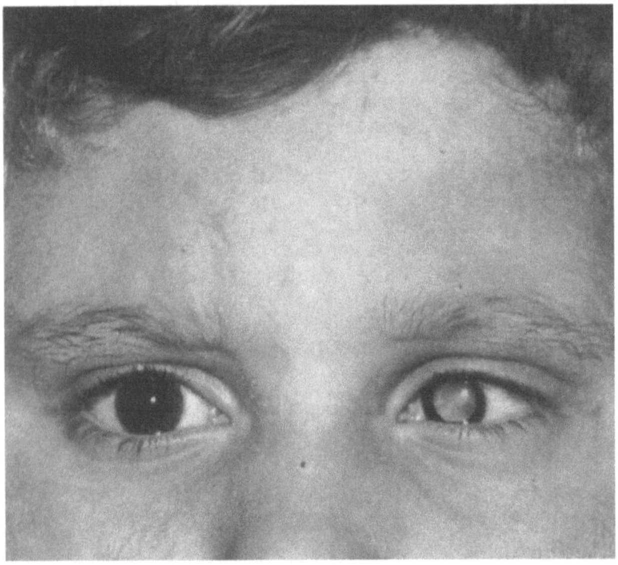

*Fig. 3. Advanced retinoblastoma presenting with squint and white pupil*

can, authors favour the alternative "leukocoria". The abnormal reflex from the pupil may be described by parents or relatives without prompting as a "cat's eye effect" but variations such as "speck", "fishtail", "glow" or "gleam" are common or, on the other hand, "one can see into the eye", "the pupil has disappeared". Initially, such reflections are noted at certain angles only and are of fleeting character so that on close inspection the eye appears normal, a fact not always properly appreciated in children's clinics. The reflex may be seen first in bright conditions but, perhaps more typically, in artificial light with the greater dilatation of the pupil. It becomes increasingly obvious and this enhancement may give a metallic lustre, frequently commented upon by earlier observers.

Nystagmus can be largely discounted, being noted in approximately 1% of the patients. It has been traditional to record the form of presentation and in reviewing 500 cases HOWARD and ELLSWORTH (1965) quote 61%, 22% and 5% for the cat's eye effect, strabismus, and visual disability respectively, though combinations frequently develop within short time intervals, mostly of course a white pupil and squint in association (Fig. 3). It is interesting to note that in this large series, as in that of BEDFORD et al. (1971), there are a number of symptomless cases examined because the hereditary pattern of this disease is known and many children at risk are examined before the tumours are large enough to produce any obvious physical signs.

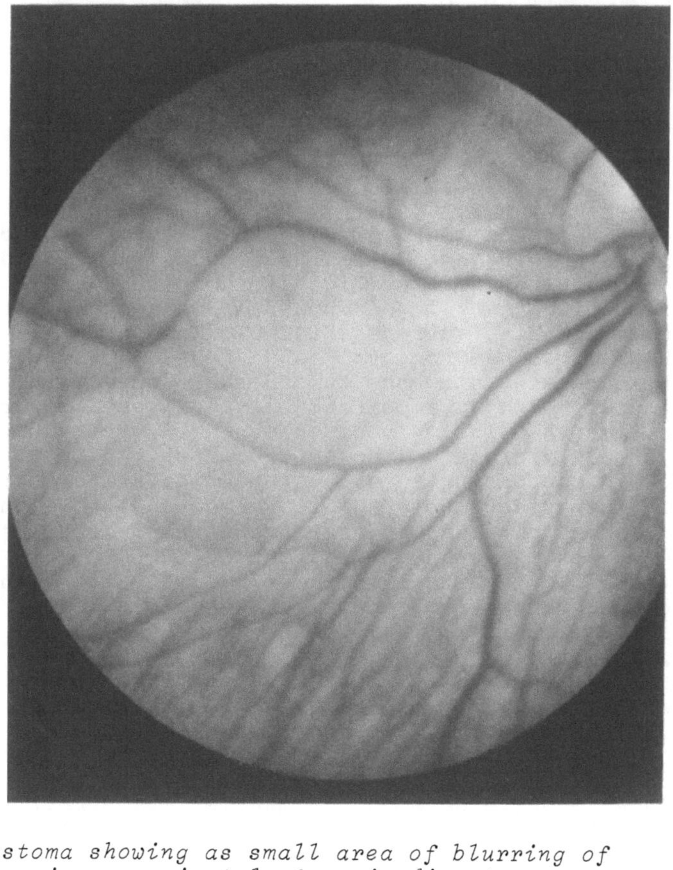

*Fig. 4. Early retinoblastoma showing as small area of blurring of choroidal pattern. Tumour is approximately 1 mm in diameter*

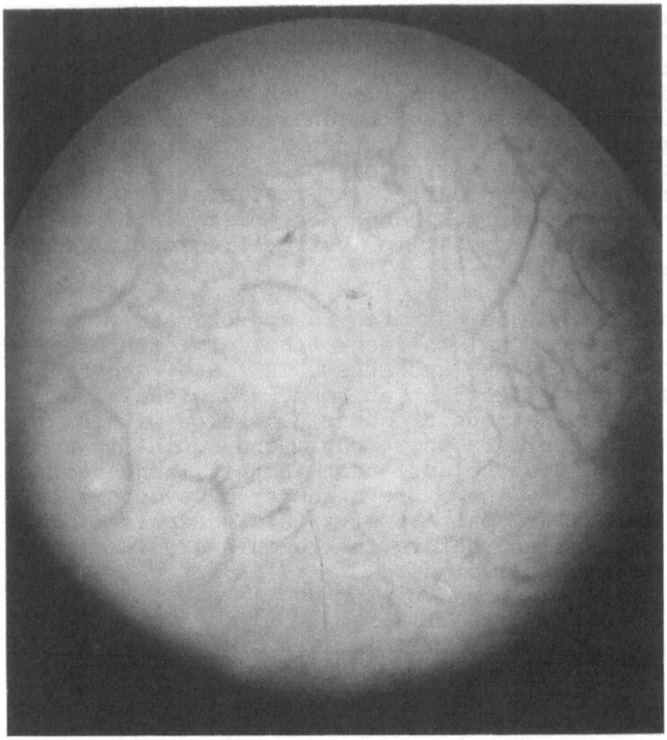

*Fig. 5. Typical surface of large retinoblastoma showing fine vessels outlined against white tumour tissue*

At its inception there is slight loss of translucency, a small retinoblastoma showing as a gelatinous nodule, barely discernible against the underlying choroid (Fig. 4). Continued growth gives the classical hemispherical swelling composed of whitish-pink tissue with fine blood vessels upon its surface (Fig. 5). The border is relatively sharp and usually of rounded or oval shape i. e. "retinoblastoma circumscriptum". With increasing size the tumour takes on a mottled aspect becoming more flocculent with an appearance often likened to cream cheese. At the same time vascularity becomes enhanced with short stretches and loops of vessels visible on the surface mostly pursuing only a short course before disappearing into the tumour substance, but superficial networks or tufts may develop. In a few cases a notable enlargement of the feeder vessels may be seen, so as to cause confusion with Von HIPPEL-LINDAU disease, as has been pointed out by BEDFORD and MacFAUL (1969). Small spots reflecting the light more brightly are found in the majority of cases and, when lying superficially, have a pearly appearance, as stressed by REESE (1963).

Anatomical considerations decree that the vascular response will be sited primarily within the inner retinal layers, continuing and successful growth being dependent upon the development of a supporting vasculature around the vessels of which much of the tumour becomes mantled as a stratified epithelium - often with palisading of the basal layer - while between the mantles lie erratically disposed zones of necrotic and disintegrating cells (Fig. 6). This lobular-dendritic or so-called tubular build was stressed first by IWANOFF (1869) and leads to unevenness of the surface, both in regard to contour and re-

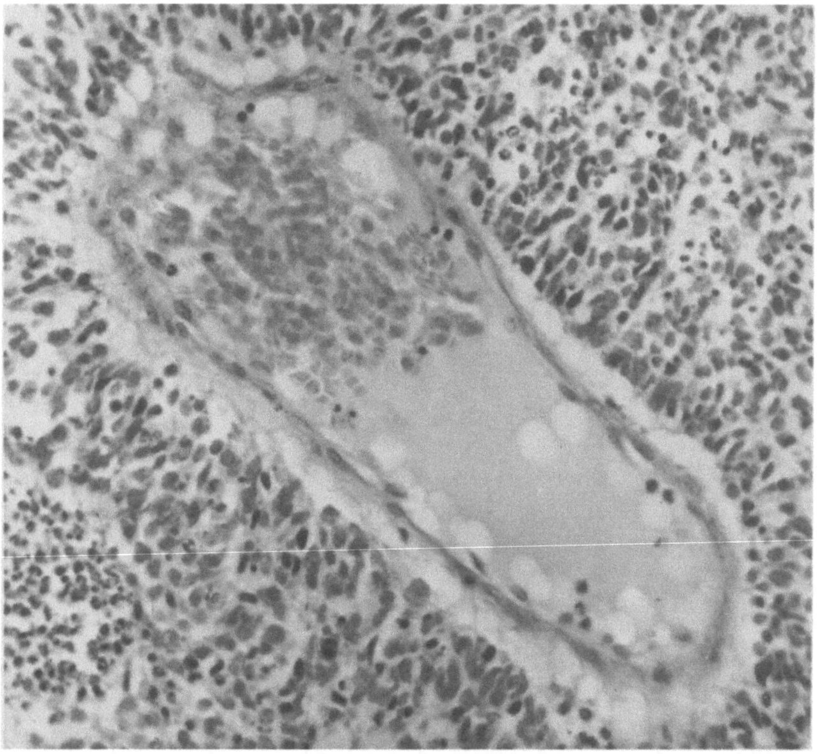

*Fig. 6. Perivascular mantles with palisading of basal cells. Necrosis in outer zone with pyknotic nuclei (X 275)*

flectance. The oldest cells migrate outwards and die off and the picture is similar to that seen in oat-cell carcinoma of bronchus, the resemblance being heightened by the deposition of basophilic material in ring fashion around the vessel walls, which appears to be accumulated DNA (MULLANEY, 1968, 1969). In these mantles the junction between the viable and dead cells is mostly sharp - causing WINTERSTEINER to postulate an invasion of necrotic areas by vessels complete with their cuffs of tumour cells - rather than a simple dependence on blood supply. He also noted the changing calibre of individual vessels which contributes to the vagaries in size and shape of vessel segments on viewing the surface. The speckling emphasized by REESE and others is due to the presence of small blocks of calcified cells, found mainly in necrotic zones but often partially enclosed by the viable cells of the mantles. This calcification is a strictly focal process with mostly a notable coherence of the cells which also stain positively with Periodic-Acid-Schiff techniques (Fig. 7) and the resultant particles are in the nature of drusen, being found in the majority of cases. Using radiographic methods PFEIFFER (1936) demonstrated their presence in 15 out of 20 enucleated eyes, a figure confirmed by FULTON 1950, though KREIBIG 1949 found an incidence of 80%. Their demonstration by X-ray is a useful adjunct in establishing the diagnosis. Clinically, SWAN and HYMAN (1952) demonstrated such calcification in 18 out of 23 patients.

Spread beneath the retina, even with this structure remaining largely in position, may be extensive giving the appearance of "miliary" tumour nodules and this has been interpreted - one imagines without good cause

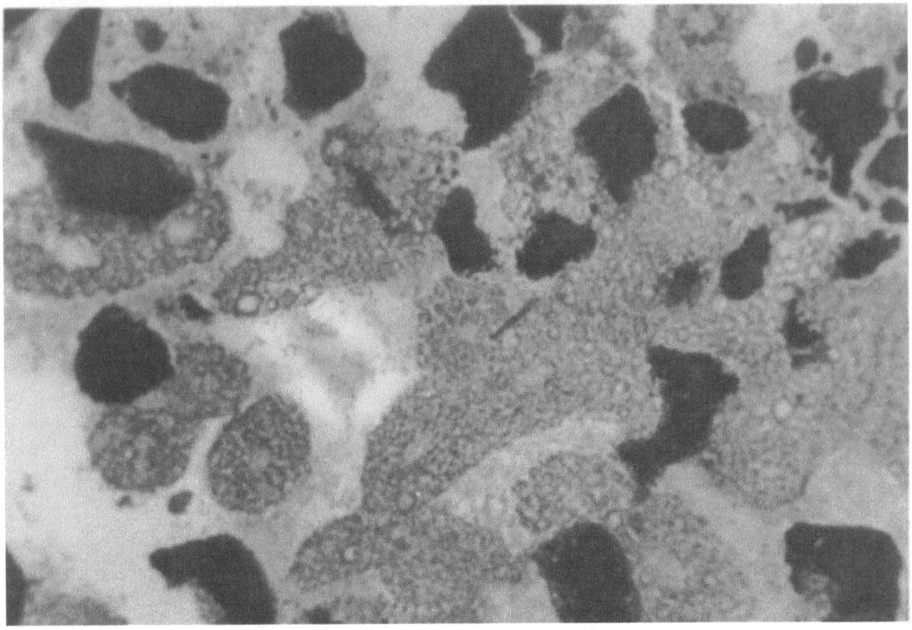

*Fig. 7. Chunks of PAS-positive, calcified cell groups (X 55)*

- as a richly multifocal origin e. g. DUKE-ELDER (1940). This seeding capacity is a most important attribute, of which one takes account in assessing the general growth pattern which, as originally noted by HIRSCHBERG (1968, 1969), takes two main forms, namely the "exophytic"

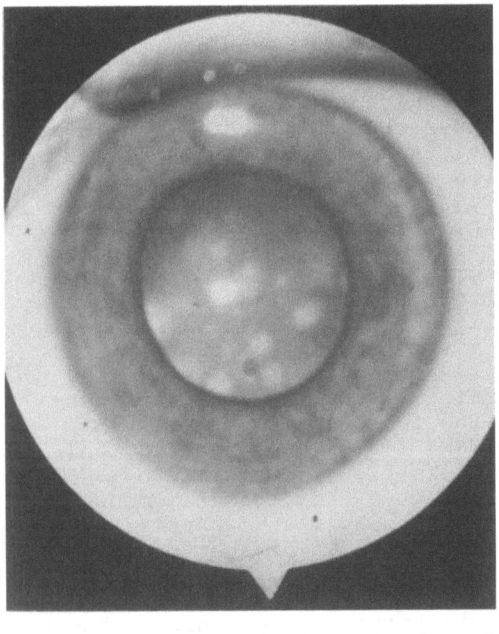

*Fig. 8. Tumour cells have broken free into vitreous and show as white balls with seeding on to retina*

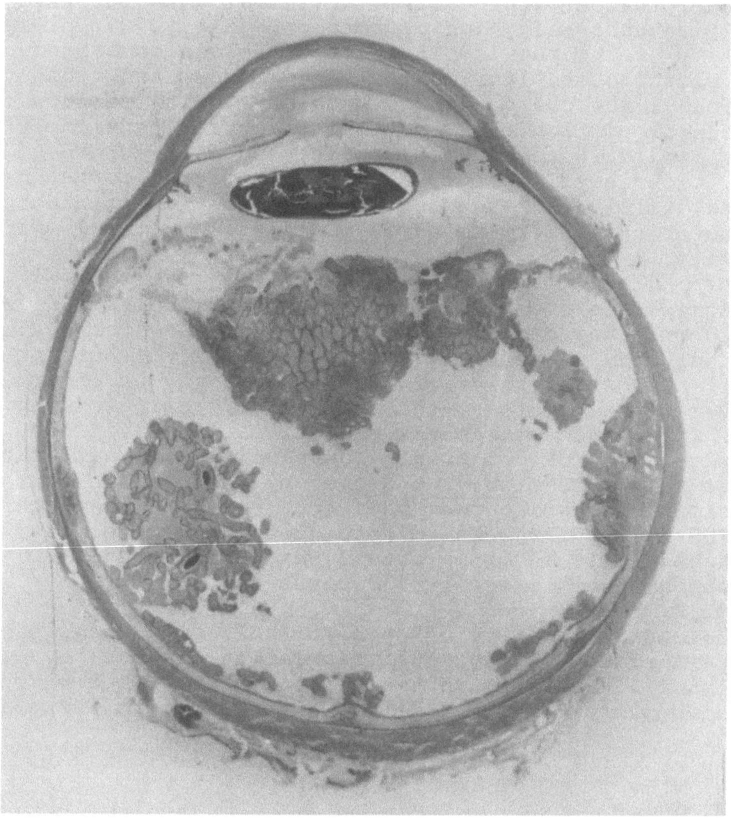

*Fig. 9. Endophytic retinoblastoma with minimal detachment with focal growth around new vessels and coarse seeding inwardly*

and the "endophytic". In the former the tumour bulges into the subretinal space with an initial, local separation of the retina which progresses to a lobulated detachment in which one can usually spot the more solid, whitish tumour from the more translucent grey of the balloons of non-neoplastic retina. In the alternative endophytic form the main direction of growth is inwardly, often with extensive spread over the internal limiting membrane to give an enhanced "cat's eye" effect and with only a shallow and delayed separation of the retina from the choroid. For the clinician the grey-white floating particles visible in the vitreous chamber establish the diagnosis with virtual certainty (Fig. 8). These seedlings vary in size and number and are often of a coarse nature (Fig. 9).

2. Stage of Ocular Complications

There may be a preceding history of a cat's eye effect, suspected blindness, or squint but often no such information is forthcoming, the disease seeming to have had a silent first stage due partly to an oversight by the child's attendants. The history, as given by the parents or other interested parties, can be interpreted almost without exception in the context of secondary glaucoma. In some eyes onset is insidious, incipient glaucoma showing itself as a partial dilatation of the pupil - which may temporarily emphasize the cat's eye reflex - and by changing colour of the iris which becomes darker than its fellow.

In the 20 cases with pertinent clinical data reported by SWAN and HYMAN (1952) an unusually high proportion, namely 50%, presented with inequality of the pupils. In others, the glaucoma produces irritability with photophobia, lacrimation and redness, and tends to be intermittent initially, the child being off colour during periods of congestion. In a small proportion the rise in intraocular tension is so severe that the child is in considerable pain, and will scream and bang his or her head. Cloudiness and increase in size of the cornea may be commented on and, rarely, enlargement of the globe itself, though such changes may be abruptly terminated by perforation with discharge of ocular contents.

On examination one finds a sluggish or fixed, semi-dilated pupil associated with angle closure and a layer of new vessels on the anterior iris surface, these being responsible for the heterochromia. The cornea is oedematous to varying degree and may be enlarged with ruptures in Descemet's membrane, the initial stretching of the globe being corneal. In advanced cases visualization of the vitreous chamber and of the retina may be hampered by developing cataract, the opacities lying in the main posteriorly, and even by dislocation of the lens. On rare occasions haemorrhage may have occurred into the anterior chamber. DOLLFUS and AUVERT were able to quote a total of four cases, two of which had followed minor trauma, and BEDFORD et al. (1971) found spontaneous hyphaema twice in 139 cases.

A substantial minority of eyes in the second stage have a special character in that they suggest inflammatory disease, i. e. endophthalmitis with marked turbidity in the vitreous cavity but beyond which one may perceive dimly the outlines of whitish tumour tissue, easily mistaken

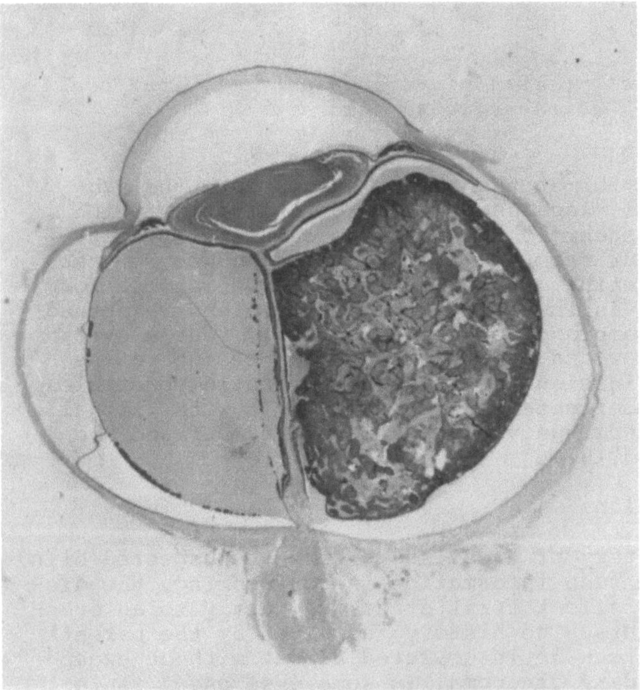

*Fig. 10. Exophytic retinoblastoma with large solitary subretinal tumour and subretinal seeding*

for active choroiditis. Haemorrhage may make visualization more difficult, but even so, seeding tumour particles may be detectable behind the lens; later on, these will extend into the anterior chamber as deposits on the iris, floating particles or sometimes massed in the lower part as a tumour "hypopyon". This pseudo-inflammatory presentation of endophytic retinoblastoma poses a serious threat to life. Since 1925 in the Manchester series, the enucleation of several eyes was inordinately delayed on such a basis with a fatal result in all. By contrast, oculists are less loath to remove eyes with the full detachments and shallow anterior chambers associated with exophytic retinoblastoma where the visual prognosis is manifestly poor, though even here the case may be mistaken for one of simple detachment if, as sometimes happens, the tumour is masked (Fig. 10).

As an uncommon alternative, shrinkage, usually temporary, of the globe may be seen. PARSONS (1904) described such a globe removed from a female aged 18 months with no evidence of perforation. Tumour was present in the other eye and he thought it pertinent that at least in 10 of 14 cases quoted in the literature the disease had been bilateral. In a series of 35 cases PARKHILL and BENEDICT (1941) found two atrophic globes, both enucleated during the second year of life for unilateral disease.

### 3. Stage of Extraocular Spread

Within the civilized communities of the world, it is almost unknown for the disease to present in a florid third stage i. e. of fungation where the eye or its remains become carried forward by an ugly, vascular mass protruding from the orbit with oedematous swelling of the lids and to which may be added local facial deformity from the now usually rapid and invasive growth. Occasionally, less advanced cases are seen with a degree of proptosis and congestion (Fig. 11). Initially the eye movements may be little impaired, as originally stressed by ROSAS (1830), but ultimately the local muscular and fatty tissues undergo complete atrophy as the growth fills the orbit.

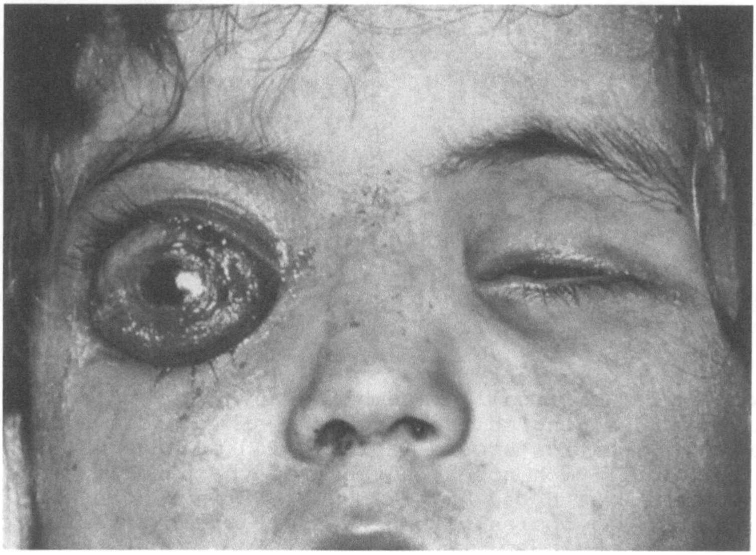

*Fig. 11. Advanced case of retinoblastoma showing extra-ocular extension and proptosis*

1. Spread by Local Propagation. Entry into the orbit is effected via the posterior scleral canals and their emissary vessels; only rarely in advanced cases is there a scleral hole, though this structure may become so thinned by glaucomatous stretching as to make enucleation without rupture a difficult procedure. Further progress under natural conditions leads to widespread involvement of the neighbouring bones of the skull including the nasal cavities and, on occasion, the opposite orbit with considerable resulting erosion and also widening of the orbital fissures with loss of the boundaries between the orbital tumour and its intracranial or retromaxillary extensions. Normally the dura mater is an effective barrier to central penetration but orbit to brain spread is recorded at autopsy, a noteworthy route being through the cribriform plate of the ethmoid, as in the two cases quoted by MERRIAM (1950) and CARBAJAL (1959), the latter modifying his classification somewhat to separate sharply, intradural from extradural secondaries. In analogous fashion and as a late manifestation, spread of tumour can occur from the anterior segment of the globe via the anterior scleral canals with the production of subconjunctival masses. Figure 12 depicts heavy involvement of the iris with tumour in the

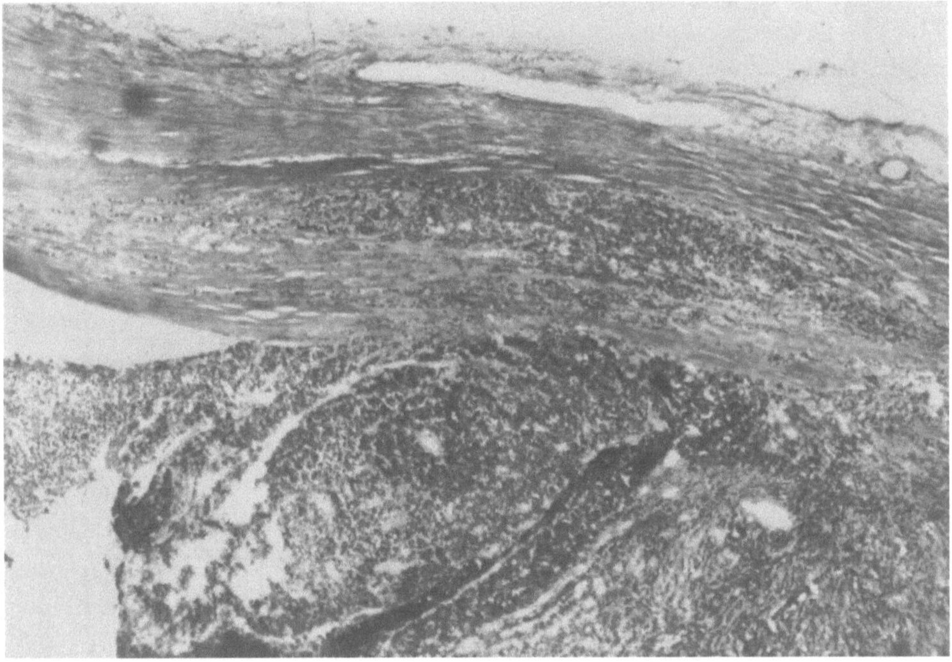

*Fig. 12. Advanced retinoblastoma with invasion of the ciliary body, iris and anterior sclera, together with tumour hypopyon (X 50)*

lower angle, clinically resembling a "hypopyon" and commencing spread into the adjoining sclera. From the orbit and conjunctiva extension via the lymphatics occurs rapidly with enlargement of the preauricular and cervical lymph nodes, notably of the parotid group. Local lymphatic enlargement was noted by WINTERSTEINER in 28 cases and by MERRIAM in 5 out of 17 autopsies with or without other affected glands.

An independent and major route of direct extension is centralwards within the optic nerve (Fig. 13). In most cases entry is effected from the optic disc through the lamina cribrosa, the tumour lying axially in the

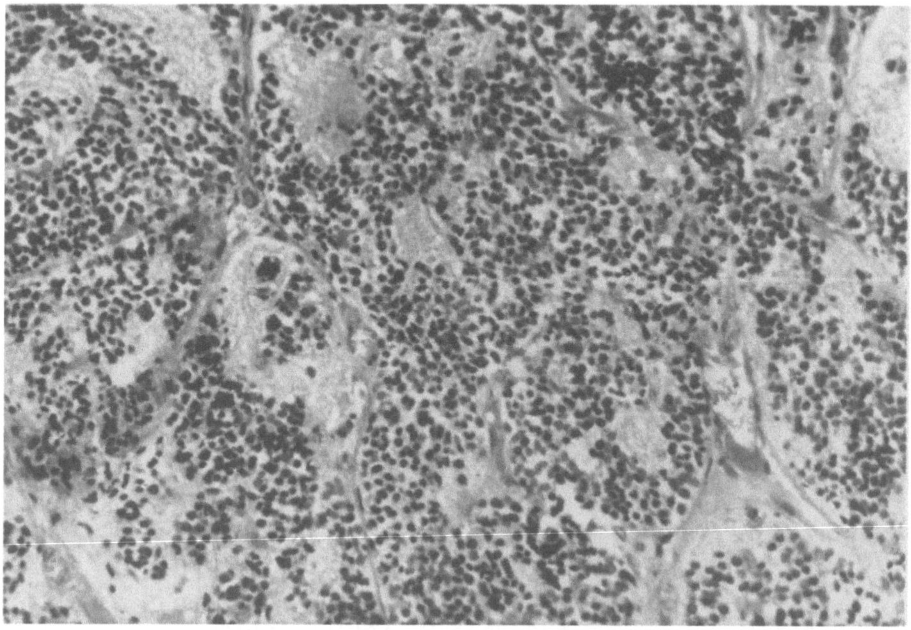

*Fig. 13. Invasion of optic nerve by retinoblastoma cells (X 250)*

nerve but complicated ultimately by spilling over into the vaginal i. e. subarachnoid space. Among the 12 post-mortem cases reported by CARBAJAL, case 2 was noteworthy in that the optic nerve was distended by tumour to the chiasm without further intracranial spread, and cases 5 and 9 in that the opposite optic nerve was involved with ampulliform enlargement behind the sclera. Blindness from involvement of the fellow optic nerve is common in the older literature - WINTERSTEINER reporting some 25 cases, and in fact intracranial spread via the optic nerve used to be the major cause of death, but in recent times has been much less of a problem due to earlier enucleation and the now well-established practice of taking a long stretch of optic nerve. This trend has been obvious for some time. REESE (1931) found optic nerve extension in 53% of 119 enucleated globes, in 43% beyond the line of section; in a further series of 116 enucleated eyes reported in 1948 the corresponding figures were 27% and 8.5%. In some cases there is early penetration of the subarachnoid space of the nerve, BROWN (1966a) illustrating such an event; the source of such tumour is usually the choroid bordering the nerve head. With spillage into the subarachnoid space widespread dissemination occurs through the meninges of both the brain and spinal cord on the basis of propagation and of seeding with often many individual tumours. The basal region is involved in particular but the neoplasm may spread widely over the hemispheres. The symptomatology is complex with neck rigidity, convulsions, stupor, pareses, and not infrequently hydrocephalus.

Following unsuccessful enucleation, orbital recurrence may be seen within a period varying nearly always from a few weeks to several months, the source of the tumour being sometimes the severed optic nerve. In modern times, due to the standard practice of orbital irradiation in suspect cases, the incidence of this complication is now low, as are the disfigurements of local extension.

2. Haematogenous Spread. Retinoblastoma never presents in metastatic form, there being always a history of preceding ocular disease. This stems from the fact that dissemination via the blood stream is a complication of local spread of retinoblastoma outwards through the ocular coats. The choroid is the major starting point for tumour emboli and neoplastic cells have been demonstrated in emissary veins. If this structure is invaded to marked degree, the outlook is usually poor and can nearly always be forecast on the basis of this finding. Choroidal involvement can occur early and at several points but provided this is restricted to small foci the prognosis is as a rule favourable. BONIUK (1964) compiled some pertinent data from the Armed Forced Institute of Pathology: 46 cases with slight choroidal involvement produced 11 deaths from metastatic tumour i. e. 25% mortality, while 85 cases with marked choroidal involvement had a 65% mortality. In the Manchester series a few patients with distant metastases have failed to develop orbital tumour though local prophylactic measures were not undertaken. The older observers tended to regard haematogenous as a sequel to local extra-global spread but this dreaded complication was to be anticipated anyhow and the presence of an orbital extension is in itself by no means always fatal. Exceptionally, in a number of reported cases exenteration has proved successful, the first example being the fifth case of NELLESSEN (1872) in which a walnut-sized orbital recurrence developed four weeks following enucleation and the patient was observed for 4 1/2 years subsequently. Most favoured would seem those cases where the orbital tumour has been derived from an infiltrated optic nerve. A possible site of tumour dissemination is the central retinal vein near its exit from the globe. WINTERSTEINER compared case 2 of LANDSBERG (1875), the child being alive and well 5 years later, with his own case 16, suggesting that in reality the neoplastic cells lay outside the endothelium. MERRIAM, however, was able to demonstrate a clump of neoplastic cells within the lumen in a patient coming to post-mortem but such an event must be the great exception as accumulated experience indicates that distant metastasis does not take place from the retina itself. PAPOLEZY (1937), quoting material from the Berlin Eye Clinic reported by ADAM together with data from Budapest, noted 100% survival rate following enucleation in the first stage of the disease, the explanation "being in the relationship of the tumour to the retinal blood vessels".

In Manchester, as elsewhere, there has been reluctance on the part of paediatricians responsible for terminal care to ask for an autopsy so that the known distribution of secondaries is often far from complete. Between the 61 autopsies reported by WILSON and THOMPSON in 1900 and his personal series of 17, MERRIAM could review only 24 other published cases - both series were very similar and in general agreement with CARBAJAL. In his 17 cases, 9 patients had died of metastatic spread, all with osseous deposits, in 7 in the calvaria and at distant sites, in one at distant sites alone and in one in the calvaria alone, though here distant bones were not examined. In regard to visceral spread, the liver is the most frequent site but tumours may be found in any of the abdominal organs often associated with enlargement of local or inguinal nodes. A notable exception is the lung, no secondaries being recorded by MERRIAM, and WINTERSTEINER could quote only one example, though TAKTIKOS (1966), analysing a series of 48 fatal cases, found involvement of the lungs on four occasions. As a dramatic event, haematogenous spread to the brain itself is possible. During the last 9 years two patients attending St. Bartholomew's Hospital have died of solitary cerebral metastases, one case histologically proven, and BRUNNER (1971) has reported one case with a late fatal outcome.

## DIFFERENTIAL GROWTH BEHAVIOUR

Retinoblastoma permits a "nicety of observation" and, rightly, investigators in this field of cancer in particular have felt it incumbent upon themselves not only to establish the order of events, but also their basis in time as the disease evolves from a localised ocular tumour to a highly invasive and widely disseminating neoplasm. In regard to onset, the maximum genesis of tumours is within the first 12 months of life and, together with the congenital tumours, accounted for nearly a third in the 467 children of WINTERSTEINER's series where the age was recorded, i. e., 34 congenital and 102 in the first year of life. Subsequently, there is a gradual but accelerating decline in incidence, almost complete by the seventh year. The figures for symptomatic onset in the Manchester series during the last 50 years are analysed in Table 2 (see page 269). The histories have been compiled carefully from interviews with the relatives, often retrospective, and, as a consequence, there is a "shift to the left" as compared with most reported series. In 40 cases of untreated retinoblastoma WINTERSTEINER estimated the total duration of the disease as an average of 17 months, noting the greatest variation in the first stage. This is an underestimate and in the majority of cases pursuing a largely natural course a fatal outcome is to be expected between 1 1/2 and 2 1/2 years. In modern times the length of history prior to clinical observation has of course tended to be less e. g. averaging some 6 months in 28 unilateral cases listed by PARKHILL and BENEDICT (1941). However, in regard to orbital recurrences, these authors found a time interval from enucleation which varied between 1 and 8 months, in full agreement with WINTERSTEINER who considered that, with few exceptions, 1 year was sufficient to assess the prognosis.

In a minority of patients the disease departs from standard behaviour in regard to delayed onset, prolonged course, or a combination of both. The first acceptable example of long duration was reported by BOWATER (1868), an 11-year-old boy presenting with secondary glaucoma and exophthalmos from orbital extension though the disease had commenced in earliest childhood. In the case of MAKIUCHI (1935) an amaurotic cat's eye was confirmed in a boy aged 10 years, enucleation being delayed a further 10 years to reveal a tumour which extended out into the orbit and contained rosettes. In bilateral retinoblastoma similar behaviour may be seen in a wide disparity of onset as between the two eyes. A well-known case is that of MAGHY (1919) with 18 years between the enucleation of the two eyes; vision failed in the second eye at the age of 20 years and it was removed nearly 4 1/2 years later. SCHRECK (see MEISNER, 1951) has quoted the case of a woman developing retinoblastoma at 19 years of age, the other eye having been removed for retinoblastoma at the age of 2 years. One Manchester patient died at 3 1/2 years from cerebral extension, two tiny white spots of retinoblastoma being found in the second eye at post-mortem.

The odd unilateral case in teenagers has been reported, as by CRESPI (1876) of a 16-year-old boy with less than a year's history. More dramatic is the occasional occurrence of unilateral tumours in adults, as in reports by TUSHAUS (1940); RASMUSSEN (1944); DEPOUILLY et al. quoted by DOLLFUSS and AUVERT (1953); MEHRA and HAMID (1961); MAKLEY (1963). The age of these five male patients ranged from 34 to 52 years, the tumours favouring an endophytic build and showing rosettes. The presence of these last suggests that growth rate was at a moderate level. Investigators such as PARKHILL and BENEDICT have concluded that rosetted retinoblastomas grow more slowly and have in general a better prognosis; there is on record at least one case of known cerebral invasion lasting a few years, the patient ultimately dying with widespread, rosetted retinoblastoma within the central nervous system. HERM and HEATH (1956) suggest that differentiation often becomes progressively less within the retina itself.

Recurrence locally in the orbit, in the glands of the neck, or very occasionally at distant sites may be slow to develop. Examples of this kind spill over into others which appear to represent reactivation after many years. REESE (1963) quotes three patients with local recurrence following treatment at intervals of 6 to 9 years. One female patient in the Manchester series lost the right eye at 6 months and the left at 2 1/2 years after unsuccessful irradiation. She remained well until the age of 15 years only to develop swellings of the left preauricular and other cervical nodes; following biopsy she was treated with a cytotoxic drug and irradiation and remains well 16 years later. A second and less fortunate male patient had his left eye enucleated at 1 1/2 years and the right eye 1 year later as a radium implant had been unsuccessful. He remained well for 15 years, developing chest symptoms in his 18th year and dying after 6 months. At autopsy, though there were widespread metastases including those in the lung, these were small apart from a mass of tumour in the paraaortic glands. Another extreme case is that of REISER (1948), the patient developing a local orbital recurrence after a period of 14 years. Cases of this kind are examples of limited metastasis at sites where the tumour has difficulty in becoming established. A period of arrest within the retina itself is a possibility and might well account for many late onset retinoblastomas. RYCHENER (1948) reported a small tumour beneath the optic nervehead in a 33-year-old woman which appeared to have developed on the scar of an "old choroiditis".

Of relevance in regard to such anomalous behaviour must be the structural changes in the neoplastic retinae. In recent years and having an obvious bearing on the subject are a number of case reports in which the morbid anatomical findings have conformed to the rare but distinctive pattern of "retinoblastoma planum". Under the title of "Diffuse Infiltrating Retinoblastoma" SCHOFIELD (1960) described 5 cases of this kind in at least 4 of which the diagnosis had been established by aspiration of fluid from the anterior chamber, as each appeared to contain a hypopyon, the known duration of which had not exceeded 4 months. In the enucleated eye from an 8-year-old boy described by MANSCHOT (1956) small clusters of cells on the iris and in the anterior chamber had been noted clinically and in conjunction with the vitreous haze had led to a provisional diagnosis of tuberculosis, the eye having been inflamed for 3 months. WEIZENBLATT (1957) recorded the tragedy of an 8-year-old boy with one year's history of defective left vision who at initial examination showed ball and strand-like opacities in the vitreous, was labelled "uveitis" and died of cerebral retinoblastoma 1 1/2 years later, a short time after enucleation. The age distribution of these seven unilateral cases is striking, being 1, 4, 6, 8, 8, 9 and 11 years and all male apart from the youngest. In all these enucleated globes the basic neoplasia had been of an in situ character, widespread and often involving much of the retina though producing little in the way of retinal thickening, but with ribbons of tumour cells both to the deep aspect from rupture of the outer layers in older lesions and in substantial amount on the inner aspect of the internal limiting membrane whence nodular masses had become detached to float in the vitreous chamber and beyond. WINTERSTEINER separated the plane or diffuse from the circumscribed tumours while HIRSCHBERG regarded them as a later stage. In effect, they are unusually flat examples of retinoblastoma which produce little in the way of retinal detachment and, as they progress, behave in endophytic fashion. The adult case of DEPOUILLY et al. so well illustrated by DOLLFUS and AUVERT, also belongs here. In a recent Manchester case the enucleated right eye contained multiple patches of retinoblastoma planum involving much of the retina (Fig. 14) and at

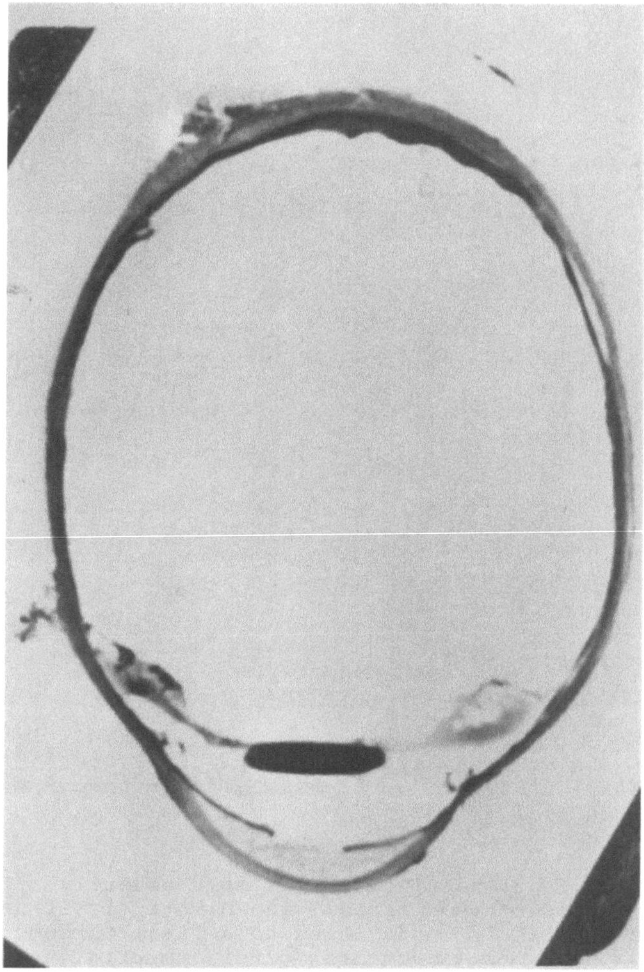

*Fig. 14. Retinoblastoma planum. Extensive multiple foci with restricted or negligible thickening of retina*

varying stages of development. Some foci show only proliferation and fusion of the nuclear layers, others are more lumpy with spread to the internal retinal face (Fig. 15) and, very occasionally, a true endophytic growth with supporting vascular skeleton. The boy was almost 5 years old at enucleation and the history, as judged by photophobia and change in the colour of the iris, dates back to an age of 6 months or less. Of significance is the still relatively lowgrade neoplasia in the main and posterior lesion and also the presence of a solitary retinoblastoma showing a few coarse drusen at the superotemporal equator in the left i. e. second eye which has remained static during 2 1/2 years of observation. HOSCH (1888) followed such a case with the ophthalmoscope, the tumour in the one eye continued to grow and eventually fungate while a lesion near the disc in the second eye with some large drusen remained unchanged. Altogether, within the Manchester series 10 patients have been discovered with functioning eyes harbouring spontaneously arrested retinoblastoma, all being adult at recognition apart from the one boy. In two patients the lesions comprised solitary unilateral tumours and, in a third, multiple ones distributed 4 : 1 between the retinae. In the re-

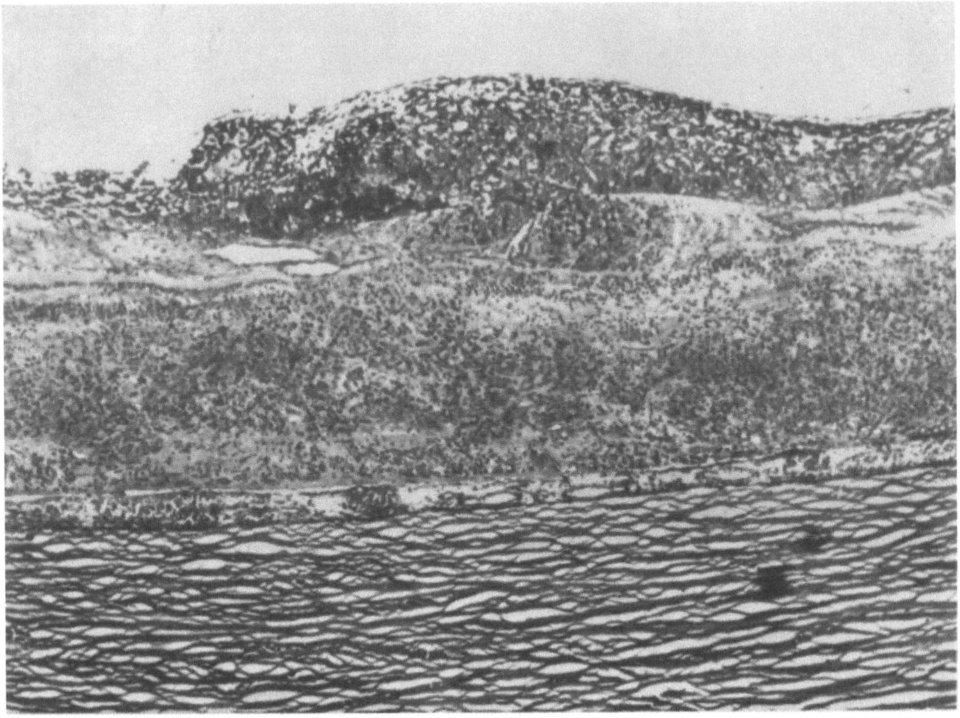

*Fig. 15. Retinoblastoma planum. Intraretinal neoplasia of variable density with focus of highly cellular tumour erupting on to internal retinal face (X 65)*

maining 7 bilateral cases the most severely affected eye had been enucleated for retinoblastoma, known in at least 5 of the patients to be active and likely to have led to a fatal outcome failing removal. Following a death from bronchial carcinoma with cerebral secondaries one of these retained eyes became available for histological examination. The neoplastic retina was thickened by an excess of neural elements with loss of the normal structure but preserving a relatively open and fibrillary pattern without necrosis apart from the odd small group of calcified cells. A Liverpool case provides one further example, the tumour being in a boy of 8 years but of long duration; it extended downwards as a relatively flat thickening of the retina beneath the disc with some coarse drusen in its lower part and was of moderate cellularity (Figs. 16 and 17). These eleven cases of spontaneous arrest in functioning eyes have been reported in some detail by one of the authors (SMITH, 1974) with the suggestion that the intraretinal proliferation has remained relatively low grade prior to arrest instead of "exploding" into a typical retinoblastoma. The "infiltrating" type of retinoblastoma appears to form a bridge between those occasional lesions destined for arrest and the usual proliferative form, and it would seem that the fundamental difference vis-à-vis the latter hinges on the relative lack of vascular response shown by the plane varieties so that the typical structure of increasing nodularity with viable tumour mantled around new vessels is avoided. In effect, natural arrest is to be correlated with an absence of vasoproliferation, prominently displayed by actively growing tumours and at times including a notable dilatation of the feeder vessels. This could well be linked with a failure to produce an angiogenic factor such as has been demonstrated in many cancers including

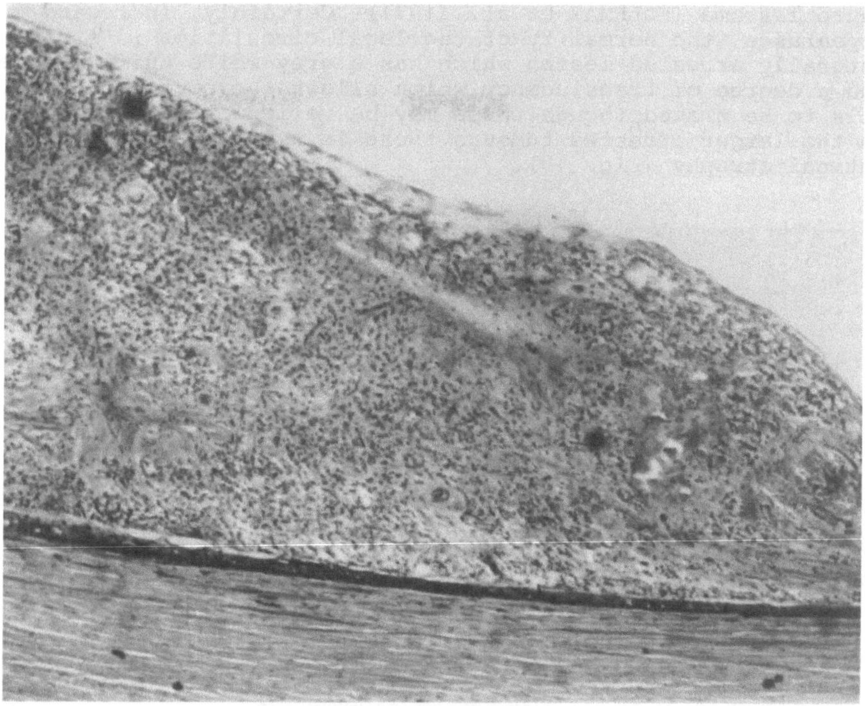

*Fig. 16. Spontaneously arrested retinoblastoma. Diffusely thickened in situ retina of moderate cellularity (X 50)*

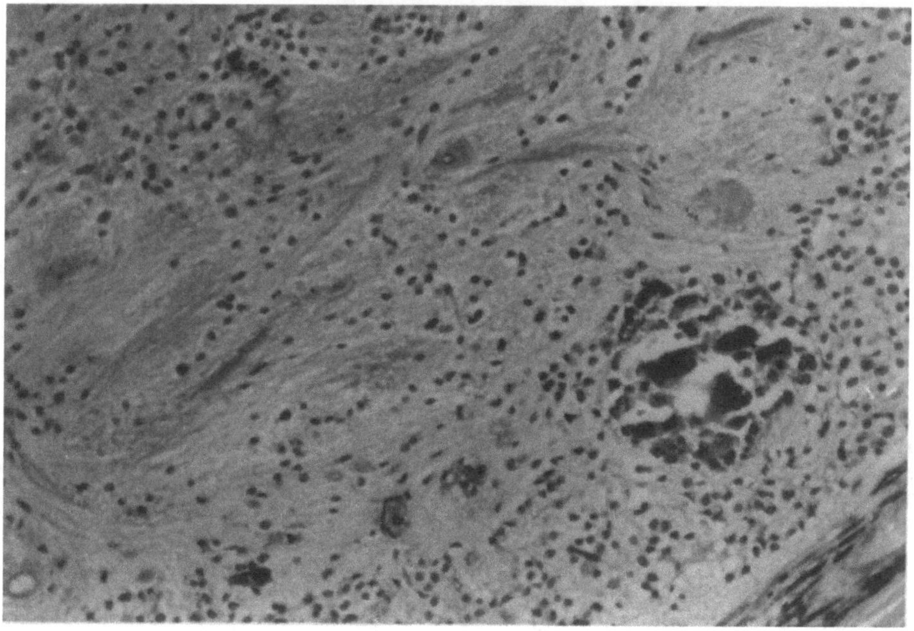

*Fig. 17. Spontaneously arrested retinoblastoma, showing low cellularity, fibrillary tissue, and calcified drusen. Reprinted from Transactions of the Ophthalmological Societies of the U.K. Volume XCIV Part IV 1974 (X 160)*

neuroblastoma (FOLKMAN et al., 1971). Certainly, in regard to fundal appearance, the normality of the local circulation is striking in the naturally arrested lesion which has a grey-white uniform appearance and a degree of translucency which allows the course of the larger vessels to be traced, though these may be veiled or even masked in part. In the larger arrested tumours there is usually a background of chorio-retinal atrophy (Fig. 18).

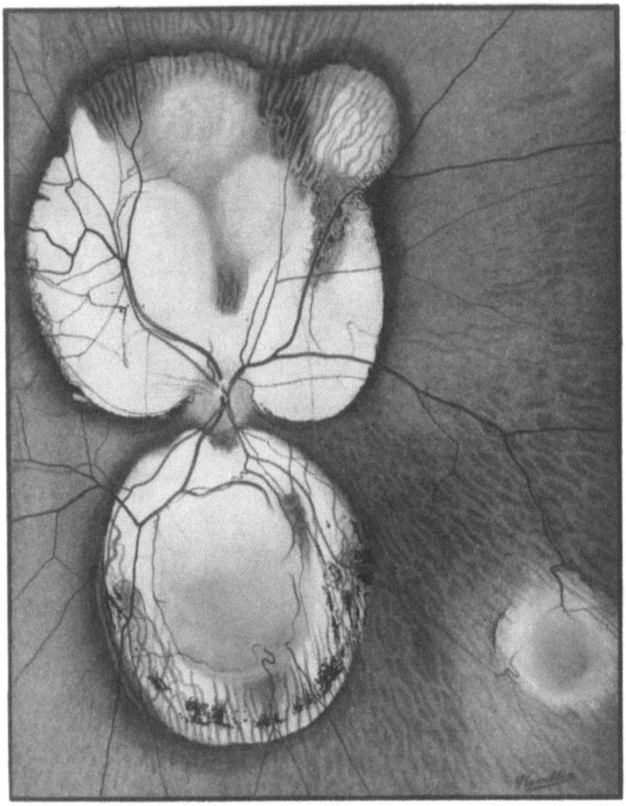

*Fig. 18. Multiple lesions of spontaneously arrested retinoblastoma with emphasized background of chorio-retinal atrophy showing some masking of vessels. Reprinted from Transactions of the Ophthalmological Societies of the United Kingdom. Volume XCIV Part IV 1974*

Out of the 7 Manchester patients retaining one functioning eye with naturally arrested retinoblastoma, the male noted above as dying of cerebral secondaries from bronchial carcinoma differed from the others in that the first and shrunken eye was not enuclated till 37 years and then on cosmetic grounds. Initially, this case was reported by STEWARD et al. (1956) with a review of the literature. A few additional examples of arrest have been reported since, including the comparable case (BONIUK and GIRARD, 1969) of a male aged 62 years with a shrunken right globe and a left one showing chorio-retinal atrophy with two elevated, chalky lesions. BONIUK and ZIMMERMAN (1962) have reviewed a unique collection of 14 shrunken eyes considered to contain arrested retinoblastoma, 6 being unilateral. The three cases where the eyes were enucleated at 8, 18, and 46 years would be fully acceptable and are, presumably, the ones where calcified clumps of tumour cells lay isolated in fibrous tissue often with local bone formation. The ages of the other 11 children at enucleation ranged from only 1 month to 3 1/2 years, 3 dying of tumour spread from the other eye and one having a recurrence. These could incorporate examples of temporary regression, a phenomenon well known to WINTERSTEINER and earlier writers and associated in particular with shrinkage of the globe following an acute congestive phase. The mechanism is one of retinal ischaemia with wholesale destruction of the tumour leaving as a residue the calcified blocks of cells which are more or less indestructible and which may also figure prominently in tumours arrested by artificial means, as by irradiation. Permanent arrest under such conditions may warrant the term "spontaneous regression" as the atrophy includes the retina itself, but it seems unlikely that this favourable result can be attributed solely to the inhibiting influence of ischaemia. On a more localised and temporary basis in a tumour projecting into the vitreous cavity, GROLMANN (1887) was able to watch shrinkage and renewed growth with the ophthalmoscope, the eye then developing a tumour hypopyon.

## GENETICS OF RETINOBLASTOMA

Retinoblastoma is a rare disorder, in general having been regarded as occurring in approximately 1 in 25,000 live births, as by ELLSWORTH (1969). FALLS and NEEL (1951) found 1 per 20,288 live births and calculated the rate of mutation to the retinoblastoma gene as $2.3 \times 10^{-5}$ per generation. SCHAPPERT-KIMMIJSER et al. (1966) have suggested the figure of 1 in 15,000. FRANCOIS (1964) has produced a summary suggesting that the incidence is becoming more common over the years, not only because of increasing success in treatment but as the spontaneous rate is also increasing. Retinoblastoma was thought to have much the same incidence throughout the world but recent data by ALBERT et al. (1974) indicate that it is unusually common in Haiti.

The familial occurrence of this tumour has attracted considerable attention since LERCHE (1821) reported 3 boys and 1 girl affected from amongst 7 siblings. Owing to the low survival rate among the earlier reported cases - as opposed to the modern figure of 80% or slightly better - no case of vertical transmission was recorded until 1896 (DE GOUVEA) when 3 out of 8 siblings were reported with the disease, the father having had a unilateral enucleation in 1872. However, a few known pedigrees had suggested this possibility. Thus, WINTERSTEINER quotes a case of GRAEFE in which several siblings of the mother had died from "eye cancer" in the first years of life and, later in 1874, THOMSON and KNAPP recorded a brother and sister together with three cousins affected by the disease.

From the large number of pedigrees now available it has become established that where retinoblastoma is familial it is inherited in dominant fashion with a high penetrance, at 80% (VOGEL, 1961; GORDON, 1974), and will include a number of unilateral cases, as for example in the recent series of BEDFORD et al. which incorporates several unilateral cases known to be hereditary. SORSBY (1972) thought penetrance might be even higher than 80% and estimated that 5%-10% of unilateral cases were incompletely expressed gonadal mutations, current theory attributing the beginnings of transmissible disease to germinal as opposed to somatic mutations. KNUDSON (1971) has developed a two-hit hypothesis by which the development of retinoblastoma is related to two successive mutational events. It is postulated that in the hereditary form the first mutation has already taken place so that the cells are already primed and this correlates with the greater risk of multiple lesions.

Even accepting such a dual origin, the frequency of the second event to produce a penetrance around 80% would seem unusually high for a mutation. The incidence of bilateral disease in second and third generations conforms closely to an 80% penetrance, but in first generations it has been at a much lower level, this difference being highlighted by retrospective reviews such as that of DOLLFUS and AUVERT (1953) who in 224 cases drawn from first generations found a unilateral to bilateral ratio of 2 : 1 i. e. similar to retinoblastoma overall. Two factors favour reduced bilaterality in the first generation. Firstly, there is a bias in favour of unilateral transmitters as they have had a somewhat better survival rate and have produced far more children than those affected with bilateral retinoblastoma; secondly, many patients of the first generation have not been subjected to the same careful observation as their descendents. This is well brought out in the Manchester series where there are 17 families with affected 1st degree relatives. In no less than 5 of these families the first affected member has shown unequivocal, spontaneously arrested retinoblastoma, on three occasions in the retained second eye and on two occasions without enucleation, these last comprising a solitary unilateral and multiple bilateral lesions respectively. This could still be an under-assessment since it has not been possible to examine the three unilateral probands born prior to 1900 as they had died. The corrected figures for first generation transmitters gives a bilaterality of 56%, much closer to the theoretical 80% but leaving a gap which could well be attributable to the difference in breeding habit. These results embracing 52 individuals with familial retinoblastoma are illustrated in Table 1. In two of the

Table 1. Hereditary retinoblastoma (17 families - Manchester series)

| Generation | | Totals | (Spont. Arrest) |
|---|---|---|---|
| 1st | Normal | 1 | |
| | Unilateral | 7 | (1) |
| | Bilateral | 9 | (4) |
| 2nd and 3rd | Unilateral | 6 | |
| | Bilateral | 27 | (1) |
| | Unknown | 3 | |

three "unknowns" of the second generation the evidence favours bilaterality. The third child died on the first day of life from a rare blood disease, the eyes being obtained post mortem. The right one contains a large tumour but, so far, histological examination of the left eye has proved negative.

Thus, analysis in regard to the first generation is misleading and it would seem more rewarding to rectify the disturbed laterality ratio by computing the numbers of potential transmitters, an exercise only possible where the patients and their close relatives have been systematically examined, as applies in the regional series assembled in Manchester. After deducting affected descendants numbering 24 there is a residuum of 108 unilateral and 58 bilateral cases presenting within the 50 years 1925 - 1974 inclusive. Accepting all such bilateral and 10% of the unilateral cases as transmitters and also allowing for slight referral bias represented by two bilateral cases presenting initially outside the region, the computed bilaterality rate for the first generation would be 84%. Based on these regional figures from the North West one may estimate that out of new cases unassociated with familial disease, two-fifths would be of the hereditary type and three-fifths would fall within the so-called "sporadic" group.

In only one of the 17 Manchester families does the first generation consist of individuals with normal fundi. In many of the earlier reported pedigrees the parents have had supposedly normal fundi, causing some investigators to favour recessive transmission, though this is at variance with the high proportion of affected siblings. In a wider context one cannot exclude the possibility of recessive inheritance which BADTKE (1940) thought might well play a major role in sporadic retinoblastoma. A number of cousin marriages have been implicated, HEMMES (1931) finding two such in a series of 48 patients together with one case resulting from a father-daughter union. In 72 families FALLS and NEEL (1951) found a blood relationship only once, the patients being first cousins once removed. A cousin of one Manchester case produced a fourth child with the disease, both of these examples being unilateral.

Familial retinoblastoma presents early, contrasting with the greater range of the sporadic forms, this being reflected in the figures for symptomatic onset as between the bilateral and unilateral cases (Table 2). Of bilateral cases 79 % had symptoms dating back to the first year of life, as compared with only 36% of the unilateral.

Table 2. Symptomatic onset (1925 - 1974 Manchester series)

| Unilateral | | | | | | | | | Total |
|---|---|---|---|---|---|---|---|---|---|
| Age (years) | -1 | -2 | -3 | -4 | -5 | -6 | -7 | -8 | |
| Number of cases | 41 | 24 | 27 | 9 | 4 | 3 | 2 | 1 | |
| | Additionally, two cases of spont. arrest at 11 and 25 yrs. | | | | | | | | 113 |
| Bilateral (based on 1st affected eye) | | | | | | | | | |
| Age (years) | -1/2 | -1 | -1 1/2 | -2 | -2 1/2 | -3 | -3 1/2 | | |
| Number of cases | 43 | 18 | 9 | 3 | 2 | 1 | 1 | | 77 |

A slow rate of growth characterises a small proportion of known familial (or bilateral) retinoblastomas, manifest in delayed onset, notably in relation to the second eye and by a prolonged course in those destined to be fatal. Two Manchester cases are worthy of mention. The first, a girl, lost her left eye at 9 months, was blind in the second eye by 5 years but survived till within a fortnight of her tenth birthday. The second concerns a boy, also a second generation case but of another family, diagnosed as bilateral retinoblastoma in the first year of life and who eventually died in his eighth year from local disease, the only distant secondaries found being in both kidneys. BROWN (1966 a) in regard to 22 unilateral cases found a postoperative survival time ranging from 2 - 17 months with an average of 9.2 months. By contrast, in 42 bilateral cases ultimately fatal, only 76% had died 3 years after enucleation. Inherent in these figures is the suggestion of two populations, the one showing a fairly standard pattern and comprising children with unilateral disease, and the other exhibiting a more variable course and comprising children with bilateral i. e. hereditary retinoblastoma. The spontaneously arrested tumours derive from those of slow growth and it seems likely that this phenomenon is a manifestation of familial retinoblastoma in particular, if not exclusively.

In 1963, a further dimension was added to the genetics of this disorder when LELE et al. reported an abnormal karyotype in a female patient with bilateral retinoblastoma in which about one-third of the long arm of a D-chromosome was missing. In 1969 ALLERDICE et al. established the concept of a specific 13q-deletion syndrome. They reviewed the wide spectrum of congenital malformation which was associated with retinoblastoma in approximately one quarter of the children. The range of abnormality has included mental retardation, microphthalmos, colobomata, ptosis, facial asymmetry, malformed ears, cleft palate, short webbed neck, clinodactyly, absent thumbs, lumbosacral agenesis, undescended testicles, hypospadias and imperforate anus. Studies in chromosome banding indicate that the syndrome may be subdivided according to the site and size of the deletion. Retinoblastoma has been related to an interstitial deletion of mainly band q21 (ORYE et al., 1974) and may be found with mild or severe manifestations of the syndrome. ORYE et al. compared their patient who had mild psychomotor retardation, a bifid uvula, and clinodactyly with those of LELE et al. and WILSON et al. (1969, 1973), both of whom had minor anomalies including a degree of mental retardation and in the latter case a cleft palate. HOWARD et al. (1974) brought the total of reported cases of retinoblastoma associated with D-deletion up to nine, five of the tumours being bilateral, three unilateral, and one unspecified.

JENSEN and MILLER (1971) analysed a large hospital series drawn from several centres, adequate information being obtained on 1077 children. In regard to anomalies, only mental retardation significantly exceeded expectations, there being 15 cases of severe mental defect, as compared with 4.7 expected on the basis of similar studies of other childhood cancers. In addition to one with Down's syndrome, 6 had anomalies outside the nervous system including colobomata, microcephaly, cleft palate and low-set ears which are features of the D-deletion syndromes. The association between mental retardation and retinoblastoma is well known and it seems likely that a proportion of children showing both characteristics will have an underlying chromosome anomaly of this type. However, the incidence of mental defect would seem higher than the above figures suggest, being recorded by FALLS and NEEL as occurring five times in their series of 73 cases, one having internal hydrocephalus. TAKTIKOS (1964) found this association in 9 out of 300 cases, the one unilateral case being a typical mongol and 3 of the others having hydrocephalus. In Manchester since 1925 there are 7 mentally retarded children out of 145 survivors of retinoblastoma, i. e. 4.8%.

## Second Primary Cancers

In the series of 1077 children investigated by JENSEN and MILLER, 11 were known to have developed second primary tumours outside the field of radiotherapy or when no radiation had been given, 3 of these being osteosarcomata of the femur. KITCHIN and ELLSWORTH (1974), based on an initial population of 1130 retinoblastoma patients seen mainly at the Institute of Ophthalmology, New York, increased this total to 9 osteosarcomas of the long bones; in addition, they found two thyroid cancers, a Wilms' tumour, and a Ewing's sarcoma, all patients having had bilateral retinoblastoma except one of those developing carcinoma of the thyroid. Over the same period 17 soft tissue and 16 bone sarcomas together with two examples of squamous epithelioma had developed within the radiation fields so that overall there were 7% second primaries after a mean latent period of 13 years. SCHIMKE et al. (1974) have reported a brother and sister who survived bilateral retinoblastoma only to develop osteogenic sarcoma of the femur at 9 and 11 years respectively. Chromosome studies carried out on the boy were normal; specifically no D-group abnormality was found. AHERNE (1974) records six examples of osteosarcoma presenting within the age group 12-17 years, three in the femur and three in the tibia. Five of these patients had been afflicted with bilateral retinoblastoma, one belonging to the Manchester series. A second Manchester case also died from sarcoma which developed at the upper end of the tibia, but described histologically as of "polymorphous cell" type. This association of hereditary retinoblastoma with non-radiogenic osteosarcoma is a most striking one and is in marked excess of other secondary cancers of the childhood period. Acute lymphoblastic leukaemia has been recorded by STRONG et al. (1972) and HOEFNAGEL et al. (1973).

Clearly, it is important to investigate the entire life span of patients who have suffered from retinoblastoma, particularly those in the hereditary group. Out of the 52 known hereditary cases in the Manchester series so far there have been 13 deaths in childhood - eight from retinoblastoma itself, two from sarcoma of tibia, two from measles at a very early age, and one on the first day of life from a blood disorder considered to be congenital dyserythropoiesis type 1. Otherwise there are 27 survivors and nine known to have died of second cancers, as listed below:

| Sex | Age at death (yrs.) | Nature of Second Cancer |
|---|---|---|
| F | 31 | Radioresistant metastatic tumour of unknown origin presenting initially in the shaft of the femur |
| F | 42 | Sarcoma botryoides of the vagina (reported by LEVENE, 1960) |
| M | 47 | Multiple sarcomatous nodules, probably leimyosarcoma but primary site unknown |
| F | 52 | Carcinoma of breast |
| M | 47 | Carcinoma of lung |
| M | 52 | Carcinoma of lung |
| M | 56 | Carcinoma of lung |
| M | 54 | Carcinoma of lung and of bladder |
| F | 61 | Carcinoma of bladder |

In these later age groups, the number of second primary cancers is far in excess of the expected frequency and it seems that the presence of a transmissible retinoblastoma gene poses an additional threat throughout life.

## CLINICAL MANAGEMENT

### Examination

There is now no doubt that the single most important instrument for the evaluation of eyes containing this tumour is the use of the indirect ophthalmoscope employing scleral indentation under full general anaesthetic (see Fig. 19). This was first stressed by REESE and ELLSWORTH (1963) and using this technique it was reported by REESE (1967) that the diagnosis is certain in over 90% of the cases. This instrument facilitates the examination of the whole fundus and enables an arbitrary classification of the disease to be made.

However, in certain other cases other techniques may be necessary and in cases of eyes suffering from uveitis or hypopyon aspiration of the anterior chamber may be necessary, whilst the presence of opaque media may necessitate the use of ultrasonography as suggested by TILL and OSSOING (1968) and in advanced cases CSF may be involved as reported by IFEKUNIGWE et al. (1966). In these cases it is usual for the optic foramina to be enlarged on X-ray investigation. The excretion of VMA and HVA as suggested by BROWN (1966b) may occasionally be useful but it does not appear to be of any routine clinical use.

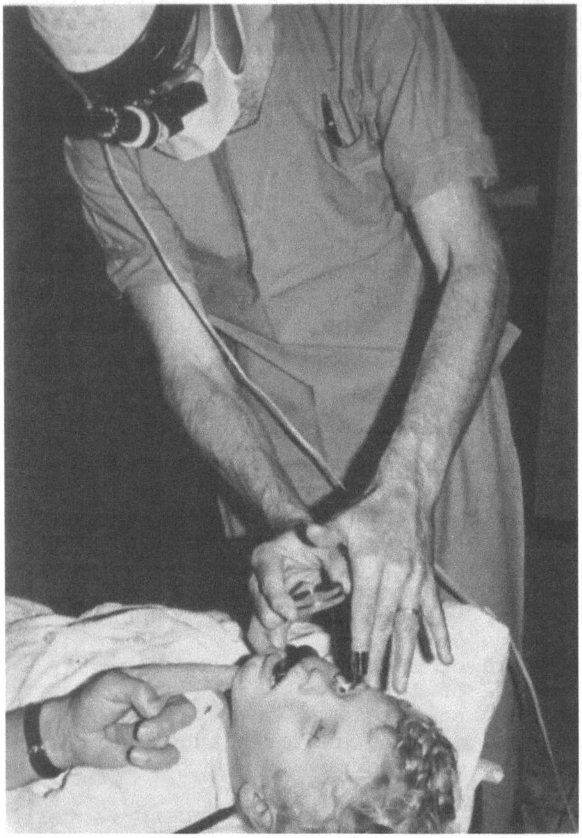

*Fig. 19. A modern indirect ophthalmoscope being used with scleral indentation. Note that this may only be accomplished correctly with child under full general anaesthesia*

In summary then, in any well-developed country where only the milder form of the disease presents, all that is required is a full examination with binocular indirect ophthalmoscopy under general anaesthesia. With most advanced cases conventional X-rays will show the spread of the disease to the various fissures of the orbit or to the optic foramen. CSF examinations may be called for as may be a brain scan or a full skeletal survey with X-rays to prove or refute the presence of metastases.

## Treatment

Since the days of bilateral enucleations treatment has progressed extensively via different avenues of approach.

In the 1940's and 1950's various centres throughout the world were perfecting their own separate techniques and for a decade each large specialised unit propounded its own methods. Nowadays, however, it is generally conceded that no single technique is suitable for all cases and most large eye tumour centres employ several, if not all, therapeutic approaches; not necessarily using them together, sometimes consecutively or singly in an attempt not only to deal with the tumour, but also reduce the number of complications which can occur.

1. "Whole-Eye" Irradiation

This can be administered by one of two routes:

a) The temporal approach with betatron as practised by the New York school and reported by ELLSWORTH (1970). Using this technique the more severely affected eye has usually been removed and with the "knife-edge" of this type of radiation directed transversely an attempt is made to spare the lens of the remaining eye and to irradiate the whole retina as a primary form of treatment. This school believes the whole retina is at risk and must be "sterilised": a theory that has not met with complete acceptance in other centres like London where it is not considered that the other, more affected eye, must always be removed (see enucleation). This technique is technically very easy and is widely recognised and used. Recurrences can be dealt with by light-coagulation, cryotherapy, or the application of a cobalt plaque.

b) The direct anterior approach utilising the cobalt beam unit as reported by SKEGGS and WILLIAMS (1966). With this technique the whole eye is deliberately irradiated. The technique is very easy and both eyes can be treated if necessary, the child being sedated under ketamine. It can be used for very large anterior tumours and is probably the only technique which will deal with free-floating neoplastic cells in the vitreous. Its only disadvantage would appear to be that all cases develop a radiation cataract, but it does seem that all do not progress and those that do can be very easily treated with modern aspiration techniques. Recurrences may be treated as in a).

Both of these "whole-eye" techniques will aim to deliver something in the order of 4000 rads over 3 to 4 weeks. At one time chemotherapy was employed routinely in those cases undergoing "whole-eye" irradiation by either a) or b) utilising TEM or cyclophosphamide. Nowadays TEM by the intra-arterial route is only used for residual orbital disease whilst cyclophosphamide together with vincristine is useful for palliation of metastases.

2. Focal Eye Irradiation

There have been several attempts with small numbers of cases suggesting the use of various forms of gamma ray emitters but the main work has been done by STALLARD (1966). The discs used can be of various shapes and sizes, the most useful being the circular ones (Fig. 20) as can be seen by the isodose curve (Fig. 21). However, the higher doses received by the base of the tumour preclude their use adjacent to the disc or macula and the large plaque (15 mm active diameter) will almost certainly produce vascular complications anywhere in the eye. Thus at present probably the largest plaque that can be used routinely is the 10 mm circular one but not nearer than, say, 10 mm from the optic disc or macula (see indications and complications). The use of beta applicators (106 Ruthenium) has been suggested by LOMMATSCH (1966). It would appear that these applicators can be very useful but it is likely that the complications may prove to be similar to those noted for cobalt plaque (see complications) and therefore they will be subject to the same limitations (see indications).

3. Light-Coagulation

In 1963 HÖPPING and MEYER-SCHWICKERATH (1964) showed how useful light-coagulation could be for certain tumours. Thus, in spite of subsequent doubts raised by other workers, there is now no doubt that it has a place in the treatment of certain small tumours (see indications).

4. Cryosurgery

LINCOFF in 1967 reported the first case of a retinoblastoma so treated. Several small series followed thereafter, culminating in a report by

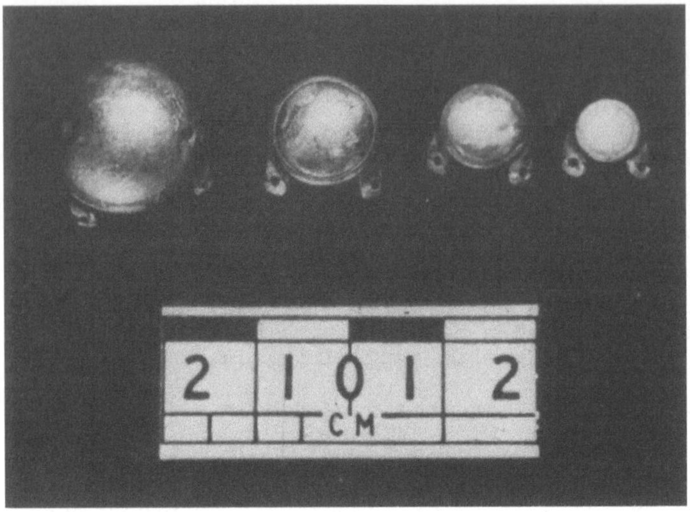


*Fig. 20. Circular radio-active applicators, 5, 7.5, 10 and 15 mm radio-active diameter*

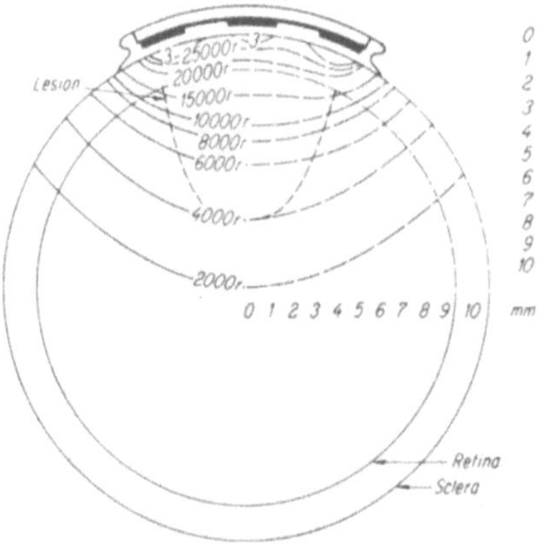


*Fig. 21. 10 mm radio-active diameter circular applicator, 1.84 mC $^{60}Co$, to show isodose curves. The interrupted line represents the outline of the neoplasm*

TOLENTINO and TABLANTE in 1972. They reported a series of five cases treated by this modality. This paper showed that there is a definite place for this form of therapy in certain forms of tumours (see indications).

Thus it can be seen that there are various forms of treatment involving either whole-eye treatment or focal treatment which can be used and the form of therapy embarked on primarily should be that which can not only deal with the neoplasm present, but produces the least complications for a tumour of any given size in any given site (see indications and complications).

5. Enucleation

In the past this was probably the treatment to save a child's life in advanced cases. Over the decades however, such advanced cases are not commonly seen in well-developed countries, but even so one of the most vexed questions still asked is "which eye should be enucleated?". In the last 10 years the answer has been changing. Thus REESE and ELLSWORTH (1963) stressed enucleation of the more affected eye in bilateral cases. Similar comments were made about unilateral cases in which case it was suggested that the eye should always be removed without any attempted therapy (LEELAWONGS and REGAN, 1968). However, STALLARD had already stated "there is no case for excision of the unilateral tumour of 10 mm".In the series of BEDFORD et al. the only indication for enucleation was involvement of the optic nerve and each eye is taken on its own merits. Because therapy is now so successful it would seem there has been a move away from the automatic removal of either a singly affected eye or the worse eye in a bilateral case. After enucleation, as stressed by BEDFORD and MacFAUL, there should be no implant whatsoever in the orbit as such a mass precludes palpation at subsequent examinations.

Prognosis of Retinoblastoma (after ELLSWORTH)

| Group | Prognosis | Characteristics | Results |
|---|---|---|---|
| I | Very favourable | Solitary and multiple tumours less than 4 disc diameters at or behind equator | 100% |
| II | Favourable | Solitary and multiple tumours 4-10 disc diameters at or behind equator | 100% |
| III | Favourable | Any lesion anterior to equator. Solitary lesion greater than 10 disc diameters behind equator | 82% |
| IV | Unfavourable | Multiple tumours greater than 10 disc diameters. Any lesion extending anteriorly beyond the limits of ophthalmoscopy | 75% |
| V | Very unfavourable | Massive tumour involving more than half the retina. Vitreous seeding | 75% |
| VI | Very unfavourable | Residual orbital disease. Optic nerve involvement and extrascleral extension | 75% |

Complications

1. Cobalt Plaques or Ruthenium Plaques
The larger retinal vessels appear most susceptible to the relatively high doses of radiation seen here and in children diffuse dense vitreous haemorrhages tend to appear some months after the plaque is placed near to the optic nerve. This will occur with even small plaques but there is a higher chance with larger plaques.

2. Light-coagulation
It has been suggested (HOWARD, 1966; HOWARD and BLODI, 1966) that light-coagulation might facilitate the spread of neoplasms into the choroid and on a general ophthalmological basis it was seen that light-coagulation posteriorly is bound to produce relatively large field defects. In addition of course it cannot be used for large tumours.

3. Cryosurgery

No undue major complications have been reported yet and it should be anticipated that their advent is unlikely, provided the indications for treatment are stringently observed (see indications).

4. "Whole-Eye" Irradiation

The most feared complication of either the cobalt beam unit or the betatron is the development of radiation-induced sarcoma. The largest relevant series reported so far is that of SAGERMAN et al. (1969). They described 21 cases, the latent period being from 4-30 years. Other smaller series have been reported and it is probably a matter of time before a case is reported from all types of radiation, either by whole-eye techniques or by the focal techniques mentioned above. A radiation cataract inevitably develops with cobalt beam therapy using the direct anterior field but this apparently does not produce a serious hazard particularly in view of modern aspiration techniques.

## Indications for Treatment

1. All tumours up to 3 mm

A single small tumour could be treated by any of the former therapies listed above but the type of therapy is not so much dictated by the size as by situation. It would appear unnecessary to deliberately irradiate the whole eye either with the betatron or cobalt beam unit as these forms are, ideally, only given once as repeated doses give an increased chance of radiation-induced sarcoma or perhaps brain necrosis. A small single tumour can easily be treated focally and if, during the initial examination, it can be seen on the dimple produced by the scleral depressor, then cryosurgery would be indicated as it is quick and effective. If however, the tumour is farther back then light-coagulation would be indicated. If it is adjacent to the optic disc or macula then the field defect so induced would prohibit this form of therapy. This situation would appear to be the ideal indication for the betatron used temporally to spare the lens.

2. Tumours from 3 mm - 10 mm

These would appear to be too large for certain cure with "light" or "cryo", so focal irradiation techniques appear to be indicated either by cobalt plaque or ruthenium plaque. However, should the tumour be adjacent to the optic disc or macula then again there would appear to be an excellent case for betatron therapy from the side because of the risks of bleeding from radiation retinopathy.

3. Tumours larger than 10 mm

These would appear to be best treated by whole-eye irradiation by either the betatron or the cobalt beam unit. However, the presence of vitreous seedlings would seem to indicate anterior cobalt beam therapy with the subsequent development of a radiation cataract. There may be a case for intra-arterial TEM in these cases although one of the largest units using cobalt beam therapy does not use any form of chemotherapy for the strictly intra-ocular form of the disease.

4. Multiple Tumours

Two tumours in one eye can be treated by the focal methods listed above provided that the largest tumour is not greater than 10 mm. If it is, then the whole eye must be irradiated. Below this size two tumours can be treated by a combination of focal irradiation to one and light or cryo to the other, or light to one and cryo to the other. It is probably unwise to put two focal radiation plaques on one eye at one time because of the ensuing vascular complications. All other types of tumours are best treated by whole-eye irradiation bearing in mind the criteria listed above.

5. Indications for Enucleation

There would appear to be a growing move away from the opinion that the excision of the worst-affected eye is necessary or one eye in a unilateral case. In view of the success of the techniques described above it is probably worthwhile treating all cases provided that the optic nerve can be seen to be free of the tumour. Thus, involvement of the optic nerve would appear to be the only indication for enucleation and this can be seen either by direct examination or would have to be assumed because of the presence of opaque media.

6. Recurrent Orbital Disease

It would appear that there is a case for the administration of intra-arterial TEM in these cases, perhaps combined with exenteration.

7. Metastatic Disease

At present it would seem that the administration of a combination of vincristine and cyclophosphamide offers some hope.

In general it would seem that there is a move towards a more conservative approach and to the rapid referral to large centres who are equipped with many, if not all, of the therapeutic approaches used in the above.

## REFERENCES


AHERNE, G.: Trans. ophthal. Soc. U.K. 94, 938 (1974)

ALBERT, D. M., LAHAV, M., LESSER, R., CRAFT, J.: Trans. ophthal. Soc. U.K. 94, 909 (1974)

ALLDERDICE, P. W., DAVIS, J. G., MILLER, O. J., KLINGER, H. P., WARBURTON, D., MILLER, D. A., ALLEN, F. H., ABRAMS, C. A. L., McGILVRAY, E.: Amer. J. hum. Genet. 21, 499 (1969)

BADTKE, G.: Klin. Mbl. Augenheilk. 105, 451 (1940)

BEDFORD, M. A., BEDOTTO, C., MacFAUL, P. A.: Brit. J. Ophthal. 55, 19 (1971)

BEDFORD, M. A., MacFAUL, P. A.: Brit. J. Ophthal. 53, 382 (1969)

BEER: Lhb. d. Augenkrankheiten, Vienna 2, 495 (1817)

BONIUK, M.: Ocular and Adnexal Tumours ed. M. BONIUK. Saint Louis: C.V. Mosby 1964, p. 200

BONIUK, M., GIRARD, L. J.: Trans. Amer. Acad. Ophthal. Otolaryng. 73, 194 (1969)

BONIUK, M., ZIMMERMAN, L. E.: Int. Ophthal. Clin. 2 (2), 925 (1962)

BOWATER, J. VERNON: Roy. Lond. ophthal. Hosp. Rep. 6, 155 (1868)

BROWN, D. H.: Amer. J. Ophthal. 61, 508 (1966a)

BROWN, D. H.: Amer. J. Ophthal. 62, 239 (1966b)

BRUNNER, H.: Klin. Mbl. Augenheilk. 159, 664 (1971)

CARBAJAL, U. M.: Amer. J. Ophthal. 48, 47 (1959)

CARTER, B.: Med. Times and Gazette, 5th December, p. 583 (1863)

COLLINS, E.T.: Researches into the Anatomy and Pathology of the Eye. London: H. K. Lewis, 1896

CRESPI: Gazetta medica Italiane-Lombardia. No. 26-28, 43, 44 (1876)

DE GOUVEA: Bull. Soc. Med. Chir. Rio de Janeiro 8, 25 (1896)

DEPOUILLY, OFFRET, LENOIR: Citation by DOLLFUS M. A. and AUVERT, B: Le Gliome de la Retine et les Pseudogliomes. Paris: Masson, 1953, p. 123

DOLLFUS, M. A., AUVERT, B.: Le Gliome de la Retine et les Pseudogliomes Paris: Masson, 1953, p. 42, 86, 132, 136

DUKE-ELDER, S.: Textbook of Ophthalmology. London: Kimpton, 1940, Vol. III, p. 2833

ELLSWORTH, R. M.: Trans. Amer. Ophthal. Soc. 67, 462 (1969)

FALLS, H. F., NEEL, J. V.: Arch. Ophthal. 46, 367 (1951)

FAVALORO, G.: An. di Ott. 65, 881 (1937)

FISCHER, B.: Zbl. allgem. Path. u. path. Anat. 29, 545 (1918)

FLEXNER, S.: Bull. Johns Hopk. Hosp. 2, 115 (1891)

FOLKMAN, J., MERLER, E., ABERNATHY, C., WILLIAMS, G.: J. exp. Med. 133, 275 (1971)

FRANCOIS, J.: Ocular and Adnexal Tumours. BONIUK, M. (ed.). Saint Louis: C. V. Mosby, 1964, p. 123

FREZOTTI, R., GUERRA, R., BONANNI, R.: Boll. Oculist. 46, 765 (1967)

FRIENDLY, D. S., PARKS, M.: Arch. Ophthal. 84, 525 (1970)

FULTON, H.: Amer. J. Roentg. 64, 735 (1950)

GEFFEN, L. B., LIVETT, B. G.: Physiol. Rev. 51, 98 (1971)

GINSBERG, S.: v. Graefes Arch. Ophthal. 48, 92 (1899)

GRINKER, R. R.: Arch. Ophthal. 5, 920 (1931)

V. GROLMANN, W.: v. Graefes Arch. Ophthal. 33, 47 (1887)

GORDON, H.: Birth Defects. Original Article Series 10, 185 (1974)

HEMMES, G. D.: Klin. Mbl. Augenheilk. 86, 331 (1931)

HERM, R. J., HEATH, P.: Amer. J. Ophthal. 41, 22 (1956)

HIRSCHBERG, J.: v. Graefes Arch. Ophthal. 14, 30 (1868)

HIRSCHBERG, J.: Der Markschwamm der Netzhaut. Berlin: A. Hirschwald (1869)

HOEFNAGEL, D., McINTYRE, O. R., STORRS, R. C., SULLIVAN, P. B., MAURER, L. H.: Lancet 1, 725 (1973)

HOPPING, W., MEYER-SCHWICKERATH, R. G.: Ocular and Adnexal Tumours. BONIUK, M. (ed.). Saint Louis: C. V. Mosby, 1964, p. 192

HOSCH, F.: Arch. Augenheilk. 18, 336 (1888)

HOWARD, R. O., BREG, W. R., ALBERT, D. M., LESSER, R. L.: Arch. Ophth. 92, 490 (1974)

HOWARD, G. M.: Arch. Ophthal. 68, 615 (1962)

HOWARD, G. M.: Trans. Amer. Acad. Ophthal. Otolaryng. 70, 984 (1966)

HOWARD, G. M.: Arch. Ophthal. 76, 7 (1966)

HOWARD, G. M., BLODI, F. C.: Klin. Mbl. Augenheilk. 148, 856 (1966)

HOWARD, G. M., ELLSWORTH, R. M.: Amer. J. Ophthal. 60, 610 (1965)

IFEKUNIGWE, A. E., PULVERTAFT, R. J., WILLIAMS, A. O.: Brit. J. Cancer 20, 250 (1966)

IWANOFF, A.: v. Graefes Arch. Ophthal. 15 (2), 69 (1869)

JENSEN, R. D., MILLER, R. W.: New Engl. J. Med. 285, 307 (1971)

KIFFNEY, G. T.: Arch. Ophthal. 72, 231 (1964)

KITCHIN, F. D., ELLSWORTH, R. M.: J. Med. Genet. 11, 244 (1974)

KNAPP, H.: Klin. Mbl. Augenheilk. 6, 428 (1868)

KNUDSON, A. G.: Proc. Nat. Acad. Sci. USA 68 (4), 820 (1971)

KOBAYASHI, S., MUKAI, N.: Cancer Res. 34, 1646 (1974)

KREIBIG, W.: Klin. Mbl. Augenheilk. 114, 84 (1949)

LANDSBERG, M.: v. Graefes Arch. Ophthal. 21 (2), 93 (1875)

LANGENBECK: Langenbeck's neue Bibliothek f. d. Chirurgie. Hannover: 1822, Vol. III

LATIES, A. M., JACOBOWITZ, D.: Anat. Rec. 156, 383 (1966)

LEELAWONGS, N. L., REGAN, C.: Amer. J. Ophthal. 66, 1050 (1968)

LELE, K., PENROSE, L., STALLARD, H. B.: Ann. Hum. Genet. 27, 171 (1963)

LERCHE: Vermischte Abhandlungen aus d. Gebiete der Heilkunde von einer Gesellschaft prakt. Ärzte in Petersburg. I. Samml. Nr. 14 (1821)

LEVENE, M.: Cancer 13, 532 (1960)

LINCKE, C. G.: Tractatus de fungo medullari oculi. Lipsiae (1834)

LINCOFF, H., McLEAN, J. M., LONG, R.: Amer. J. Ophthal. 63, 389 (1967)

LOMMATSCH, P., VOLLMER, R.: Klin. Mbl. Augenheilk. 148, 682 (1966)

MAGHY, C.: Brit. J. Ophthal. 3, 337 (1919)

MAKIUCHI, S.: Chio Ganka Ito. 27, 38 (1935)

MAKLEY, T. A.: Arch. Ophthal. 69, 325 (1963)

MANSCHOT, W. A.: Ophthalmologica 132, 162 (1956)

MARCHESANI, O.: Ber. dtsch. ophthal. Ges. 48, 269 (1930)

MEHRA, K. S., HAMID, S.: Amer. J. Ophthal. 52, 405 (1961)

MEISNER, W.: Ber. dtsch. ophthal. Ges. 57, 129 (1951)

MERRIAM, G. R.: Arch. Ophthal. 44, 71 (1950)

MIDDLEMORE, R.: Observations on fungus hematodes of the eye. London: Medical Gazette 6, 878 (1830)

MULLANEY, J.: Lancet 2, 918 (1968)

MULLANEY, J.: Arch. Ophthal. 82, 454 (1969)

NELLESSEN, J.: Casuistische Beiträge zur Kenntnis des Glioms d. Netzhaut. Inaug. Dissert. Halle-Wittenberg (1872)

O'GRADY, R. B., ROTHSTEIN, T. B., ROMANO, P. E.: Amer. J. Ophthal. 77, 40 (1974)

ORYE, E., DELBEKE, M. J., VANDENABEELE, B.: Clin. Genet. 5, 457 (1974)

PARKHILL, E. M., BENEDICT, W. L.: Amer. J. Ophthal. 24, 1354 (1941)

PAPOLEZY, F.: Klin. Mbl. Augenheilk. 99, 355 (1937)

PARSONS, J. H.: Roy. Lond. ophthal. Hosp. Rep. 16, 141 (1904)

PFEIFFER, R. L.: Arch. Ophthal. 15, 811 (1936)

PINTO, J. R. da GAMA: Untersuchungen über intraoculäre Tumoren. BERGMANN, Netzhautgliome. Wiesbaden: 1886

RASMUSSEN, K.: Acta. Ophthal. 21, 210 (1944)

REESE, A. B.: Arch. Ophthal. 5, 269 (1931)

REESE, A. B.: Arch. Ophthal. 40, 533 (1948)

REESE, A. B.: Tumours of the Eye, New York - Evanston - London: Harper &Row, 1963, p. 107, 146

REESE, A. B.: Arch. Ophthal. 77, 293 (1967)

REESE, A. B., ELLSWORTH, R. M.: Trans. Amer. Acad. Ophthal. 67, 164 (1963)

REISER, K. A.: Klin. Mbl. Augenheilk. 99, 350 (1937)

ROSAS, A.: Handbuch d. theoret. u. prakt. Augenheilk., Vienna 2, 1004 (1830)

RYCHENER, R. O.: Trans. Amer. Ophthal. Soc. 46, 318 (1948)

SAGERMAN, R. H., CASSADY, J. R., TRETTER, P., ELLSWORTH, R. M.: Amer. J. Roentgen 105, 529 (1969)

SCHAPPERT-KIMMIJSER, J., HEMMES, G. D., NIGLAND, R.: Ophthalmologica (Basel) 151, 197 (1966)

SCHIMKE, R. N., LOWMAN, J. T., COWAN, G. A. B.: Cancer 34, 2077 (1974)

SCHOFIELD, P. B.: Brit. J. Ophthal. 44, 35 (1960)

SICHEL, J.: Iconographie ophthalmologique p. 562. Paris: J. B. BAILLIÈRE (1859)

SKEGGS, D. B. L., WILLIAMS, I. G.: Clin. Radiol. 17, 169 (1966)

SMITH, J. L. S.: Trans. ophthal. Soc. U.K. 94, 953 (1974)

SORSBY, A.: Brit. Med. J. 2, 580 (1972)

STALLARD, H. B.: Ophthalmologica 151, 214 (1966)

STALLARD, H. B.: Tumours in Children. MARSDEN, H. B., STEWARD, J. K. (ed.). Berlin-Heidelberg-New York: Springer-Verlag, 1968, p. 174

STEWARD, J. K., SMITH, J. L. S., ARNOLD, E. L.: Brit. J. Ophthal. 40, 449 (1956)

STRAUB: v. Graefes Arch. Ophthal. 32 (1), 205 (1886)

STRONG, L. C., KNUDSON, A. G.: Amer. J. hum. Genet. 24, 48 (1972)

SWAN, K. C., HYMAN, S.: Arch. Ophthal. 47, 416 (1952)

TAKTIKOS, A.: Brit. J. Ophthal. 48, 495 (1964)

TAKTIKOS, A.: Brit. J. Ophthal. 50, 225 (1966)

TILL, P., OSSOING, K.: Ber. dtsch. ophthal. Ges. 69, 209 (1968)

THOMPSON, J., KNAPP, H.: Arch. f. Augen. Ohrheilk. 4 (1), 79 (1874)

TOLENTINO, F. I., TABLANTE, R. T.: Arch. Ophthal. 87, 52 (1972)

TS'O, M. O. M., FINE, B. S., ZIMMERMAN, L. E., VOGEL, M. H.: Arch. Ophthal. 82, 57 (1969)

TS'O, M. O. M., ZIMMERMAN, L. E., FINE, B. S.: Am. J. Ophthal. 69, 339 (1970)

TS'O, M. O. M., FINE, B. S., ZIMMERMAN, L. E.: Am. J. Ophthal. 69, 350 (1970)

TUSHAUS, R.: Klin. Mbl. Augenheilk. 105, 41 (1940)

VERHOEFF, P. H.: Trans. Amer. Ophthal. Soc. 10, 351 (1904)

VERHOEFF, P. H.: Arch. Ophthal. 51, 120 (1922)

VETSCH, U.: Arch. Augenheilk. 11, 413 (1882)

VETSCH, U.: v. Graefes Arch. Ophthal. 12 (1), 43 (1883)

VIRCHOW, R.: Die krankhaften Geschwülste. Berlin: Hirschwald, 1864, Vol. II, p. 151

VOGEL, F.: Lhb. d. allg. Humangenetik, Berlin: Springer 1961

WARDROP, J.: Observations on fungus haematodes, or soft cancer. Edinburgh: A. Constable 1809

WEIZENBLATT, S.: Arch. Ophthal. 58, 699 (1957)

WILLIS, R. A.: Pathology of Tumours. London: Butterworth, 1948, p. 881

WILSON, M. G., MELNYK, J., TOWNER, J. W.: J. med. Genet. 6, 322 (1969)

WILSON, M. G., TOWNER, J. W., FUJIMOTO, A.: Amer. J. Hum. Genet. 25, 57 (1973)

WILSON, F. N., THOMSON, E. S.: Arch. Ophthal. 29, 91 (1900)

WINTERSTEINER, H.: Das Neuroepithelioma Retinae. Vienna: Deuticke 1897

WOLFF, E.: Brit. J. Ophthal. 28, 448 (1944)

WOLTER, J. R.: Amer. J. Ophthal. 52, 497 (1961)

# Chapter 9
# Connective Tissue Tumours

One hundred and ninety-one children with connective tissue tumours were included in the Registry between 1954 and 1968. This figure certainly is less than the actual number of cases in the Region during this period since many children with these tumours are not treated by paediatricians or radiotherapists and therefore are less likely to be reported to the Registry. Although connective tissue tumours are an important group in children there has been considerable confusion about their clinical management and classification. There are two reasons for this:

a) The children initially often come under the care of a variety of specialists (such as ophthalmologists, otologists, orthopaedic or genitourinary surgeons) because the tumours arise in situations such as the orbit, ear, bones or bladder. Consequently there is little uniformity of treatment and clinical trials can rarely be organised.

b) There has been some doubt about the precise classification of a significant number of connective tissue tumours. One group comprised those malignant tumours which occur in such sites as the orbit, neck, middle ear and genito-urinary tract and histologically show a variety of forms but sometimes contain striped muscle. These tumours presented an urgent clinical problem since the results of treatment have been poor. The essential histological difficulty was to know whether they are best regarded as belonging to one group and designated "embryonic sarcomas" or whether they represented a number of distinct tumour types. On the evidence of the Registry cases we believe that they should all be grouped together, just as all Wilms' tumours, even though

Table 1. Connective tissue tumours 1954 - 1968 (assessed 1972)

| | Alive | Dead | Total |
|---|---|---|---|
| Embryonic sarcomas | 12 | 56 | 68 |
| Malignant bone tumours (excluding Ewing's tumours) | 9 | 30 | 39 |
| Benign bone tumours | 18 | 1 | 19 |
| Soft tissue fibroblastic tumours | 33 | 5 | 38 |
| Synoviomas | 5 | 6 | 11 |
| Lipomatous tumours | 8 | 2 | 10 |
| Malignant mesenchymoma | 0 | 1 | 1 |
| Myxoma | 1 | 1 | 2 |
| Leiomyosarcoma | 1 | 0 | 1 |
| Uncertain | 2 | 0 | 2 |
| | 89 | 102 | 191 |

the histological appearance varies, are considered to be variations of one neoplasm. Another group which presented considerable difficulties in classification comprised fibroblastic tumours. However, the problem here was not nearly so urgent clinically since their prognosis was, on the whole, good.

## Histological Classification

The frequency and prognosis of the connective tissue tumours included in the Register are shown in Table 1.

It will be seen that, although the 191 cases could be divided into thirteen groups, two tumour types - embryonic sarcomas and osteosarcomas - accounted for 80% of the fatalities. Malignant synoviomas, although rare, also had a bad prognosis. One other group - the fibroblastic tumours - were quite common but had a comparatively good prognosis. All the other tumour types were uncommon and had a good prognosis.

## EMBRYONIC SARCOMAS

The term "embryonic sarcoma" rather than "rhabdomyosarcoma" (which might be preferred by other authors) has been used because clear evidence of maturation towards striped muscle was not seen in every instance. Nevertheless, these 68 tumours did appear to constitute one definite group. Before considering them it is necessary to discuss the characteristics of rhabdomyosarcomas as described in the literature.

It has been known for many years that two tumours of children - the nephroblastoma and the sarcoma of the lower genito-urinary tract - may contain striped muscle. STOUT (1946) described the occurrence of rhabdomyosarcomas in other sites when he reviewed 121 cases in adults and children - 107 derived from the literature and 14 observed by STOUT himself. STOBBE and DARGEON (1950) drew attention to the fact that in children and adolescents the head and neck was a comparatively common site for rhabdomyosarcomas. They described 15 examples of these tumours seen at the Memorial Hospital, New York, between 1931 and 1949, while MOORE and GROSSI (1959) added a further 37 cases at the same hospital during the next 7 years. RIOPELLE and THERIAULT (1956), and ENTERLINE and HORN (1958) described a histological variant - the so-called "alveolar rhabdomyosarcoma". PATTON and HORN (1962) reviewed 30 cases of rhabdomyosarcoma and compared their appearance with normal human embryonic muscle. Thus the picture of this neoplasm has been built up by a study of tumours occurring in different situations in adults and children.

HORN and ENTERLINE (1958) and LAWRENCE et al. (1964) correlated the various reports and described the different forms which the rhabdomyosarcoma can take. Most of the cells are usually too undifferentiated to betray any relationship to striped muscle. They may be pointed, stellate, or spindle-shaped. Areas which contain such cells can be seen in many malignant neoplasms and it is not surprising that, especially if only a small biopsy is available, the rhabdomyosarcoma may be confused with such tumours as the reticulosarcoma or neuroblastoma. The diagnosis of rhabdomyosarcoma depends on the observation of cells with one or more of the following characters:

a) a markedly eosinophilic cytoplasm
b) a long strap-like shape with blunt ends

c) "tadpole" or "tennis-racket" forms in which the cytoplasm is drawn out in a short tail
d) cross-striations

It will be appreciated that there is a spectrum of probability in the diagnosis of embryonic sarcomas and the size of the biopsy and quality of the histological preparation are important. The presence of cross-striations puts the matter beyond doubt while in those tumours where there are less definite and more primitive rhabdomyoblasts it is difficult to be certain by light microscopy. The site of the tumour may support the diagnosis - embryonic sarcomas tend to occur in the lower genital tract, orbit, middle ear, pterygoid fossa and beside the anus. In such sites the pathologist may be justified in suspecting a striped muscle origin in a largely undifferentiated sarcoma.

## Primary Sites

The primary sites of the 68 Manchester embryonic sarcomas are shown in Table 2. It will be seen that tumours in three sites - the head

Table 2. Embryonic sarcomas primary sites

| | Alive | Dead | Total |
|---|---|---|---|
| Orbit | 6 | 3 | 9 |
| Perineum or buttock | 1 | 6 | 7 |
| Pharynx or mouth | 0 | 11 | 11 |
| Preauricular region | 2 | 0 | 2 |
| Middle ear | 1 | 3 | 4 |
| Genital | 0 | 4 | 4 |
| Bladder | 0 | 6 | 6 |
| Abdomen | 0 | 9 | 9 |
| Pelvis | 0 | 4 | 4 |
| Chest | 1 | 3 | 4 |
| Limbs | 0 | 4 | 4 |
| Paravertebral | 0 | 3 | 3 |
| Scapular region | 1 | 0 | 1 |
| | 12 | 56 | 68 |

and neck, perineum and genito-urinary system - accounted for 63% of the cases. The great mass of skeletal muscle in other sites was much less likely to become neoplastic. The involvement of the trigone, urethra, prostate, epididymis or vagina has led to the suggestion that such tumours are related to the mesonephric duct system. The tumours in the head and neck are probably associated with the development of branchial clefts in this region and the orbital neoplasms have been thought to arise particularly from the superior oblique muscle. The orbital tumours in our series were compatible with such a site of origin and one tumour in particular clearly originated in this muscle.

## Age

Embryonic sarcomas usually occur in young children (Table 3). Sixty percent of the patients were under 5 years old.

## Pathological Findings

Apart from the botryoid sarcomas there were no characteristic gross features. These "grape-like" tumours showed the gelatinous or white

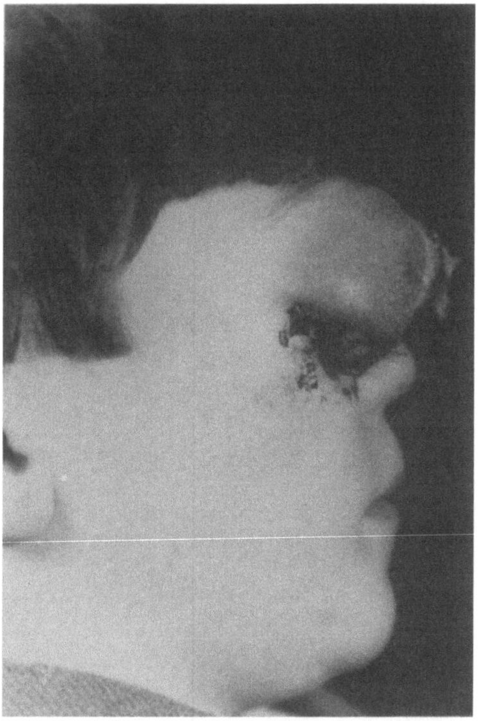

*Fig. 1. Orbital embryonic sarcoma in 7-year-old boy. Orbit was exenterated and patient is alive and well 19 years later*

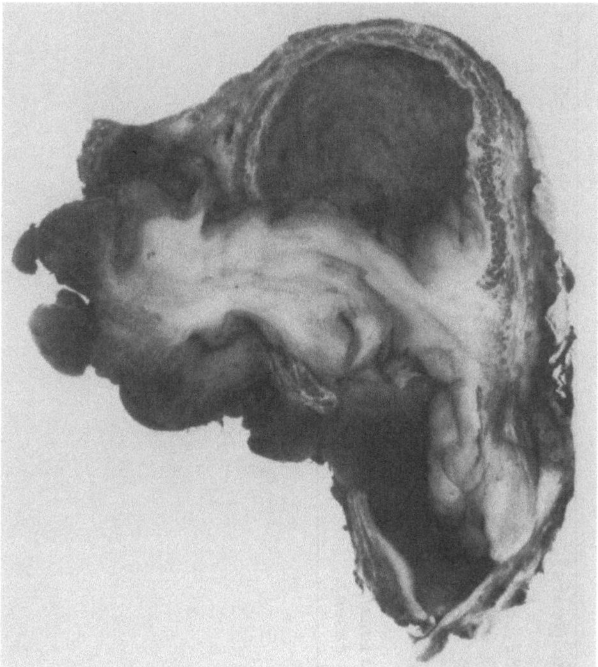

*Fig. 2. Sarcoma botryoides arising from posterior bladder wall and herniating through cystostomy incision*

Table 3. Age at first consultation

| Age (years) | -1 | -2 | -3 | -4 | -5 | -6 | -7 | -8 | -9 | -10 | -11 | -12 | -13 | -14 | -15 |
|---|---|---|---|---|---|---|---|---|---|---|---|---|---|---|---|
| Embryonic sarcomas (68 cases) | 7 | 12 | 9 | 10 | 4 | 7 | 3 | 5 | 3 | 1 | 0 | 2 | 2 | 2 | 1 |
| Osteosarcomas (28 cases) | 0 | 0 | 0 | 0 | 1 | 0 | 1 | 1 | 0 | 4 | 4 | 4 | 3 | 4 | 6 |
| Malignant synoviomas (8 cases) | 1 | 0 | 0 | 0 | 0 | 0 | 1 | 1 | 1 | 1 | 1 | 1 | 0 | 0 | 1 |

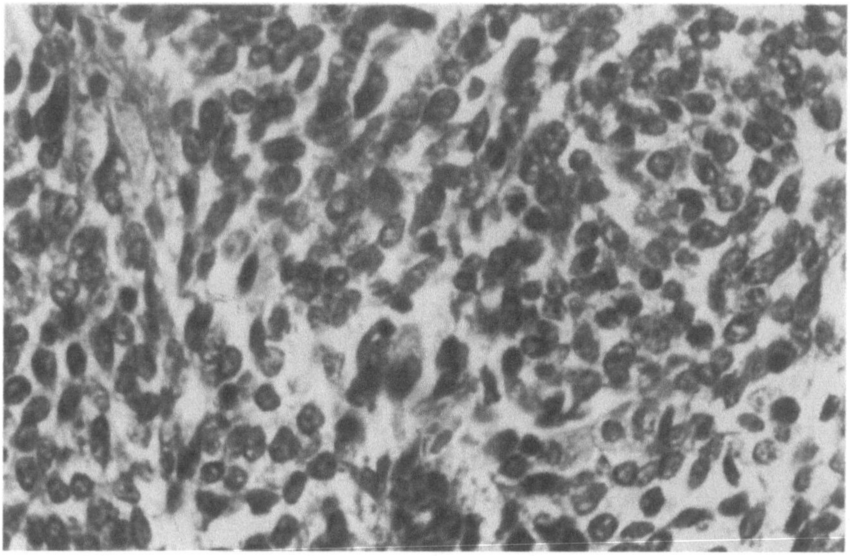

*Fig. 3. Embryonic sarcoma showing small spheroidal, polygonal and ovoid cells with little intervening stroma (H. & E. X 500)*

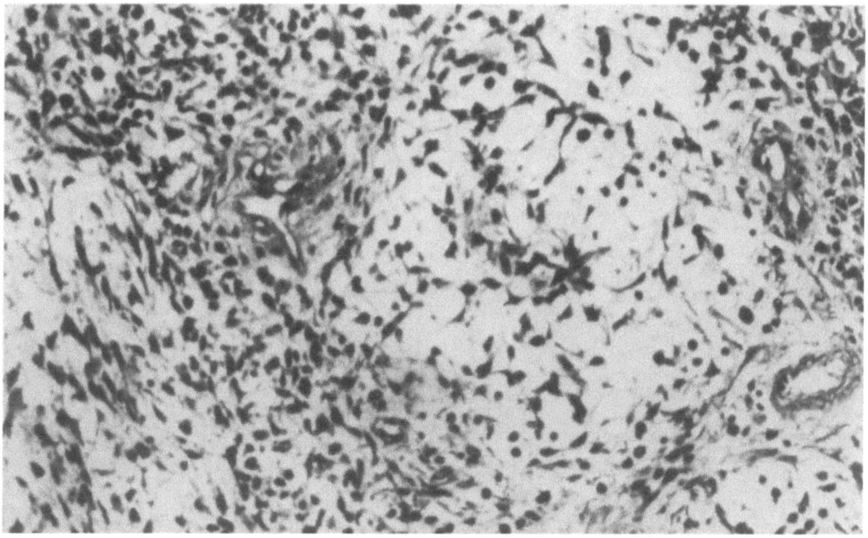

*Fig. 4. Embryonic sarcoma with loosely arranged stellate and spindle cells (H. & E. X 250)*

club-shaped fronds which have been well described. However, it is noteworthy that not all the bladder tumours showed botryoid formation, and in some cases there was merely white tumour infiltrating the wall. This might indicate a more deeply situated neoplasm, as the grape-like sarcoma is particularly associated with cellular areas of submucosal tumour. Grape-like tumours were not confined to the bladder, and polypoid formation was seen in tumours of the middle ear. Apart from the botryoid forms, the embryonic sarcomas varied in consistency between gelatinous, fleshy and firm. The colour was grey, white or pink,

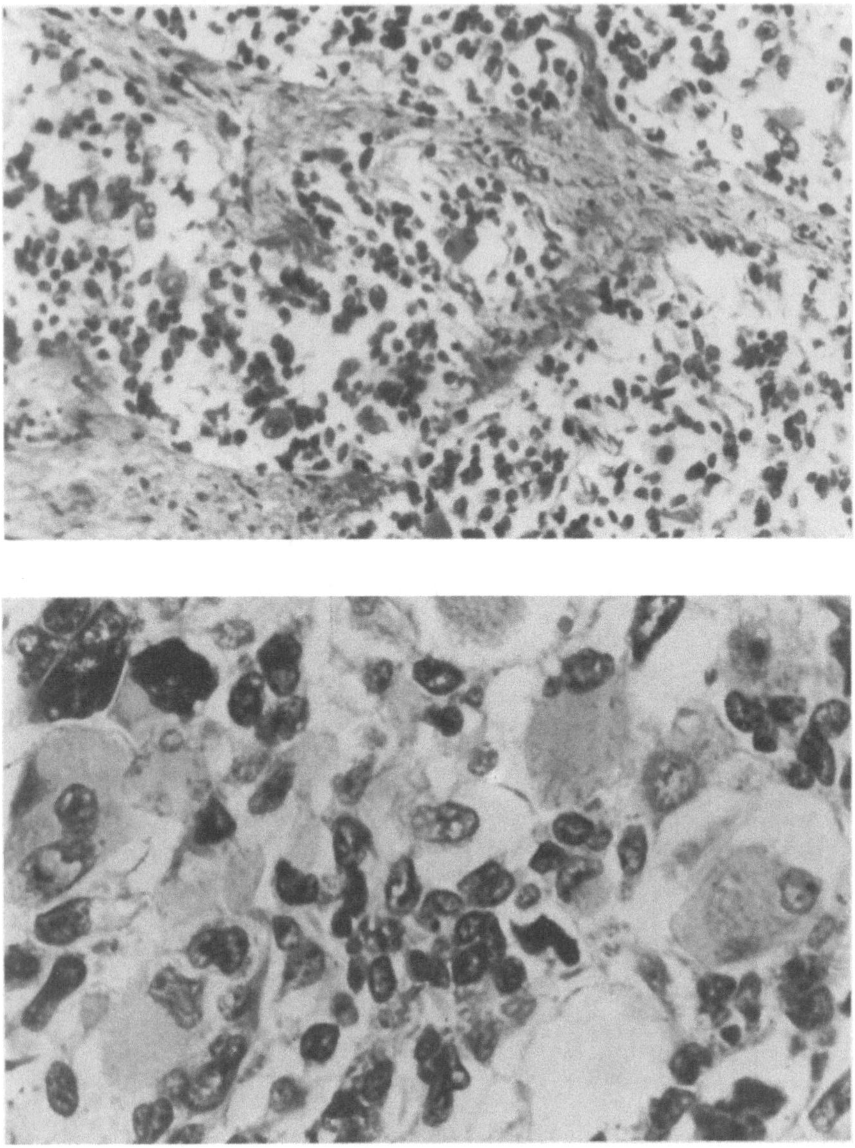

*Fig. 5. Embryonic sarcoma showing pleomorphism with development of variable amounts of eosinophilic cytoplasm (a) H.&E.X250; (b) H.&.E. X 750*

sometimes with areas of haemorrhage. There was a lobulated appearance in some cases and others were uniformly invasive.

Microscopically, variation in appearance was noted from one tumour to another and also in different parts of the same tumour. However, a basic pattern was seen consisting of immature mesenchyme with various degrees of differentiation of connective tissue, striated and possibly smooth muscle.

The various appearances encountered were as follows:

1. Cellular areas of small spheroidal, ovoid or polygonal cells, with little intervening stroma. There was minimal cytoplasm, the nuclei were moderately hyperchromatic and many showed nucleoli with nuclear degeneration and fragmentation.

2. Loosely arranged slender fusiform or stellate spidery cells with loose intervening myxomatous tissue which did not stain or had a slightly basophilic nature. Specific stains for mucin were negative. This tissue alternated with islands of greater cellularity.

3. Spindle-cell connective tissue, sometimes with reticulin formation and collagen production.

4. The cellular areas sometimes showed pleomorphism, with enlargement of nuclei and the development of variable amounts of eosinophilic cytoplasm which was well shown with Masson's trichrome stain. The cytoplasm was frequently granular or vacuolated.

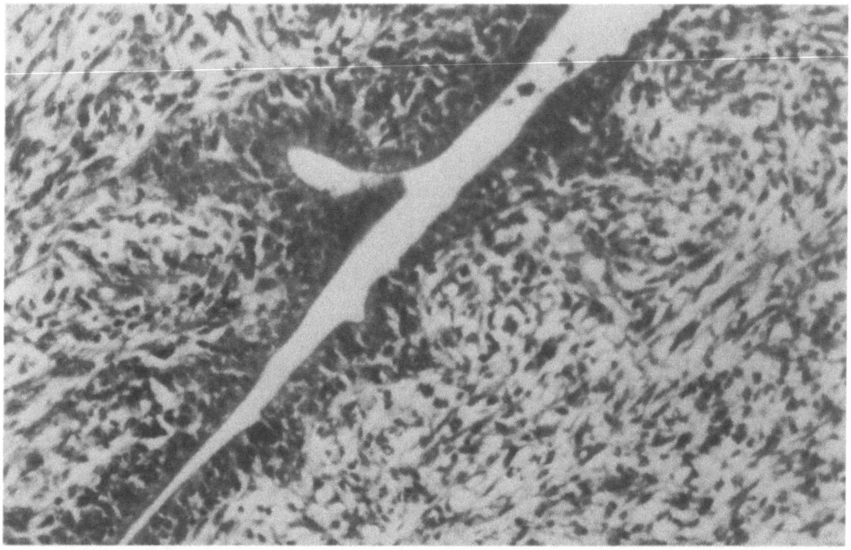

*Fig. 6. Sarcoma botryoides with increased cellularity of submucosal region (H. & E. X 250)*

5. The spindle-cell areas were sometimes more pleomorphic with nuclear enlargement, and showed "strap", "racket" and "tadpole" forms. The nucleus was central or peripheral and when it was peripheral the cell might be swollen at this point. Longitudinal myofibrils notably at the periphery of the cell were sometimes noted and cross-striation seen in the cytoplasm. This was particularly well demonstrated in PTAH preparations. However, striations were only seen in some of the tumours.

6. There were sometimes giant cells with bilobed horseshoe-shaped or even more bizarre nuclei. Occasionally such giant cells were numerous and characteristically their cytoplasm was markedly eosinophilic.

7. Alveolar arrangement with spaces of varying size and cells sometimes lying along connective tissue trabeculae. The appearance suggests degeneration of central cores or separation of cell clusters to produce this picture.

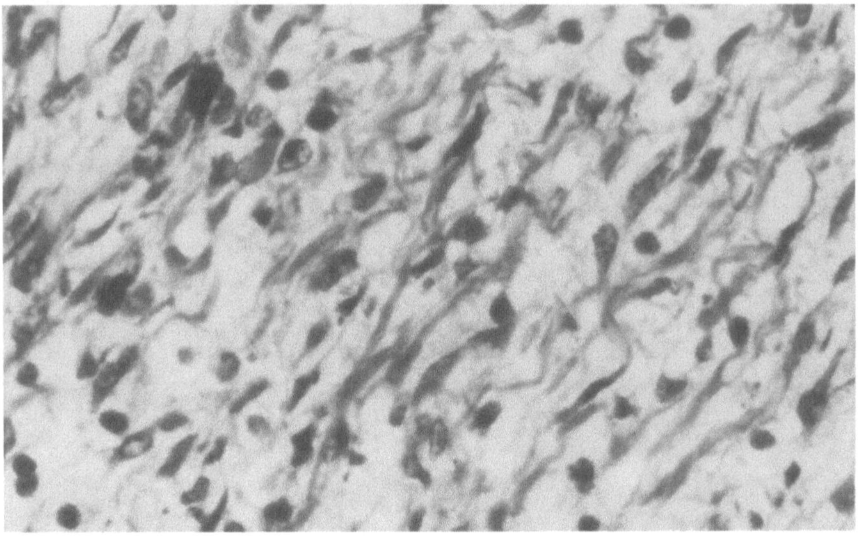

*Fig. 7. Embryonic sarcoma with "strap" formation (H. & E. X 500)*

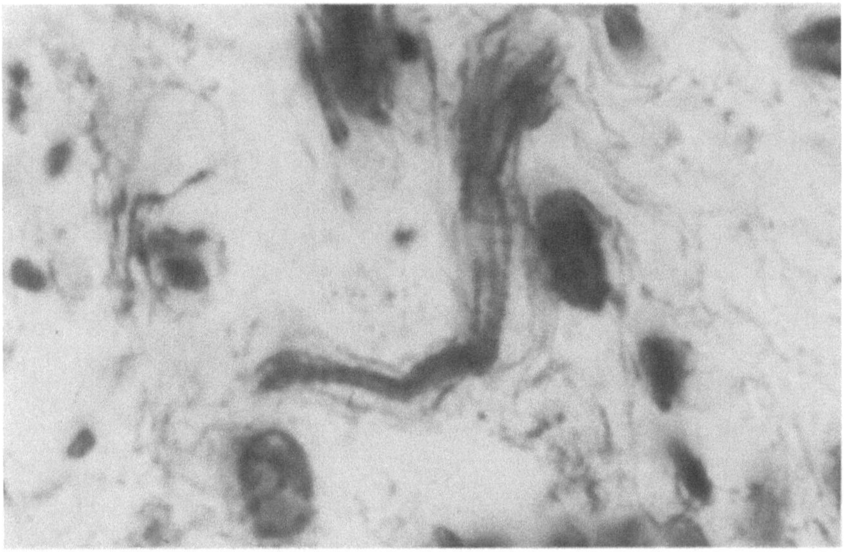

*Fig. 8. Embryonic sarcoma showing cross-striation (PTAH X 1250)*

Table 4. Histological types of embryonic sarcomas 1954 - 1968 (assessed 1972)

| | Alive | Dead | Total |
|---|---|---|---|
| Dense embryonic | 6 | 25 | 31 |
| Loose embryonic | 2 | 2 | 4 |
| Pleomorphic | 0 | 7 | 7 |
| Botryoid | 1 | 4 | 5 |
| Alveolar | 2 | 10 | 12 |
| Myoblastic | 1 | 8 | 9 |
| | 12 | 56 | 68 |

Using the above criteria together with the naked-eye appearance of the tumours, the Manchester cases could be classified into six types (Table 4).

The loose embryonic and botryoid tumours are essentially similar with a difference in the naked eye appearance and the histological finding of increased submucosal cellulartiy in the botryoid cases. Myoblastic differentiation is variable in these tumours but is not a prominent feature. The dense embryonic tumours have a more cellular uniform appearance without the loose mesenchymal areas seen in the previous types. Embryonic and loose mesenchymal features are not seen in the pleomorphic

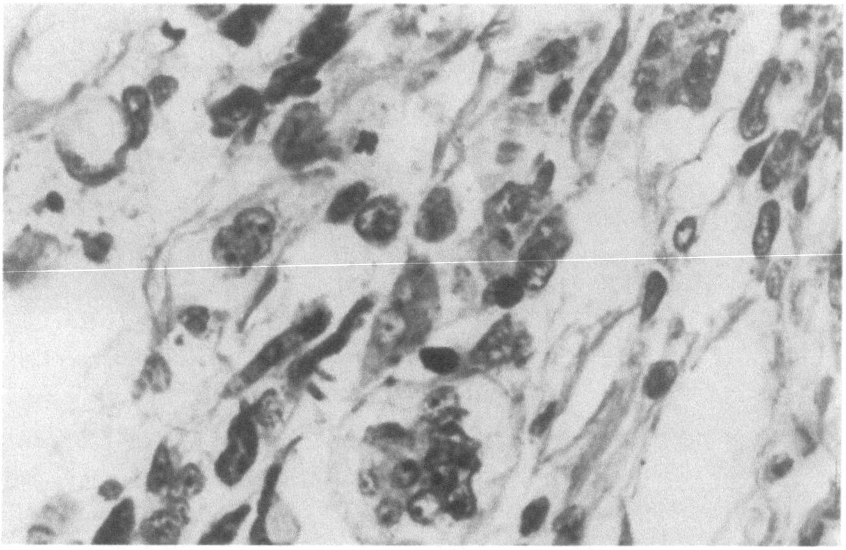

*Fig. 9. Embryonic sarcoma with marked pleomorphism, "straps" and giant cells (H. & E. X 750)*

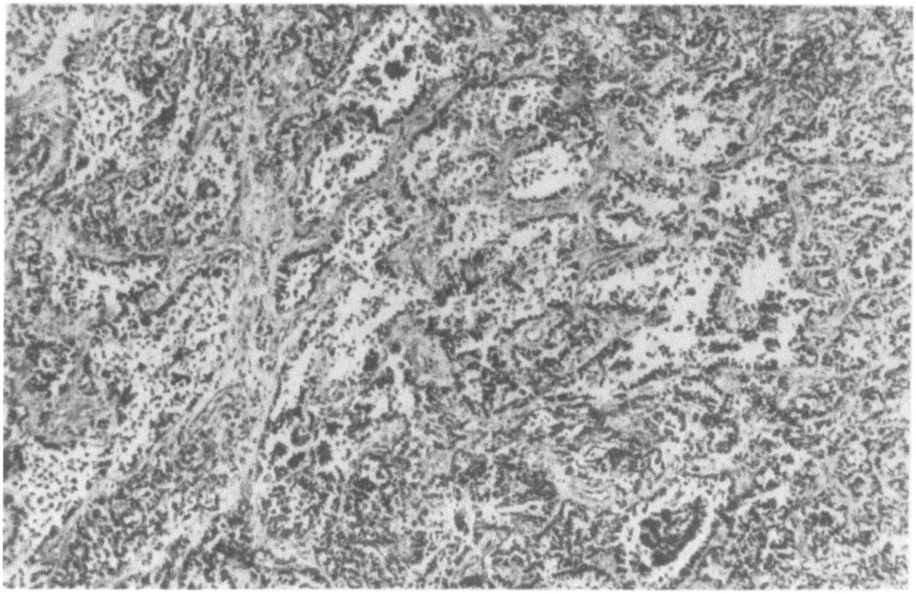

Fig. 10 a

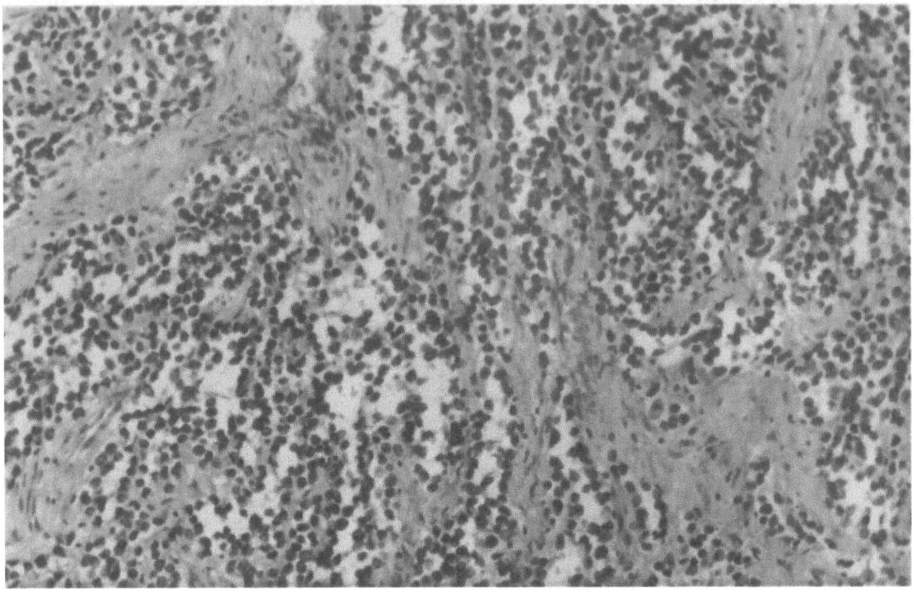

*Figs. 10a and b. Embryonic sarcoma showing alveolar formation a) H. & E. X 100; b) H. & E. X 250*

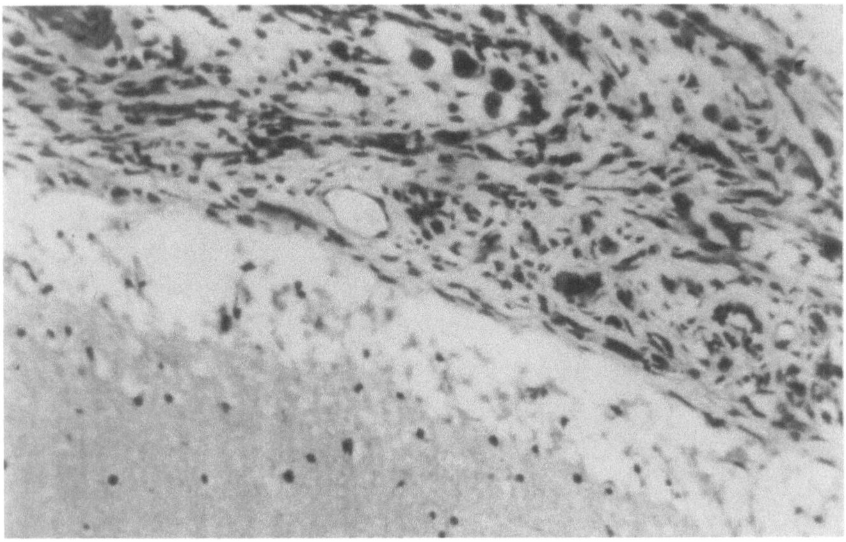

*Fig. 11. Embryonic sarcoma in meninges having spread from middle ear (H. & E. X 250)*

tumours in which the cells show considerable variation in size and morphology with bizarre atypical forms. Myoblastic differentiation is variable in the pleomorphic tumours but those in which muscle differentiation is the predominating feature have been classified in a separate "myoblastic" group. A tumour was classified as "alveolar" if this feature was prominent and the presence of only occasional spaces which may be seen in other types was not considered sufficient to place it under this heading.

## Fetal Rhabdomyoma

Benign skeletal muscle tumours are encountered particularly in the head and neck region in childhood, although these are rare and no examples have been seen in the Registry. The tumour is more superficial than the rhabdomyosarcoma and the microscopic appearances are more uniform. An analysis of nine cases is reported by DEHNER et al. (1972).

## Prognosis and Mode of Spread

In considering the clinical progress of the 68 cases, the fact that chemotherapy was rarely used in the Manchester children prior to 1969 must be taken into account. It will be seen in Table 5 that only 14

Table 5. Treatment given to children with embryonic sarcomas

| | Alive | Dead | Total |
|---|---|---|---|
| Excision only | 1 | 6 | 7 |
| Excision and XRT | 9 | 12 | 21 |
| XRT only | 0 | 18 | 18 |
| XRT and CT | 0 | 7 | 7 |
| Excision and XRT and CT | 1 | 4 | 5 |
| Excision and CT | 1 | 1 | 2 |
| Nil | 0 | 8 | 8 |
| | 12 | 56 | 68 |

out of the 68 children were given chemotherapy and, furthermore, the dosage and duration of treatment were much less than are used in present day regimes.

Following this treatment policy the following pattern emerged:

a) The disease usually progressed rapidly (Table 6). Sixty-one percent of the children had died by the end of one year and 85% by the end of 2 years. Four children died between 2 and 7 years after diagnosis and none has so far died thereafter.

b) In fatal cases, growth and recurrence of the primaries were much more in evidence than metastatic spread (Table 7). This was probably due to the fact that the primary tumours were very often not brought under control and killed the patients before metastases could develop. Metastases were seen in lungs, bones, lymph nodes, liver, skin and spleen. The main danger of embryonic sarcomas in the middle ear appeared to be spread into the brain.

c) Eleven of the 12 survivors had tumours in superficial sites (orbit, preauricular area, perineum, middle ear or back), where total or subtotal excision was possible (Table 2). The one exception was a tumour in the chest which was treated with a prolonged course of cyclophosphamide.

In order to explore further the factors influencing prognosis, 67 of the 68 cases were divided into two categories, depending on whether they arose in deep or in superficial (subcutaneous) structures. One case was excluded from this analysis because it was an incidental autopsy finding in a child who had died from another disease. The 67

Table 6. Fatal embryonic sarcomas, osteosarcomas, and malignant synoviomas. Time from diagnosis to death

| Time from diagnosis to death (years) | -1/4 | -1/2 | -1 | -2 | -3 | -4 | -5 | -6 | -7 | -8 | -9 | -10 |
|---|---|---|---|---|---|---|---|---|---|---|---|---|
| Embryonic sarcomas (56 cases) | 12 | 15 | 15 | 10 | 2 | 1 | 0 | 0 | 1 | 0 | 0 | 0 |
| Osteosarcomas (25 cases) | 0 | 8 | 5 | 10 | 0 | 0 | 1 | 1 | 0 | 0 | 0 | 0 |
| Malignant synoviomas (6 cases) | 0 | 0 | 1 | 1 | 1 | 0 | 1 | 0 | 0 | 1 | 1 | 0 |

cases were also clinically staged using a modified version of the following method proposed for the Intergroup Rhabdomyosarcoma Study MAURER (1975)

Stage 1. Localised disease, completely resected (regional nodes not involved).

Table 7. Fatal embryonic sarcomas (56 cases)
Sites of tumours at death

| | |
|---|---|
| Local | 40 |
| Lungs | 13 |
| Bones | 7 |
| Lymph nodes | 6 |
| Liver | 5 |
| Brain | 2 |
| Skin | 2 |
| Spleen | 1 |

Stage 2. a) Incomplete resection with microscopic residual disease (Tumour involvement microscopically at tissue margin. Regional nodes may be involved. No gross residual tumour).
b) Regional disease completely resected (Regional nodes involved and/ or extension of tumour into contiguous tissues other than the site of origin).

Stage 3. Incomplete resection or biopsy with gross residual disease.

Stage 4. Distant metastatic disease present at onset (lungs, liver, bones, bone marrow, brain, and distant muscles and nodes).

In trying to stage the Manchester cases which occurred prior to 1969 it was not possible to separate Stages 1, 2a and 2b. Therefore they were classified into three groups - Stage 1 and 2, Stage 3, Stage 4. Their frequencies are shown in Table 8.

Table 8. Embryonic sarcomas; frequency of clinical stages at diagnosis

| Clinical stage | Number of cases |
|---|---|
| Stages 1 and 2 | 23 |
| Stage 3 | 39 |
| Stage 4 | 5 |
| | 67 |

The effect of the following factors on the length of survival of the 67 children with embryonic sarcomas was examined: age, clinical stage, sex, histological type, site (as shown in Table 2), and whether the tumour arose in superficial or deep structures.

a) Clinical stage. Children presenting with tumours in an earlier clinical stage survived longer ($\underline{P} < 0.001$).

b) Site. Children with tumours in superficial sites, such as the orbit or perineum, survived longer than those with tumours in deep sites ($\underline{P} < 0.001$). However, it was not possible to correlate in greater detail the length of survival with the sites of the tumours as shown in Table 2.

c) Age. Younger children survived for a shorter time than older children ($\underline{P} < 0.05$) but this correlation was not directly significant because deep tumours were more frequent in younger children ($\underline{P} < 0.05$).

d) Histological type. It was not possible in this series to find any correlation between histological type and length of survival. However, there was a significantly higher proportion ($\underline{P} < 0.025$) of the loose and dense embryonic histological types amongst those children who presented in clinical stages 3 and 4 (see Table 9). Possibly, therefore, these types represent the more malignant end of the spectrum.

e) Sex. No correlation between sex and survival time could be found.

Table 9. Embryonic sarcomas; relationship between histological type and clinical stage at diagnosis

| Clinical stage | Number of children with histological type | | | | | All types |
|---|---|---|---|---|---|---|
| | Embryonic (dense and loose) | Pleomorphic | Botryoid | Alveolar | Myoblastic | |
| 1 and 2 | 6 | 3 | 3 | 5 | 6 | 23 |
| 3 | 25 | 3 | 2 | 7 | 2 | 39 |
| 4 | 4 | 1 | 0 | 0 | 0 | 5 |
| Total | 35 | 7 | 5 | 12 | 8 | 67 |

## Treatment of Embryonic Sarcomas

Over recent years the picture regarding survival in childhood embryonic sarcomas has changed very considerably due to the introduction of multimodal therapy. In the past the prognosis of these tumours depended very largely on the site of origin. From 1940 - 1969 the survival rate at the Christie Hospital was 50% for orbital tumours and 0% for retroperitoneal and abdominal tumours of this type. It is now clear that cure at that time depended on the stage at which the tumour presented and the associated possibility of total macroscopic removal prior to radiotherapy. The introduction of chemotherapy has now made possible preoperative and preradiation reduction in the size of lesions so that they are more amenable to attack.

The wide variety of primary sites makes it difficult to discuss surgery in general terms, but nevertheless, in situations where total macroscopic removal is possible, surgery would be considered the first line of approach, except perhaps in orbital lesions (vide infra). Embryonic sarcomas are less easy to stage than some other tumours and subclassifications dependent on site are necessary. There is as yet no international agreement, but we have attempted to emulate the American Intergroup Rhabdomyosarcoma Study Grouping with the Manchester cases. These groups have been outlined earlier in the chapter. This classification places some potentially good prognostic cases in Group III - e. g. orbital tumours biopsied and then treated by radiotherapy. It is also possible that in Group II there should also be included a group in which total regional lymph node removal has been carried out.

Despite the difficulties an attempt should be made to classify each case into a stage on a clinical and histological basis and then gear therapy appropriately to the site and stage of disease. Any child suspected of having an embryonic sarcoma should have the usual routine investigations carried out. These should include FBC, ESR, Chest X-ray, skeletal survey, bone marrow biopsy and whenever possible liver and brain scans. If the primary is in the orbit or head and neck, a lumbar puncture should be done to look for tumour cells in the CSF. In the case of abdominal and bladder primaries IVP, inferior vena cavagrams and, whenever possible, lymphangiography are indicated, as these investigations will help establish the extent of disease prior to surgery.

Biochemical investigations should include blood urea, uric acid, liver function tests and alkaline phosphatase.

## Orbital Tumours

These usually present with symptoms and signs at an early stage and remain localised. Some authors advocate complete exenteration and only employ other modalities of treatment for recurrent disease (JONES et al., 1965). In other centres reliance has been placed on primary radiation after diagnostic biopsy (CASSADY et al., 1968), and the results are comparable; there are, however, complications of high dose irradiation to the orbit and the involved eye often develops cataract in addition to hypoplasia of the orbit. It remains to be seen whether combinations of surgery, radiotherapy and chemotherapy will improve the outlook further and allow for less deforming therapy.

## Facial Tumours

These primaries behave in an aggressive way and often show evidence of local spread and regional node involvement at presentation. Complete surgical removal is often impossible and very deforming and, because of the large volume , radiation dosage has been limited and rarely curative. With the development of effective chemotherapy used after biopsy it is now possible to achieve considerable shrinkage of the primary and thus allow for a higher dose of radiation to a smaller field, and hopefully, better long-term results will be achieved. Other centres advocate the use of radium needles rather than XRT.

## Nasopharyngeal Tumours

This group does not usually present in a localised stage and is usually not amenable to surgery. A very good improvement in results has been achieved by triple therapy.

## Retroperitoneal Tumours

Clinically these tumours are very difficult to differentiate from neuroblastomas. They are usually very advanced at diagnosis and again the primary use of chemotherapy may well improve the efficacy of subsequent radiotherapy and surgery.

## Genito-urinary Tumours

Botryoid tumours of the bladder usually present with symptoms related to obstruction of ureters or urethra. Primary surgery will usually be necessary to relieve obstruction, but while very radical procedures have been advocated in the past, the use of chemotherapy in association with more limited surgery and radiotherapy is now being investigated. Vulval, vaginal and uterine tumours can usually be managed in a similar way, but need to be assessed on an individual basis. Prostatic tumours are a greater problem and are very difficult to control. Very few cures have been described. It has been suggested that radiation therapy and radium seeds might be utilised to bring the primary under control while chemotherapy was employed to control spread. Testicular and paratesticular tumours have a good prognosis if diagnosed early and if treated by radical orchiectomy and removal of the spermatic cord. Some centres believe that radical node dissection should also be carried out routinely, but there is no evidence as yet that the results are better, although it is necessary to ascertain whether or not the nodes are involved and postoperative therapy should include pelvic and para-aortic lymph node irradiation in all but Stage I cases.

## Limb Tumours

Tumours of the extremities have often been treated with amputation in the past but it may well be that wide excision with associated high dose radiation and chemotherapy can achieve similar and even better results without mutilation.

## Radiotherapy

The following regimes are used at the Christie Hospital for the treatment of children with embryonic sarcomas.

## Cheek, Orbit, Middle Ear or Post-Nasal Spaces

With small lesions, small field beam directed XRT; dose 5500 rads in 3 weeks. With larger lesions the fields are those which will cover the lesion with a margin and the dose will depend on size, but at least 3000 - 3500 rads are given in 3 weeks. If the tumour has shrunk, an extra 1500 - 2000 rads may be delivered to a smaller volume in a further week. Alternatively the extra dose can be given by a radium implant.

Abdomen or Paratesticular

The whole abdomen usually needs to be treated. If the kidneys can be safely shielded throughout, 3000 rads in 4 weeks is given. Additional irradiation to the primary area may be considered in individuals but will depend on the reaction of the patient to the initial treatment. If the kidneys cannot be shielded, 2000 rads are given to the whole abdomen in 3 weeks with an extra 1000 - 1500 rads locally to the primary area in 1 week.

Chest

Radiation dose to the whole chest is limited by lung tolerance and therefore is restricted to 2000 rads in 3 weeks, perhaps 2500 rads in 4 weeks. If the primary can be treated, while sparing the lungs so that they receive little or no radiation, a higher dose should be aimed for. This will usually not exceed 3000 - 3500 rads in 3 weeks. If radiation is being used for the treatment of chest metastases, the first doses quoted are used. Correction should be made for lung transmission.

Limbs

Where it is possible to radiate only one portion of a limb a dose of 4500 rads in 3 weeks should be given to the muscle groups concerned, and another 1000 rads in 1 week should be considered to a small remaining primary focus.

It may sometimes be better to sacrifice the limb and have amputation only, followed by chemotherapy.

Perianal

Radiation in this instance may be X-ray therapy or a radium implant or a combination of the two. If a small lesion, the appropriate radium implant should be done to a dose 5500 - 6000 rads in 7 days. With larger lesions X-ray therapy is used, the size of the field being enough to cover the lesion with a good margin, and the dose to be given should be 3000 rads in 3 weeks, and extra to the remaining tumour mass, say another 1000 - 1500 rads in a week. A half dose radium implant could be carried out instead of the extra X-ray dose. Each case would need to be judged individually.

Full blood (including platelet) counts are done twice weekly during radiation. If WBC falls below 2500 or platelets below 120,000, daily counts are done. Treatment may need to be interrupted if WBC is less than 1500 or the platelets less than 75,000.

Chemotherapy Regimes

Several chemotherapy regimes have now been established and shown to be effective in preventing spread, in reducing the size of primary

tumours and in controlling metastatic disease. The report of HEYN and HOLLAND (1970) of a Group A study of 58 children, Stage I-IV, indicates that actinomycin D and vincristine used continuously for 1 year after surgery are valuable in patients in whom there is total removal or only microscopic residual disease. HOLTON et al. (1973) have recently reported on the treatment of 19 cases of variable stage and site, in whom, in addition to surgery and radiation, combination chemotherapy with vincristine, cyclophosphamide and actinomycin D was given for 1 year in Stage I and II, and 2 years in Stage III and IV. Complete response was seen in 17 cases. At the time of the report 11 patients were free of disease at 4 - 49 months from diagnosis. CUNNINGHAM and KING (1972) report a single case of an embryonic sarcoma of the middle ear treated with surgery, radiation and chemotherapy and they comment on the usual rapidly fatal course of the disease at this site. In Manchester there is one survivor similar to the one quoted by CONTE and SAGERMAN (1971).
CTR.24/59. Boy, aged 2 years, who attended hospital in March 1959 with a discharging right ear and an aural polyp which proved to be an embryonic sarcoma. There was extensive destruction of the right petrous bone and right facial palsy. XRT (4170 rads in 14 days) and adenopterin were given and the facial palsy became much less marked. Five months later the lesion was explored thoroughly but histological examination of the excised tissue revealed no residual neoplasm. However the child was left with a facial palsy. The tumour has not recurred during the past 15 years but the patient is very small for his age, presumably due to pituitary dysfunction secondary to the treatment.

The reports from the Children's Unit of the M.D. Anderson Hospital (WILBUR et al., 1971; DONALDSON et al., 1973) using the VAC chemotherapy regime (see below) are also very encouraging and our experience has largely been with this combination.

## Manchester Results

Prior to 1968 children in Manchester had only been given small doses of drugs usually at the time of recurrence (see Table 5) and the overall survival was 18%.

Since that time actinomycin D, 15 micrograms/kg daily for 5 days every 12 weeks for 2 years has been given; or, more recently, the VAC regime has been used - starting on day 1 vincristine 1.5 mg/m$^2$ is given weekly for 12 weeks, actinomycin D, 15 micrograms/kg for 5 doses over 5 - 8

Table 10. 18 Manchester children with embryonic sarcomas since 1968

| Site | No. of cases | Clinical stage | Survival |
|---|---|---|---|
| Orbit | 1 | 3 | Died 2 months |
| Head and neck | 3 | 3, 3, 1 | Died 9 months; alive at 5 years; alive at 4 years |
| Nasopharyngeal | 1 | 3 | Died 1 year |
| Retroperitoneal | 3 | 3, 3, 4 | Died 2 months; died 6 months; died 2 months |
| Bladder | 2 | 2b, 3a | Alive at 4 years; alive at 2 years |
| Vagina | 1 | 3 | Alive at 4 years |
| Prostate | 1 | 3 | Died 15 months |
| Paratesticular | 4 | 1, 1, 2b, 2b | Alive at 4 years; alive at 2 years; died 2 years; died 16 months |
| Extremity | 2 | 4, 3 | Alive at 2 years; alive at 3 years |

days every 12 weeks for 6 courses and cyclophosphamide 10 mg/kg daily for 7 days every 6 weeks for 2 years. A total of 18 children have been treated with one or other of these regimes and at the present time nine survive at 15 to 60 months from diagnosis. The sites and stages are outlined in Table 10. Thus at present there is 50% survival, but two children have disease, one recurring 6 months and the other 1 year after the completion of 2 years chemotherapy.

The toxicity has been found to be minimal unless radiation is given at the same time and, for this reason, when initial surgery is possible the first course of chemotherapy is given paraoperatively and cyclophosphamide should not commence until 6 weeks after the start of radiation. If the chemotherapy is given first in the case of inoperable tumours, 6 weeks of chemotherapy is completed and the second course of cyclophosphamide omitted while giving radiation. Mucositis and epilation still occur but the former can be dealt with by nasogastric feeding and the use of frequent oral toilet with mouth washes. This chemotherapy regime should not be attempted unless first-rate supportive care is available. Nevertheless, the results suggest a very marked improvement in overall prognosis.

## MALIGNANT PRIMARY BONE TUMOURS

There were 69 children with malignant primary bone tumours and these with the embryonic sarcomas accounted for the majority of fatal cases amongst children with connective tissue tumours. The frequency of the various types is shown in Table 11. Ewing's tumours, which are considered separately in Chapter 13 because their histogenesis is uncertain, present somewhat similar clinical problems and are therefore also included in Table 11.

Table 11. Malignant primary bone tumours 1954 - 1968 assessed 1972

| | Alive | Dead | Total |
|---|---|---|---|
| Osteosarcomas | 3 | 25 | 28 |
| Chondrosarcomas | 1 | 2 | 3 |
| Fibrosarcomas | 2 | 2 | 4 |
| Osteoclastomas | 3 | 0 | 3 |
| Reticulum cell sarcoma | 0 | 1 | 1 |
| Ewing's tumours | 2 | 28 | 30 |
| | 11 | 58 | 69 |

### Osteosarcoma

There were 29 tumours in 28 children in this group. One boy died from osteosarcoma of the fibula and ulna preceded by a periosteal fibrosarcoma in the temporal region which had recurred on a number of occasions necessitating the removal of a plate of bone before local treatment was effective. The patient had an identical twin who appeared healthy but whose son developed an embryonic sarcoma in the pterygoid region. In the other 27 children the tumours arose as single bone lesions in the sites shown in Table 12. Since the most common sites were the lower end of the femur and upper end of the tibia, two-thirds of the osteosarcomas in the Manchester series arose in the region of the knee. The

Table 12. Sites of osteosarcomas

| | Alive | Dead | Total |
|---|---|---|---|
| Femur | 3 | 13 | 16 |
| Tibia | O | 5 | 5 |
| Humerus | O | 4 | 4 |
| Clavicle | O | 2 | 2 |
| Fibula and Ulna (multiple primaries) | O | 1 | 1 |
| | 3 | 25 | 28 |

age incidence (Table 3) shows that only occasional tumours occurred before the tenth year. The youngest child was aged 4 years.

## Histology

The histological features of osteosarcomas are well known. The tumours of the present cases showed irregular spindle and polygonal cells with varying degrees of osteogenesis. Although strictly speaking the diagnosis of osteogenic sarcoma requires the certain recognition of tumour bone which must be preceded by osteoid, the histological material available in the Manchester cases made it often necessary to make the diagnosis on the general cellular pattern rather than on the presence of

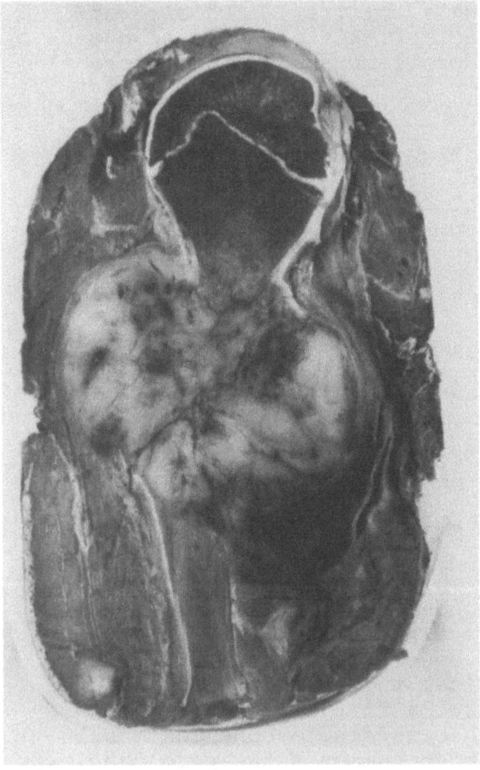

*Fig. 12. Osteosarcoma of humerus with pathological fracture*

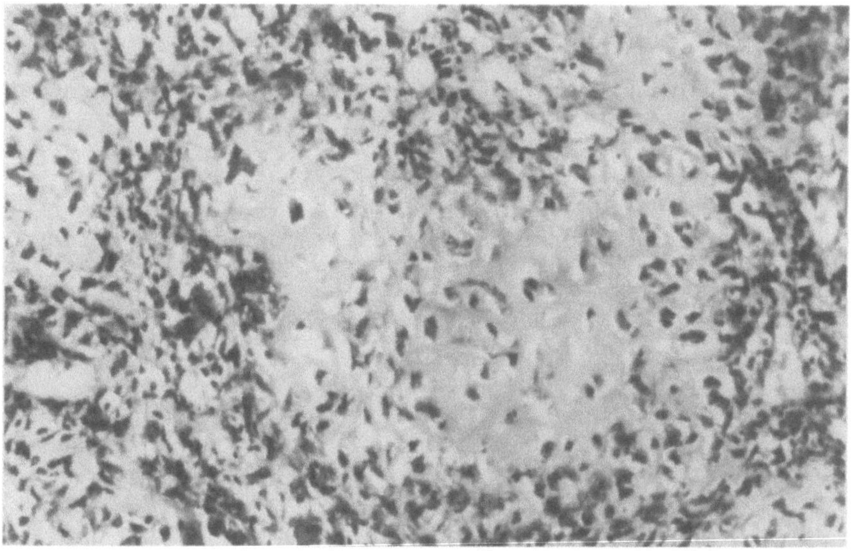

*Fig. 13. Osteosarcoma with marked osteoid production (H. & E. X 250)*

osteoid which was only seen in sections of 10 of the 28 tumours. In some tumours there was calcification and it was sometimes difficult to distinguish new bone formation from partially destroyed non-neoplastic trabeculae. The variation in ossification was marked and in two cases there was such extensive bone formation that the tumours could be called "sclerosing osteosarcomas". The variation in osteogenesis may make the distinction between osteogenic sarcoma and fibrosarcoma of bone difficult and one Manchester tumour which appeared to be a fibrosarcoma at biopsy proved to be an osteosarcoma at autopsy. However, the diagnosis of osteosarcoma can be established by the demonstration of alkaline phosphatase in smears or frozen sections of unfixed tumour tissue even when the cells appear to have a fibroblastic appearance. Frequently, giant cells were present, sometimes with one bizarre nucleus and sometimes with many nuclei either arranged in a "horse-shoe" manner or in an "osteoclast" fashion, although there were fewer nuclei than in a typical osteoclast. One variant comprised those tumours in which islands of cartilage were present in addition to osteoid and this was seen in four cases. This so-called chondroblastic osteosarcoma may form predominantly atypical sheeted matrix intermediate between cartilage and osteoid. In the Bristol Registry figures and in reports from the Mayo Clinic this tumour has had a bad prognosis (PRICE, 1974) and responds poorly to irradiation.

## Prognosis

The results of treatment of the Manchester osteosarcomas prior to 1969 were very bad - only 3 survivors remained in 1972 amongst the 28 children who had had this tumour (Table 12). The progress of the disease was usually rapid - 46% died within 1 year and 85% within 2 years of diagnosis (Table 6). Twenty-two of the 25 children who died had lung metastases and 3 children had deposits in other bones. All 3 survivors had femoral primaries. Two were treated in 1955 and 1960 by amputation only and the tumours have not recurred since then. The other survivor had an osteosarcoma of the greater trochanter in 1956. A biopsy was taken, the tumour irradiated (3000 rads in 3 weeks)and adenopterin was given for a month. The femoral tumour responded well with deposition of new bone. However, multiple lung metastases appeared and these were treated with chest irradiation (2500 rads in 43 days) and adenopterin. Since then there has been no evidence of growth of either the primary or the metastases, which have calcified.

## Chondrosarcoma

There were three chondrosarcomas. These tumours are considered to be less malignant than osteosarcomas but the three Manchester cases showed considerable variation in malignancy. One tumour arose from the pelvis of a 13-year-old boy and had a very malignant histological appearance.

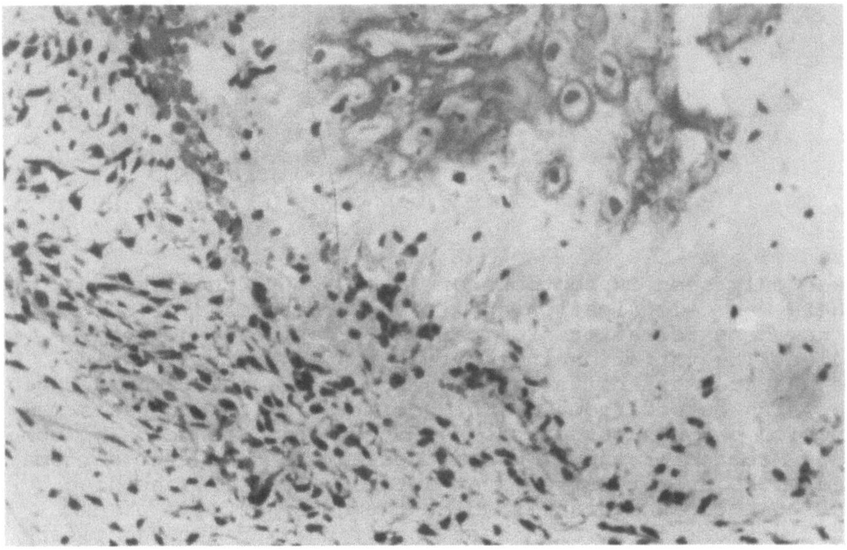

*Fig. 14. Chondrosarcoma (H. & E. X 250)*

No treatment could be given and the boy died 5 months after diagnosis without any metastases being apparent. The second tumour was of intermediate malignancy and arose in the os calcis of a 13-year-old boy who was treated with a below-knee amputation. He remained well for 3 1/2 years and then developed lung metastases and died 4 1/2 years after diagnosis. The third tumour was a very low grade chondrosarcoma in the upper end of the tibia in a 10-year-old girl. The leg was amputated in 1968 and the tumour had not recurred 4 years later.

## Fibrosarcoma of Bone

Fibrosarcomas arising in association with bones have a much worse prognosis than fibrosarcomas of soft tissues in children. Histologically they consist of fibroblastic cells without the polygonal osteoblast-like cells and osteogenesis seen in an osteosarcoma. Some authors have separated periosteal and endosteal fibrosarcomas but this distinction may be difficult to make in individual cases. There were 4 Manchester cases in this group - 3 in the femur and one arising on the outer surface of the vault of the skull. The tumour of the skull was definitely periosteal and has not recurred since it was excised in 1957. One child had a femoral fibrosarcoma treated by amputation in 1966 and has remained well since that time. At the time of amputation the tumour was both endosteal and periosteal. The other 2 femoral fibrosarcomas were endosteal and these 2 patients died, one with lung metastases and one with a tumour in the base of the skull.

## Osteoclastoma

Three children with osteoclastomas were included in the Registry. Their ages ranged from 8 to 10 years and the tumours were in the lower end of

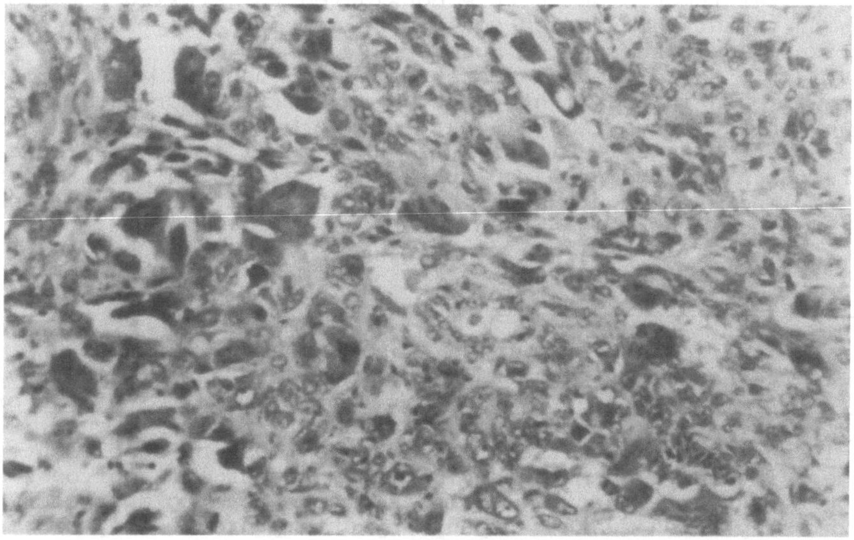

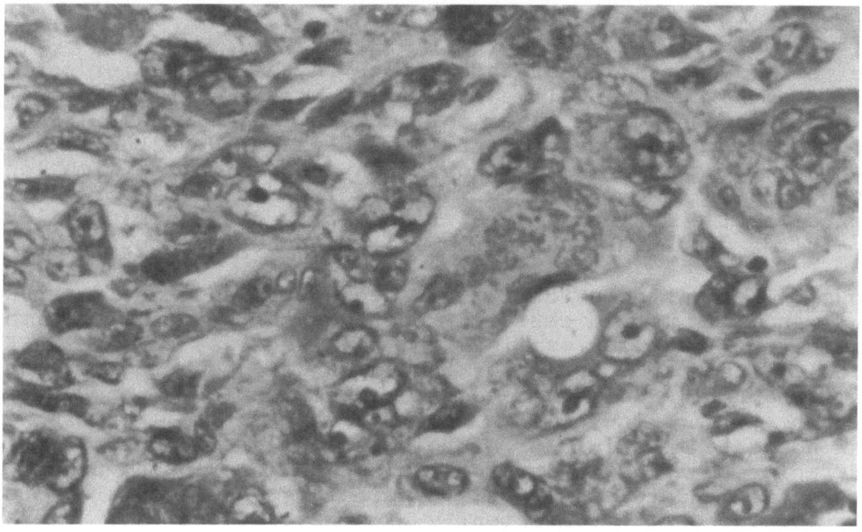

*Fig. 15a. Osteoclastoma of lower end of radius (H. & E. X 250)*
*b. Detail of (a) (H. & E. X 750). In spite of pleomorphism patient remains well 9 years after excision*

the radius, the upper end of the humerus and the lower end of the femur. All of them showed mitotic activity indicating their malignancy. The radial tumour was treated in 1957 by local excision and a bone graft and amputation was performed in the other two cases in 1958 and 1960. All of these 3 patients are still alive and well without any sign of recurrence of their tumours.

## Reticulosarcoma of Bone

The relationship of this tumour to Ewing's sarcoma of bone is not clear and is discussed in Chapter 13. One child had a non-osteogenic malignant tumour of the femur which differed histologically from the other Manchester tumours which were considered to be Ewing's sarcomas. It was felt that this lesion could most appropriately be described as a reticulum cell sarcoma of bone.
CTR.74/64. Girl, aged 13 years, attended hospital with a month's history of pain in the right thigh. X-rays showed increased density of the lower third of the femoral shaft. There were also 3 subcutaneous nodules over the skull. Biopsies of the femoral lesion and a scalp nodule were taken and showed large spheroidal cells with prominent nucleoli resembling the picture seen in reticulum cell sarcomas elsewhere. The child died 1 month later. No autopsy.

## Treatment of Bone Sarcomas

For bone sarcomas (e.g. osteo-, fibro-, chondro-, Ewing's) as with soft tissue sarcomas (e. g. embryonal, synovial) the essential first principle of effective curative treatment is complete control of the primary tumour. Often this can only be obtained with radical surgery: where this is inexpedient or declined, radiotherapy must be supplemented by prolonged intensive chemotherapy. Ewing's tumour and embryonal sarcoma are two obvious and important examples of the need to appreciate fully this first step which must accompany any attempt to destroy or restrain clinically occult micrometastases.

### Osteosarcoma

The terrible mortality of this tumour in the Manchester series with only 3 of 28 children alive at 4 years agrees with the results from a larger series of 125 cases collected by PRICE et al. (1975), who reported only 12% free of disease at 5 years. Nevertheless, the fact that 90% of osteosarcomas in children present in the limb long bones may be a significant point of potentially favourable prognosis if and when effective antimetastatic treatment is devised. In children about two-thirds of all osteosarcomas arise in the knee region.

Biopsy. There is no evidence that open biopsy adversely affects prognosis and this method certainly provides the pathologist with the maximum of tissue for examination. Nevertheless, LEE and MACKENZIE (1964) illustrate the risk of tumour fungation through a long biopsy incision. LEE (1973) advocates the employment of a punch technique through a 1 cm skin incision. In most cases a drill biopsy will furnish adequate material for histological diagnosis but calls for considerable expertise in interpretation when sectioned. Chondroblastic, anaplastic and telangiectatic types of osteosarcoma are more ominous, likewise those with consistently high mitotic activity (over 15 mitoses per square mm of cellular tumour tissue). It must be emphasized that the absence of these unfavourable histological features does not eliminate the need for active treatment both of the primary and of the occult micrometastases which probably already exist.

Primary Treatment. The bad results, with 50% of patients showing evident metastases at 5 months after treatment, has almost inevitably led to two divergent methods of management:

1. Megavoltage irradiation of the primary to the maximum permissible dose, followed at 6 months by amputation if free of evident disease. In the series reported by LEE and MACKENZIE (1964) the dosage employed ranged from 6000 to 8000 rads given over 6-8 weeks. Some children were included, but the patients were mostly teenagers over 15 years of age. Some modification of the treatment plan may therefore be required according to age of the patient and size of the tissue volume to be treated.

2. Prompt amputation following biopsy and diagnosis.

For osteosarcoma the results of these two regimes leave but little to choose in terms of survival.

Five years results for patients of all ages

| | | |
|---|---|---|
| Irradiation with or without delayed amputation | - 119/501 | = 23.8% alive |
| Radical surgery | - 191/903 | = 21.0% alive |

These data were collected from the world literature by TRIFAUD and MEARY (1972).

The former method, introduced at the Westminster Hospital, has no curative advantage, but does avoid mutilating operations for the majority of patients. Its usage is contraindicated for fungating tumours, or with complications such as fracture or flexion contracture, or tumours containing a great deal of cartilage, and for sarcomas of very young children. Its most useful application has been for tumours of the arm (usually in the proximal humerus). Even with the dose of radiation mentioned above, seemingly viable residual tumour tissue may persist in about one-third of tumours treated (LEE and MACKENZIE, 1964).

The similar failure of prompt amputation to control the disease indicates that probably as many as 90% of children have occult micrometastases at the time of operation, if not before this. The obvious conclusion follows that until there is efficient antimetastatic treatment no real improvement in the overall results can be anticipated. Preoperative irradiation before biopsy or immediately preceding amputation has not been of significant value, likewise for tumours of the leg bones there is little to choose between the results of disarticulation and transfemoral amputation. Past failures have stimulated a wider concept of essential treatment of osteosarcoma adjuvant to the application of either Method 1 or 2 supra. Radiotherapy combined with surgical excision as may be expedient is usual for tumours arising elsewhere in the skeleton.

Adjuvant Treatment. Several new methods are now undergoing trial:

A. "Prophylactic" irradiation of lungs (i. e. before evident metastases). This has been carried out by NEWTON (1973) and consists of giving 1950 rads of megavoltage radiation to the lungs in 13/18 days during the latter weeks of irradiation of the primary tumour. With 17 patients of all ages, the results are encouraging and the median disease-free interval has been at least tripled. This method has been applied to adults and may need considerable modification for children. Its drawback is that it can only destroy or restrain the growth of pulmonary micrometastases. A recent study of 123 long bone osteosarcoma patients of all ages in the records of the Bristol Bone Tumour Registry shows that 27 of 83 patients known to have died with pulmonary secondaries also had metastases elsewhere (JEFFREE et al., 1975). This problem may possibly be resolved by sequential chemotherapy. There can be no doubt that lung irradiation is beneficial during the 2 years following treatment of the primary tumour and the 5 year results of NEWTON's series are awaited with interest.

B. Adjuvant Chemotherapy

A number of reports have shown that overt metastases of osteosarcoma may respond to chemotherapy - notably to regimes including adriamycin (Doxorubicin) and high dose methotrexate with citrovorum rescue (CORTES et al., 1973; JAFFE et al., 1973; GOTTLIEB et al., 1972; ROSEN et al., 1973). It is thus reasonable to suppose that clinically occult micrometastases may likewise be sensitive to these cytotoxic drugs given early in the treatment planned for any patient. This may be either:

1. Ten to 14 days after amputation or as soon as clinically expedient
2. Commencing during the course of radiotherapy for the primary if this method is preferred or site conditioned
3. Following "prophylactic" irradiation of the lungs if metastases appear

In connection with this, several protocols of pulsed multidrug chemotherapy are under current trial at different centres with varied combinations of cytotoxic drugs. Possibly the most promising are regimes which employ adriamycin, Dimethyl-triazeno-imidazole-carboxamide (DTIC), and high dose methotrexate with leucovorin rescue. The reports cited by ROSEN et al. (1973, 1974) give information specifically about children. Chemotherapy is rapidly moving and the current literature should be consulted for up-to-date information, but the treatment plan described by CORTES et al. (1974) seems worthy of a careful trial. Encouraging early reports have been published also by PRATT et al. (1974) and SUTOW et al. (1974).

The usage of these methods entails a careful and close watch for cardiotoxicity, marrow depression, and upon kidney and liver function. Two undesirable side effects are temporary loss of hair and sterilization. They are also of value for patients with evident metastases, but so far no beneficial effect has been noted for secondaries in the brain.

It must be emphasized that these new adjuvant methods of treatment are to some extent "experimental medicine" with attendant ethical and statistical overtones. They are stages in the ultimate development of curative therapy for osteosarcoma. Hence, it is essential to collect and analyse all records of patients so treated. Moreover, whilst treatment of the primary tumour may well be undertaken by many hospitals, the complicated adjuvant treatment (whichever form is decided) should be given in selected regional centres only with special experience in all aspects of chemotherapy. Concentration of cases in a limited number of treatment centres would be of practical benefit to patients and more rapidly lead to evaluation of the results of treatment. The total incidence of osteosarcoma in the United Kingdom is about 150 new cases annually (excluding those complicating Paget's disease). Of these not more than 50 new cases annually will be in children. This lack of clinical material underlines the difficulty in assessing the precise benefit of any advances in management.

C. Immunotherapy
Early reports from the Memorial Sloan-Kettering Hospital Group have shown some benefit from active immunotherapy using an autogenous lysed-cell vaccine prepared from UV irradiated tumour cells (MARCOVE et al., 1973). Likewise, beneficial results are claimed by ENNEKING and MARSH (1973) for a method of adoptive immunotherapy based upon crosstransfusion of sensitised leucocytes obtained from volunteers who received heterografts of viable tumour tissue from patients so treated. The final results of these investigations will indicate their antimetastatic value and the possible role of adjuvant specific immunotherapy for a small residual tumour cell population. Evidence from several sources, however, suggests that adoptive immunotherapy attempted by intravenous infusion of allogeneic or xenogeneic sensitised cells acts mainly upon pulmonary metastases, with but little effect upon secondaries elsewhere.

Non-specific immunotherapy has no present clinical application in the treatment of osteosarcoma, although providing an active research field with this and other solid tumours. Studies of bone sarcomas and their cells in tissue culture have revealed the presence of tumour specific antigens (MOORE et al., 1973) but much more basic work is required to establish the value and techniques of practical immunotherapy. Brief lucid accounts of tumour immunology are given by MOORE (1971) and by HERSCH et al. (1974).

D. Other New Methods
Mention should also be made of the work of OHNO (1971) who claimed 36% 5-year survival (all ages) for cases treated by a combined regime including bronchial artery infusion with mitomycin C, nitromin and 5-fluorouracil. The sophisticated technique includes aortic catheterization and again is unlikely to destroy extrapulmonary metastases. MARTINI et al. (1971) describe multiple thoracotomies for pulmonary metastases attended by some success. The original papers should be consulted.

## Chondrosarcoma

This tumour is rare during childhood so that one can only generalise and extrapolate from its known behaviour in adults. In children, however, it tends to be more aggressive and one should distinguish between tumours which are predominantly cellular and likely to metastasize and those which are well differentiated and sometimes histologically referred to as "low grade". The former rather resemble chondroblastic osteosarcoma and should be treated as such. The latter provide a problem almost entirely surgical since, although metastatic spread is unusual, they require complete and utter removal. Spillage of cells at any operation or residual tumour tissue will almost certainly regrow ultimately, and may prove fatal from damage to adjacent vital organs. Cartilage tumours are notoriously radio-resistant, although palliative irradiation may be required for relief of pain.

## Fibrosarcoma

Again rare during childhood, this tumour has a slightly better prognosis than osteosarcoma but tends to behave in a fashion similar to osteosarcoma of like age of patient. Since it, too, is radio-resistant primary treatment should be planned along lines similar to osteosarcoma - amputation when possible, otherwise local surgical removal and radiotherapy. This should be followed by adjuvant chemotherapy, since metastatic spread is at least as extensive as with osteosarcoma and with a slightly higher proportion of extrapulmonary deposits. An extended course of pulsed multidrug treatment may be given to include adriamycin, cyclophosphamide and vincristine. In children, fibrosarcoma may occasionally complicate a simple bone cyst.

## Reticulosarcoma

For patients of all ages the prognosis and results of treatment are influenced by at least 2 factors:

1. A favourable result at 5 years may be anticipated for 40% or so of cases for tumours which are restricted to one bone only. Otherwise, in multicentric cases the results are bad (PRICE, 1973).

2. Tumours responding well to treatment are histologically well reticulated and devoid of intracellular glycogen (cf. Ewing's sarcoma).

In the Bristol Bone Tumour Registry records 1 child (BTR/1135. Girl, aged 7 years) is alive and well 12 years after treatment. Three other children with multifocal lesions have died respectively at 2, 4, and 9 months. Tumours with a confusing histological pattern intermediate between reticulosarcoma and Ewing's tumour are sometimes seen and usually behave like the latter. In children it is advised that the treatment given should be similar to that applied for Ewing's tumour of bone - radiotherapy with adjuvant pulsed multidrug chemotherapy. Good recent reports on the treatment of osseous reticulosarcoma of all ages are given by MILLER and NICHOLSON (1971) and also by DAHLIN (1973). In the former paper, treatment included non-specific immunotherapy additional to radiotherapy and surgery.

## Giant Cell Tumour

This is a rare tumour in bone before the time of skeletal epiphyseal fusion. Although usually amenable to conservative treatment in an adult, in a child a giant cell tumour tends to be quite atypical and to behave in an aggressive, sometimes frankly malignant manner. In a rapidly progressive osteolytic tumour which has been shown to have the histological appearances of a giant cell tumour, it is probably prudent to give treatment based upon the regime advocated for osteosarcoma. These cases are uncommon, and each must be evaluated and managed according to its individual problems.

## BENIGN PRIMARY BONE TUMOURS

There were 5 types in this group (Table 13).

Table 13. Benign primary bone tumours

| | Alive | Dead | Total |
|---|---|---|---|
| Fibroma of bone | 6 | 1 | 7 |
| Osteoid osteoma | 7 | 0 | 7 |
| Giant cell lesion of jaw | 3 | 0 | 3 |
| Chondroblastoma | 1 | 0 | 1 |
| Osteoma | 1 | 0 | 1 |
| | 18 | 1 | 19 |

Fibroma of Bone

The term "non-osteogenic fibroma of bone" was introduced by JAFFÉ and LICHTENSTEIN (1942). These authors point out that a neoplastic origin was not universally accepted and WILLIS (1962) regards the lesion as a variant of fibrous dysplasia. Seven children were included in this group. Their ages ranged from 6-14 years. The lesions presented with localised pain and behaved as benign cysts expanding the cortex rather than invading it. Pathological fractures occurred. A cystic appearance was seen on X-ray and biopsies showed the spindle cell fibrous nature of the lesions, sometimes with foam cells. The cellularity was variable

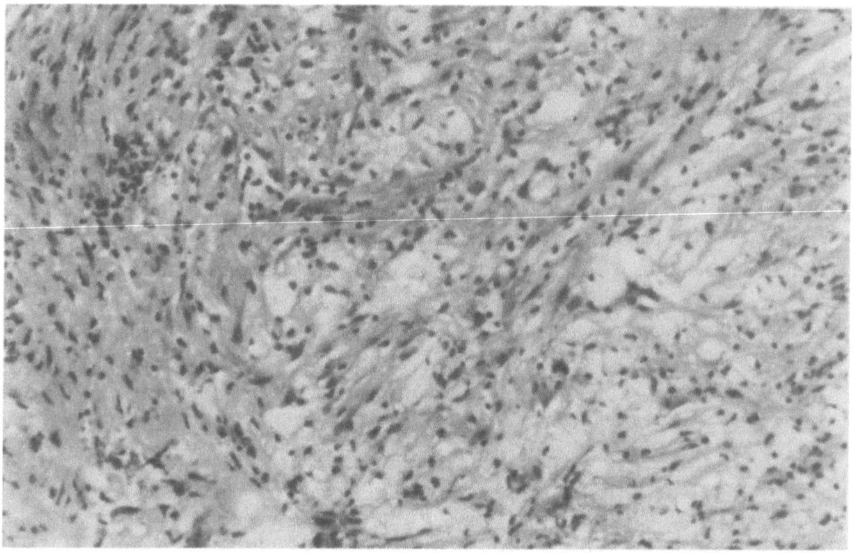

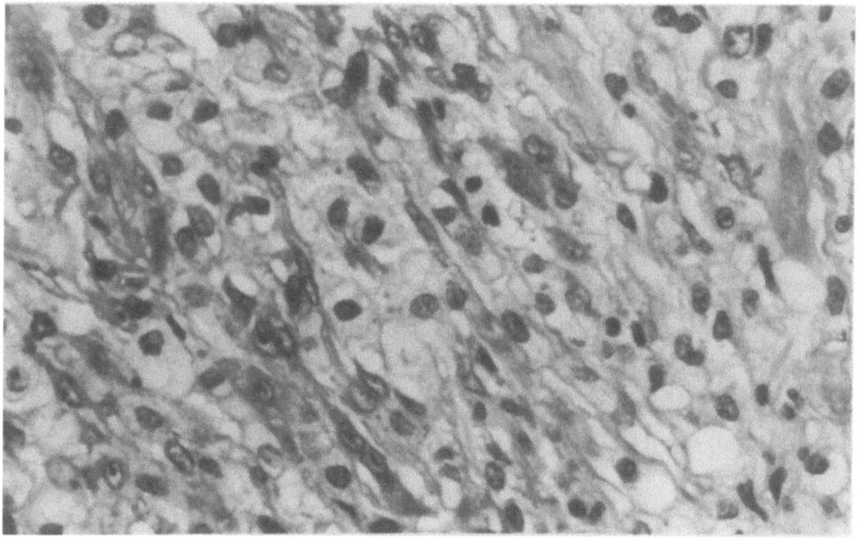

*Fig. 16a. Fibroma of bone with spindle and vacuolated cells (H.&E. X 175)*
*b. Detail of (a) (H. & E. X 500)*

with areas of more plump cells and giant cells, and hypocellular portions where elongated spindle cells were separated by swollen vacuolated cells. Three of the lesions occurred in the tibia, two in the femur, one in the fibula, and one involved several lumbar vertebrae. The tumours responded well to curetting. The only fatality was in the case of the child with involvement of the vertebrae who developed paraplegia and died from haemorrhage during an operation to relieve this.

## Osteoid Osteoma, Osteoblastoma and Chondroblastoma

There is some difference of opinion concerning the nature of the osteoid osteoma and chondroblastoma. WILLIS (1962) considered that both may be seen as variants of fibrous dysplasia and some chondroblastomas may be chondrifying osteoclastomas. Both these tumours, however, appear to have characteristic features. Osteoid osteoma and osteoblastoma are variants of one benign osteoblastic process, the type depending on whether the compacta or spongiosa are involved (DIAS and FROST, 1974). In some cases the chondroblastoma may show invasive tendencies (COPELAND and GESCHICKTER, 1949).

The findings of the 7 cases of the osteoid osteoma/osteoblastoma group in this series add little to what is already known about this tumour. In 4 children the lesions were in the tibia, 1 in the fibula, 1 in the talus, and 1 in the femoral neck. The ages of the patients were between 6 and 12 years. Pain referable to the tumour was the presenting symptom in all cases. Initially the pain tended to occur at night. There was tenderness at the sites of the lesions and bone thickening was detected on palpation. A red or purple nodule, up to 1 cm in diameter, was described in several of the cases and treatment was by excision. However, 1 patient was initially thought to have chronic osteomyelitis, and a satisfactory cure was obtained merely by curetting the lesion. In one of the tibial tumours bony sclerosis was seen on X-rays of the opposite tibia. There was, however, no central translucency and in the absence of surgery the presence of a second osteoblastoma cannot be proven.

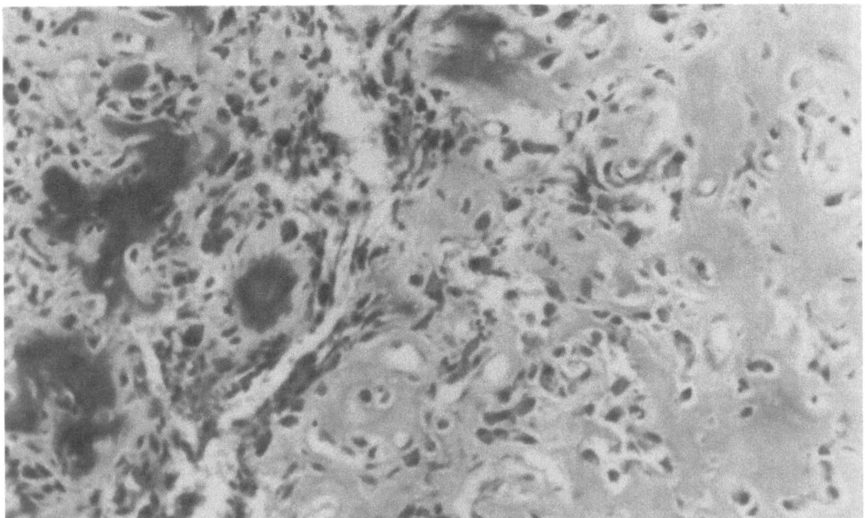

*Fig. 17. Osteoid osteoma showing part of central nodule and surrounding sclerotic bone (H. & E. X 250)*

The chondroblastoma was in the tibia of a 13-year-old girl who gave a history of pain in the knee for 6 months. The upper end of the tibia

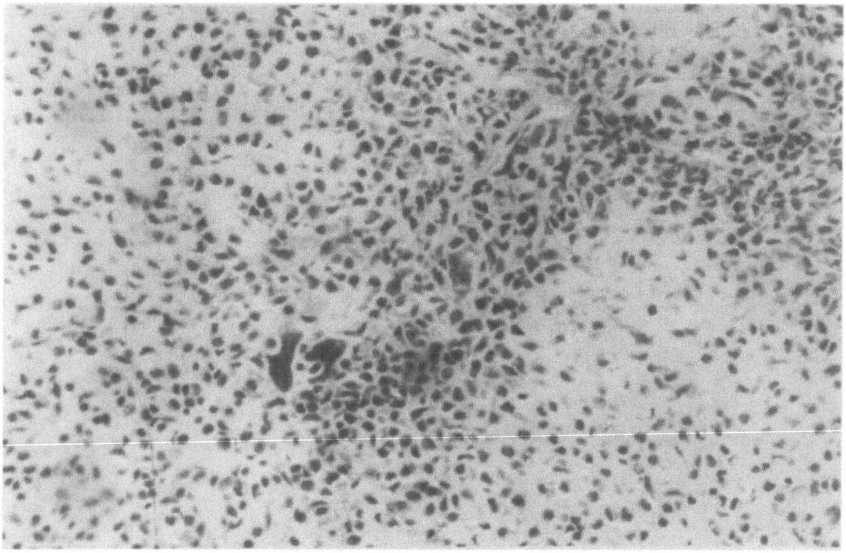

*Fig. 18. Benign chondroblastoma removed from upper end of tibia (H. & E. X 250)*

contained a large cavity without any surrounding bone sclerosis. Curetting of the cavity resulted in healing of the lesion and the patient was well 10 years later. Histologically the tumour contained cartilage with polygonal cells and giant cells resembling osteoclasts.

## Giant Cell Lesions of the Jaw

The 3 Manchester cases classified under this heading consisted microscopically of a spindle cell matrix and scattered giant cells of osteoclast type with, in one case, osteoid formation. The spindle cells although varying between relatively short forms with small nuclei and long fibroblastic cells showed little variation between individual cells in the different areas. The appearance was that of an essentially benign lesion and it is considered that they should be separated from the osteoclastomas of long bones where pleomorphism was encountered. These jaw lesions have been considered to be giant cell granulomas (ANDERSON, 1971).

## SOFT TISSUE FIBROBLASTIC TUMOURS

In the preface to his comprehensive monograph on the differential diagnosis of fibroblastic disorders, MACKENZIE (1970) stresses the diversity of fibroblastic behaviour and the need for relating histological appearance to biological behaviour. The difficulty of doing this accurately was seen in the 38 children with soft tissue fibroblastic tumours included in the Register. They could be divided into 3 groups (Table 14).

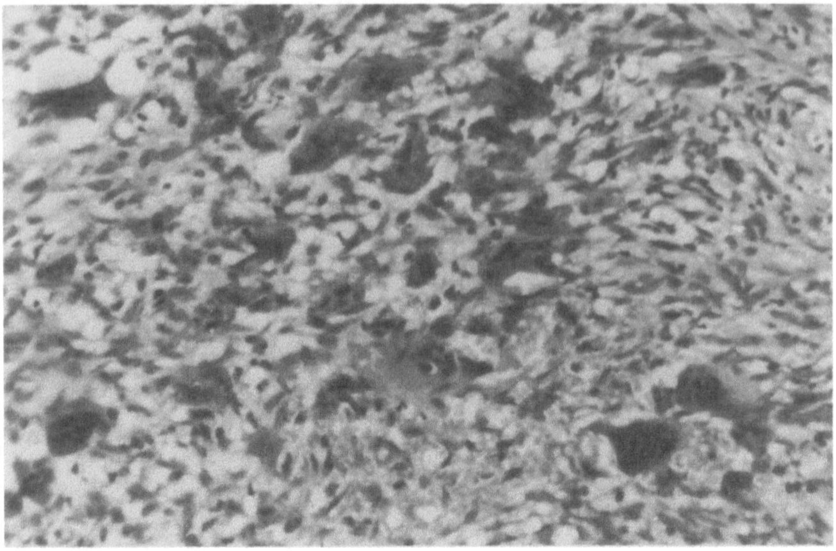

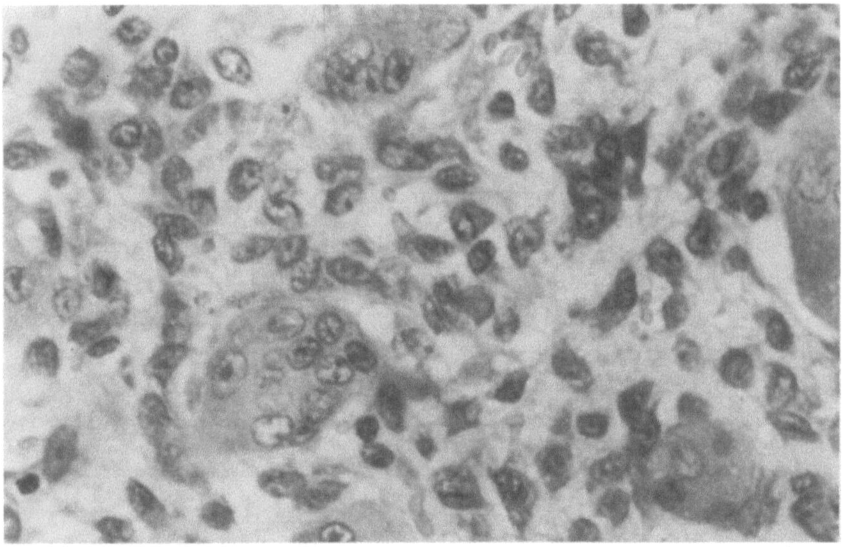

*Figs. 19a and b. Giant cell lesion of jaw (a) H.&E. X 250; (b) H.&E. X 625*

Table 14. Soft tissue fibroblastic tumours

| | Alive | Dead | Total |
|---|---|---|---|
| Fibroma/Fibromatosis/Fibrosarcoma | 26 | 4 | 30 |
| Nasopharyngeal angiofibroma | 4 | 0 | 4 |
| Meningioma | 3 | 1 | 4 |
| | 33 | 5 | 38 |

Fibroma/Fibromatosis/Fibrosarcoma

It is recognised that the present series does not include all the children with these tumours in the Manchester region, since many of the lesions would not be considered to be of sufficient severity to be referred to the Registry. Therefore the Manchester cases can only be regarded as a sample of this group.

In reviewing a large series of children with fibroblastic tumours STOUT (1954 and 1962) stresses the following points:

a) These tumours rarely metastasise.
b) They are locally invasive.
c) It may be difficult or impossible to predict their future behaviour from their histological appearance.
d) Other mesenchymal tumours such as malignant synoviomas or liposarcomas may contain areas of fibroblastic tumour tissue derived from other mesenchymal cells becoming transformed into fibroblasts.

STOUT (1954) used the term "juvenile fibromatosis" to include a fibrous growth which could not be assigned to any other category. Forty-one of the 44 cases in his series arose in the areas - neck, shoulder, hands and feet, buttocks thighs and legs. In this review and in a later survey of juvenile fibrosarcomas (STOUT, 1962) he could neither make a clear-cut histological distinction between fibromatosis and fibrosarcoma, nor could he pick out those few tumours which eventually metastasised.

The 30 Manchester tumours were much more widely scattered throughout the body than in STOUT's series. They arose in such situations as the hands and feet, buttocks, legs, scalp, abdominal cavity, bronchus, and duodenum. However both series suggested that fibroblastic tumours in children have a special tendency to occur in the shoulder region - this occurred in 6 of the 30 Manchester cases. Histologically, the tumours varied between being frank sarcomas and having such a benign appearance that some could almost be described as "fasciitis". Calcification was present in one case and lymphocytic infiltration in another. One fibroma in the nose had a myxomatous appearance.

The prognosis of this group is good. By 1972 only 3 of the 30 Manchester children had died of their tumours. Two were retroperitoneal and the other was in the face. One of the retroperitoneal tumours appeared to be histologically benign but the other 2 were frank fibrosarcomas. Lung metastases developed in the child with the retroperitoneal fibrosarcoma but there was no evidence of metastatic spread in the other 2 children who died prior to 1972. Although these results are encouraging, late recurrences can occur and one Manchester child has died since 1972.
CTR.23/61. Boy aged 1 1/2 years who developed a large mass medial to the left scapula in May 1960. This was thought to be a cyst but in February 1961 exploration revealed it to be a low grade fibrosarcoma which could not be removed. Six months after adenopterin and irradiation (4000 rads in 20 days) were given the tumour had become much smaller and could be excised in April 1962. Sections showed that it was invading the surrounding muscle but it appeared histologically low-grade. The child remained well for the next ten years but in August 1972 a mass in the region of the original tumour appeared and a biopsy showed a highly malignant sarcoma. Lung metastases developed, irradiation and chemotherapy had little effect and the child died in November 1973.

Soft tissue fibroblastic tumours may occur in the newborn and show evidence of rapid growth and histological malignancy. One such fibro-

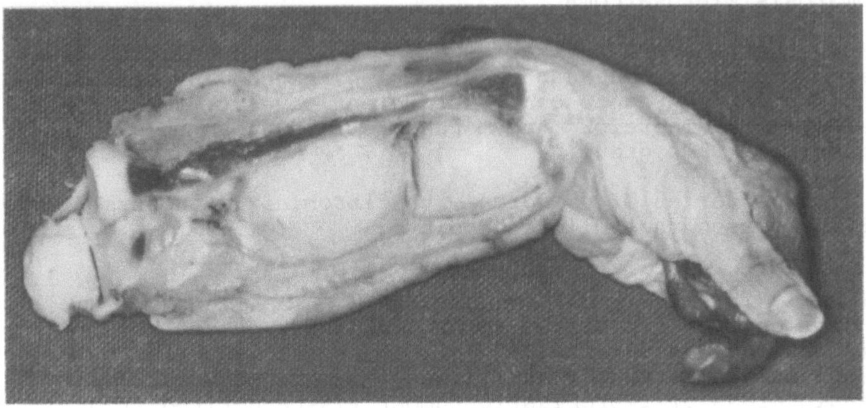

*Fig. 20. CTR.111/69. Interosseous fibrosarcoma of forearm in premature infant*

sarcoma was seen in a Manchester infant in 1956 involving most of the leg below the knee. Following amputation the tumour has not recurred. Another Manchester infant - a premature baby weighing 2 lbs 9 ozs - developed a fibrosarcoma of the forearm at the age of 6 weeks in 1969. Following biopsy, conservative treatment was attempted but rapid growth occurred and the arm was amputated. The tumour had not recurred 4 years later. BALSAVER et al. (1967) describe 5 cases of congenital fibrosarcoma and review the literature.

Although the 30 Manchester cases of fibroma/fibromatosis/fibrosarcoma form a comparatively small and incomplete group, the findings are in agreement with STOUT's conclusions. Only 2 of these 30 tumours have metastasised, whereas 10 showed evidence of local invasion and some required re-excision. It was difficult to predict the subsequent behaviour of the tumours from their histological appearance. Therefore

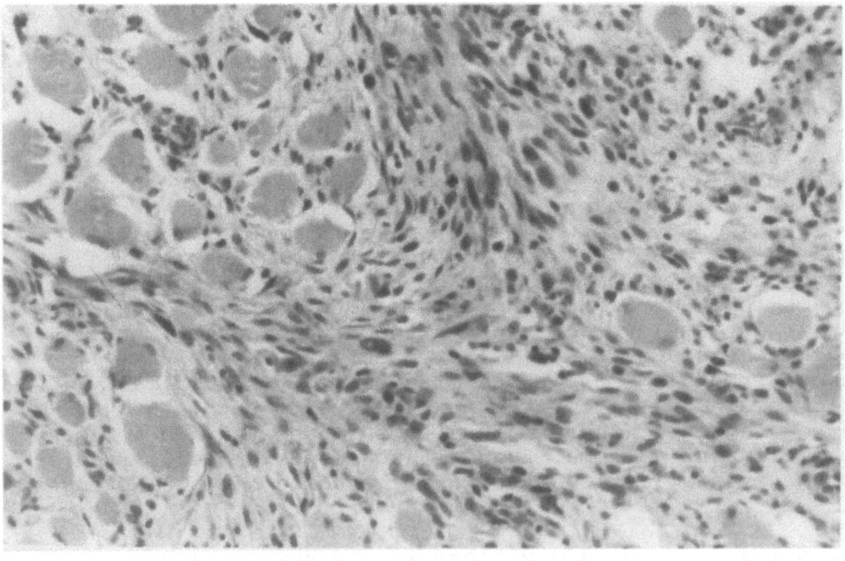

*Fig. 21. Fibrosarcoma invading muscle (H. & E. X 250)*

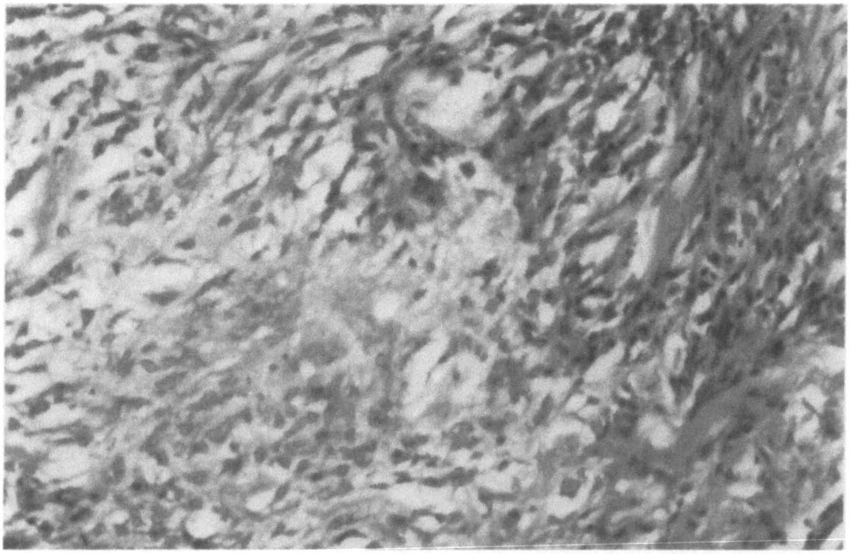

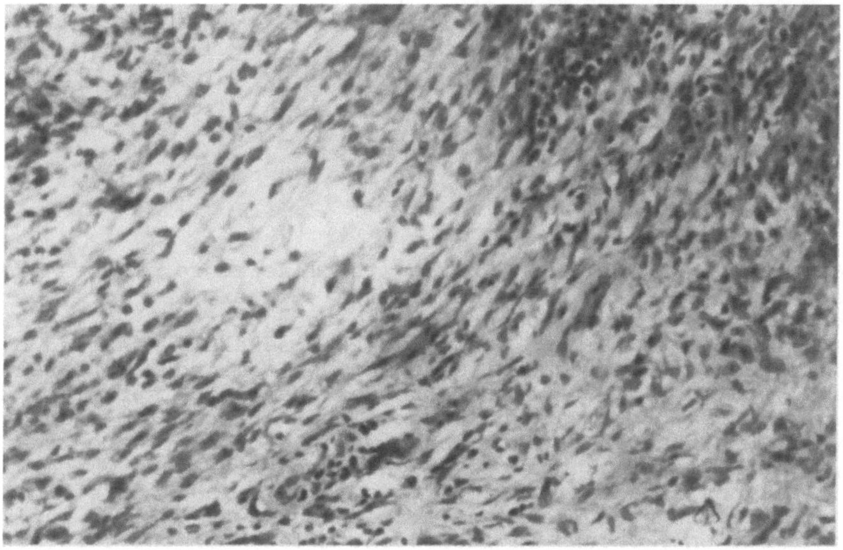

*Fig. 22. Giant "rheumatic" nodule showing (a) prominent collagen degeneration and (b) more cellular proliferative tissue. The mass was excised from the pretibial region of a 3 1/2-year-old girl. It was firm and white and was thought to be a neoplasm at operation (a) and (b) H. & E. X 250*

STOUT's recommendation that every effort should be made to excise these tumours widely is still valid and reliance should not be placed on any residual tumour being destroyed by irradiation or chemotherapy. In view of the possibility of fibrosarcomas recurring after many years the value of any new form of treatment would be very difficult to assess.

## Nasopharyngeal Angiofibromas

Four examples of this tumour were encountered and as in previous reports, the patients were all boys. Their ages ranged from 9 to 13 years. The loose hypocellular fibrous tissue with large thin-walled vessels makes severe haemorrhage likely both before and during operation. Excision alone was carried out in 1 case and excision combined with radiotherapy in the other 3. All are alive and well.

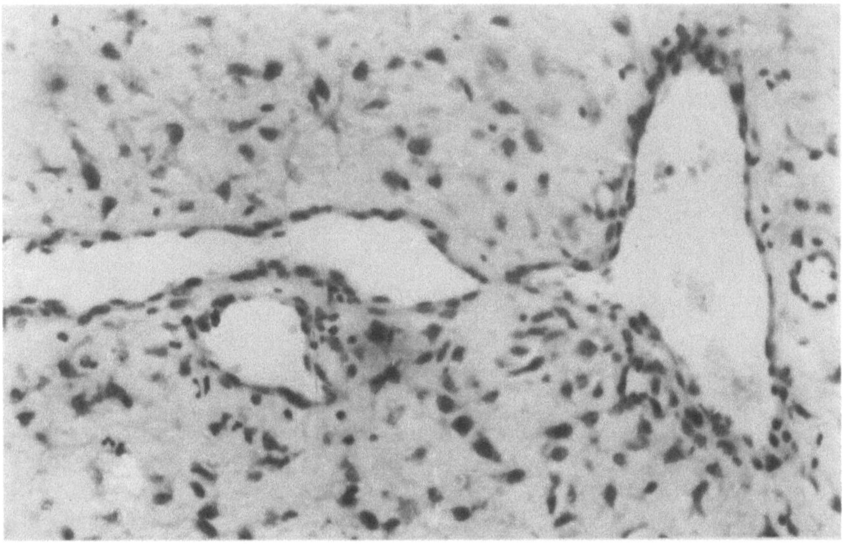

*Fig. 23. Nasopharyngeal angiofibroma (H. & E. X 250)*

APOSTOL and FRAZELL (1965) review the literature of this tumour and describe 40 cases seen at the Memorial Center, New York, between 1932 and 1963. All were males between the ages of 8 and 27 years. Only 2 died from the tumour and 1 survivor was severely disabled by it. Five others had some residual disease and the remainder appeared to be completely cured. These authors consider that total surgical excision is the preferred treatment and suggest that irradiation should not be given. They note that the 3 cases which did badly were treated by X-rays. This view is supported by one Manchester case which was treated initially by irradiation (2000 rads, 4 MeV, in 11 days) in 1964, but continued with nosebleeds until the tumour was excised in 1969. Since the tumour only occurs in adolescent males, hormone treatment has been tried - either testosterone or stilboestrol. APOSTOL and FRAZELL state that testosterone was unsuccessful in their experience but note that SCHIFF (1959) and MacCOMB (1963) report good results with stilboestrol.

## Digital Fibrous Tumours in Infants and Young Children

These tumours, which may be multiple, were described by JENSEN et al. (1957). They may be attached to, but do not invade, the periosteum of the phalanx. McKENZIE et al. have shown that they tend to regress spontaneously and recur only if incompletely excised.

Cytoplasmic inclusions which may not be detected in ordinary H & E preparations have suggested a viral origin, but MEHREGAN et al. were unable to isolate viruses in culture in 2 cases. Metastasis does not occur.

## Meningiomas

The 4 meningiomas included in the Manchester series are described in Chapter 6.

## SYNOVIOMAS

These tumours include benign (giant cell tumours of tendon sheath) and malignant synoviomas. Three benign tumours were encountered in children aged 6, 11 and 12 years; one on the extensor aspect of the ankle, another on the thumb and a third on the middle finger.

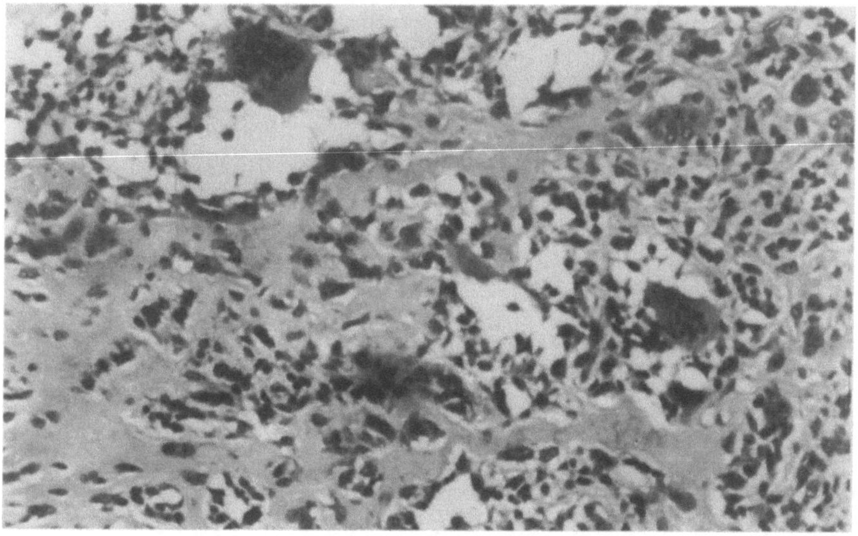

*Fig. 24. Benign synovioma (giant cell tumour of tendon sheath) (H. & E. X 250)*

Malignant synoviomas were seen in 8 children, 2 in the foot and 1 each in the groin, elbow, thigh, hand, scapular region and knee. Histologically, the tumours showed a spindle- or spheroidal-cell structure with mesothelial clefts and sometimes giant cells. STOUT (1962) points out that the differential diagnosis between malignant synovioma and fibrosarcoma may be difficult or impossible, because parts of a synovioma may contain only fibroblastic elements. Furthermore, it may be very difficult to be certain whether a cleft is truly mesothelial or not. Thus, although the 8 examples of malignant synovioma in the Manchester series have been diagnosed with reasonable confidence, the diagnosis has been seriously considered in other cases which were ultimately otherwise classified e. g. as fibrosarcoma or embryonic sarcoma of alveolar type.

The results of treatment of the malignant synoviomas in the Manchester series have been poor - 6 out of the 8 children have died from their tumours. In general the disease progressed much more slowly than occurred with embryonic sarcomas or osteo- and chondrosarcomas (see Table 6), and in 2 cases death did not occur until between 6 and 8 years after diagnosis. On the other hand, one 14 year old boy with

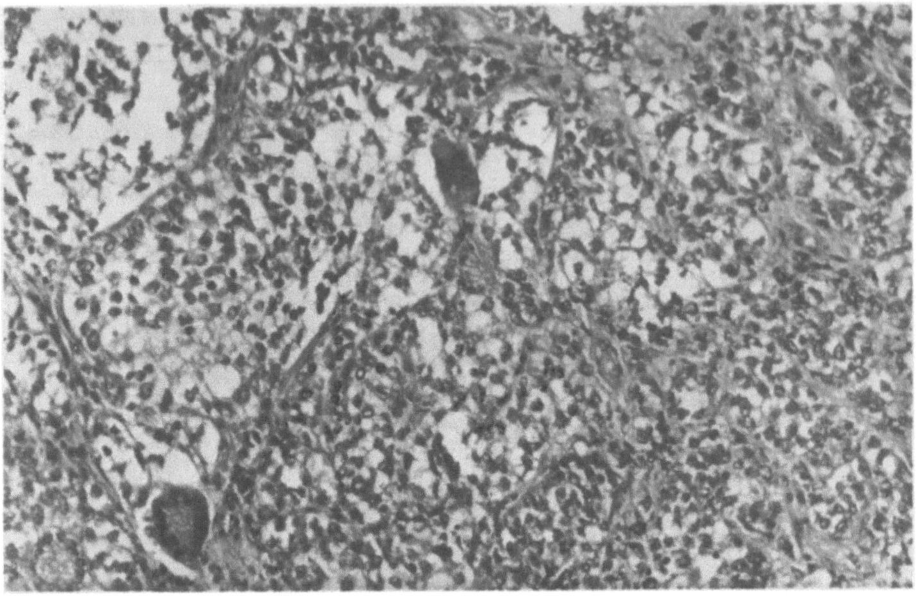

*Fig. 25. Synovial sarcoma. Metastasis in lymph node showing lobular arrangement with vesicular and giant cells (H. & E. X 250)*

a primary in the foot, presented with generalised neoplastic invasion of the bone marrow and death occurred within 6 months. CROCKER and STOUT (1959) from a study of 43 malignant synoviomas in children stress the value of wide local excision and 1 of the Manchester children with a tumour of the forearm is alive and well 9 years after amputation without any other treatment being given. The other survivor was treated by excision and irradiation of a synovioma in the groin and has remained well for 18 years. In view of the long time before it is possible to consider that a child who has had a malignant synovioma is cured, the value of chemotherapy and irradiation is difficult to assess. It would seem, therefore, that wide surgical excision should still be considered to be the main method of treatment. This means that, if a malignant synovioma is in a limb, amputation should not be delayed in the hope of controlling the tumour by irradiation or chemotherapy.

## LIPOMATOUS TUMOURS

Many examples of lipomatous masses of childhood, for example, in association with spina bifida, have not been included in the Register. However, there were 10 cases - 2 retroperitoneal, 2 intracranial, 2 in the arm and 1 each in the hand, buttock, chest wall, and scapular region - which, because of their size, difficulty of removal or local invasiveness, are referred to here. One of the retroperitoneal tumours was diagnosed at laparotomy. Although it was histologically not very cellular, no attempt was made to remove it and the patient - a 14-year-old boy - died 10 months later. At autopsy the tumour weighed 17,600 g and it was felt that with greater surgical boldness the tumour might have been removed at the initial operation. A similarly massive retroperitoneal lipoma was successfully removed from a 2-year-old girl. The children with lipomas of the arm, hand, chest wall and scapular region

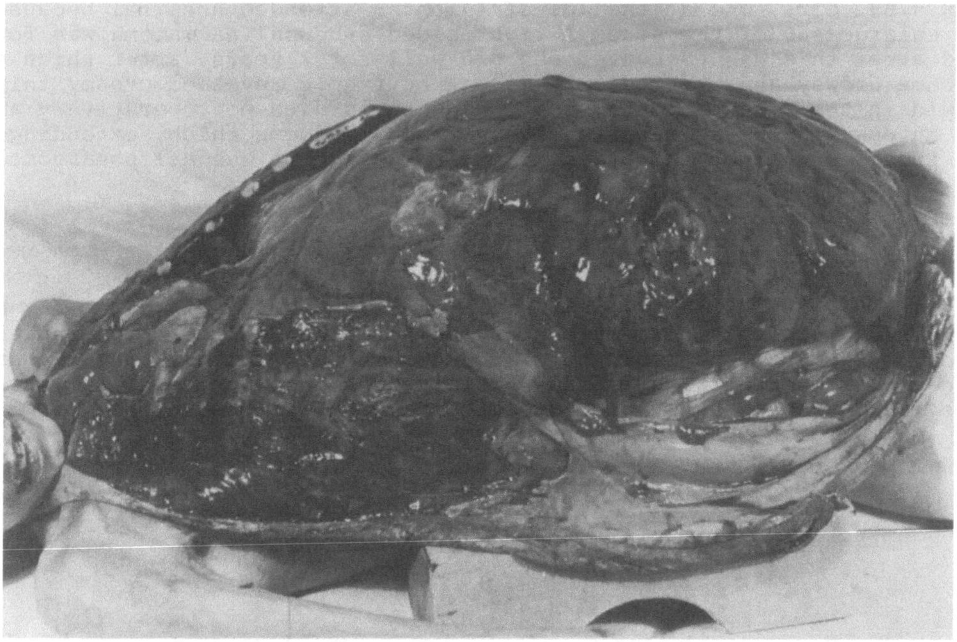

*Fig. 26. Massive abdominal lipomatous tumour (COURTESY Dr. R. C. WOODCOCK)*

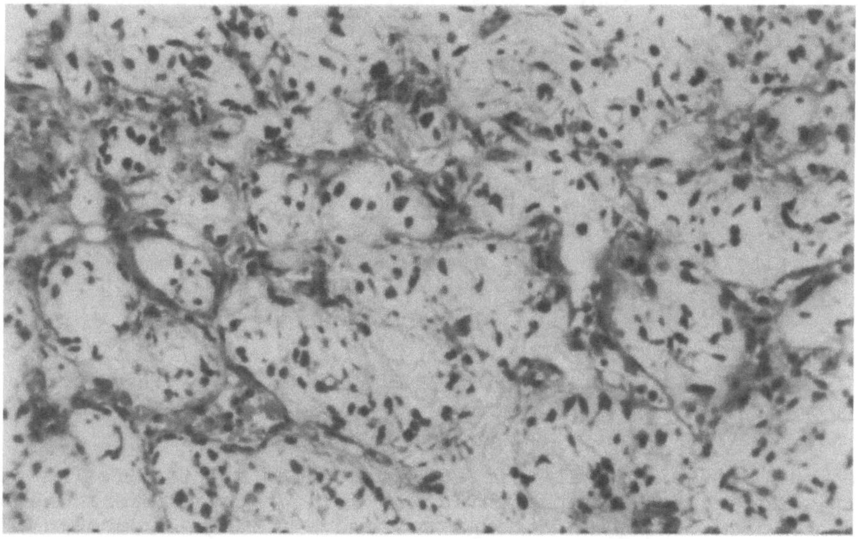

*Fig. 27. Photomicrograph of tumour shown in Fig. 26 with lipoid-filled cells and rather more cellular tissue (H. & E. X 250)*

are all alive and well, but considerable surgical difficulty was experienced in their treatment because the tumours tended to spread widely into surrounding tissues. One girl, who had a large lipoma of the hand, has since given birth to a child who developed on orchioblastoma. One of the children with an intracranial lipoma is alive 10 years after excision of the tumour; the history of the other is as follows:

CTR.9/69. Girl, who at the age of 4 months attended hospital because of enlargement of the head. A right-sided subdural haematoma was found and after this was evacuated she did well for 2 years, after which she became drowsy and started to vomit. A burr hole revealed creamy thick fluid in the right subdural space. The child died postoperatively and at autopsy there was a white fleshy tumour 3-4 cms thick, extending into the bone but not the brain. Histologically it was a liposarcoma.

OTHER TUMOURS

Single examples of a myxoma on the medial aspect of the thigh and an ivory osteoma of the skull were included in the Register. One 3-year-old girl presented with a 3 day history of a lump in the groin which was found to be due to a leiomyosarcoma 1" in diameter arising from

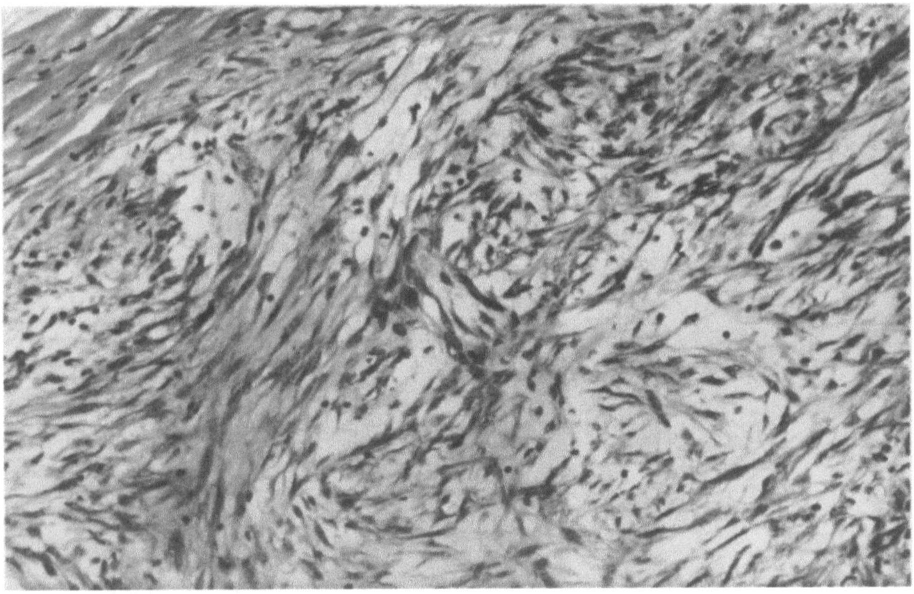

*Fig. 28. Leiomyosarcoma of femoral vein referred to in text (H. & E. X 275)*

the wall of the femoral vein and distending its lumen. The tumour and vein were excised and the child was well 7 years later. One 5-year-old boy died during an attempt to remove a large hypocellular myxomatous tumour of the liver. Another 5-year-old child was found to have a retroperitoneal malignant mesenchymoma consisting of cartilage and embryonic connective tissue, and died 5 months later.

Two tumours were encountered which were thought to be mesenchymal in origin but did not fit into any of the above groups. One case presented with a lump on the flexor aspect of the forearm in a 10-year-old girl. The tumour was excised and was described as being 1 inch in diameter, haemorrhagic, not encapsulated, and to be infiltrating the flexor muscles. The other case was a 13-year-old boy with a lesion on the lower leg which was curetted, but recurred and 20 months later a

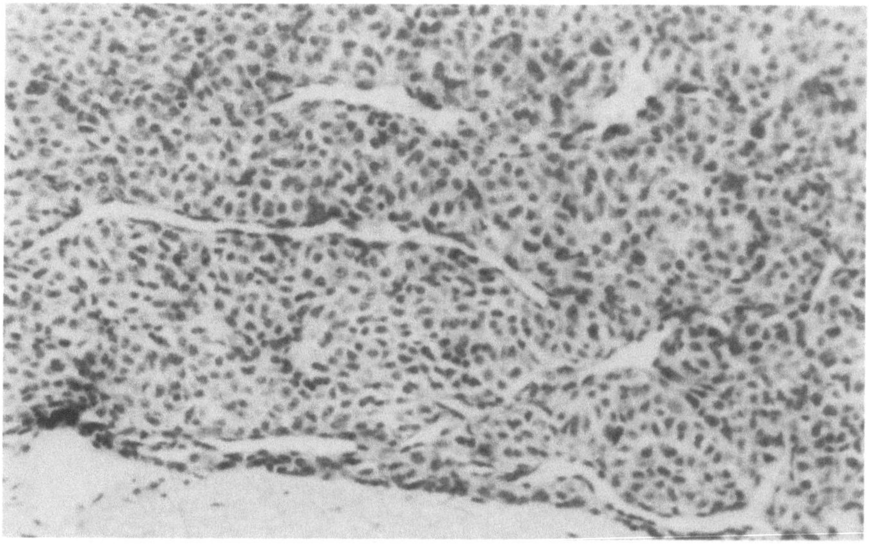

*Fig. 29. Mesenchymal tumour of uncertain nature removed from leg of 13-year-old boy referred to in text. There are polygonal cells and thin-walled vascular channels (H. & E. X 250)*

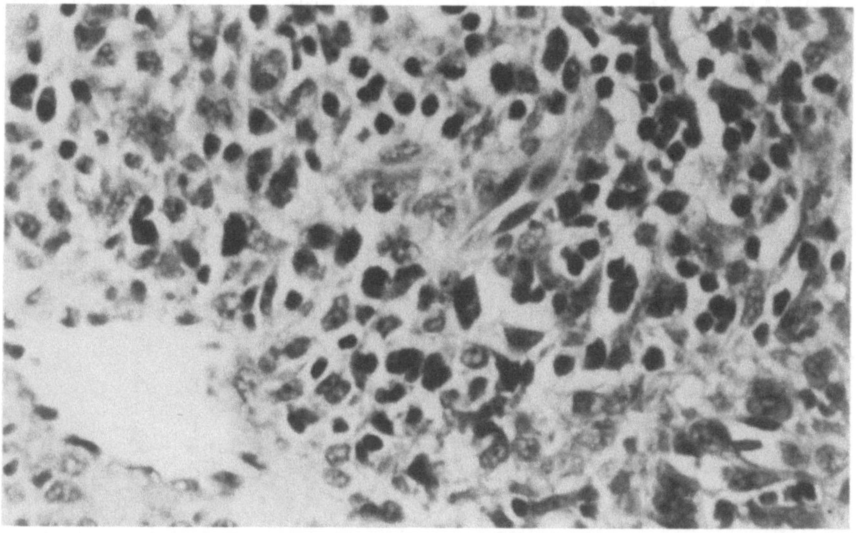

*Fig. 30. Mesenchymal tumour of uncertain nature removed from forearm of 10-year-old girl referred to in text. Plasma and spindle cells are seen in addition to vascular spaces (H. & E. X 500)*

well-defined vascular mass, 1" in diameter, was excised from the subcutaneous tissue. Both children have remained well ever since.

The histological features were similar in the 2 cases, showing sharply defined cellular lobules approximated to muscle in 1 case but not invading between individual fibres. The cells were moderately uniform in size and polygonal with occasional mitotic figures. Thin-walled capillary channels and large blood-filled spaces were prominent and a suggestion of perivascular arrangement was noted in some places.

A diagnosis of haemangiopericytoma was considered in these cases while some features suggested a relationship to non-chromaffin paraganglioma. The presence of haemosiderin with lymphocytic or plasma cell infiltration together with some spindle-cell areas was reminiscent of a Kaposi nodule in the tumour of the forearm. KAUFFMAN and STOUT (1960) applied the term haemangiopericytoma to 31 tumours of childhood from the newborn period up to 13 years.

## REFERENCES


ANDERSON, W. A. D.: Pathology 6th ed., St. Louis: C. V. Mosby, 1971, p. 1087

APOSTOL, J. V., FRAZELL, E. L.: Cancer 18, 869 (1965)

BALSAVER, A. M., BUTLER, J. J., MARTIN, R. G.: Cancer 20, 1607 (1967)

CASSADY, J. R., SAGERMAN, R. H., TRETTER, P., ELLSWORTH, R. M.: Radiology 91, 116 (1968)

CONTE, P. J., SAGERMAN, R. H.: New Eng. J. Med. 284, 92 (1971)

COPELAND, M. M., GESCHICKTER, C. F.: Ann. Surg. 129, 724 (1949)

CORTES, E. P., HOLLAND, J. F., WANG, J. J., GLIDEWELL, O.: Proc. Am. Soc. Clin. Onc. 15, 170 (1974)

CORTES, E. P., HOLLAND, J. F., WANG, J. J., SINKS, L. F.: The Colston Papers No. 24. Bone - Certain Aspects of Neoplasia. PRICE, C.H.G., ROSS, F. G. M. (eds.). London: Butterworths, 1973, p. 265

CROCKER, D. W., STOUT, A. P.: Cancer 12, 1123 (1959)

CUNNINGHAM, M. D., KING, F. H.: Amer. J. Dis. Child. 124, 401 (1972)

DAHLIN, D. C.: The Colston Papers No. 24. Bone - Certain Aspects of Neoplasia. PRICE, C. H. G., ROSS, F. G. M. (eds.). London: Butterworths, 1973, p. 207

DEHNER, L. P., ENZINGER, F. M., FONT, R. L.: Cancer 30, 160 (1972)

DIAS, L. de S., FROST, H. M.: Cancer 33, 1075 (1974)

DONALDSON, S. S., CASTRO, J. R., WILBUR, J. R., JESSE, R. H. Jr.: Cancer 31, 26 (1973)

ENNEKING, W. F., MARSH, B.: The Colston Papers No. 24. Bone - Certain Aspects of Neoplasia. PRICE, C. H. G., ROSS, F. G. M. (eds.). London: Butterworths, 1973, p. 431

ENTERLINE, H. T., HORN, R. C. Jr.: Amer. J. Clin. Path. 29, 356 (1958)

GOTTLIEB, J. A., BAKER, L. H., QUAGHANA, J. M., LUCE, J. K., WHITECAR, J.P. Jr., SINKOVICS, J. G., RIVKIN, S. E., BROWNLEE, R., FREI, E.III: Cancer 30, 1632 (1972)

HERSCH, E. M., GUTTERMAN, J. U., MAVLIGIT, G. M.: Cancer Treatment Reviews 1, 65 (1974)

HEYN, R., HOLLAND, R.: Proc. Amer. Assoc. for Cancer Research Abstracts 11, 36 (1970)

HOLTON, C. P., CHAPMAN, K. E., LACKEY, R. W., HATCH, E. I., BAUM, E. S., FARARA, B. E.: Cancer 32, 1310 (1973)

HORN, R. C. Jr., ENTERLINE, H. T.: Cancer 11, 181 (1958)

JAFFÉ, H. L., LICHTENSTEIN, L.: Amer. J. Path. 18, 205 (1942)

JAFFE, N., FARBER, S., TRAGGIS, D., GEISER, C., KIN, B. S., DAS, L., FRAUENBERGER, G., DJERASSI, I., CASSADY, J. R.: Cancer 31, 1367 (1973)

JEFFREE, G. M., PRICE, C. H. G., SISSONS, H. A.: Brit. J. Cancer 32 (I), 87 (1975)

JENSEN, A. R., MARTIN, L. W., LONGINO, L. A.: J. Ped. 51, 566 (1957)

JONES, I. S., REESE, A. B., KROUT, J.: Trans. Am. Oph. Soc. 63, 223 (1965)

KAUFFMAN, S. L., STOUT, A. P.: Cancer 13, 695 (1960)

LAWRENCE, W. Jr., JEGGE, G., FOOTE, F. W. Jr.: Cancer 17, 361 (1964)

LEE, E. S.: The Colston Papers No. 24. Bone - Certain Aspects of Neoplasia. PRICE, C. H. G., ROSS, F. G. M. (eds.). London: Butterworths, 1973, p. 163

LEE, E. S., MACKENZIE, D. H.: Brit. J. Surg. 51, 252 (1964)

MacCOMB, W. S.: Amer. J. Surg. 106, 754 (1963)

McKENZIE, A. W., INNES, F. L. F., RACK, J. M., BREATHNACH, A. S., GROSS, M.: Brit. J. Derm. 83, 446 (1970)

MACKENZIE, D. H.: The differential diagnosis of fibroblastic disorders. Oxford: Blackwell Scientific Publications 1970

MARCOVE, R. C., MIKÉ V., HUVOS, A. G., SOUTHAM, C. M., LEVIN, A. G.: The Colston Papers No. 24. Bone - Certain Aspects of Neoplasia. PRICE, C. H. G., ROSS, F. G. M. (eds.). London: Butterworths, 1973, p. 313

MARTINI, N., HUVOS, A. G., MIKÉ, V., MARCOVE, R. C., BEATTIE, E. J. Jr.: Ann. Thor. Surg. 12, 271 (1971)

MAURER, H.M., J. Ped. Surg. 10, 977 (1975)

MEHREGAN, A. H., NABAI, H., MATTHEWS, J. E.: Arch. Derm. 106, 375 (1972)

MILLER, T. R., NICHOLSON, J. T.: Cancer 27, 524 (1971)

MOORE, M.: J. Bone and Joint Surg. 53-B, 13 (1971)

MOORE, M., WITHEROW, P. J., PRICE, C. H. G., CLOUGH, S. A.: Int. J. Cancer 12, 428 (1973)

MOORE, O., GROSSI, C.: Cancer 12, 69 (1959)

NEWTON, K. A.: The Colston Papers No. 24. Bone - Certain Aspects of Neoplasia. PRICE, C. H. G., ROSS, F. G. M. (eds.). London: Butterworths, 1973, p. 307

OHNO, T.: Cancer 27, 549 (1971)

PATTON, R. B., HORN, R. C. Jr.: Surgery 52, 572 (1962)

PRATT, C. B., HUSTU, H. O., SHANKS, E.: Proc. Amer. Ass. Cancer Res. 15, 19 (1974)

PRICE, C. H. G.: The Colston Papers No. 24. Bone - Certain Aspects of Neoplasia. PRICE, C. H. G., ROSS, F. G. M. (eds.). London: Butterworths, 1973, p. 177

PRICE, C. H. G.: Personal communication (1974)

PRICE, C. H. G., ZHUBER, K., SELZER-KUNTSCHIK, M., SELZER, M., WILLERT H. G., GROH, P., MATEJOVSKY, Z., KEYL, W.: J. Bone and Joint Surg. 57 B, 341 (1975)

RIOPELLE, J. L., THÉRIAULT, J. P.: Ann. d'Anat. Path. 1, 88 (1956)

ROSEN, G., TAN, C., EXELBY, P., BEATTIE, E. J. Jr., MURPHY, M. L.: Proc. Amer. Ass. Cancer Res. 15, 172 (1974)

ROSEN, G., TAN, C., SUWANSERIKUL, S., MURPHY, M.L.: Proc. Amer. Ass. Cancer Res. 14, 95 (1973)

SCHIFF, M.: Laryngoscope 61, 981 (1959)

STOBBE, G. D., DARGEON, H. W.: Cancer 3, 826 (1950)

STOUT, A. P.: Ann. Surg. 123, 447 (1946)

STOUT, A. P.: Cancer 7, 953 (1954)

STOUT, A. P.: Cancer 15, 1028 (1962)

SUTOW, W. W., SULLIVAN, M. P., FERNBACH, D. J.: Proc. Amer. Ass. Cancer Res. 15, 20 (1974)

TRIFAUD, A., MEARY, R.: Pronostic et traitement des sarcomas ostéogéniques. Paris: Masson, 1972, p. 123

WILBUR, J. E., SUTOW, W. W., SULLIVAN, M. P.: Paper read before American Pediatric Society and Society for Pediatric Research, Atlantic City (1971)

WILLIS, R. A.: The pathology of the tumours of children. London: Oliver and Boyd, 1962, p. 131

# Chapter 10
# Renal Tumours

There were 87 renal tumours included in the Manchester Children's Tumour Registry from 1954 to 1968 (Table 1).

Table 1. Renal Tumours 1954 - 1968 (assessed 1972)

| Type | Alive | Dead | Total |
|---|---|---|---|
| Wilms' tumours (including polycystic nephroblastoma) | 26 | 56 | 82 |
| Mesoblastic nephromas | 1 | 1 | 2 |
| Carcinomas | 1 | 1 | 2 |
| Angiosarcoma | 0 | 1 | 1 |
| | 28 | 59 | 87 |

## WILMS' TUMOUR

The Wilms' tumour (nephroblastoma) was first described a century ago by EBERTH (1872). In a review of early literature on the subject WILLIS (1962) pointed out that there were many excellent descriptions of this neoplasm prior to the account by WILMS (1899). EBERTH used the term "myoma sarcomatodes renum" and ever since then pathologists have been struck by the fact that this tumour contained elements (especially striped muscle) which were foreign to normal kidney. WILMS considered that this was due to the presence of mixed foci of myotome, nephrotome and sclerotome in the developing kidney. Other writers, notably MUUS (1899) and NICHOLSON (1931) were unable to accept this view and the controversy is reviewed by WILLIS (1958). Although it is practically impossible to be certain of the cells of origin, the most reasonable explanation of the diversity of tissues is that advocated by MUUS who considered that the neoplasm is derived from embryonic cells capable of differentiating not only into renal elements but also into connective tissue and muscle.

Not only because it has been recognised for so many years, but also because there is practically never any difficulty in its histological diagnosis, the numerical importance of the Wilms' tumour has sometimes been over-emphasised. The 82 children with this neoplasm - 41 boys and 41 girls - represent 7% of all non-leukaemic cases included in the Register. This is slightly lower than the proportion reported by BODIAN and RIGBY (1964) who state that 11% of 1167 children with non-leukaemic tumours treated at the Hospital for Sick Children, Great Ormond Street, London, had Wilms' tumours. Obviously, it is not so common as its prominence in text books would suggest.

## Aetiological Factors

The existence of clusters of Wilms' tumours in certain families and the association of this neoplasm with aniridia, renal malformations and congenital overgrowth of part of the body were discussed in Chapter 2. Unlike retinoblastoma, the familial nature of Wilms' tumours has been obscured in the past by the high mortality of the disease. However, the reports by BROWN et al. (1972) and KAUFMAN et al. (1973) leave little room for doubt that this tumour may occur in siblings and in several generations of certain families. Presumably with improved treatment the number of such families will increase.

## Site

All the Manchester cases were renal in origin - 38 were in the right kidney, 41 in the left kidney, and 3 were bilateral. THOMPSON et al. (1973) describe 2 children with extrarenal Wilms' tumours and quote reports of 3 other cases in the literature. The ectopic tumours arose in the mediastinum (1 case), near a normal kidney (1 case), near the isthmus of a horseshoe kidney (1 case), and in the inguinal region (2 cases). The possibility of a primary Wilms' tumour arising in the inguinal region calls into question reports of metastases occurring in the spermatic cord.

## Macroscopic Appearance

The Wilms' tumour induces little fibrous reaction and is usually white, soft and friable. Cysts may occur and areas of necrosis are common. Since it lies deeply in the abdomen it has commonly grown to a very large size before it is diagnosed. In the Manchester series the tumours

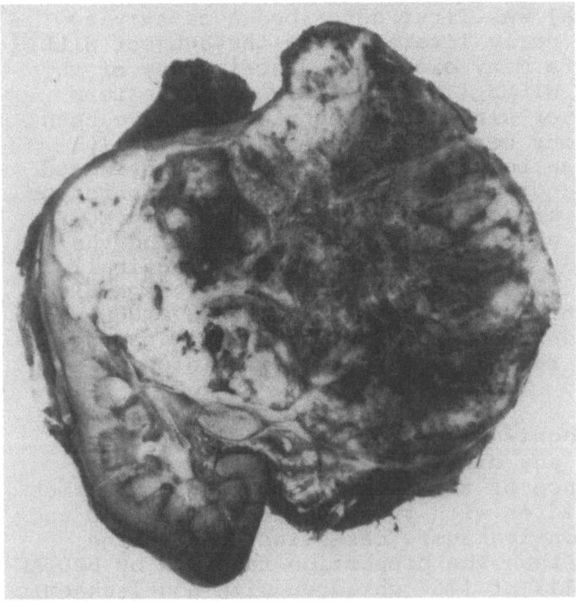

*Fig. 1. Wilms' tumour showing white fleshy tissue with areas of haemorrhage*

removed before irradiation measured between 5 and 18 cm in their long axis - the average being 12 cm . The highest recorded weight was 1500 g. The effect on the kidney depends on the site of the tumour. If it arises near the surface of the kidney it will expand extrarenally and the organ will be displaced rather than distorted. If it arises in the pelvis it tends to grow down the ureter. Usually, however, it expands the renal parenchyma and the kidney becomes stretched over the surface of the tumour. The covering of the neoplasm may be very thin and easily torn during removal, and when this happens, the soft tumour tissue oozes out.

## Microscopic Appearance

The varied histological picture seen in a Wilms' tumour is in keeping with the concept that it arises from embryonic tissue not definitely committed to one mode of differentiation. The rounded or polygonal hyperchromatic cells with stellate myxomatous tissue are reminiscent of the embryonic (rhabdo) sarcoma. Striated muscle fibres are seen in varying stages of development from pleomorphic cells with eosinophilic cytoplasm to more mature forms. In addition, occasional giant cells with bizarre nuclei may be present and are probably differentiating towards muscle cells. In general, the striated muscle appears to be more mature in Wilms' tumours than in embryonic sarcomas - perhaps this is due to the fact that at the time of diagnosis, Wilms' tumours are usually larger, and therefore older, than embryonic sarcomas. Mature striped muscle is most prominent in irradiated Wilms' tumours. The most characteristic histological features of the Wilms' tumour is the presence of tubules which were seen in two-thirds of the Manchester cases. There is considerable variation in the degree of tubule formation not only in different tumours, but in various parts of the same tumour (Figs. 5 - 7). The tubular differentiation is represented by a rosette appearance, by occasional poorly formed tubules without basement membranes blending with the surrounding structures or by numerous tubules

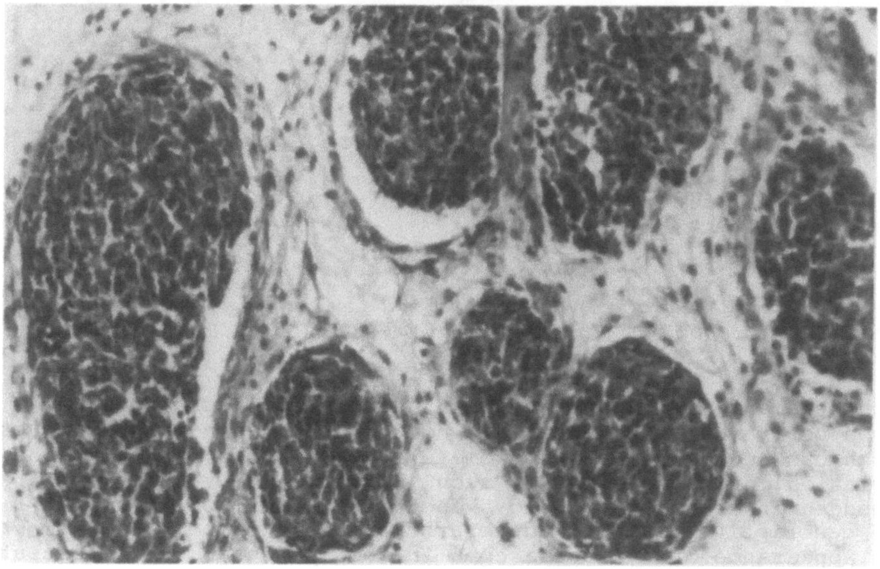

*Fig. 2. Wilms' tumour with islands of undifferentiated cells separated by loose mesenchyme (H. & E. X 250)*

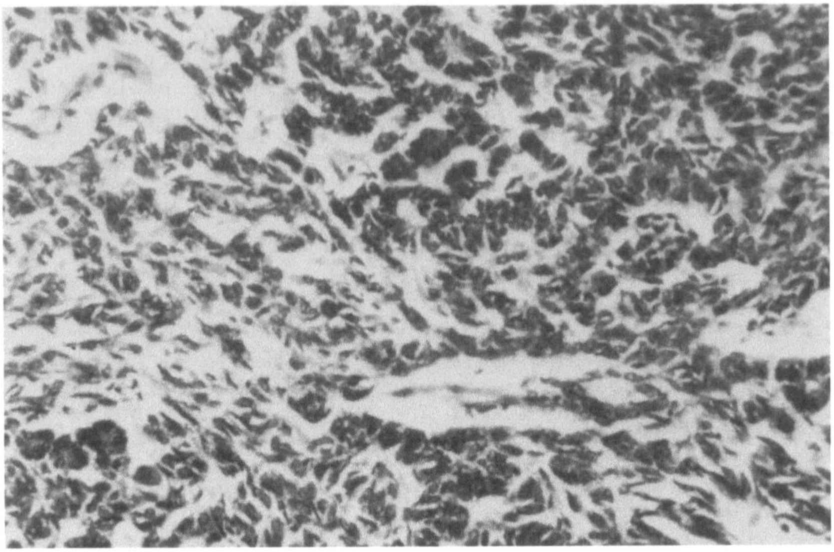

*Fig. 3. Anaplastic Wilms' tumour with polygonal cells showing little evidence of differentiation (H. & E. X 250)*

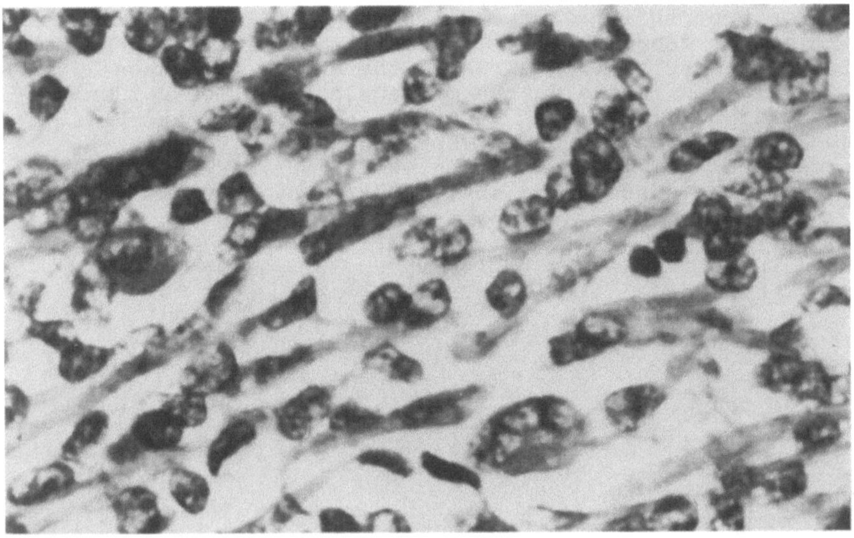

*Fig. 4. Wilms' tumour (non-irradiated) with polygonal cells and muscle fibres, some showing faint striation (H. & E. X 625)*

with basement membranes giving an adenosarcomatous appearance. Sometimes perivascular rosettes are noted. Other adenomatous structures which can be recognised as glomeruli are, in contrast with the tubular formation, only occasionally seen (Fig. 8). The tubules are frequently embedded in areas of spindle-shaped mesenchymal cells giving rise to the descriptive title of adenosarcoma. These spindle cells may have the appearance of a fibrosarcoma in some parts and differentiation into fibrous tissue elements was encountered in about one quarter of the Manchester tumours. Cartilage and bone which has been found by other authors in Wilms' tumours was not seen in the present series.

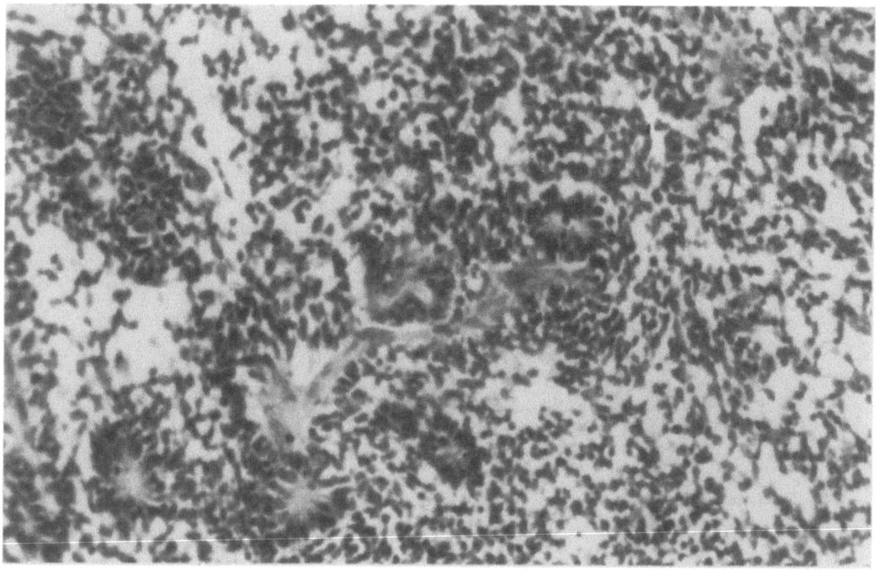

*Fig. 5. Wilms' tumour with early tubule formation (H.&E. X 250)*

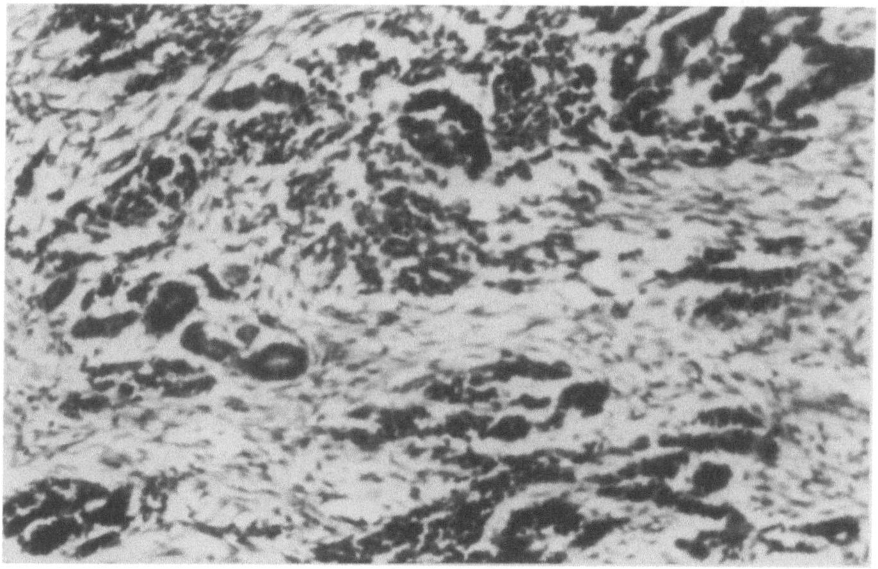

*Fig. 6. Wilms' tumour with more abundant tubules separated by spindle-celled mesenchyme (H. & E. X 250)*

The histological diagnosis of nephroblastoma is not difficult in the great majority of the tumours. In a few neoplasms, however, differentiating features are minimal and a diffuse arrangement of polygonal cells is noted with scanty pleomorphic spindle cells and occasional large cells which suggests muscle origin. Calcification is rarely encountered.

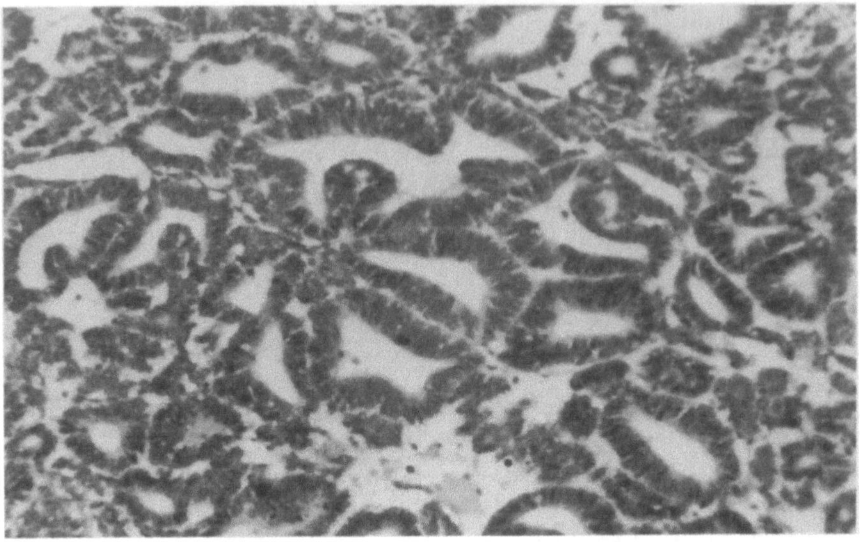

*Fig. 7. Wilms' tumour with extensive tubular differentiation (H. & E. X 250)*

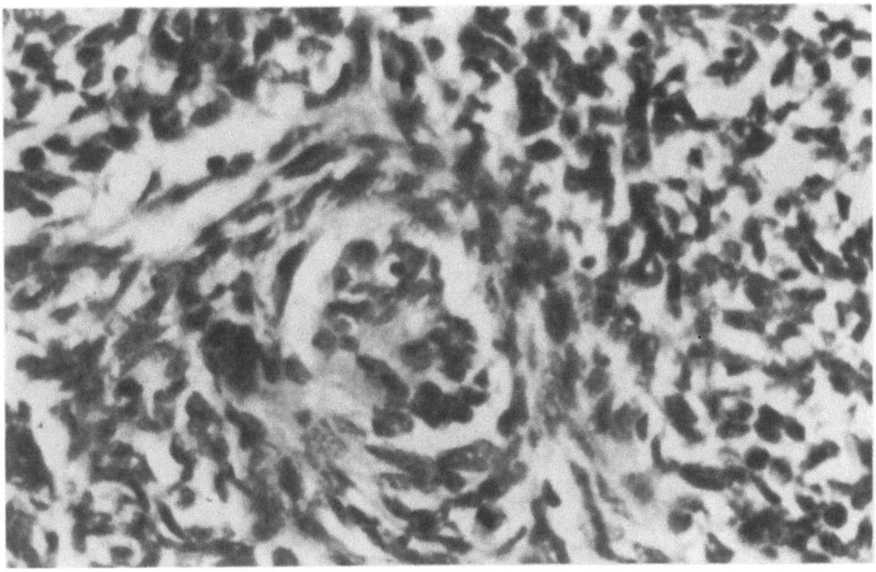

*Fig. 8. Wilms' tumour showing glomerular structure (H.&E.X500)*

A number of studies have been carried out in an attempt to relate the histological appearance to the prognosis in nephroblastoma. HARDWICK and STOWENS (1961) devised a classification in which each tumour was rated on the basis of its resemblance to the normal or developing kidney and survival was found to be better in the cases where more differentiated elements predominated. BODIAN and RIGBY (1964) divided the tumours into 7 groups based on reniform, tubular, papillary, and various types of mesenchymal and blastemal appearance. Better prognosis was seen in the tubular and papillary subtypes. Tubular structures were not regarded by TINAZTEPE (1973) as a favourable feature, although the presence of glomerular structures was a good prognostic finding. JEREB and SANDSTEDT (1973) placed the tumours in 3 groups, i. e. highly differentiated with glomerular and tubular structures, tubules but no glomeruli, and poorly differentiated. There was 75%, 25%, and 19% survival in the 3 groups, respectively. PEREZ et al. (1973) found a higher cure rate in differentiated than in undifferentiated tumours, although the degree of differentiation did not appear to be significant and the best results were seen in the small atypical group with leiomyomatous, myxomatous or haemangiomatous features.

The Wilms' tumours in the Registry during the 15 year period under review were studied by LAWLER et al. (1975). Out of 75 cases, eight could not be classified due to insufficient material or bilateral tumours in different histological groups. The remaining 67 were assessed for the presence of tubules, glomerular structures, smooth and striated muscle, nests of blastema and differentiation of blastema. The only significant feature related to the prognosis was the tubular differentiation, not only as regards the presence or absence of tubules, but also as regards the degree of tubular differentiation. There was also close correlation between the histological tubular grading and the clinical stage of the patient.

The degree of epithelial differentiation appears to be important in assessing the prognosis in a Wilms' tumour. This may include the tubular features, cystic or papillary structures, and possibly the glomerular formation. In the Manchester material glomeruli were not found to be significant, and it may be noted that the tubules appear to be relatively radiosensitive whereas the glomeruli are less so. However, the numbers are small and further assessment is required in this field. Although the tumours from patients in whom hypertension was reported did not show any definite distinguishing features, glomerular structures were seen in 2 of the 4 such cases in the Register. Sympathetic nervous tissue as described by MASSON (1957) was not encountered.

## "Polycystic Nephroblastoma"

Pseudocysts due to local degeneration are often seen in Wilms' tumours. More rarely, true cysts, either macroscopic or microscopic, have been reported. BOGGS and KIMMELSTIEL (1956) describe a case under the title of benign multicystic nephroma and regarded multilocular cystic disease of the kidney as being a neoplastic condition related to Wilms' tumours. CHRIST (1967) reported a case in which he considered the cysts to be part of the tumour and used the term polycystic nephroblastoma.

One tumour in the Manchester series appears to come in the category of polycystic nephroblastoma.
CTR.85/55. Girl, aged 5 years, presented with abdominal pain, vomiting and a mass in the right loin. Laparotomy revealed a tumour of the lower pole of the kidney and nephrectomy was performed. The specimen consisted of a firm, white, lobulated tumour, 13 cm in diameter, with some haemorrhage and necrosis. Compressed, but otherwise normal kidney tissue, was medial to the tumour. No cysts were apparent on naked eye examination but microscopically many were seen. They were lined by flattened epithelium with areas of proliferation and papillary projections. Other parts of the tumour had the appearance of a tubular nephroblastoma and this gave some support to there being an association between cystic disease and nephroblastoma. Postoperative abdominal irradiation was given and the patient remains well 17 years later. This satisfactory outcome is in keeping with the suggestion that the polycystic nephroblastoma is a relatively benign condition.

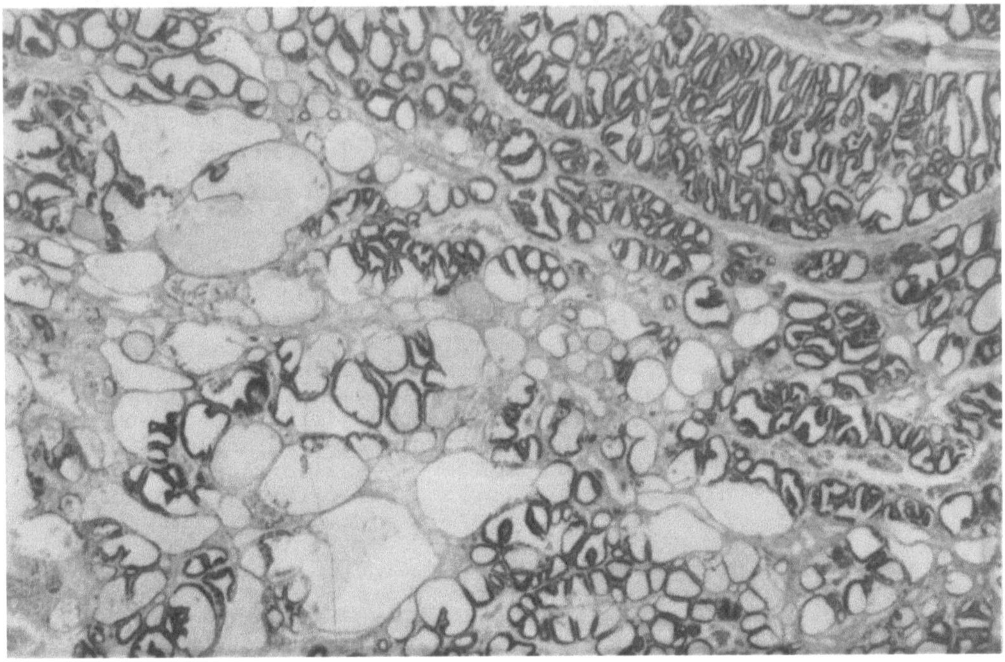

*Fig. 9a. Polycystic nephroblastoma showing cysts with flattened lining and epithelial proliferation in addition to nephroblastic tubular formation (H. & E. X 35)*

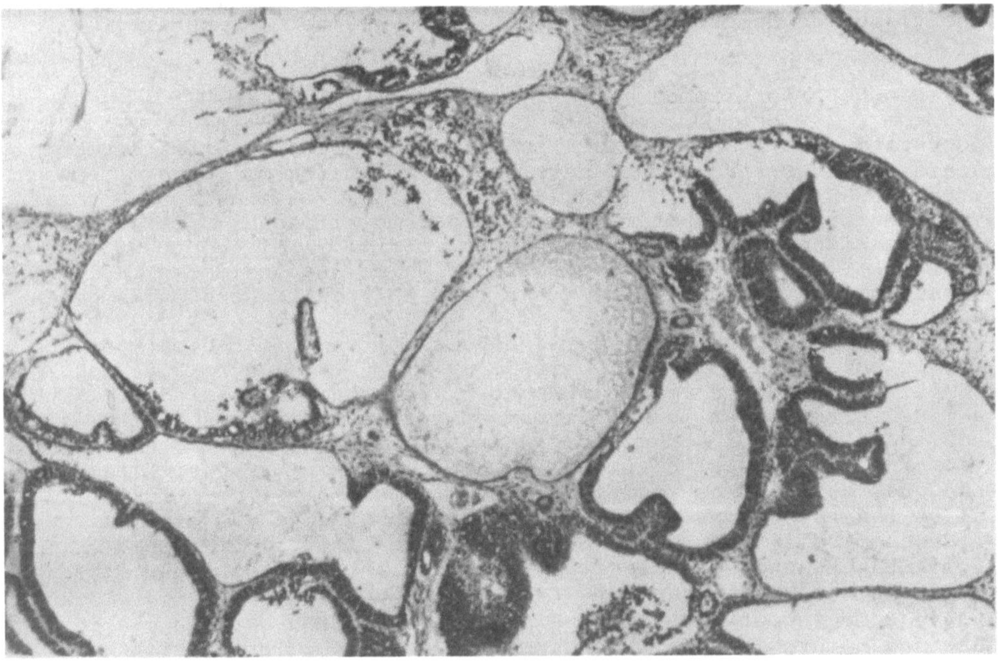

*Fig. 9b. Detail of cyst formation and epithelial proliferation (H. & E. X 125)*

Mode of Spread

Wilms' tumours spread to lymph nodes, lungs, liver and, rarely, bones. In the untreated cases described by earlier writers (LOUGHNANE, 1914; KRETSCHMER and HIBBS, 1931; BRADLEY and PINCOFFS, 1938) the unrestrained growth in the abdomen dominated the picture, but since the introduction of treatment by nephrectomy and abdominal X-rays, extra-abdominal metastases have increased in importance. In 50 of the 56 fatal Manchester cases tumour deposits were present at the time of death. The sites of these are shown in Table 2.

Table 2. Sites of recurrence and metastases in fatal Wilms' tumours

| | |
|---|---|
| Abdomen only | 16 |
| Lungs only | 15 |
| Lungs and abdomen | 12 |
| Lungs and bones | 3 |
| Abdomen and bones | 3 |
| Thorax (? lungs, ? mediastinum) | 1 |

In addition, 1 child who was treated for pulmonary metastases in 1962 still survives. Thus the frequency of spread to lungs and abdomen was approximately equal. Spread in the abdomen in the Manchester cases was most commonly to the local lymph nodes. Less commonly, growth along the renal vein was noted at operation. Rather surprisingly, hepatic deposits were observed in only 1 child at the initial operation and in none of the 7 children who had autopsies. It is likely, however, that spread to liver is more frequent than these figures would suggest since it was quite common in the reports of earlier writers. Possibly a number of the abdominal recurrences noted in Manchester children represented liver metastases but there was no positive evidence on this point. It is very difficult to be sure about the importance of direct spread

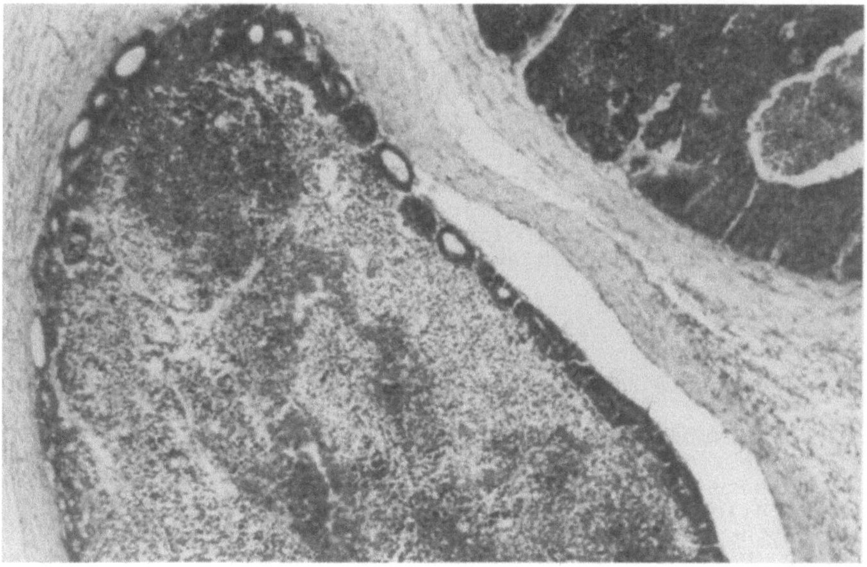

*Fig. 10. Wilms' tumour extending along renal vein (H.&E. X 60)*

of the Wilms' tumour in the peritoneal cavity. Mention has been made of the liability of the capsule to rupture with spill of the soft neoplastic contents and it is easy for the surgeon to liberate this tumour tissue into the peritoneal cavity at operation.

## CLINICAL MANIFESTATIONS

The age of diagnosis of the Manchester children is shown in Table 3.

Table 3. Wilms' tumours. Age at diagnosis

| Age (years) | 0- | 1- | 2- | 3- | 4- | 5- | 6- | 7- | 8- | 9- | 10- | 11- | 12- | 13- | 14- |
|---|---|---|---|---|---|---|---|---|---|---|---|---|---|---|---|
| No. of cases | 10 | 22 | 12 | 15 | 10 | 9 | 0 | 1 | 1 | 1 | 0 | 1 | 0 | 0 | 0 |

The age distribution of the Manchester cases is compared with that of 422 cases derived from the literature by COLLINS (1958) in Table 4. The fact that the age distribution in these two unrelated series is similar, suggests that it represents the true situation in Wilms' tumours.

### Symptoms and Signs

One child was brought to hospital with a history of injury and an abdominal mass was noted at routine examination. Preadmission symptoms and signs in the other 81 patients are shown in Table 5.

Although abdominal swelling was the commonest abnormality noted, it was surprising that a mass was felt by only twenty parents before medical advise was sought. By the time the children were admitted to hospital, however, the tumour could be felt in 75 of the 82 cases. Six of the 7 children in whom no mass could be felt after hospital admission had presented with haematuria.

Since the Wilms' tumour commonly manifests itself in a striking fashion either by an abdominal swelling or haematuria, it is not surprising that there is seldom any delay in diagnosis. Half of the Manchester children with this tumour were referred to hospital within a few days and 90% within 3 months of clinical onset. Once they were in hospital 80% were diagnosed straightaway.

### Hypertension

There was evidence of hypertension in 4 children in the Manchester series.
CTR.82/58. Boy, aged 4 months, admitted to hospital with a right-sided abdominal mass. He died 4 days later before treatment was started. The blood pressure was not taken. At autopsy the left ventricle was hypertrophied. Bilateral Wilms' tumours were found, the right 6 cm in diameter and the left 2 cm in diameter.
CTR.82/62. Boy, aged 2 years. Admitted to hospital with haematuria. B P 210/120. Diagnosed as acute nephritis for 3 weeks during which time the blood pressure gradually fell to 120/75. By then an abdominal

Table 4. Age distribution of Wilms' tumours (expressed as a percentage of total cases for each year)

| Age (years) | 0- | 1- | 2- | 3- | 4- | 5- | 6- | 7- | 8- | 9- | 10- | 11- | 12- | 13- | 14- |
|---|---|---|---|---|---|---|---|---|---|---|---|---|---|---|---|
| Manchester cases | 12.2 | 26.8 | 14.6 | 18.3 | 12.2 | 11.0 | 0 | 1.2 | 1.2 | 1.2 | 0 | 1.2 | 0 | 0 | 0 |
| COLLINS (1958) | 12.8 | 17.1 | 17.1 | 19.4 | 12.4 | 7.6 | 4.3 | 2.9 | 1.5 | 1.5 | 1 | 1 | 0.4 | 0.4 | 0.2 |

Table 5. Preadmission symptoms and signs of Wilms' tumours

| | |
|---|---|
| Abdominal swelling | 43 |
| Abdominal pains | 22 |
| Haematuria | 15 |
| Vomiting | 8 |
| Anorexia ) | |
| Lassitude ) | 7 |
| Loss of weight ) | |
| Fever | 3 |
| Scrotal swelling | 1 |
| Umbilical hernia | 1 |
| Swelling of feet | 1 |

mass had become palpable and a Wilms' tumour (6 cm in diameter) in the upper pole of the right kidney was removed. Five months after a course of X-rays the BP was 95/50, and 2 months later a lung metastasis was noted. The child died 7 months later.
CTR.16/63. Girl, aged 1 1/2 years, with left-sided abdominal mass. Preoperative BP 160/100. During nephrectomy systolic BP varied between 250 and 100. During the 3 days following operation BP 125/60, 160/100, 140/85. Postnephrectomy - abdominal X-rays (tumour dose 2500 rads was given in 39 days). No further BP readings taken. Four months after completion of the course of X-rays the child died. At autopsy there was left ventricular hypertrophy and the lungs showed evidence of heart failure. The right kidney showed a florid glomerulonephritis. There was no residual tumour.
CTR.18/63. Boy, aged 11 months. No preoperative blood pressure readings taken but during the removal of a large left-sided Wilms' tumour the systolic blood pressure varied between 250 and 130. During the 3 postoperative days BP 140/85, 180/?, 155/120. The child died on the fourth day. No autopsy.

It is likely that hypertension due to Wilms' tumour is more common than is suggested by the number observed in this series, since the blood pressures of these children were seldom recorded. SILVER (1947) reported hypertension in 7 out of 8 cases; BRADLEY and DRAKE (1949) in 10 out of 12 cases, and SUKAROCHANA et al. (1972) in 22 of 46 cases.

BRADLEY and PINCOFFS (1938) first noted the association of hypertension and Wilms' tumour and since then, cases have been reported by DANIEL (1939), KOONS and RUCH (1940), SMITH (1946), HUGHES et al. (1949) and COX and SMELLIE (1955-56). Several of these authors suggested that the hypertension is due to renal ischaemia caused by pressure of the tumour on the renal arteries. This theory received support from the careful investigation of SUKAROCHANA et al. who found raised renin levels in 5 children with renal tumours. They stated that the hypertension was relieved by nephrectomy and did not recur when metastases appeared. However, BRADLEY and DRAKE reported 1 child who had the primary removed and in whom severe hypertension was later noted in association with lung metastases.

Hypertension is a feature of Wilms' tumour which has been largely ignored by clinicians. Since death may be caused by this complication, the investigation of any case should always include blood pressure readings.

## Clinical Examination

The most constant feature is a renal swelling which can be felt deep in the flank using bimanual palpation with one hand behind in the lumbar region. The mass is usually irregular, solid, and feels heavy. Frequently it causes abdominal distension. The child may be pale but polycythaemia occasionally occurs (THURMAN et al., 1966). Metastases can rarely be detected by clinical examination. Right-sided tumours may distort and displace the liver so that it becomes clearly palpable and this may lead to diagnostic difficulty. The size and fixity of the mass and the degree to which it extends across the midline gives some guidance to the ease of surgical removal. The initial diagnosis depends on careful abdominal palpation and an awareness of the mode of presentation of the Wilms' tumour. Abdominal distension in infants demands serious consideration and Health Visitors and Child Welfare clinics have a part to play. However, excessive palpation must be avoided and there should be no delay in referring the child for diagnostic procedures and treatment.

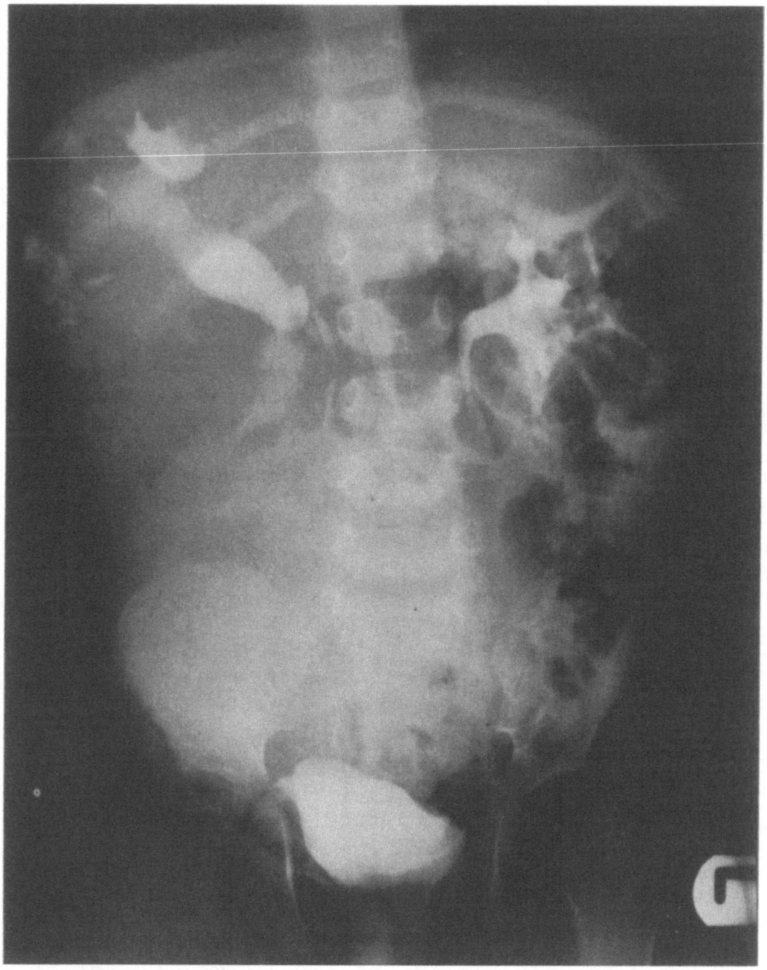

*Fig. 11. Intravenous pyelogram in case of right-sided Wilms' tumour. There is good dye excretion, with some delay in drainage from right renal pelvis which is distended and distorted and displaced upwards. In addition there is a relative opacity below the pelvis indicating presence of tumour lying in lower pole of kidney. Courtesy of Dr. F.P.A. CAPPS of Shrewsbury and Dr. J.R. MANN of Birmingham.*

Intravenous pyelography and chest X-rays must be undertaken immediately. Calcification is rarely seen in the tumour and does not have the diffuse stippled pattern seen in neuroblastoma. When it does occur it may form plaques round the periphery of the tumour. Typically, the affected kidney excretes dye and gross distortion of the pelvicalyceal pattern is obvious. The calyceal system is elongated and compressed, but occasionally, due to compression and obstruction, local or general dilatation is seen. Injection of the dye into the internal saphenous system allows the inferior vena cava to be outlined and may show displacement or obstruction of the vein, or invasion of the lumen by tumour. Apparent complete obstruction of the vein does not preclude successful excision of the tumour (McDONALD and HILLER, 1968). The opposite kidney must be meticulously examined because of the possibility of bilateral disease, and the association with developmental renal disorders must be remembered.

LALLI et al. (1966) recorded that intravenous pyelography failed to show any excretion on the affected side in 10% of cases. Therefore retrograde pyelography or aortography are occasionally needed. The latter is most useful in the further elucidation of the nature of an intrarenal mass. Displacement of the aorta and displacement and stretching of the intrarenal branches of the artery will be seen in many Wilms' tumours. The nephrographic phase shows displacement of the kidney substance by tumour which contains vessels with pools of dye beside them. Definite arteriovenous malformations are not seen.

A 24h urine specimen should have catecholamine estimations carried out to exclude neuroblastoma. Microscopy may show some excess of red cells or even malignant cells. However, in the majority the urine is normal and of no value in excluding Wilms' tumour.

Percutaneous needle biopsy is contraindicated because of the risk of rupturing the tumour capsule and of producing spread of malignant cells. Ultrasonic scanning has only a small place in the investigation. Its main value is to separate cystic masses, such as hydronephrosis, from solid tumours. Occasionally Wilms' tumours may be cystic.

Although an abdominal mass is palpable in the vast majority of children with Wilms' tumours when medical advice is sought, there are a few patients who may present before the tumour is large enough to be felt. Nearly all such children have haematuria as the initial symptom. No tumour could be felt on hospital admission in 7 of the 82 Manchester cases.

## Differential Diagnosis

The Wilms' tumour has to be distinguished from other tumours in the renal area and non-neoplastic conditions of the kidney.

1. Neuroblastomas often show a stippled calcification on X-rays. On the pyelogram or arteriogram the kidney and pelvic outline will be seen to be relatively unchanged but will be displaced as a whole, usually downwards and outwards. Metastases will generally occur in bones and may be palpable in the skull. Bone metastases are rare in Wilms' tumours. The detection of increased catecholamine excretion in the urine has helped in the diagnosis of neuroblastoma.

2. A teratoma may also show calcification on X-rays but this is usually more differentiated and bone and tooth formation may be seen.

3. Leukaemic infiltration of the kidneys may render them palpable. The diagnosis will be obvious from a blood or marrow examination.

4. Benign renal lesions which present as masses include hydronephrosis, cystic kidneys, pyonephrosis, renal cysts and renal vein thrombosis. Multicystic kidneys usually fail to show any dye excretion on the descending pyelogram and arteriography reveals severe attenuation of the blood supply. It might be thought that pyonephrosis could be diagnosed by the presence of the signs of sepsis but real confusion may occur and the possibility of a Wilms' tumour must always be kept in mind. In pyonephrosis, arteriography does not show a tumour but there is a diffuse abnormal vascular pattern. Arteriography will also differentiate the renal cyst in which the branches of the renal artery are distorted and stretched over an avascular filling defect. In thrombosis of a renal vessel the history is characteristic and X-rays show a large non-functioning kidney with a poor vascular pattern.

In summary, therefore, the following investigations should be carried out on all children suspected of having Wilms' tumours:

Full blood count, including platelets
Chest X-ray
Skeletal survey
Urinalysis including catecholamine estimation
Blood electrolytes and urea
Intravenous pyelogram and cavogram
Liver scan
Blood pressure estimation

## TREATMENT

If a child is suspected of having a Wilms' tumour, there should be no delay in carrying out the necessary investigations and initiating treatment. However, since the prognosis depends so much on the familiarity of the surgeons, radiotherapists and chemotherapists with this tumour, it is always worthwhile to transfer the child immediately to a centre specialising in paediatric oncology. Once the patient is admitted to such a centre it should always be possible to start treatment within 24h. Surgery, irradiation and chemotherapy all have a place in the treatment of Wilms' tumour. Since it has not been possible to cure a large number of cases by one method alone, it is generally agreed that combined treatment is necessary. Up to recent years the therapeutic history of this disease was one of gradual evolution rather than of controlled clinical trials and although various authors (GROSS and NEUHAUSER, 1950; LATTIMER et al., 1959; WILLIAMS, 1964; HOWARD, 1965) reported improvement in survival rates over the years, it was difficult to be certain which alterations in technique had been responsible. The better results might well have been due to the growth in experience of those who were particularly interested in this disease and not solely to radical alterations in therapy. The setting up of a number of collaborative clinical trials has now provided a more scientific basis for therapy evaluation in Wilms' tumours.

### Clinical Staging

As with other tumours, the clinical staging of Wilms' tumours has permitted more accurate therapy evaluation. Although other methods have been suggested (FLEMING and JOHNSON, 1970), the following system of staging is at present applied in Britain to all patients included in the Medical Research Council Clinical Trial (1970). This system is essentially the same as that used in the American National Wilms' tumour study (D'ANGIO, 1972).

Stage I. A well encapsulated tumour which is entirely removed at operation. Spillage of the tumour does not take place at operation and there is no involvement of the para-aortic nodes on biopsy.

Stage II. There is extension of the tumour beyond capsule either by:

1. Local infiltration or
2. Extension along the renal vein or
3. Involvement of the para-aortic glands

but where the surgeon believes total removal of macroscopic disease is possible.

Stage III. There is extension of the tumour beyond the capsule and:

1. Spillage of tumour at operation or
2. Tumour is felt to have been left at time of operation or
3. There are peritoneal metastases.

Stage IV. Spread to liver, lungs, bones or brain found at diagnosis.

Stage V. Tumours of both kidneys.

Most protocols stipulate initial surgical removal of the main tumour mass together with paraoperative chemotherapy as it is logical to assume that at the time of tumour manipulation dissemination may occur. Radiation should begin as soon after surgery as possible and certainly within 2 weeks. In most large American centres irradiation is begun within 72h of operation and this may be a significant factor in the high cure rate in some of their reported series.

## Surgery

In most cases surgical excision should be undertaken as soon as possible. All the preparations for bold and radical surgery should be made. The loin approach is inadequate and a liberal transperitoneal incision is necessary with early ligation of the renal pedicle. Some Wilms' tumours are enormous and can only be safely removed with minimal handling if a large incision has been made.

After the peritoneum is opened the abdominal cavity is examined for possible spread and the other kidney for a second tumour. The peritoneum lateral to the colon on the side of the tumour is then incised and the colon is displaced medially until the inferior vena cava and aorta are plainly seen. The renal pedicle must be isolated and tied as soon as possible. However, in some cases the distortion of the renal veins and arteries is so marked that it is advisable to see the aorta and opposite renal vessels before dividing those to the affected side. The dissection on the medial side must then be taken upwards and downwards clearing tissue in front of the major vessels with due regard

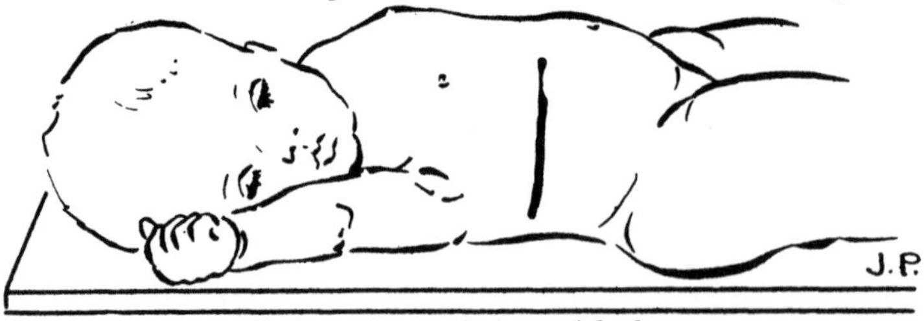


*Fig. 12a. Incision for right-sided tumour*

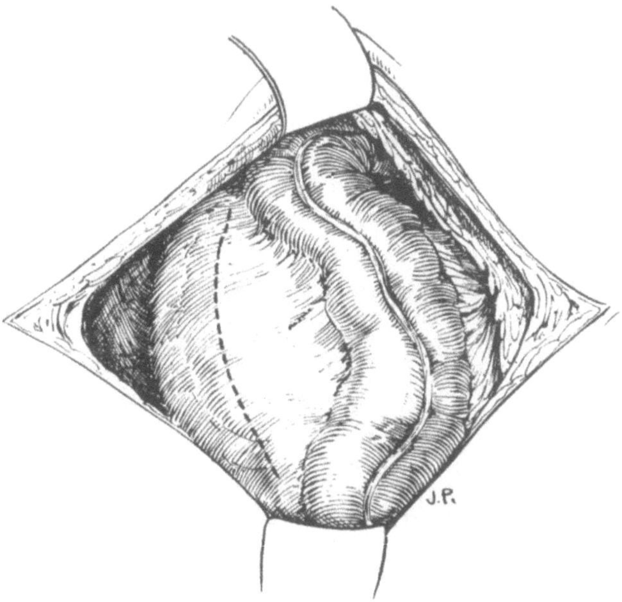


*Fig. 12b. Peritoneal incision to right of ascending colon*

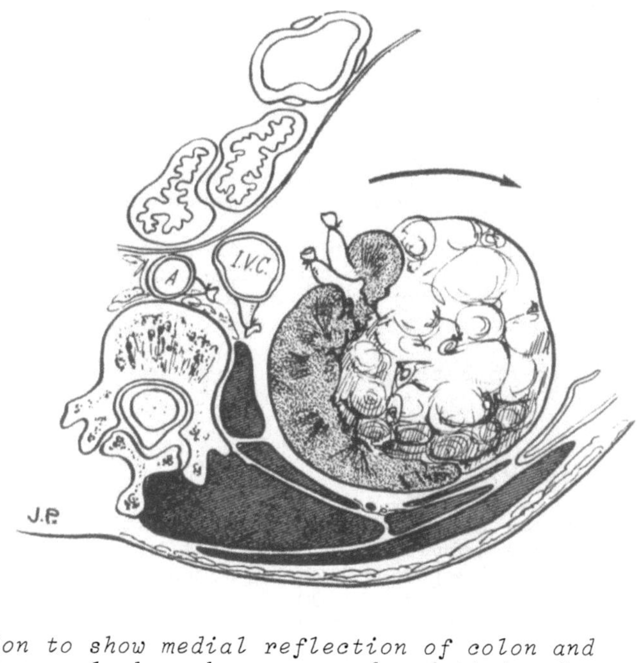


*Fig. 12c. Transverse section to show medial reflection of colon and parietal peritoneum. Renal vessels have been exposed and tied and kidney and tumour are being rolled laterally*

to the superior mesenteric artery. The kidney is removed with any overlying peritoneum, as much fat as possible and generally with the adrenal gland. Any adherent structures such as the diaphragm or tail of the pancreas must be excised as far as necessary. The advisability of dissection of the para-aortic glands is debatable. Obviously involved glands must be removed, but other glands should be left because of dangers inherent in prolonging the operation and because of possible diminution of tumour resistance.

Extension of the tumour into the large veins must be pursued if at all practicable. Lengths of vena cava have been resected and replaced. Suitable vascular clamps must always be available and it is advisable to mobilise the large vessels early if there seems any danger of tearing them.

Surgery may be necessary to resect localised secondaries. This is rarely necessary in the abdomen but single liver metastases can be successfully removed. The removal of lung deposits either during the initial phase of treatment or later is sometimes required.

## Chemotherapy

Actinomycin D (FARBER, 1966; BURGERT and GLIDEWELL, 1967; WOLFF et al., 1968) was the first drug shown to have any effect on Wilms' tumour, and it was soon clear that vincristine (SULLIVAN et al., 1967; VIETTI et al., 1970) was also active and perhaps even more efficacious in metastatic disease. Cyclophosphamide has a more limited effect. Recently, adriamycin has been shown to be active in significant numbers of patients resistant to the other agents (WANG et al., 1971).

Actinomycin D has usually been given in a dosage of 15 micrograms/kg/day for 5-day courses at 6 or 12 week intervals.

Vincristine sulphate is usually given in doses of 1.5 mg/m$^2$ weekly in pulses for 3 in every 12 weeks or at 14-day intervals over a prolonged period.

Cyclophosphamide may either be administered orally on a daily basis of 3 mg /kg or in a weekly intravenous high dose schedule 300-600 mg/m$^2$.

Adriamycin is also given in pulses, the dose most frequently used having been 20 to 30 mg/m$^2$ per day for 3 days every 7-14 days. However, there is now evidence accruing that a larger dose 60 - 75 mg/m$^2$ given once every 21 days may be more satisfactory.

In most co-operative studies chemotherapy schedules have been continued for 1 - 2 years.

## Radiotherapy

It has been common practice to give some form of abdominal irradiation after nephrectomy in most cases of Wilms' tumour. Until the last few years in Manchester the whole abdomen was treated using parallel opposed fields either at 300 KV or latterly at 4 MeV. The femoral heads were shielded throughout and the opposite kidney after 2000 rads. The dose used was 2500 rads at 300 KV in 5 weeks or 3000 rads at 4 MeV in the same time. More recently the volume irradiated in Manchester has been reduced so that, now, treatment is given from the diaphragm to the sacral promontory on the involved side and as far laterally as the kidney hilum on the opposite side leaving the remaining kidney out completely. The dose delivered midway between the two parallel opposed fields is 3000 rads in 4 weeks using 4 MeV irradiation. At present, if the whole abdomen has to be treated because there has been spread across the midline or down into the pelvis, the opposite kidney is

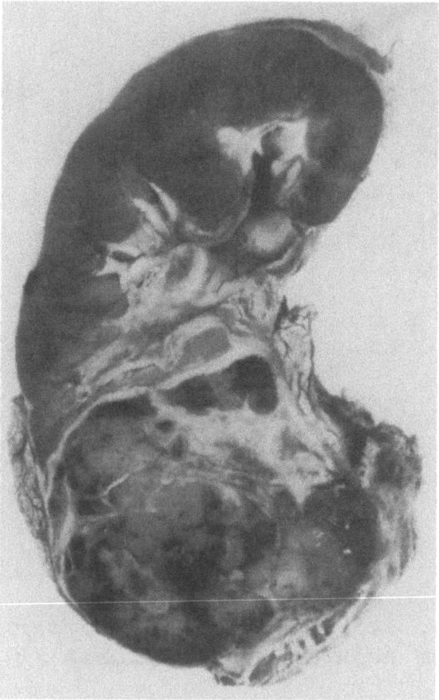

*Fig. 13. Wilms' tumour after irradiation*

shielded throughout from the back field and the dose should still be 3000 rads, which can be given in 4 weeks but is probably more safely given in 5 weeks.

Because it is important to cover all known disease with a margin, there is very little place for irradiating the kidney bed alone. The present policy in Manchester is to give the smaller volume treatment in Stage I

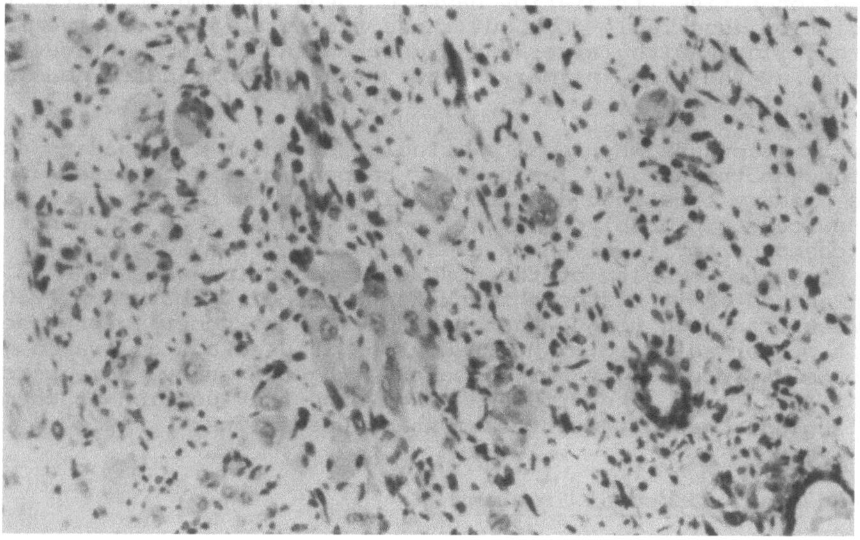

*Fig. 14a. Wilms' tumour after irradiation. There is extensive destruction and the surviving cells are largely muscle (H. & E. X 250)*

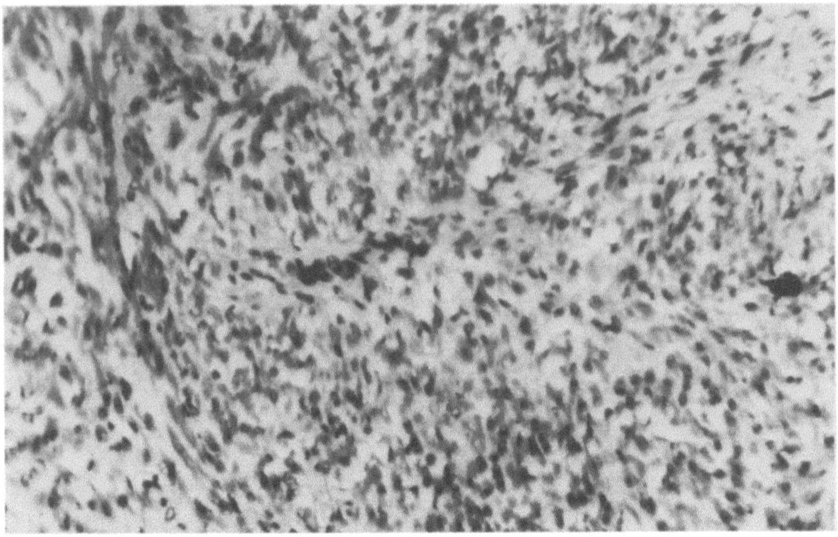

*Fig. 14b. Wilms' tumour after irradiation. The tissue consists of uniform regular muscle fibres (H. & E. X 250)*

and II cases, but to increase it, if necessary, in Stage III where the disease is more widespread. Possibly radiotherapy may not be needed in Stage I, but at present this is not certain and the American Group Trial may answer this question. It would obviously be a great advantage, particularly in very young children, if both radiotherapy and chemotherapy could be omitted since this would reduce the possibility of the late effects of treatment.

In other centres - notably the Institut Gustav Roussy - both pre- and postoperative radiotherapy have been advocated and have given results equal to those reported in most other series. In Manchester the results of preoperative irradiation have not been as good as postoperative irradiation (see Table 10), but those receiving preoperative irradiation were children with larger and almost certainly later stage tumours for which, at the time, primary surgery was not considered feasible (PEARSON et al., 1964).

Chest metastases may require irradiation which is nowadays usually given with chemotherapy. If, as usually happens, the metastases appear after the primary treatment and are multiple, radiotherapy alone can produce a few cures (probably about 14%), and it does seem that this is improved if chemotherapy is given in addition. However, the giving of chemotherapy poses the problem of the dose of irradiation which can be tolerated. In Manchester it has been found that without chemotherapy 2500 rads in 4 weeks can be given to the whole chest, the humeral epiphyses being left out or shielded. 4 MeV radiation is used and allowance made for lack of absorption in air in calculating the tumour dose percentage from each field. The problems concerning the addition of chemotherapy will be discussed under treatment complications.

## Management of Special Problems

Stage IV Disease. The commonest form of Stage IV disease involves metastatic spread to the lungs only and at the time of presentation the primary tumour within the kidney is often operable. In these circumstances removal is indicated with paraoperative chemotherapy of combination type. In most instances there will be a response to this treatment with complete regression of pulmonary disease. Removal of the primary should be followed by the appropriate radiotherapy which, if the chest is not likely to be immediately troublesome or has responded well to chemotherapy, can consist first of abdominal irradiation as appropriate for the clinical staging. Irradiation to the chest can be given later on when the child has recovered from the abdominal therapy or, alternatively, if there has been a good response to chemotherapy, the chest irradiation can be delayed in case there is a recurrence. If there is need to proceed immediately to irradiation to the chest and abdomen at the same time, a dose of 2000 rads in 5 weeks using 4 MeV radiation can be delivered or the dose can be correspondingly higher in a longer time. Alternatively, the chest can be treated alone and the abdominal irradiation left until a later date. In some cases the primary tumour may be considered inoperable and in these circumstances the initial use of chemotherapy will usually reduce tumour size and render it operable, thus leaving a much smaller volume of malignant tissue for subsequent irradiation therapy. It may even be decided to rely entirely on chemotherapy for the treatment of a small primary.

## Single or Localised Pulmonary Metastases

Single or multiple metastases confined to one lobe may be removed surgically. The problem of whether or not they represent the only radiologically discernible evidence of otherwise widespread disease must, however, be faced and it is advisable for continued chemotherapy to be given if surgery is carried out.

Bone metastases. The incidence of bone metastases is low and little experience has been gained in their management. There is evidence that they are more resistant to chemotherapy and radiotherapy than lung and liver metastases. Although radiotherapy will not cure these children, it can be used in short courses for pain relief. For spine and long bones the doses employed have been 1250 rads at 300 KV or 1500 rads at 4 MeV in a single treatment or 2500 rads (300 KV) or 3000 rads (4 MeV) in 4 days.

Stage V disease. The children with bilateral Wilms' tumours pose an interesting but by no means hopeless problem (RAGAB et al., 1972). The incidence of bilateral tumours varies considerably in different reported series (LEEN and WILLIAMS, 1971). It seems that lung metastases seldom occur in this group and that the behaviour of the tumour is atypical. Treatment requires to be individualised dependent on the findings at diagnosis. In a proportion of cases total resection of both tumours is possible with retention of good renal function. The majority of cases fall into a category where removal of the larger tumour and kidney is necessary and where either resection is possible on the other side or where chemotherapy and radiation have to be used to control the residual disease. In some instances resection of tumour may be feasible after radiation and chemotherapy.

Bilateral nephrectomy and renal transplantation has been advocated but this should probably be reserved for cases not amenable to more conventional approach (DE LORIMER et al., 1968).

## Follow-up of Children Treated for Wilms' Tumours

The following investigations should be carried out:

Chest X-rays monthly for 6 months, then 3-monthly while chemotherapy is being continued and at least 6-monthly for 2 years thereafter.

| | |
|---|---|
| Liver scans ) <br> Liver function tests ) <br> Blood urea ) <br> Urinalysis ) | 3-monthly while chemotherapy is being continued |

## Complications of Treatment

The use of combined therapy has resulted not only in a higher survival rate in children with Wilms' tumours, but also in an increase in complications. It is, of course, very necessary to recognise the symptoms and signs of these complications and not to assume that any deterioration in the patient's condition is necessarily due to progress of the tumour.

### Liver Damage

In the past the development of abdominal distension and diarrhoea with associated anorexia during the course of radiation to the abdomen has been thought to be due to the effect of the treatment on the bowel. This plays some part but there is now definite evidence of hepatic damage shown by enlargement of the liver, deterioration in liver function tests, and in the more severe cases the development of ascites and even liver failure. Serial liver scans will show a pattern of damage often confined to the left lobe when the original Wilms' tumour was left-sided and radiation has not involved the right lobe of the liver. There is no doubt, however, that this syndrome is due to the combined effect of chemotherapy and radiation and is seen as frequently in Manchester with the use of vincristine as with actinomycin D. The majority of cases recover with appropriate management but there is a mortality in the children with severe liver failure. The histology shows degeneration and haemorrhage extending out from the centre of the lobule.

### Pneumonitis

When radiation was first given to both lungs, it was considered that fairly high doses would be tolerated. However, many patients developed both acute pneumonitis and later radiation fibrosis, which eventually led to heart failure and death. Children with acute pneumonitis have sudden onset of severe dyspnoea. They often become cyanosed and auscultation of the chest reveals fine râles throughout the lung fields. The patients are improved by being put in high oxygen concentrations and in the Manchester cases there has also been improvement with short courses of steroids in high doses. There is no evidence to suggest that antibiotics are helpful. In children who have had acute radiation pneumonitis the symptoms have recurred with subsequent chemotherapy although they are less severe.

Radiation pneumonitis and fibrosis do not seem to occur at 4 MeV radiation with a dose of 2500 rads in 4 weeks provided that, in calculating the depth doses, allowance is made for the less absorption in air. If, however, chemotherapy is used as well, there may be some enhancement or similar effect from the drugs which makes this dose unsafe. Indeed, in Manchester acute radiation pneumonitis has been seen at 2000 rads in 5 weeks when both actinomycin D and vincristine have been used. In the case of actinomycin D the symptoms recurred with a subsequent course of the drug. If chemotherapy is to be used, the dose to the lungs should be less than the previously stated safe dose and probably 1500 rads in 3 - 4 weeks would be safe. It is to be hoped that radiobiological experiments may indicate the maximum radiation dose which is safe, and yet is also most likely to be of curative value.

## Growth Retardation

Bone growth within a field radiated to the doses used in the treatment of Wilms' tumour will usually be less than normal. In the Manchester cases the only abnormalities have been shortening of the length of the spine and narrowing of the pelvis and, if chest irradiation had to be given, the whole bone structure of the chest has been smaller than usual. The changes have always been symmetrical, but scoliosis can occur if only half the spine is irradiated and therefore it is better that any treatment should include both sides of the vertebrae, as whilst a short symmetrical spine is acceptable, a scoliosis should be avoided if possible.

In addition to bone growth retardation, the abdominal wall tends to show an absence of subcutaneous fat. This resembles the situation seen in the neck following irradiation usually for lymph node neoplasms such as Hodgkin's disease.

## Sexual Development

Because of the Manchester policy of treating the whole abdomen, the ovaries in girls have been irradiated and a variety of situations has occurred in sexual development, which has by no means been predictable. The dose to the ovaries has in the main been at the same biological dose for many years. There have been three groups:

1. No development at all, meaning no secondary sex characteristics and no menstruation.

2. Secondary sex characteristics have developed but menstruation has not occurred.

3. Both secondary sex characteristics and menstruation have occurred and the girl may appear normal, but although 1 girl has twice been pregnant, she has been unable to carry to term and has lost each baby at about 5 months. There has been no detectable cause for this and the 1 foetus studied had no apparent abnormality. As she has an additional congenital deformity of the left arm, there may in her case be other genetic reasons for the problem. Most of the others in this group have been sterile.

The boys on the other hand appear to have developed normally. The problems which the girls have, due to little or no ovarian function, can be helped by replacement hormones, so that secondary sex characteristics develop, and monthly withdrawal bleeding can occur.

## Second Primaries

Although a second primary in a child cured of a Wilms' tumour has been reported (REGELSON et al., 1965), none has occurred amonst the 82 Manchester children with this disease in the Register. However, 1 Liverpool child irradiated in Manchester for bilateral Wilms' tumours (RICKHAM, 1957), developed acute myelomonocytic leukaemia 12 years later.

## Inherited Disease

With increased survival due to better treatment, the fact that Wilms' tumour, like the retinoblastoma, may sometimes be inherited, has become apparent (BROWN et al., 1972; KAUFMAN et al., 1973). Therefore the children of those who have been cured of Wilms' tumours should be considered to have an increased risk of developing this neoplasm.

## PROGNOSIS

### Manchester Cases 1954 - 1968

When a recurrence of a Wilms' tumour develops it is nearly always obvious within 2 years of the onset of the clinical disease (GROSS and NEUHAUSER, 1950). Fifty-one (90%) of the 56 fatal cases in the Manchester series died within 2 years of the original diagnosis and 54 (94%) died within 3 years. The other 2 children died 5 years after the initial treatment. The proportion surviving at various times after diagnosis is shown in Figure 15. The overall 3 years survival rate of the Manchester cases was 34%. COLLINS (1958) put forward a method of estimating the period after treatment during which recurrence might happen. The period of risk was defined as the age of the child plus 9 months - i. e. the actual time from conception to the date when the tumour was diagnosed. Assuming that each tumour had a constant growth rate, even one viable cell left after treatment would produce a mass the size of the original tumour within this period of risk. COLLINS tested this hypothesis in a review of 422 cases derived from the literature and found only 2 children in whom recurrence was deferred beyond the period of risk. However, this does not prove the

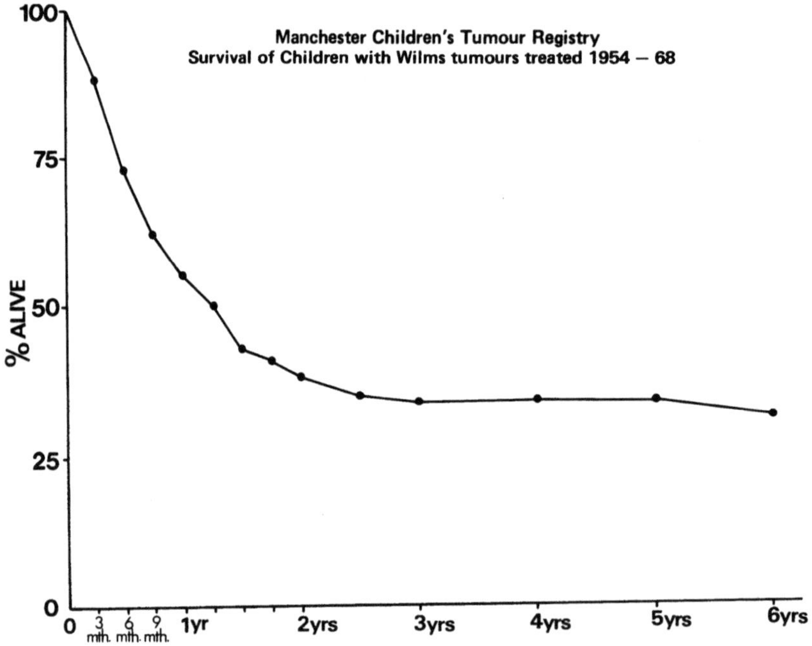


*Fig. 15. Survival times of children with Wilms' tumours 1954 - 1968*

value of the method. To do this, it would be necessary to demonstrate that Wilms' tumours in older children grew more slowly than in younger ones and COLLINS brought forward no evidence that this is so. Over half of the children with Wilms' tumours are over 3 years old so that the period at risk calculated by COLLINS' method is usually much longer than that which is found to be necessary in practice. PLATT and LINDEN (1964) found that the 2 year survival rate was almost identical with COLLINS' variable period survival rate.

Table 6. Wilms' tumours. Sex of patient

| | Alive (3 years) | Dead | Total |
|---|---|---|---|
| Boys | 13 | 28 | 41 |
| Girls | 15 | 26 | 41 |

Sex. This did not appear to have any influence on prognosis (Table 6).

## Site

The prognosis of right-sided tumours appeared to be somewhat better than those in the left side, but this was not statistically significant (Table 7).

Table 7. Wilms' tumours. Site of tumour

| | Alive (3 years) | Dead | Total |
|---|---|---|---|
| Right | 16 | 22 | 38 |
| Left | 12 | 29 | 41 |
| Bilateral | 0 | 3 | 3 |

## Haematuria

Five of the 15 children presenting with haematuria are still alive, giving a survival rate of 33%. Thus this sign did not appear to affect the outcome.

Table 8. Wilms' tumours 1954 - 1968. Effect of age on prognosis

| Age (years) | Survival rate (3 years) | | |
|---|---|---|---|
| 0- | $\frac{4}{10}$ | $\frac{11}{32}$ | (34%) |
| 1- | $\frac{7}{22}$ | | |
| Over 2 | $\frac{17}{50}$ | | (34%) |

## Age

In the first edition of this book it was reported that the prognosis in Manchester children was better in those under 2 years old and this agreed with the experience of GROSS and NEUHAUSER (1950) and WILLIAMS (1964). However, in the Manchester series from 1954 to 1968 age does not seem to have any influence on prognosis (Table 8).

## Clinical Stage

Accurate clinical staging of children with Wilms' tumours requires the cooperation of surgeons who understand the classification used. The fact that the Manchester children were operated upon in many hospitals by many different surgeons and that the operation notes were often inadequate meant that the accuracy of clinical staging could not always be guaranteed. However, it was possible to stage 69 of the 82 cases with reasonable certainty. In Table 9 it will be seen that there is a correlation between clinical stage and survival rate.

Table 9. Wilms' tumours. Clinical stage and survival rate

| Clinical stage | Survival rate (3 years) | |
|---|---|---|
| 1 | $\frac{12}{17}$ | (70%) |
| 2 | $\frac{4}{10}$ | (40%) |
| 3 | $\frac{6}{32}$ | (19%) |
| 4 | $\frac{0}{7}$ | (0%) |
| 5 | $\frac{0}{3}$ | (0%) |

## Treatment

The initial treatment given is shown in Table 10. Up to the end of 1968 the treatment policy in the Manchester area consisted mainly of initial nephrectomy followed by abdominal irradiation (without chemotherapy) and most of the survivors were treated in this way. However, this regime rarely succeeded when there was evidence of tumour spread

Table 10. Wilms' tumours. Effect of treatment

| | Alive (3 years) | Dead |
|---|---|---|
| Nephrectomy and XRT | 13 | 23 |
| XRT and nephrectomy | 5 | 11 |
| Actinomycin D, nephrectomy, and XRT | 10 | 9 |
| Nephrectomy alone, XRT alone, or no treatment | 0 | 11 |

- 8 of the 13 3-year survivors so treated had Stage I disease, 2 Stage II, 2 Stage III, and in 1 case the Stage was not known. The addition of actinomycin D resulted in 10 survivors, 4 of whom had had Stage I disease, 2 Stage II, and 4 Stage III.

## Centralisation

The overall survival rate of 34% of children with Wilms' tumours in the Manchester Region from 1954 to 1968 is not as good as the 47.3% survival at the Boston Children's Hospital from 1940 to 1947 (GROSS and NEUHAUSER, 1950) or the 50% survival at the Hospital for Sick Children, London, from 1952 to 1959 (WILLIAMS, 1964). Although it would be virtually impossible to determine how far these differences are real and how far they are due to case selection, there is no doubt that children with Wilms' tumours have the best chance of survival if they are treated in centres which have a special interest in paediatric oncology. In the Manchester Region between 1954 and 1968, 74 of the children with Wilms' tumours had some form of operative treatment which was carried out by 28 different surgeons, 17 of whom saw only 1 case during the 15 years under review. In these circumstances the surgeons could not have acquired the experience to have removed these tumours with the skill which this operation demands. Since 1964 an increasing proportion of these patients has been operated upon by two paediatric surgeons working in conjunction with a paediatric oncologist. Although the number of cases is not yet sufficient to be statistically significant, the difference in the results achieved by this central team compared with those of the general surgeons in the Region is striking (Table 11). The removal of a Wilms' tumour is a difficult procedure

Table 11. Wilms' tumours 1964 - 1969

| | Survival rate (3 years) |
|---|---|
| Operated upon by paediatric surgeons | 12/20 (60%) |
| General surgeons | 4/16 (25%) |

which should only be undertaken by those who have the opportunity to acquire experience in this operation. The radiotherapy requires the skill of those specialising in paediatric tumours and the patients can only benefit from the development of better chemotherapy if the drugs are given by paediatric oncologists who are treating children with cancer all the time. Clinicians who are not in a position to acquire these very specialised skills should not treat children with Wilms' tumours, but should refer them whenever possible to a children's cancer centre.

## MESOBLASTIC NEPHROMA

Although reports of non-malignant renal masses - variously described as leiomyomas or hamartomas - have appeared in the literature for many years, these lesions were regarded as rareties of little practical importance. However, KAY et al. (1966) drew attention to the fact that they may be large enough to present as palpable abdominal masses and therefore be confused with Wilms' tumours. The terms neonatal fibromatosis, fibroma, fibrosarcoma, leiomyosarcoma, fibrous and leiomyomatous hamartoma have been applied to this spindle-cell tumour. We are in favour of the name mesoblastic nephroma, to imply a relationship between this tumour and the nephroblastoma, with however unilateral growth of mesodermal elements.

Among the more recent cases in the Register which are not included in the period covered by this review there is a tumour showing features of nephroblastoma, mesoblastic nephroma and polycystic nephroblastoma. The tubules seen in the mesoblastic nephroma have been considered as either remnants from the existing kidney structure or as representing part of the tumour itself, and we favour the latter interpretation.

Two infants with this condition were included in the Register up to the end of 1968.
CTR.34/61. Boy, aged 3 months, presented with abdominal distension for 2 weeks. Laparotomy revealed a mass (16 x 14 x 8 cm ) confined to the left kidney, which was removed. Postoperative irradiation to the abdomen was given and the child remains well 15 years later.
CTR.2/64. Boy, who was noted to have an abdominal mass at the age of 10 days. Laparotomy revealed a lesion 8 x 6 x 5 cm in the left kidney. There was no extrarenal spread and the kidney was removed. The infant was then given actinomycin D, 30 μg daily for 10 days. Abdominal irradiation was started, but 3 days later the platelets had fallen to 70,000/cm, and the child died the following day. At autopsy there was no residual tumour, but a coliform septicaemia was found.

Connective tissue, smooth muscle and islands of cartilage have been reported in these tumours, although in the 2 Manchester cases seen up to 1968 the lesions were entirely fibromatous. The naked eye appearance is uniform pale grey, or yellow and fleshy and does not show the lobulation or necrosis of the Wilms' tumour. Haemorrhage is unusual but was noticed in a recent Manchester case. The mesoblastic nephroma is more

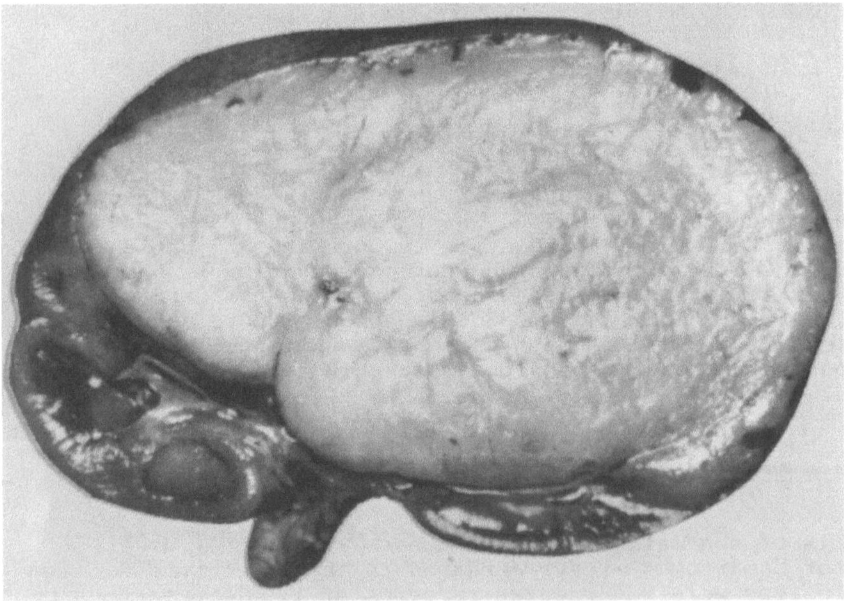

*Fig. 16. Mesoblastic nephroma. The structure is uniform and pale without lobulation or necrosis*

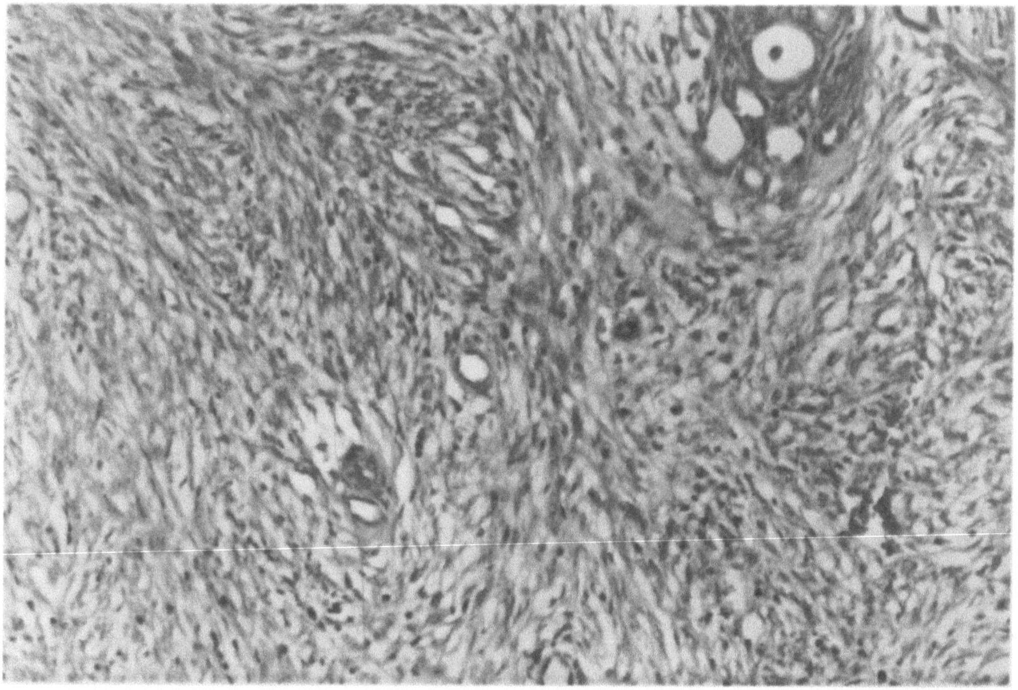

*Fig. 17. Mesoblastic nephroma showing fibroblastic proliferation. The nuclear chromatin is delicate and there are embedded renal tubules*

common in infants but recently a similar tumour was seen in a 10-year old girl.

Microscopically the absence of malignant epithelial and undifferentiated mesenchymal tissue distinguishes this condition from the Wilms' tumour. Embedded renal tubules may be present. It shows no tendency to form distant metastases, although local recurrence and extension are possible, so that in general irradiation or chemotherapy are neither necessary nor desirable. Indeed, since it usually occurs in infancy, the patients may die from marrow depression if actinomycin D is given. This happened in the case described by KAY et al. and in one of the Manchester children.

## RENAL CARCINOMAS

There were 2 Manchester children with renal carcinomas up to the end of 1968 - one had a clear cell carcinoma and the other a papillary tumour.

The child with the clear cell carcinoma was a girl (CTR.40/59) aged 4 years, who had a primary in the left kidney which was considered inoperable and was treated by irradiation. Three months later the tumour had spread to the mediastinum and cervical nodes from which a biopsy was taken. The abdominal mass did not respond to irradiation and the child died 2 months later. Since 1968 2 other Manchester children with clear cell carcinomas have been seen, one being shown in Figure 18.

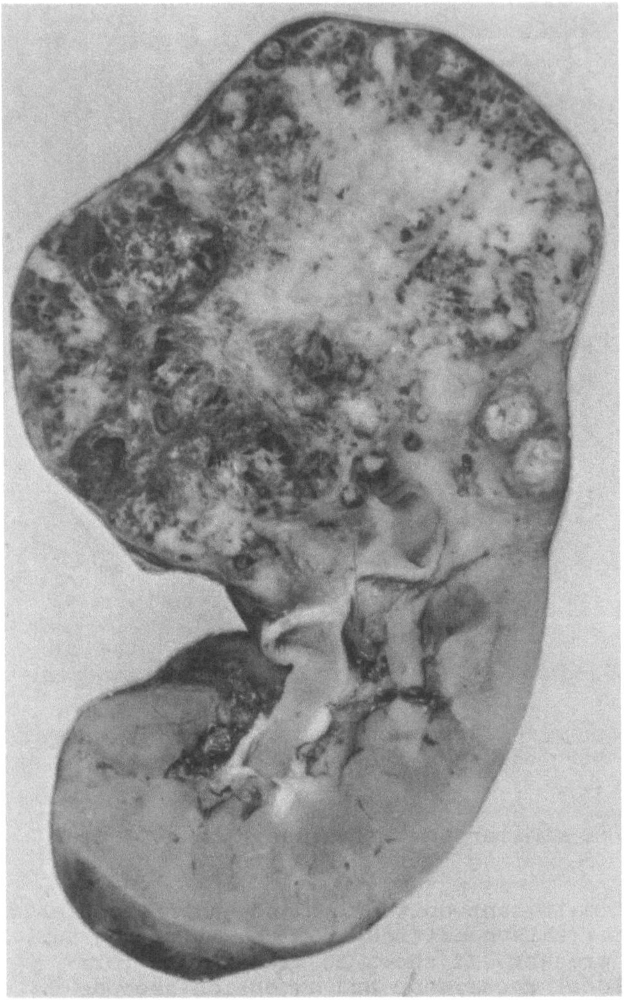

*Fig. 18. Renal carcinoma of predominantly clear cell type. The structure is more variegated than the nephroblastoma. Haemorrhage, necrosis, and cyst formation are prominent*

The child with the papillary carcinoma was a 9-year-old boy (CTR.108/68) who had an encapsulated tumour, 7 cm in diameter, in the cortex of the left kidney. Nephrectomy was performed, irradiation was given, and the patient remains well 4 years later.

According to PALMA et al. (1970), there are about 50 reports of renal carcinomas in children in the literature. DEHNER et al. (1970) collected records of 15 cases in children between 3 and 14 years old. These authors consider that those tumours with clear cells showing a mixed trabecular and tubular pattern have a better prognosis than those with papillary formation made up of granular cells.

The presentation and findings in renal carcinoma are similar to Wilms' tumour although there is a greater tendency to haematuria. In Manchester, treatment policy has been identical with that in Wilms' tumours ex-

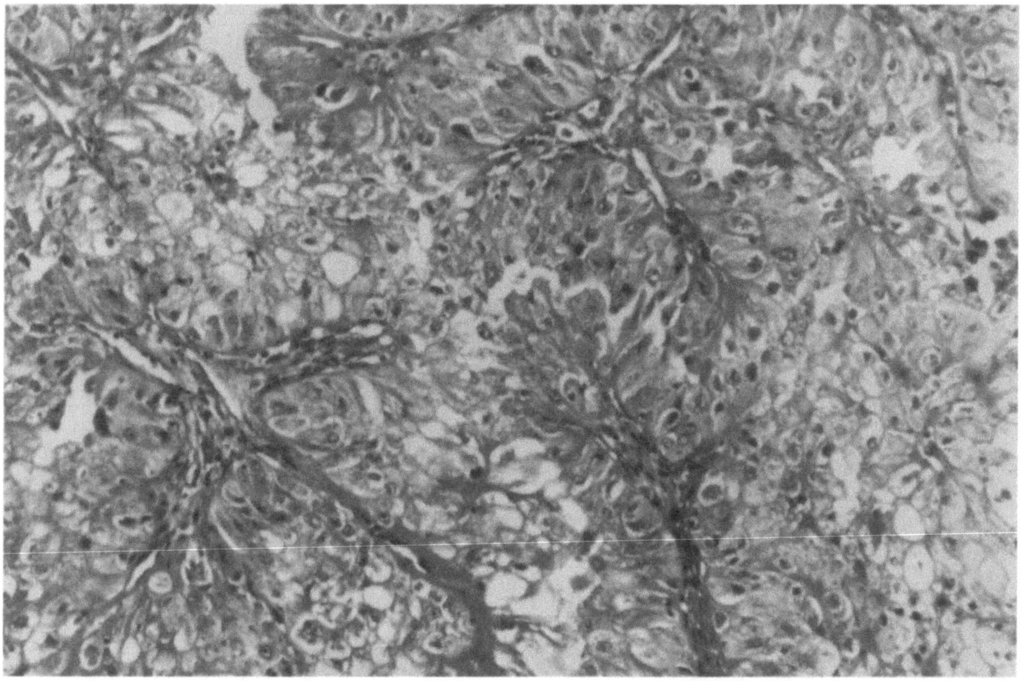

*Fig. 19. Renal carcinoma of predominantly clear cell type (H. & E. X 250)*

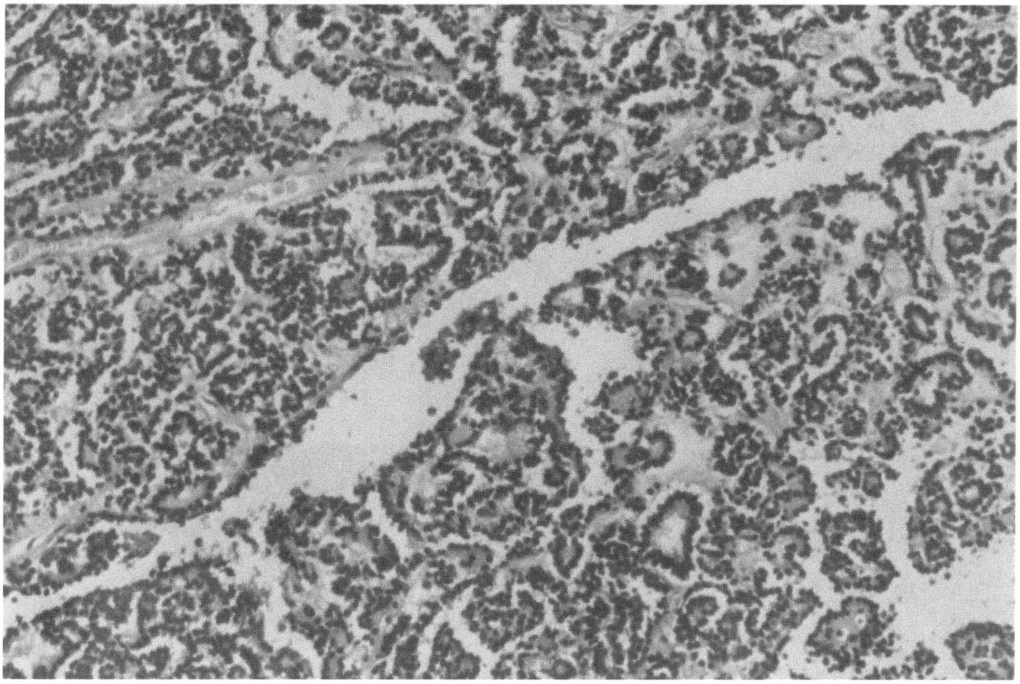

*Fig. 20. Renal carcinoma of papillary type (H. & E. X 125)*

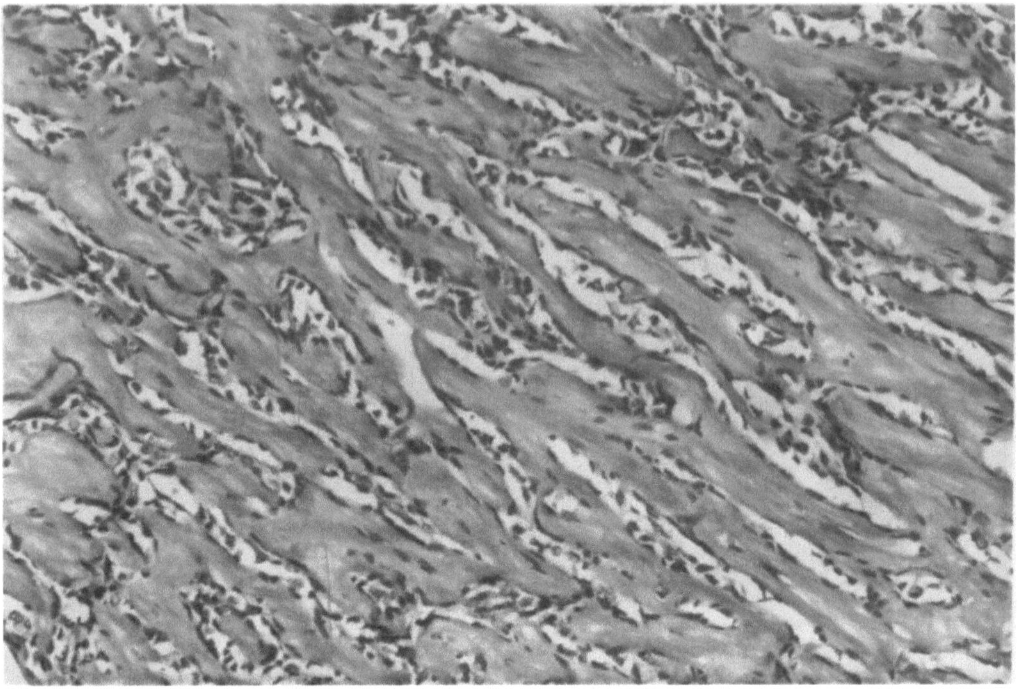

*Fig. 21a. Renal angiosarcoma showing blood-filled endothelial-lined channels separated by fibrous stroma (H. & E. X 125)*

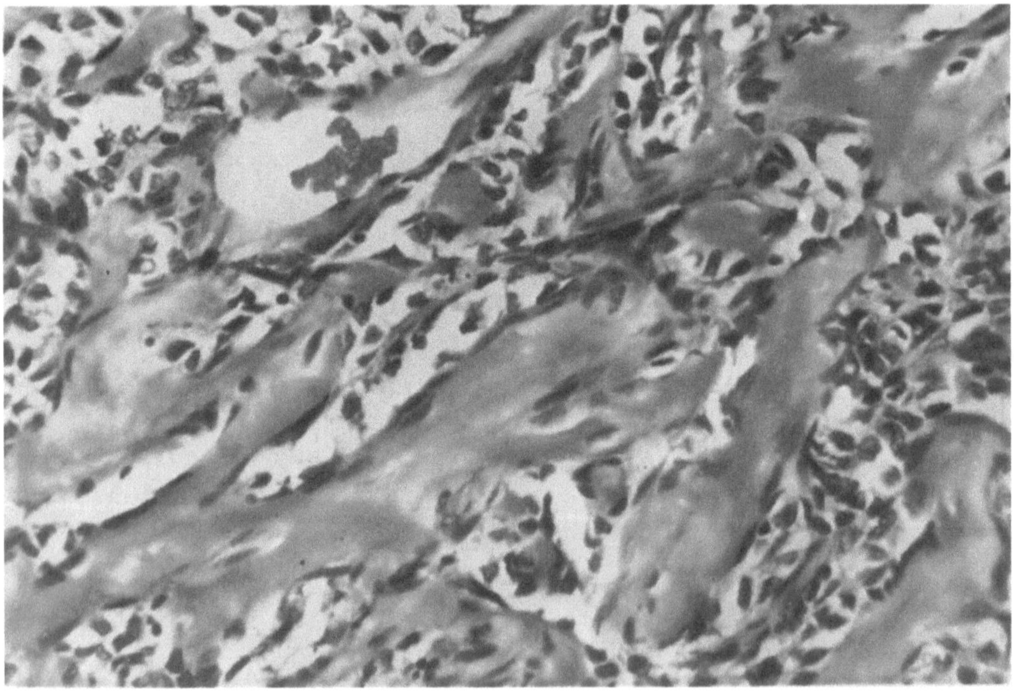

*Fig. 21b. Detail of vascular channels (H. & E. X 500)*

cept that, where indicated, second-look operations are undertaken after radiotherapy and chemotherapy.

## ANGIOSARCOMA OF THE KIDNEY

The one example of this tumour occurred in a 4-year-old boy (CTR.114/57), the son of a Jamaican father and a British mother. He had a tumour 11 cm in diameter in the left kidney with spread to the adjacent lymph nodes. Following removal of the primary mass, abdominal irradiation was given. A year later metastases occurred in the bones of the skull and later in the right femur and humerus. There was no evidence of lung metastases. The disease progressed slowly and the child died 4 1/2 years after diagnosis. There were no stigmata of tuberous sclerosis (GOLJI, 1961).

## REFERENCES


BOGGS, L. K., KIMMELSTIEL, P.: J. Urol. 76, 530 (1956)

BODIAN, M., RIGBY, C. C./ Tumours of the Kidney and Ureter. E. RICHES (ed.). London: Livingstone, 1964, Chap. 18

BRADLEY, J. E., DRAKE, M. E.: J. Ped. 35, 710 (1949)

BRADLEY, J. E., PINCOFFS, M.: Ann. Int. Med. 11, 1613 (1938)

BROWN, W. T., PURANIK, S. R., ALTMAN, D. H., HARDIN, H. C.: Surgery 72, 756 (1972)

BURGERT, E. O., GLIDEWELL, O.: J. Amer. Med. Ass. 199, 464 (1967)

CHRIST, M. L.: J. Urol. 98, 570 (1967)

CÔLLINS, V. P.: Cancer 11, 89 (1958)

COX, P. J. N., SMELLIE, J. M.: Gt. Ormond St. J. 10, 112 (1955-56)

D'ANGIO, G. J.: Cancer 30, 1528 (1972)

DANIEL, W. E.: Sth. Med. J. 32, 1014 (1939)

DEHNER, L. P., LEESTMA, J. E., PRICE, E. B.: J. Ped. 76, 358 (1970)

DE LORIMER, A. A., BELZER, F. O., KORINTZ, S. L., KUSHNER, J. H.: Surgery 64, 850 (1968)

EBERTH, C. J.: Virchow's Arch. 55, 518 (1872)

FARBER, S.: J. A. M. A. 198, 826 (1966)

FLEMING, I. D., JOHNSON, W. W.: Cancer 26, 660 (1970)

GOLJI, H.: J. Urol. 85, 919 (1961)

GROSS, R. E., NEUHAUSER, E. B. D.: Ped. 6, 843 (1950)

HARDWICK, D. F., STOWENS, D.: J. Urol. 85, 903 (1961)

HOWARD, R.: Arch. Dis. Childh. 40, 200 (1965)

HUGHES, J. G., ROSENBLUM, H., HORN, L. G.: Ped. 3, 201 (1949)

JEREB, B., SANDSTEDT, B.: Cancer 31, 1423 (1973)

KAUFMAN, R. L., VIETTI, T. J., WAHNER, C. I.: Lancet 1, 43 (1973)

KAY, S., PRATT, C. B., SALZBURG, A. M.: Cancer 19, 1825 (1966)

KOONS, K. M., RUCH, M. K.: J. A. M. A. 115, 1097 (1940)

KRETSCHMER, H. L., HIBBS, W. G.: Surg. Gyn. and Obst. 52, 1 (1931)

LALLI, A. F., ÅHSTRÖM, L., ERICSSON, N. O., RUDHE, H.: Radiology 87, 495 (1966)

LATTIMER, J. K., MELICOW, M. M., USON, A. C.: N. Y. St. J. Med. 59, 415 (1959)

LAWLER, W., MARSDEN, H. B., PALMER, M. K.: Cancer 36, 1122 (1975)

LEEN, R. L. S., WILLIAMS, I. G.: Cancer 28, 802 (1971)

LOUGHNANE, F. M.: Brit. J. Surg. 2, 77 (1914)

MASSON, P.: Ann. d'Anat. path. 2, 133 (1957)

McDONALD, P., HILLER, H. G.: Clin. Radiol. 19, 1 (1968)

Medical Research Council. The working party in embryonal tumours in childhood and protocol for a therapeutic trial in the treatment of nephroblastomas, 1970

MUUS, N. R.: Virchow's Arch. 155, 401 (1899)

NICHOLSON, G. W.: J. Path. Bact. 34, 711 (1931)

PALMA, L. D., KENNY, G. M., MURPHY, G. P.: Cancer 26, 1321 (1970)

PEARSON, D., DUNCAN, W. B., POINTON, R. C. S.: Brit. J. Radiol. 37, 154 (1964)

PEREZ, C. A., KAIMAN, H. A., KEITH, J., MILL, W. B., VIETTI, T. J., POWERS, W. E.: Cancer 32, 609 (1973)

PLATT, B. B., LINDEN, G.: Cancer 17, 1573 (1964)

RAGAB, A. H., VIETTI, T. J., CRIST, W., PEREZ, C., McALLISTER, W.: Cancer 30, 983 (1972)

REGELSON, W., BROSS, I. D. J., HANANIAN, J., NIGOGOSYAN, G.: Cancer 18, 58 (1965)

RICKHAM, P. P.: Brit. J. Surg. 44, 492 (1957)

SILVER, H. K.: J. Ped. 31, 643 (1947)

SMITH, N. J.: Arch. Path. 42, 549 (1946)

SUKAROCHANA, K., TOLENTINO, W., KIESEWETTER, W. B.: J. Ped. Surg. 7, 573 (1972)

SULLIVAN, M. P., SUTOW, W. W., CANGIR, A., TAYLOR, G.: J. A. M. A. 202, 381 (1967)

THOMPSON, M. R., EMMANUEL, I. G., CAMPBELL, M. S., ZACHARY, R. B.: J. Ped. Surg. 8, 37 (1973)

THURMAN, W. G., GRABSTALD, H., LIEBERMAN, P. H.: Arch. intern. Med. 117, 280 (1966)

TINAZTEPE, K.: Turkish Journ. of Ped. 15, 82 (1973)

VIETTI, T. J., SULLIVAN, M. P., HAGGARD, M. E., HOLCOMB, T. M., BERRY, D. H.: Cancer 25, 12 (1970)

WANG, J. J., CORTES, E., SINKS, L. F., HOLLAND, J. F.: Cancer 28, 837 (1971)

WILLIAMS, D. I.: Tumours of the Kidney and Ureter. E. RICHES (ed.). London: Livingstone, 1964, Chaps. 19, 22

WILLIS, R. A.: The Borderland of Embryology and Pathology. London: Butterworth, 1958, p. 422

WILLIS, R. A.: The Pathology of the Tumours of Children. London: Oliver and Boyd, 1962, p. 51

WILMS, M.: Die Mischgeschwülste der Niere, Leipzig, 1899. A. Georgi

WOLFF, J. A., KRIVIT, W., NEWTON, W. A. Jr., D'ANGIO, G. J.: New Eng. J. Med. 279, 290 (1968)

# Chapter 11
# Teratomas and Other Genital Tumours

N. J. BROWN and F. A. LANGLEY

The tumours reviewed in this chapter are derived from three sources - the Manchester Children's Tumour Registry, the Manchester Ovarian Tumour Registry, and the Testicular Tumour Panel. The Ovarian Tumour Registry covers 26 years, 1947-1973, but its purpose is mainly diagnostic and the "follow-up" is not as comprehensive as that of the Children's Tumour Registry. The tumours included from the Ovarian Registry are from girls of 16 years and less in age. The various types of tumour included in the Manchester registers are listed in Table 1, those of the Testicular Tumour Panel in Table 5. The frequency with which a particular tumour is seen is no indication of its true inci-

Table 1. Teratomas and genital tumours

| | a | b |
|---|---|---|
| **Teratomas and allied tumours** | | |
| Intracranial | 4 | 0 |
| Cervical | 2 | 0 |
| Intrathoracic | 3 | 0 |
| Spinal axis | 3 | 0 |
| Sacrococcygeal | 17 | 0 |
| Bladder | 1 | 0 |
| Para-ovarian | 0 | 1 |
| Ovarian | 37 | 9 |
| Testicular | 11 | 0 |
| Vaginal | 1 | 0 |
| **Other ovarian tumours** | | |
| Serosal | 0 | 1 |
| Sex-cord [c] | 5 | 5 |
| Lipoid | 1 | 0 |
| Rhabdomyosarcoma | 1 | 0 |
| Undiagnosed | 2 | 4 |
| Extra-ovarian disease | 2 | 2 |
| **Testicular** | | |
| Yolk sac tumour (orchioblastoma) | 5 | 0 |
| Other possible nephrogenital tumours | 2 | 0 |

[a]: Tumours occurring in children in the Manchester Hospital Region since 1953

[b]: Tumours occurring in children living outside the Manchester Region but included in the Ovarian Tumour Register

[c]: Granulosa cell tumours and androblastomas

dence in the population. Nevertheless, the two most common sites are the gonad and the sacrococcygeal region and in the gonad, teratomas far outnumber any other tumour at this age.

## TERATOMAS AND ALLIED TUMOURS ARISING OUTSIDE THE GONADS

"A teratoma is a true tumour or neoplasm composed of multiple tissues of kinds foreign to the part in which it arises" (WILLIS, 1958). This definition distinguishes a teratoma from non-neoplastic heterotopia but not from mixed tumours such as the mixed mesodermal tumour of the uterus. The distinction between teratomas and mixed tumours lies in their origin; teratomas are germ cell tumours whilst mixed tumours are not. The chief components of teratomas are skin and skin appendages, central nervous system tissue, respiratory, or alimentary tract mucosa and glands. Less common components are cartilage, bone, teeth, smooth, and striated muscle. The tissues form an unorganised mass, without axial arrangement, which may be cystic or solid. Occasionally the tumour may be composed of a single type of tissue e. g. the struma ovarii; such tumours are termed monophyletic. Teratomas arise most commonly in the gonads but they can occur elsewhere in the body from the brain to the sacrococcygeal region - their distribution being axial or nearly so.

### Histogenesis

A detailed discussion of the various theories of histogenesis is out of place but an outline is necessary in order to offer an explanation of the relationship which exists between some tumours and teratomas. NICHOLSON (1950) and WILLIS (1958) have criticised and rejected the idea that a teratoma is an abnormal conceptus. WILLIS accepts ASKANAZY's (1907) suggestion that teratogenesis occurs by morphogenesis of undifferentiated cells. BUDDE (1926) was of the opinion that teratomas probably represented misdirection of the action of the primary embryonic organiser and that these tumours originated in cells released from normal developmental control. Thus teratomas appear to arise from tissues close to the embryonic axis which differentiate along independent lines according to their own labile determinations. Apparent exceptions such as cervical and anterior mediastinal teratomas are discussed by WILLIS in terms of the changes in anatomical position of the head and neck during development.

It must, however, be remembered that the only totipotential cell normally present in the body is the germ cell and there seems no reason why this should not sometimes be the origin of a tumour which would conform to a teratoma in structure. There is evidence to support the view that the germ cells arise in the yolk sac and migrate to the gonads by way of the mesentery. WITSCHI (1948) has also shown that many germ cells in the course of migration are distributed along the embryonic axis as well as to the gonad. The extragonadal germ cells disappear as development advances. If, on occasion, some of these cells did not disappear but persisted in extragonadal sites, such cells might become the focus from which teratomas could arise. Such an origin would also account for the rare teratomas of the umbilical cord and placenta (KREYBERG, 1958; FOX and BUTLER-MANUEL, 1964; FUJIKURA and WELLINGS, 1964) which cannot be explained on the BUDDE-WILLIS hypothesis. Moreover, tumours arising in germ cells might be expected to give rise to structures of either intra- or extra-embryonic type or of both, which would readily account for the simultaneous occurrence of a choriocarcinoma or an endodermal sinus (yolk sac) tumour (TEILUM, 1965) with a teratoma. The mechanism whereby germ cells become neoplastic is not clear. GALTON and BENIRSCHKE (1959), investigated one ovarian teratoma and showed that it possessed 46 chromosomes. Germ cells are, however, haploid, and therefore either two cells must fuse or a cell must reduplicate its chromosomes. Studies of sex chromatin in these tumours have been reviewed by TAYLOR (1965). She writes "Both these hypotheses required the occurrence of meiosis during early embryogenesis when the teratoma rudiment originated. Current studies of human meiosis suggest that in females the cells undergo first meiotic prophase during foetal development and are stored in the dictyate condition from around the time of birth until ovulation, and that in males there is apparently no meiosis until puberty".

LINDER and POWER (1970) and LINDER et al. (1975) have used isoenzymes of ovarian teratomas as gene markers and correlated these observations with studies of chromosome banding. They concluded that a teratoma most probably arises from a germ cell after meiosis I, there being either suppression of meiosis II or suppression of the second polar body, or re-entry of the second polar body.

A high proportion of the extragonadal teratomas in children are found in the sacrococcygeal region and there is a great preponderance of females in this group. This sex difference would fit in with the hypothesis that teratomas arise from cells which have undergone meiosis since girls have a store of such cells from an early age whereas boys normally have them only after puberty. GROSS et al. (1951) offer an alternative explanation for the preponderance of females with sacrococcygeal teratomas. According to them, teratomas may be expected to occur more frequently in those locations where there is the greatest concentration of primitive cells, namely in the reproductive gland anlage and in the region of primitive knot (Hensen's node). The primitive knot moves caudally until it is ultimately located in the region of the coccyx. Among the many structures which arise from the primitive knot are the "genital cells". These cells migrate anteriorly and become concentrated in the developing urogenital ridge. The cephalad part of the ridge develops first but atrophies as early as 14-24 days. The caudal portion forms an undifferentiated reproductive gland at 27-35 days. The longer persistence of the caudal portion of the ridge gives a greater chance for regional sequestration of cells and the formation of teratomas in the abdomen and pelvis rather than in the thorax. In the male the anlage differentiates to form the testis during a comparatively short period at 31-34 days. However, the ovary differentiates later and over a longer period of 39-50 days. Evidently the genital cells have a shorter time to become ectopic in the male than in the female and this may account for the higher incidence of sacrococcygeal teratomas in the female.

TAYLOR (1965) points out that teratomas may occur in patients with the testicular feminisation syndrome and also in patients with Kleinfelter's syndrome. This, she suggests, raises the possibility that the association between abnormal sex differentiation and a teratoma may not be fortuitous

## Intracranial Teratomas

These tumours have been discussed by RUSSELL and RUBINSTEIN (1963) and by KOOS and MILLER (1971); a further discussion will be found in chapter 6. Two types may be found, (a) typical and teratoid, (b) atypical. Tumours of the first group occur most commonly in the pineal body or its immediate neighbourhood but may sometimes be found in the pituitary, third ventricle, or posterior fossa; midline situations being favoured. They may be composed of a mixture of mature tissues with an organoid pattern derived from all three germinal layers, or a variety of tissue elements which, although individually mature, do not recapitulate the structure of any recognisable organ. These latter are termed teratoid tumours because derivatives of all three germinal layers are not present. Atypical teratomas also occur most commonly in the region of the pineal body but the hypothalamus and pituitary are also commonly involved and the tumour may spread outside the skull (DAYAN et al., 1966). Microscopically, they are composed of large polygonal or spheroidal cells arranged in lobules separated by connective tissue trabeculae infiltrated with lymphocytes. Multinucleated giant cells of foreign body type may be present in the stroma. The structure of the tumour is like that of the seminoma of the testis or dysgerminoma of the ovary. These atypical teratomas often contain elements of a teratoid appearance; likewise, typical teratomas may contain areas composed of large spherical cells and lymphocytes. These tumours may produce a variety of clinical pictures such as diabetes insipidus, pubertas praecox, emaciation, and mental and visual disturbances. Males are more commonly affected than females.

The Children's Tumour Register includes 4 children with intracranial teratomas. These are summarised in Table 2. All proved fatal soon after operation. The tumour of CTR.119/59 surrounded the vein of Galen; it was inoperable and only a biopsy was available. It contained a mixture of tissues: an epidermoid cyst filled with keratin and other cysts lined by low columnar and cubical epithelium. There were groups of large cells separated from each other by lymphocytes and closely resembling a seminoma. There was a marked granulomatous reaction in this area (Fig. 1). The tumour of CTR.128/68 metastasized in the dorsal spine some 3 months after piecemeal removal of the primary tumour. At the time of necropsy, a month later, recurrent tumour was found both intracranially and at the site of metastasis.

Table 2. Intracranial teratomas

| | CTR.120/68 | CTR.52/61 | CTR.27/60 | CTR.119/59 |
|---|---|---|---|---|
| Age | 7 1/2 years | 9 1/2 yrs. | 7 years | 6 years |
| Sex | F | M | F | M |
| Length of history | 15 days | 5 days | 2 weeks | 9 months |
| Diabetes insipidus | Yes | None | Yes | Yes |
| Local neurological signs | Yes | Yes | No | Yes |
| Site | Floor of 3rd ventricle | Pineal | Extended down to hypophysis | Midbrain |
| Tumour | Teratoma | Teratoma | Teratoma with seminoma-like foci | Teratoma with seminoma-like areas |

In the central nervous system difficulty may sometimes be experienced in distinguishing between a malformation and a teratoma, especially if the "tumour" is in the region of the foramen magnum where reduplications can occur. Such reduplications are discussed by WILLIS (1958). Intracranial dermoid and epidermoid cysts should cause no confusion (RUSSELL and RUBINSTEIN, 1963).

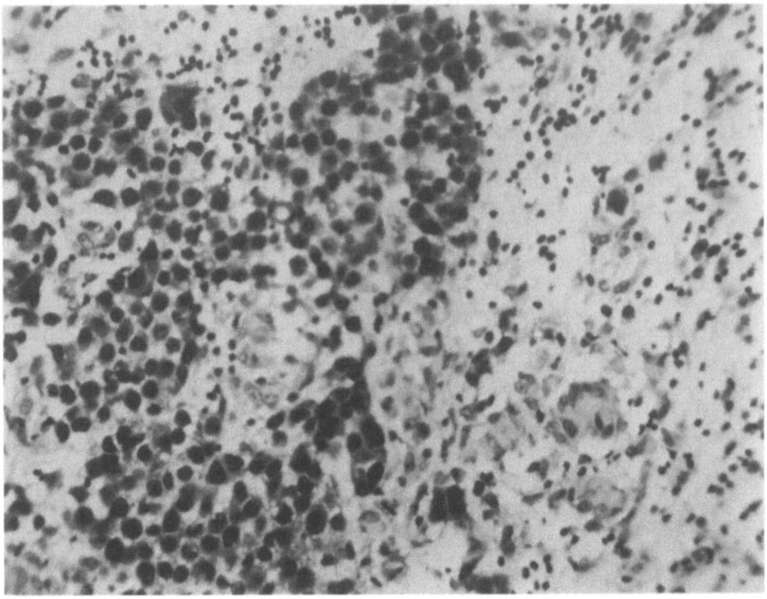

*Fig. 1. CTR.119/59 Intracranial teratoma. There is a marked similarity to seminoma (dysgerminoma) and a granulomatous reaction is present (H. & E. X 210)*

## Teratomas of the Neck

The Children's Tumour Register does not include any epignathic teratomas. Teratomas of the neck are comparatively rare but SILBERMAN and MENDELSON (1960) reviewed 80 cases and added 2 of their own. One of their cases is included in the Children's Tumour Register and is of interest in that it presents a diagnostic problem. The tumour was found in a newborn full-term male infant. It was excised and the child was alive and well 15 years later. The tumour extended from the midline of the neck anteriorly to the left ear, lying behind the sternomastoid and attached to the trachea. It was 7.5 cms in diameter and shelled out easily. The tumour consisted largely of nodules of cartilage. In the intervening stroma there were small islands of epithelial cells, the largest showing squamous epithelium centrally (Fig. 2). Thyroid tissue was stretched over the tumour as in POTTER's case (1961). SILBERMAN et al. recorded the opinion of six pathologists. Two considered it to be a malformation, one considered it a "benign teratoid tumour" and the other three considered that it might be either a teratoma or malformation, most probably the latter. The present writer views the tumour as most probably a hamartoma, possibly arising as a maldevelopment of respiratory tract. Curiously, the mother had previously had an ovarian cystic teratoma removed.

The register includes a second tumour found in a newborn girl at the time of birth and causing stridor. The right lobe of the thyroid was enlarged and the trachea pushed to the left. About half the left lobe and two-thirds of the right lobe were removed. Histologically, the tumour consisted of bronchial epithelium some of which showed squamous metaplasia, small mucin-secreting glands, smooth muscle, nodules of cartilage, and mature central nervous system tissue. The surrounding tissues included thyroid vesicles. The presence of brain tissue would indicate that this is not a hamartoma but a true teratoma.

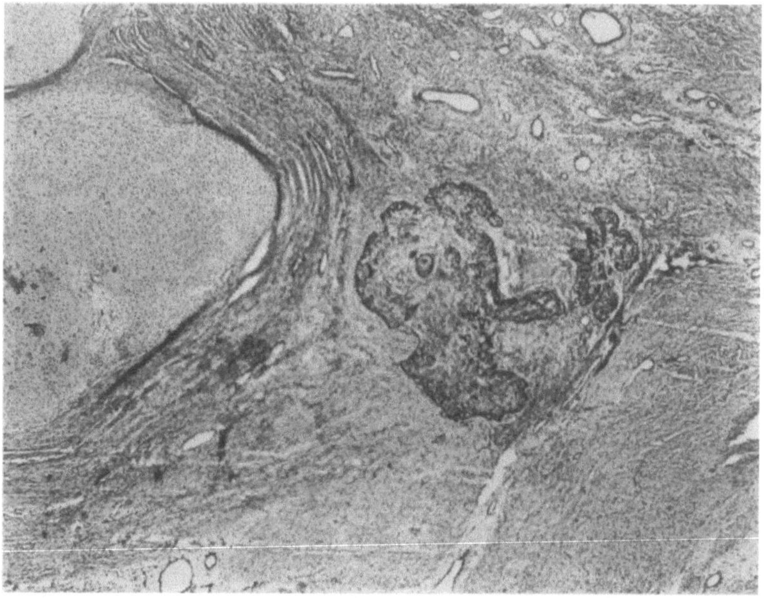

*Fig. 2. CTR.42/52 Cervical hamartoma. An island of epithelial tissue is seen adjacent to a nodule of cartilage. Epithelium is keratinized in centre (H. & E. X 30)*

Attempts have been made to distinguish teratomas of the thyroid gland from cervical teratomas (SAPHIR, 1929; BALE, 1950). Such distinctions seem unnecessary. An interesting cervical teratoma not included in SILBERMAN and MENDELSON's review is the one of the tonsil causing respiratory obstruction in the newborn, described by BAUGH and O'DONOGHUE (1955). The majority of teratomas of the neck are present at birth and they are rare after the age of 1 year. They are equally divided between the sexes. All varieties of tissue from the three germinal layers have been found in these tumours. About three-quarters of them contain brain tissue and half contain thyroid tissue. On histological examination they are usually benign but the prognosis is difficult to assess since many of the children die soon after operative removal of the tumour. Among the few found in adults some have metastasized.

## Intrathoracic Teratomas

Mediastinal teratomas are most commonly located in the anterior mediastinum but may be intrapericardial. Two anterior mediastinal teratomas are included in the Manchester series. One occurred in a girl of 6 months of age. It was a typical cystic teratoma. The girl is alive and well 16 years later. Another was seen in association with a solid ovarian teratoma and is discussed below. A third intrathoracic tumour occurred in a girl, 1 1/2 years old, and presented as dyspnoea of acute onset. Thoracotomy revealed an extensive tumour involving the left lower lobe, pleura, and diaphragm. She died 2 months later of bronchopneumonia and metastases were found in the opposite lung, coeliac lymph nodes, and ovaries. Histologically, the tumour was a malignant teratoma consisting of sheets of undifferentiated cells, "embryonic" mesenchyme, and small spaces lined by squamous epithelium or mucin-secreting cells. Because of the extent of the primary tumour its site of origin in the thorax could not be determined. POUND and WILLIS (1969) have described a similar tumour in a 10-month-old male infant. They think the genesis of such tumours is like that of intracardiac and intrapericardial teratomas, being rare outlying congeners of the more common mediastinal teratomas.

A fourth intrathoracic teratoma was found in a male infant who was cyanosed after birth and remained so until he died in congestive heart failure at 20 days. The tumour ran down the anterior wall of the interventricular septum, projected into the right ventricle, and entered the

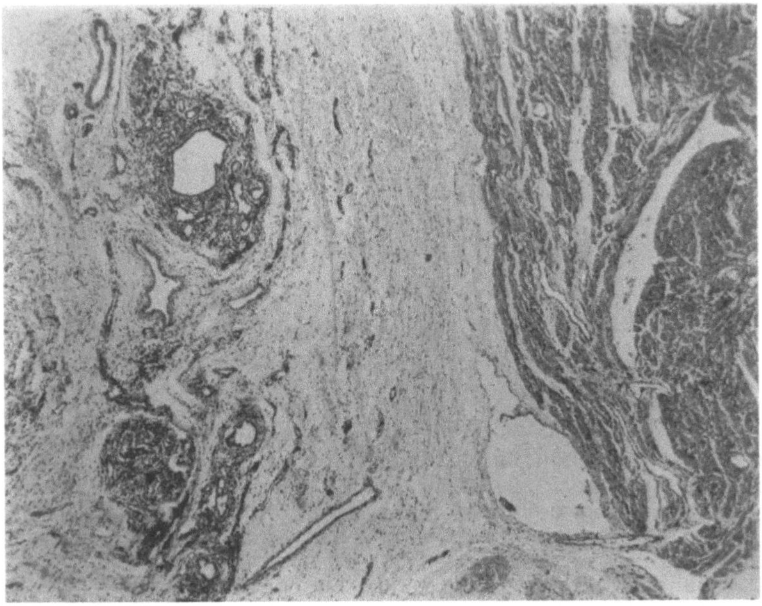

*Fig. 3. CTR.28/60 Intracardiac teratoma. Myocardium lies to right and tumour on left lies just beneath epicardium (H. & E. X 30)*

anterior cusp of the tricuspid valve. The tumour was polycystic and derivatives of all three germinal layers could be identified (Fig. 3). Although the child was a boy the tumour was sex-chromatin positive. There was no evidence of malignancy. WILLIAMS (1961) considered that this case together with the tumours of DE CHÂTEL (1932), ANDERSON and DMYTREKY (1946), LEIGHTON et al. (1950), and SOLOMON (1951) form a group of intracardiac teratomas characteristically occurring to the right of the midline, near the tricuspid ring. They are distinct from the more common benign subepicardial teratomas of which he found fourteen in the literature. These latter commonly arise near the roots of the great vessels (WILLIS, 1946; CLAIREAUX, 1951). The intracardiac teratomas must be distinguished from rhabdomyosarcomas (KIDDER, 1950) and intramural fibromas (CLAY and SHORTER, 1957) which are also found in children.

WILLIS suggests that an intrapericardial teratoma is only a peculiarly situated variety of a mediastinal teratoma. Whether a tumour arising at the level of the base of the heart assumes an anterior or intrapericardial position may depend on the main direction of growth. This hypothesis cannot explain the origin of the intracardiac teratomas which WILLIAMS suggests may be related to certain epithelial inclusions reported in the same area. He found reports of 21 cases with such inclusions in the heart. Whereas mediastinal teratomas often do not produce symptoms until adult life most of the intrapericardial and intracardiac teratomas are found in very young children. This is probably because even a small tumour in the pericardium and heart can easily interfere with the circulation.

## Teratomas of the Spinal Axis

Teratomas in the vertebral canal are rare and must be distinguished from enterocysts and epidermal cysts.

Three spinal teratomas are included in the Children's Tumour Register. One occurred in a girl of 11 years. She was perfectly well until a week before admission to hospital when she complained of low backache which was severe at night. On laminectomy a thick-walled cyst was found at the level of L 1 and a tumour at the level of L 2. The cyst was opened and drained of mucous material and the tumour was partially excised. The girl was well 15 years later although she had had some inversion of the right foot which was corrected surgically. The tumour included certilage, plain muscle, mucous glands, transitional epithelium, Pacinian corpuscles, and central nervous tissue.

The other two cases were seen in the neonatal period. One appeared as a defect in the thoracic spine through which protruded a hard mass. It measured 1.75 x 0.5 cms and consisted of bone, cartilage, and various types of epithelium. Subsequent whole-body X-ray showed craniolacunia and multiple congenital abnormalities of the vertebrae. Hydrocephalus developed. The second case presented a lumbar meningocoele. A sac was excised which contained a variety of tissues: enteric, nephric, and squamous epithelium. This child was also hydrocephalic.

The problem posed by intraspinal cysts is well illustrated by the case of KNIGHT et al. (1954-55). Their cyst was lined partly by gastric mucosa, partly by squamous and partly by ciliated epithelium. The authors state that WILLIS examined the cyst and considered that it was not a teratoma but similar to enterocysts and gastrocysts found in the abdomen and thorax. Intraspinal enteric cysts are associated with malformation of the vertebral bodies. They have been discussed at length by BREMER (1957), RHANEY and BARCLAY (1959), BENTLEY and SMITH (1960) and MORISON (1963). The ventrally situated yolk sac herniates through a defect in the notochord and may give rise to a variety of malformations such as a posterior enteric sinus, intraspinal enteric cyst, or a prevertebral enteric cyst. CAMERON (1957) has pointed out that spinal teratomas are fairly frequently associated with spina bifida, which is usually of occult type, and regards this combination as not fortuitous. In his own case of intraspinal teratoma CAMERON found, besides the spina bifida, a myelocoele, Arnold-Chiari malformation, and a partial splitting of the spinal cord. It is very probable that in both intraspinal enteric cysts and teratomas the primary defect is a relatively simple deviation from normal embryological development similar to that seen in experimental embryology caused by artificially delayed insemination of the ova of fish and frogs. If an enteric vestige remains in the spinal canal an enteric cyst will develop but, because of its close association with the yolk sac, ectopic germ cells may be included in which case a teratoma may develop.

## Sacrococcygeal Teratomas

There have been a number of extensive reviews of these teratomas. KEEN and COPLIN (1906) summarised the older literature. HANSMAN and BERNE (1932) described a teratoma in a girl of 1 month and collected reports of 12 others occurring in children. GROSS et al. (1951) gave an account of 40 such tumours studied at the Children's Hospital, Boston. BODIAN and WHITE (1952) and BERRY et al. (1969) have reviewed the cases seen at the Hospital for Sick Children, London. These tumours can occur at any age but predominantly in early life. BALARD (1923) records one in a 3-month-old foetus, HANSMAN and BERNE (1932) in an 8-month-old foetus, and we have seen one in a stillborn infant, causing obstructed labour. These tumours are found more frequently in females than in males - for example, HANSMAN et al. (1932) found them in the ratio of 5 females to 2 males and GROSS et al. (1951) in the ratio of 4 females to 1 male. BERRY et al. (1969) found 41 females to 17 males and in this Manchester series 14 females to 3 males. The reason for this distribution is uncertain and has been discussed earlier in this chapter. The tumours are usually retrorectal in situation but when large may extend well beyond this site. In 2 of the cases described by GROSS et al. (1951) they extended into the spinal canal and grew upward outside the dura as finger-like projections. The tumour described by KEEN and COPLIN (1906) was unusual because it was associated with a fistula joining the rectum and the skin.

GROSS et al. (1951) stress that for reasons of prognosis it is important to place in separate categories those teratomas which are noted

Table 3. Sacrococcygeal teratomas

| CTR numbers | Age of presentation | Sex | Sex chromatin | Size of tumour | Diagnosis | Follow-up |
|---|---|---|---|---|---|---|
| 72/54 | Birth | F | + ve | 5 cm | Benign | well 16 yrs. later |
| 66/56 | Birth | M | - ve | 2.5 cm | Benign | well 15 yrs. later |
| 127/56 | Birth | F | + ve | 17 cm | Benign | well 15 yrs. later |
| 22/59 | Birth | M | - ve | 3.5 cm | Benign | well 10 yrs. later |
| 48/59 | Birth | F | + ve | 7.5 cm | Benign | well 13 yrs. later |
| 79/60 | Birth | F | + ve | 28 gms | Benign | well 10 yrs. later |
| 125/65 | Birth | F | | 4 and 6 cm | Benign | well 7 yrs. later |
| 76/67 | Birth | M | | 10 cm | Benign | well 4 yrs. later |
| 120/69 | 5 1/2 months | F | | 6 cm | Benign | well 2 yrs. later |
| 61/70 | 4 months | F | | 20 cm | Benign | |
| 85/54 | Birth | F | ? | 12.5 cm | Carcinoma | Died age 2 years |
| 24/56 | 2 years | F | ? | ? | Malignant teratoma | Died age 2 years 3 months |
| 46/58 | Birth | F | ? | 7.5 cm | Carcinoma | Died age 21 months |
| 63/58 | 3-4 months | F | + ve | 4 cm | Malignant teratoma | Died age 13 months |
| 73/60 | 1 year | F | ? | Biopsy only | Endodermal sinus | Died age 15 months |
| 65/62 | 3 years | F | ? | Biopsy only | Papillary carcinoma | Died age 3 years 11 months |
| 119/68 | Birth | F | | 4 cm | Benign | Died age 16 days |

at birth and those which are initially discovered later in childhood. This is well illustrated in our material (Table 3). All the benign tumours, except one, presented as lumps at the time of birth. The exception (CTR.79/60) presented as a sacrococcygeal sinus at birth. At the age of 2 months the sinus and surrounding cysts were excised and at 1 year a large teratoma was removed. Two malignant tumours showed abnormalities at birth. One child (CTR.85/54) had a dimple behind the anus followed by a sacrococcygeal tumour 5 months later. In the second child (CTR.46/58) the natal cleft came further up the back than is usual and curved to the left. About 18 months later she had difficulty in sitting down and a bluish mark like a varicose vein appeared 2.5 cms behind the anus. On removal the benign tumours were soft and solid but contained cystic areas. Histologically, they were unremarkable benign teratomas. The malignant tumours presented a variety of patterns. The tumour CTR.63/58 occurred in a child suffering from mucoviscidosis, two sisters having previously died of this disease. At the time of her death metastases were found in her liver. The sacrococcygeal tumour was predominantly an adenocarcinoma but small areas of respiratory tract epithelium could be identified. The tumour CTR.73/60 had the structure of an endodermal sinus (yolk sac) tumour as described by TEILUM (1959) in the ovary (Fig. 4). HUNTINGTON et al. (1963) have described an endodermal sinus tumour (yolk sac tumour) in association with a sacrococcygeal teratoma and we have seen another situated in the presacral region. The three remaining tumours presented difficulties in diagnosis. Two were carcinomas of non-specific type but with some papillary areas not unlike ependyma; in 1 case the tumour had metastasized to the lung. Only a small biopsy specimen was available from the third tumour (CTR.65/62) and this showed a papillary pattern and some cystic spaces. The diagnosis of teratoma in these three tumours was by exclusion and in each case the possibility

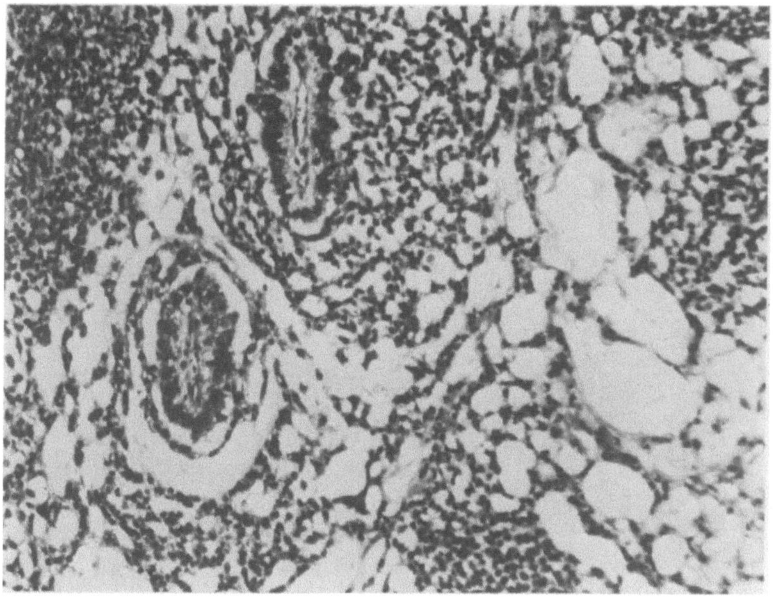

*Fig. 4. CTR.73/60 Sacrococcygeal teratoma with endodermal sinus pattern. Each of the perivascular structures on left consists of a mesodermal core with a central capillary and is covered by a visceral layer of cylindrical cells. On right there is a meshwork with wide cystic spaces. Compare this with TEILUM's (1965) figures (H.&E. X 120)*

of chordoma was considered and rejected. Likewise 2 were examined by a neuropathologist who excluded a diagnosis of ependymoma.

Only 1 child (CTR.119/68) with a benign tumour died; she had a number of congenital abnormalities and an examination of the peripheral blood showed a trisomy in the 13-15 group.

GROSS et al. (1951) discussed the differential diagnosis of sacrococcygeal tumours and indicated that, apart from teratomas, the following should be considered: 1) meningocoele, 2) chordoma, 3) ependymoma, and 4) pilonidal cysts and sinuses. Prior to surgery they found radiological evidence of calcification in 43 percent of their tumours and regarded this finding as very helpful in differentiating teratomas from other retrorectal masses such as duplication of the colon.

BERRY et al. (1969) pointed out that the commonest site of a teratoma in infancy is in the sacrococcygeal region. However in childhood (under the age of 15 years) ovarian and testicular teratomas are more common than sacrococcygeal tumours (see Table 1). Indeed there is very little overlap in the age of presentation of these tumours probably because the intra-abdominal ovarian tumours are not conspicuous externally. It is not necessary to suppose that the ovarian tumours originate later than the sacrococcygeal tumours.

## Teratoma or Hamartoma of the Bladder

The Children's Tumour Register includes one possible teratoma of the bladder. It was removed from a boy of 3 months of age who soon after birth passed blood in the urine. The bladder was excised and the ureters transplanted into the colon. He died at the age of 16 months with uraemia and hyperchloraemic acidosis. The tumour formed a cystic mass in the anterior wall of the bladder extending from 1.5 cms above

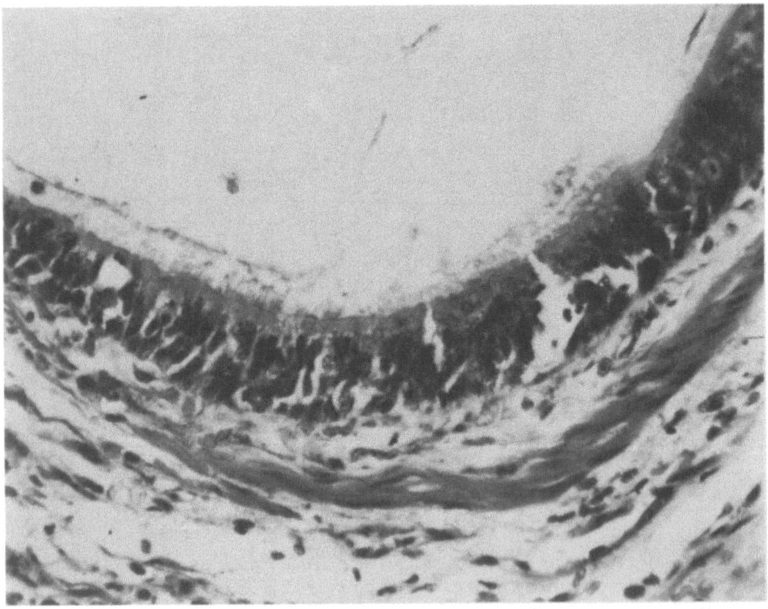

*Fig. 5. CTR.79/91 Teratoma or hamartoma of the bladder showing ciliated respiratory tract epithelium (H. & E. X 380)*

the prostate to the urachus. The cysts contained gastric mucosa which seemed to be in continuity with the surrounding bladder mucosa; an area of ulceration may well have been peptic. Respiratory tract epithelium was also present (Fig. 5). GORDON (1963) has described intestinal metaplasia of the urinary tract. It seems probable that the changes here are hamartomatous rather than teratomatous but this is not certain.

## Endodermal Sinus (Yolk Sac) Tumour of the Vagina

The Manchester register includes one vaginal tumour (68/67). The girl was born prematurely at 28 weeks gestation. At the age of 2 years and 3 months she developed a brown vaginal discharge. On examination a tumour, resembling profuse granulation tissue, was noted on the mucosa of the right labium majus and extended into the lateral vaginal wall. A biopsy revealed the neoplasm to be an endodermal sinus (yolk sac) tumour. Following X-ray and chemotherapy (adenopterin) the tumour regressed for a time but she died at the age of 3 years and 2 months with multiple metastases in the lungs and a large abdominal mass.

Endodermal sinus (yolk sac) tumours of the vagina are rare and usually diagnosed before the age of 2 years (VAWTER, 1965; TEILUM, 1971). They must not be confused with adenocarcinomas of the vagina occurring in adolescent girls and young women resulting from steroid therapy having been given to their mothers during pregnancy (HERBST et al., 1970).

## OVARIAN TERATOMAS AND RELATED GERM CELL TUMOURS

The tumours reviewed here are listed in Table 4. This Table does not indicate the relative incidence of the various tumours. In recent

Table 4. Germ cell tumours of the ovary

| | |
|---|---|
| Cystic teratomas | 22 |
| Solid teratomas | 6 |
| Struma ovarii | 1 |
| Dysgerminomas | 10 |
| Gonadoblastomas | 3 |
| Chorioncarcinomas | 2 |
| Endodermal sinus (yolk sac) tumours | 7 |

Note: Some of these tumours are combined

years many cystic teratomas have probably been seen by gynaecologists rather than paediatric surgeons and thus have not been referred to the tumour registry. Nevertheless, cystic teratomas both in this series and in others (COSTIN and KENNEDY, 1948), are by far the commonest ovarian tumours in childhood.

### Cystic Ovarian Teratomas

The age at the time of diagnosis varied from 2 1/2 to 16 years except for one microscopic tumour found incidentally in a child dying at 7h. Usually there was abdominal pain with a palpable abdominal or rectal mass. In 2 patients abdominal swelling was the presenting sign, whilst a third child, aged 16 years, had 3 months amenorrhoea and abdominal swelling. The abdominal pain was often recurrent: once, in a girl of 10 years, it had occurred from time to time over a period of 6 years. More often, there were attacks of pain over a period of months or days, sometimes ending in a severe attack of pain and vomiting. Once a diagnosis of appendicitis was made. In 5 children the presenting signs were those of an abdominal crisis, in 2 the tumour had ruptured and in another 2 it had undergone torsion. One child, aged 13, had a recurrent urinary tract infection. All the children, with the exception of the 1 dying at 7h, were alive and well at the latest follow-up which varied from 3 to 19 years. Of the 17 who are now over 18 years old 12 are known to be married and of these, 7 have children of their own. Thus the preceding ovarian disease does not seem to have significantly affected their fertility.

Ten of the tumours were in the right ovary and four in the left; one tumour was bilateral. On histological examination all were sex chromatin positive. There was much variation in the size of the tumours but their mean diameter in children under 7 years was about half that of children over that age. It is interesting to note that torsion occurred in younger children with smaller tumours and rupture in older girl with larger tumours.

## Solid Ovarian Teratomas

It is usual to divide solid teratomas into two histological types: 1) adult, composed of mature structures, which are usually benign, and 2) embryonal, composed of immature structures, which are usually malignant. The problem for the diagnostic pathologist is to decide whether such a tumour is benign or malignant. This is particularly true in children, since it is undesirable to expose the other ovary to unnecessary radiation. In a tumour which is mostly of mature type an extensive examination may be necessary to exclude malignancy and because such a tumour may be large the search is very laborious. If immature structures are found it may be difficult to decide whether these are malignant or whether they have not yet fully differentiated. This problem arises particularly in those tumours containing nervous tissue. Sometimes these tumours may be combined with other types of germ cell tumours such as endodermal sinus (yolk sac) tumour, choriocarcinoma, or dysgerminoma.

There are six solid teratomas in this study. The children's ages ranged from 2 to 14 years but all except one were 10 years old or over, thus the tumours occur in somewhat older children than those with teratomas at other sites. Two of the tumours were combined, one with a dysgerminoma and choriocarcinoma and the other with a dysgerminoma and an endodermal sinus (yolk sac) tumour. All the tumours were large. Five were malignant and one was probably benign.

This last case was previously described briefly by WILLIS (1962) and more recently by us in the previous edition of this monograph. It is now possible to give the final account. The patient was aged 10 years and had a right-sided ovarian tumour weighing 430 gm. It contained squamous epithelium, hair, skin, ependyma, and brain tissue together with undifferentiated mesenchyme. The tumour was regarded as probably malignant but the patient was not given radiotherapy at that time. Initially no X-ray photograph was taken of the child's chest, but a year later a mass was found in the superior mediastinum. This was thought to be a metastasis and it was irradiated and watched for a year when a thoracotomy was performed. A mass 8 x 6 x 6 cm was removed from the mediastinum; it contained cartilage, plain muscle, fibrous tissue, and squamous epithelium. This was regarded as benign and as an example of an independent teratoma rather than a metastasis. She was followed up regularly in the ensuing years and remained well, married, and had a child. However, at the age of 25 years, following a road accident she was found to have a mammary carcinoma with spinal metastases from which she died. Since this tumour was in the irradiated area it was counted, for statistical purposes, as a radiation-induced lesion. Whilst this may be true the possibility that it was not iatrogenic but an independent primary tumour cannot be excluded. We have seen a benign cystic teratoma in a woman of 19 years followed shortly by a carcinoma of the colon from which she died.

BREEN and NEUBECHER (1967) summarised 11 cases, described as malignant teratomas. Five of the patients died within the year, one was still surviving at 8 years and 7 months and another at 4 years and 7 months. They regarded solid teratomas as resistant to radiotherapy and offering a chance for a good prognosis only when limited to one ovary with no evidence of extension or metastasis. They advocate surgical conservation as the treatment of choice in unilateral disease because it makes little difference to survival if the opposite adnexae and uterus are removed. Occasionally, and especially in children, solid teratomas may be associated with diffuse glial implants on the peritoneum. ROBBOY and SCULLY (1970) have reviewed a number of such cases and concluded that it is justifiable to spare the ovary opposite the primary ovarian tumour unless it is involved by embryonal neoplasia or is totally replaced by a benign tumour and that therapy directed against the peritoneal implants of mature glia is not required.

## Struma Ovarii

There was one example of struma ovarii in this series. This occurred in a girl of 12 years who had a 3 weeks history of abdominal pain, severe at times and sometimes associated with vomiting. There was no clinical evidence of thyrotoxicosis. A smooth round swelling, 9 cm in diameter, was found in the abdomen. It was multiocular and had undergone torsion. On microscopic examination it was found to be composed of thyroid tissue.

## Dysgerminoma

A dysgerminoma is composed of large cells, with vesicular cytoplasm, arranged in islands or strands separated by a variable amount of connective tissue infiltrated by lymphocytes and sometimes by plasma cells and eosinophils. Giant cells and granulomatous foci may be present. Electron-microscopic studies indicate that the tumour cells closely resemble "germ cells" (LYNN et al., 1967; OVERBECK and PHILIP, 1969). Morphologically these tumours are closely similar to the "atypical teratoma" of the pineal gland and hypothalamic region. Some dysgerminomas are associated with congenital abnormalities of the genital tract but the genetic status of patients with such tumours may need reassessing in the light of recent work on intersexes and dysgenetic gonads (FATHALLA et al., 1966; TAYLOR et al., 1966; JONES, 1971). Thus FETTIG et al. (1968) and DEWHURST et al. (1971) have described dysgerminoma in XY phenotypic females and I have seen one in an XXX patient.

This series includes ten girls with dysgerminomas, their ages ranging from 10 to 17 years. In 2 cases (referred to above) these were associated teratomatous elements. In one girl the symptoms were those of an acute abdomen caused by torsion of the tumour. A more typical his-

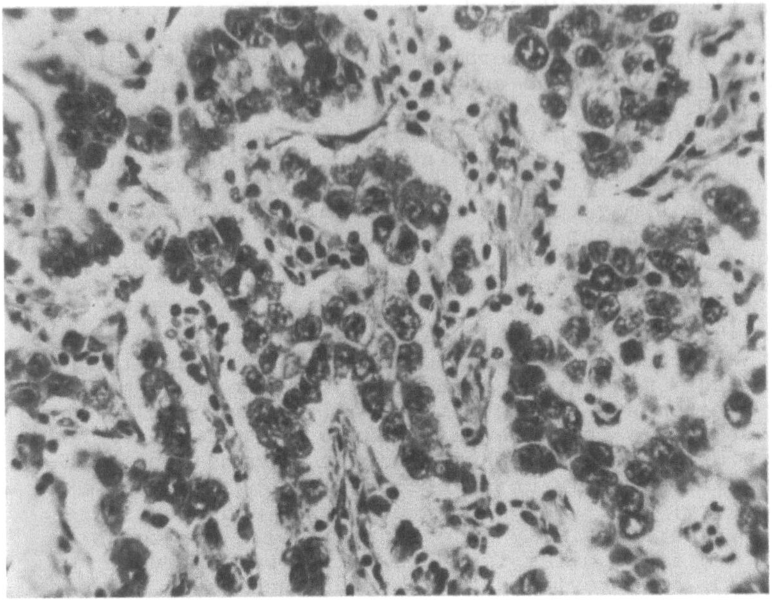

*Fig. 6. CTR.91/63 Ovarian dysgerminoma. There are cords of large tumour cells separated by connective tissue septa infiltrated with lymphocytes (H. & E. X 380)*

tory is that of a girl of 12 years. She had had abdominal pain for 4 months. Although she had started to menstruate 10 months before admission to hospital there had been no menses since the onset of the pain. The abdomen was distended by a large palpable mass. At laparotomy a large ovarian tumour was found on the left side, about 17.5 cms in diameter. Microscopically it was a typical dysgerminoma (Fig. 6). Small para-aortic glands were palpable and the right ovary was thought to contain a neoplastic nodule. X-ray therapy was instituted and the child was alive and well 9 years later. Only 2 other children with dysgerminomas were adequately followed up and both were alive and well after 6 and 7 years.

BREEN and NEUBECKER (1967) in a series of 68 patients with dysgerminoma found a 5-year survival rate of 84.8 percent and a 10-year survival of 81.8 percent. They suggest that because of this low degree of malignancy, and provided the tumour is unilateral and free, conservative surgery without postoperative radiation is adequate therapy in the childbearing years. Radiotherapy is effective if there is extension or metastasis. However, if there is an associated malignant germ cell neoplasm the tumour will fail to respond to treatment by irradiation. It is therefore of considerable importance to make an extensive histological examination of such tumours to determine whether or not any other germ cell tumour is present. SCULLY (1970 a) quotes four studies of unilateral encapsulated dysgerminomas. The 5-year survival rate ranged from 90 to 95 percent and the recurrence rate from 10 to 22 percent.

The Manchester Ovarian Tumour Register contains an atypical dysgerminoma associated with precocious puberty. This case was previously described by HAIN (1949). The girl aged 8 years looked like one of 12, there had been a growth of axillary and pubic hair for 2 years and her breast development was that of a girl of 16 or 17. She had had intermittent vaginal bleeding for 6 months. No signs of virilism were seen. The 17-ketosteroid excretion was only slightly in excess of normal for a child of 8 years but there was a strongly positive Aschheim-Zondek reaction. There was abdominal swelling and ascites. Following removal of a pedunculated tumour from the left ovary the signs of precocity gradually diminished and, after a time, the excretion of gonadotrophin ceased. The tumour appeared to be a typical dysgerminoma and this was confirmed by Emil Novak. Included in the tumour were Graafian follicles in various stages of maturation and some eosino-

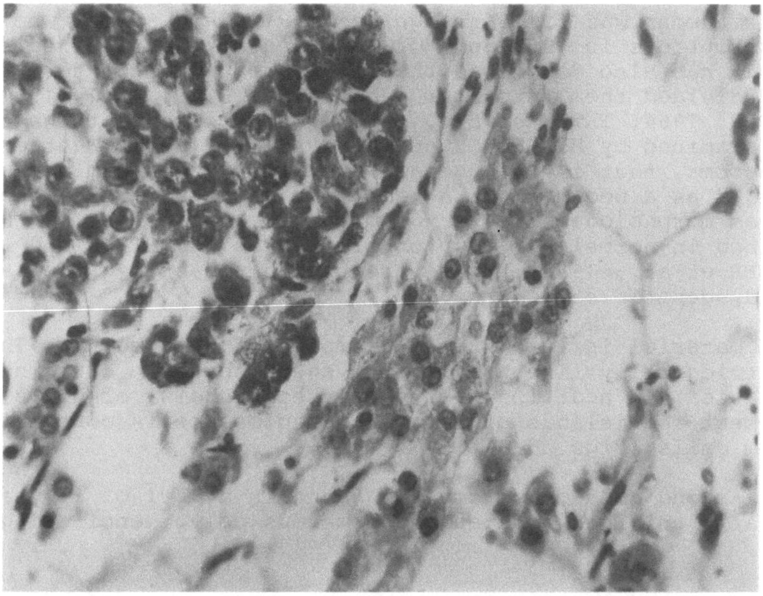

*Fig. 7. OTR.127 Atypical ovarian dysgerminoma. Tumour cells are seen on left. These have large nuclei and a little, illdefined cytoplasm. On right there is a group of Leydig-like cells, with smaller nuclei and abundant eosinophilic cytoplasm (H. & E. X 380)*

philic cells which might be of Leydig type (Fig. 7). The nuclei of the stromal cells were sex chromatin positive. SCULLY (1953) in his original paper noted that this was one of four tumours in the medical literature diagnosed morphologically as a dysgerminoma but appearing to produce sex hormones. In this case the excessive urinary gonadotrophin cannot have been of neoplastic origin since it did not immediately disappear after removal of the tumour. Probably, therefore, it arose in the pituitary. It is interesting to speculate on the nature of the stimulus which, presumably, arose in the tumour and whether the Leydig-like cells were primary constituents of the tumour or a reaction to pituitary hormones.

## Gonadoblastoma

The gonadoblastoma, which can arise in an abnormal testis as well as in a dysgenetic ovary, occurs most frequently in phenotypic females who often show virilization. Histologically, it is composed of two principal types of cell a) large cells like those of a dysgerminoma, and b) small cells of the granulosa-Sertoli cell type, but often the stroma contains a third type of cell resembling the Leydig cell. Calcified foci are often present. SCULLY (1970 a) describes three patterns in which these elements may be arranged. The Sertoli-granulosa like cells may surround the germ cells in a coronal fashion and may enclose rounded hyaline bodies (Fig. 13) or they may line the periphery of discrete nests occupied by germ cells. In some tumours the neoplastic foci may be circumscribed but in others the germ cells may spread out diffusely giving the appearance of a dysgerminoma. Occasionally, the tumour may present itself as a dysgerminoma with only a small focus of granulosa-Sertoli cell tissue to reveal its true nature.

This tumour was first recognised in 1953 by SCULLY who gave typical descriptions in 1963 and 1970 a and a comprehensive review in 1970 b. TETER has also described these tumours under the term "gonocytoma" and divided them into four subgroups (TETER, 1961, 1962; PHILIP and TETER, 1964; TETER et al., 1964). TETER's concepts have been critically examined by HUGHESDON and KUMARASAMY (1970). Whether a pure gonadoblastoma, that is one unassociated with a dysgerminoma, should be regarded as a neoplasm or a hamartoma remains an open question but structures morphologically very similar to gonadoblastomas have been described in normal and cryptorchid testes (HORSTEIN and HEDINGER, 1965; HUBER et al., 1968); these are probably best regarded as hypoplastic or dysgenetic structures.

Our material includes three examples of this tumour. The first appeared histologically like a typical dysgerminoma but contained foci of calcification. In addition groups of theca-lutein, or hilus, cells were present and islands of Sertoli-granulosa cells containing pale staining germ cells (Figs. 8-11).

The second gonadoblastoma was found in a girl of 14 years. She had a greatly enlarged abdomen and numerous polypi encircling the external

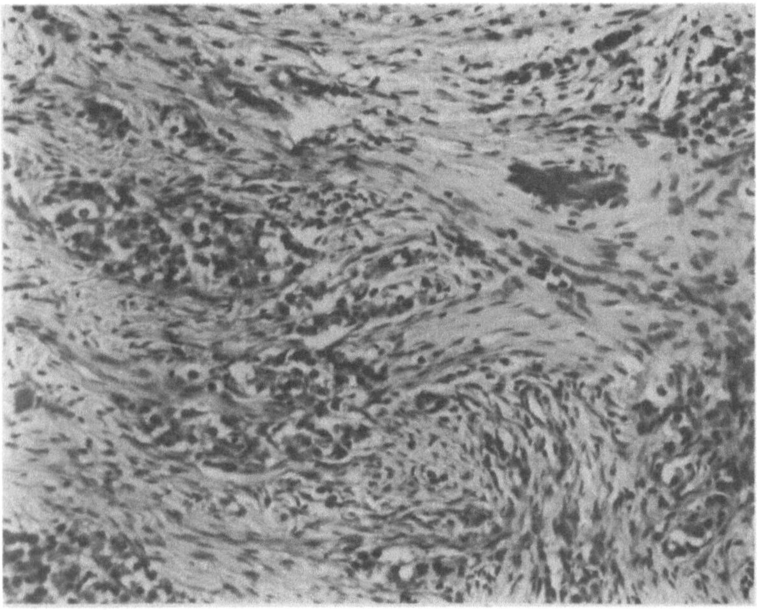

*Fig. 8. OTR.664 (By courtesy of Mr. A. C. MUIR and Dr. L.A.D. TOVEY). Gonadoblastoma showing groups of cells like those of a dysgerminoma embedded in dense connective tissue containing foci of calcification (H. & E. X 140)*

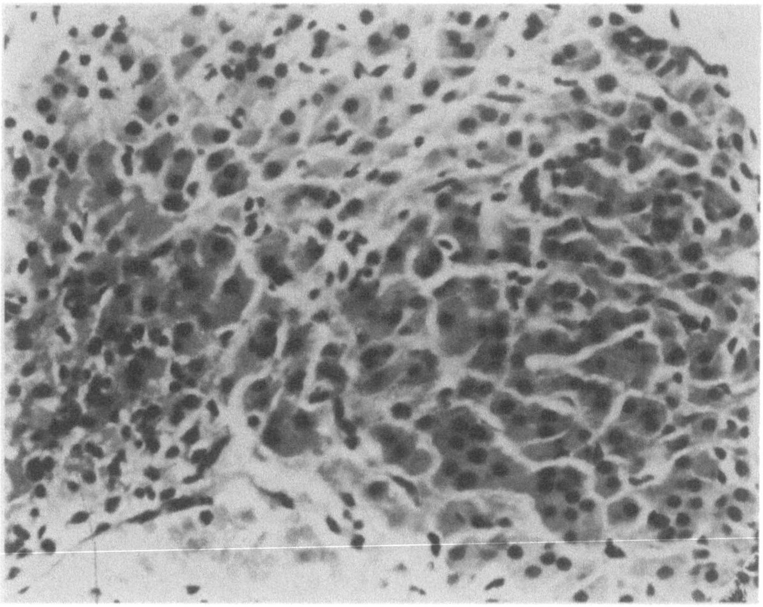

*Fig. 9. OTR.664 Groups of Leydig-like (Hilus) cells in a gonadoblastoma (H. & E. X 380)*

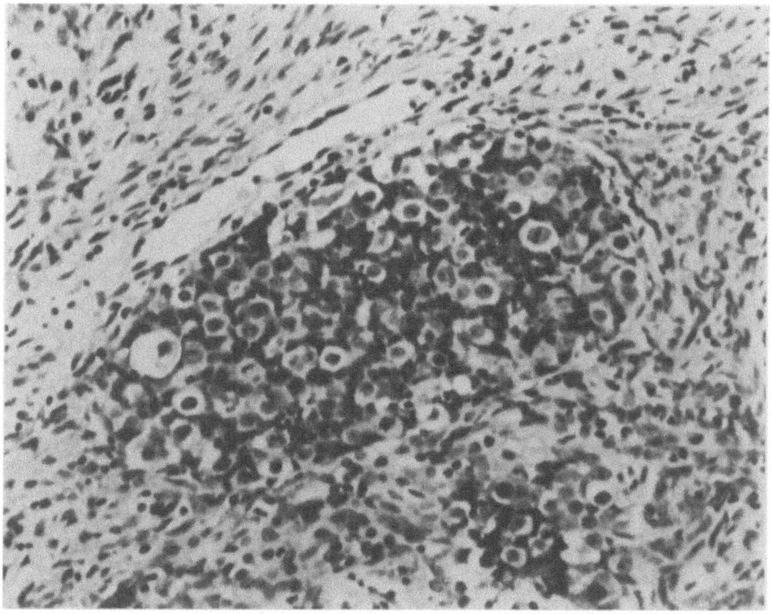

*Fig. 10. OTR.664 Gonadoblastoma showing a group of granulosa-like cells arranged round pale germinal cells (H. & E. X 240)*

cervical os. She died suddenly from a haemothorax resulting from a pulmonary metastasis. At necropsy the left ovary was found to be replaced by a large tumour (16 x 12 x 5 cms) which was freely mobile, well encapsulated, and not adherent. It was greyish, lobulated, and

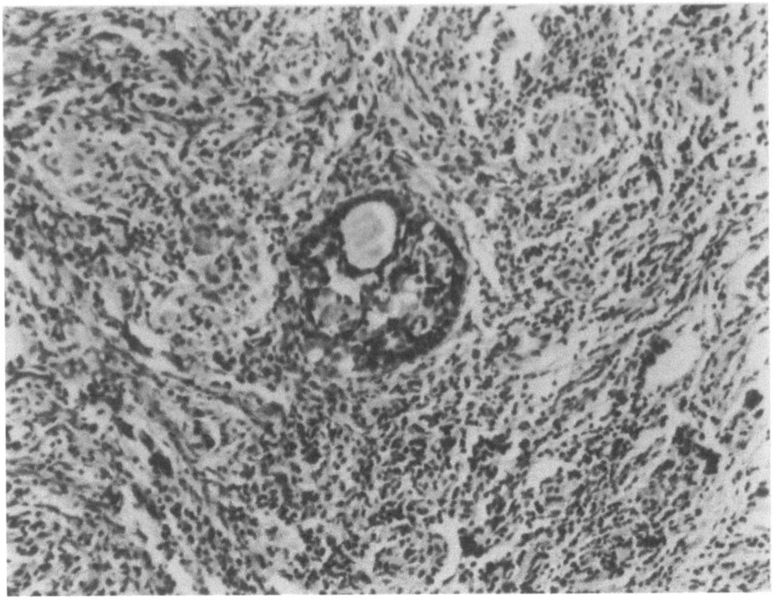

*Fig. 11. OTR.664 A group of cells similar to those in Fig. 10 in which the germinal cells are swollen and degenerate (H. & È. X 140)*

of rubbery consistency. Multiple haemorrhagic metastases were found in the lungs, liver, pancreas, and spleen. These were typical deposits of choriocarcinoma. No choriocarcinoma was found in the tumour itself, possibly because the search was not sufficiently extensive, but num-

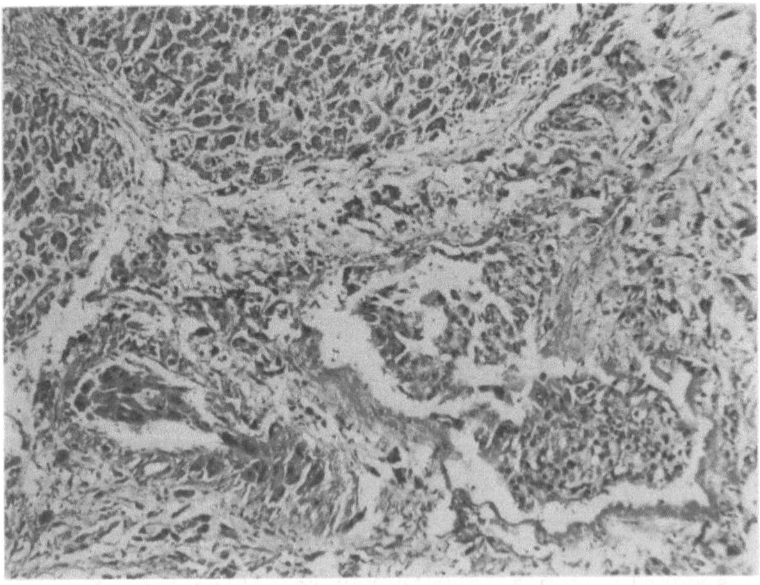

*Fig. 12. OTR.155 A metastasis in pancreas from a chorioncarcinoma of ovary. Pancreatic tissue is seen above and trophoblastic tissue in blood vessels in lower part of field (H. & E. X 75)*

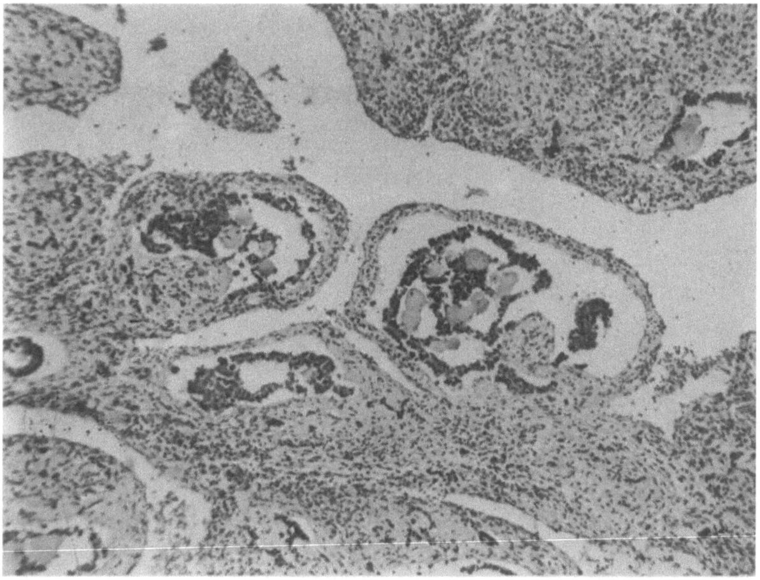

*Fig. 13. OTR.155 The ovarian tumour corresponding to Fig. 12. Structures are present similar to that in Fig. 11 (H. & E. X 75)*

erous structures were found resembling some seen in gonadoblastoma (Fig. 12, 13).

The third, referred to below, occurred in a girl of 16 years with an endodermal sinus (yolk sac) tumour in the contralateral ovary.

## Choriocarcinoma

This is a rare tumour which may occur in association with fairly well differentiated teratomas, dysgerminomas and seminomas, and other germ cell tumours. The present material includes only the 2 cases referred to above viz: one associated with a solid teratoma and the other with a gonadoblastoma.

## Endodermal Sinus (Yolk Sac) Tumours

This is a tumour which TEILUM (1959, 1965) has separated from the mesonephric tumours of the ovary with which it is often confused. It may occasionally occur in association with or form part of a teratoma, a dysgerminoma, a choriocarcinoma, or a gonadoblastoma. These associations together with its architecture which TEILUM (1971) regards as resembling extraembryonic structures such as extraembryonic mesoblast and yolk sac endoderm put it in the class of germ cell tumours. The histological appearances are: 1) a loose network of cystic spaces the meshes of which often contain hyaline, PAS positive globules, 2) a myxoid reticulum resembling the "magma reticulare", or extraembryonic mesoderm, of the exocoelum, 3) perivascular formations of endodermal sinus pattern, 4) cystic structures like yolk sac vesicles, and 5) aggregates of undifferentiated embryonal cells. Many of these features are illustrated in Figures 14 and 15. The perivascular formations and yolk sac structures occur in about two-thirds of the cases, the other features are present in almost all the tumours.

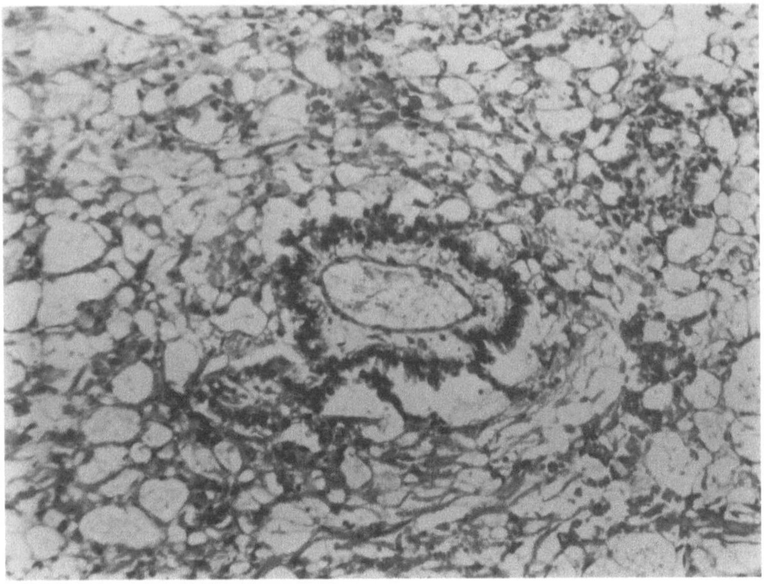

*Fig. 14. OTR.527 Endodermal sinus (yolk sac) tumour of ovary. Centrally there is a perivascular formation sourrounded by a loose vacuolated meshwork resembling the "magma reticulare" of the exocoelom. Compare with Fig. 4 (H. & E. X 120)*

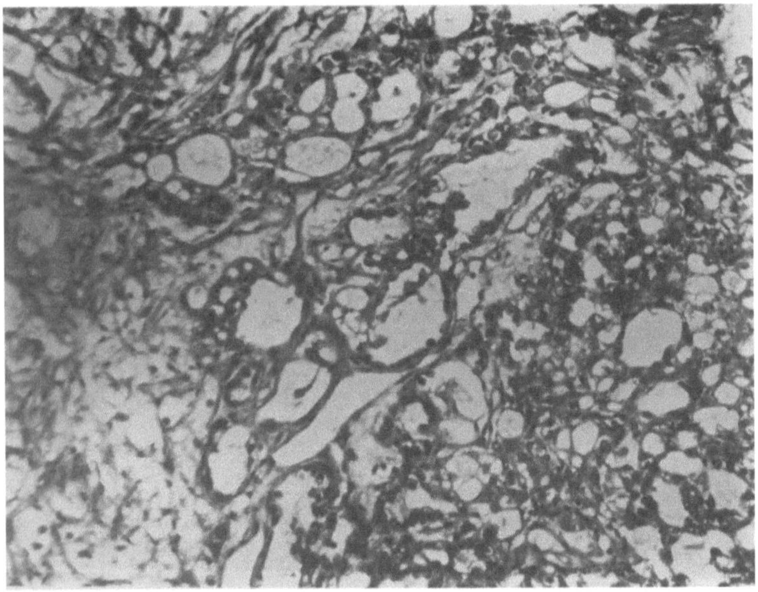

*Fig. 15. OTR.527 Endodermal sinus (yolk sac) tumour showing cysts lined by flat cells with protruding muclei. These cysts are thought to be equivalent to yolk sac vesicles of early embryo (H.&E. X 120)*

The age distribution of these tumours is of some importance since, as NORRIS and JENSEN (1972) point out, critical evaluation of "carcinomas" reported in premenarchial patients suggests that most have an endodermal sinus pattern erroneously considered to be of epithelial rather than of germ cell origin.

The Manchester series includes seven of these tumours one of which was associated with a gonadoblastoma in the contralateral "ovary". This series forms part of a larger group of 22 cases which are available for analysis. The age range of this group was from 6.5 to 35.0 years with a mean at 16 years. The clinical history is usually short (3-4 months). An abdominal mass was the presenting sign in a third of the girls, abdominal pain in about a quarter and in others nausea and vomiting, febrile attacks, menorrhagia, hirsutes, and amenorrhoea. The tumours had no predilection for either side. They were solid and varied in size from 8 to 22 cm in diameter; the outer surface was smooth and the cut surface showed necrosis, haemorrhages, and often gelatinous cysts. Sometimes there were adhesions to adjacent structures. In 1 case the tumour spread from the right to the left ovary and in 2 cases at necropsy pulmonary metastases were present. Surgery was the primary treatment in each case often supplemented by X-ray or chemotherapy. Of those followed up, all but 1 has died. The mean duration of survival of those who died was 4.5 months, the longest survival being 10 months.

BREEN and NEUBECKER (1967) stress that endodermal sinus tumours are the most lethal of all ovarian malignancies. However, 1 child treated by Dr. Martin Mott at the Bristol Royal Hospital for Sick Children has responded to intensive treatment and we are indebted to Dr. Mott for permission to publish an account of this case.

L. M., aged 9 years, attended hospital in February 1972 with anorexia and intermittent colicky abdominal pain. She was found to have an abdominal mass. Chest X-ray normal, IVP showed mild bilateral hydronephrosis. At laparotomy on 27th May 1972 a large tumour arising from the left ovary was removed by Professor A. Riddell, together with metastastic nodules on the sigmoid colon and posterior wall of the bladder. Histology showed this to be a mixed dysgerminoma-endodermal sinus tumour.

She was treated with abdominal radiotherapy 2600 rads in 4 weeks, vincristine 2 $mg/_{m}2$ weekly for 12 doses, actinomycin D 75 mcg/kg per 5 day course 3 monthly, and cyclophosphamide orally 2.5 mg/kg per day between actinomycin courses. Two further injections of vincristine were given on days 1 and 4 of each course of actinomycin which had to be reduced to 60 mcg/kg over 4 days because of profound thrombocytopenia. Other toxic side-effects have included alopecia, though hair regrowth is now largely complete, and hepatotoxicity manifested by raised liver enzymes after each course of actinomycin. Each course provoked a week's vomiting and did not settle with any antiemetic, but otherwise she attended school full-time, engaged in all normal activities, and height and weight progressed at a normal rate.

After 21 months therapy there was no evidence of disease. Treatment was therefore discontinued and 3 months later exploratory laparotomy was undertaken to look for residual disease. There was no evidence of disease macroscopically or on biopsy and serum $\alpha$-fetoprotein was negative.

Recently, $\alpha$-fetoprotein has been demonstrated in the serum of a patient with an endodermal sinus tumour (BALLAS, 1972) as well as in other cases of childhood malignancy (FINKLESTEIN et al., 1972) and we have also found it in the serum of 2 older patients with endodermal sinus tumours of the ovary. TEILUM et al. (1974) have identified $\alpha$-fetoprotein in the cells and in the hyaline droplets in a pure endodermal sinus tumour of the testis, suggesting that this protein is synthesized by the tumour cells.

Tumours of endodermal sinus pattern may occur elsewhere in the body in the sacrococcygeal region and vagina (see above) in the thorax (TEILMAN et al., 1967), and the pineal region (BESTLE, 1968). The "adenocarcinoma of the infant testis" (TEOH et al., 1960), the endodermal sinus tumour of the adult testis (TEILUM, 1971), and the orchioblastoma (BROWN, 1964) have a similar histological pattern to these tumours with only minor variations from case to case, and to that of the endodermal sinus tumour of the ovary and should therefore be considered to be of similar origin or nature.

## OTHER OVARIAN TUMOURS

Our material included 67 ovarian tumours, 45 of which were teratomas or related germ cell tumour (Table 1). Only one was an epithelial tumour, a papillary serous cystadenoma in a girl of 15 years. A number of workers have reported 1 or 2 cases of epithelial ovarian tumours in young girls (HUFFMAN, 1960; WILLIS, 1962) thus suggesting the rarity of these neoplasms. However, WITZBERGER and AGERTY (1937) found simple or multilocularcystadenomas in 32 percent of 186 ovarian tumours in children less than 10 years of age. GROEBER (1963), in a series of 220 such tumours in children under 15 years, found 8 percent to be epithelial. MOORE et al. (1967) found 19 epithelial tumours in 93 ovarian tumours in girls under 15 years and ABELL and HOLTZ (1965) found 28 percent of 188 ovarian tumours in girls under 20 years to be epithelial. NORRIS and JENSEN (1972) found that the incidence of epithelial tumours increased with the ages of the girls. In each of these studies a few of the tumours were regarded as malignant or showed borderline malignancy. FOX (1942) described a bilateral Brenner tumour in a girl of 5 years.

The term sex-cord stromal (or mesenchymal) tumours covers a range extending from granulosa cell tumours to androblastomas and including theca cell tumours. If the latter are androgenic they are commonly called arrhenoblastomas. Sex-cord stromal tumours constituted 18 percent of the series of ovarian tumours collected by NORRIS and JENSEN (1972).

### Granulosa-Theca Cell Tumours

Granulosa-theca cell tumours can occur at almost any age from infancy to the ninth decade. In a review of 250 such tumours VARANGOT (1937) found 12 in the first decade. Our material includes 7 examples in children, the youngest being 7 months old, and the oldest 17 years and all were premenarchial except this last girl. They most commonly presented with precocious puberty as in a child aged 16 months, who had episodic bleeding, her breasts were slightly enlarged, fine hair was visible over the pubis, she was tall for her age, and had a palpable abdominal mass arising from the pelvis. After removal of the tumour the signs regressed and a year later hormone assays (which had not been done previously) were normal for the age. In another girl, aged 10 years and 8 months, the presenting sign was abdominal swelling for several months before admission; concurrently she had an intermittent aching pain. Three weeks before admission a brown vaginal discharge appeared. A partly solid and partly cystic tumour was removed from the left ovary. Subsequently she developed normally. Both these tumours consisted of islands of granulosa cells surrounded by theca-like stroma. The thecal component of these tumours seems to be more conspicuous in young girls than in older women.

The following case presented a histological problem. The initial signs in this girl, aged 6 years, were enlargement of the breasts followed

4 months later by vaginal bleeding. At laparotomy the uterus was found to be the size of an adult, non-pregnant uterus, and there was a large cyst of the left ovary. The right ovary could not be found. Following removal of the ovarian cyst the breasts regressed and vaginal bleeding ceased. Subsequently she commenced to menstruate at the age of 14. The

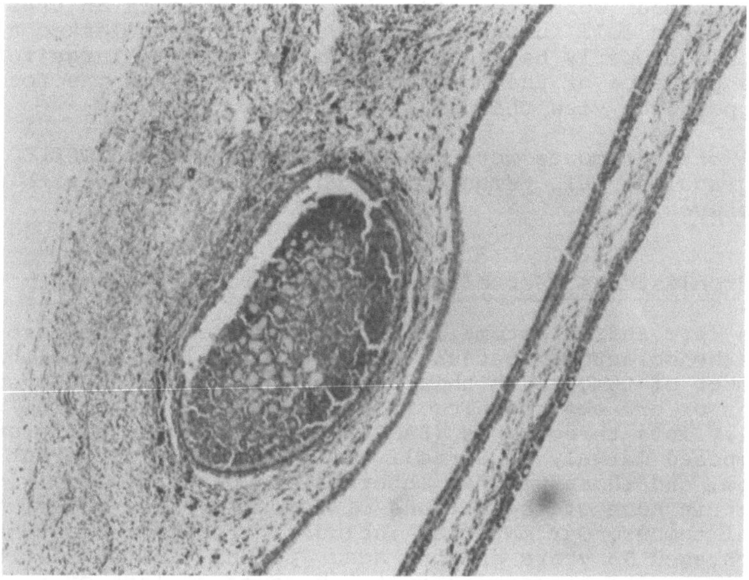

*Fig. 16. CTR.64/58 Granulosa cell tumour showing a cyst on right lined by granulosa cells. On left there is an island of granulosa cells containing numerous Call-Exner bodies (H. & E. X 50)*

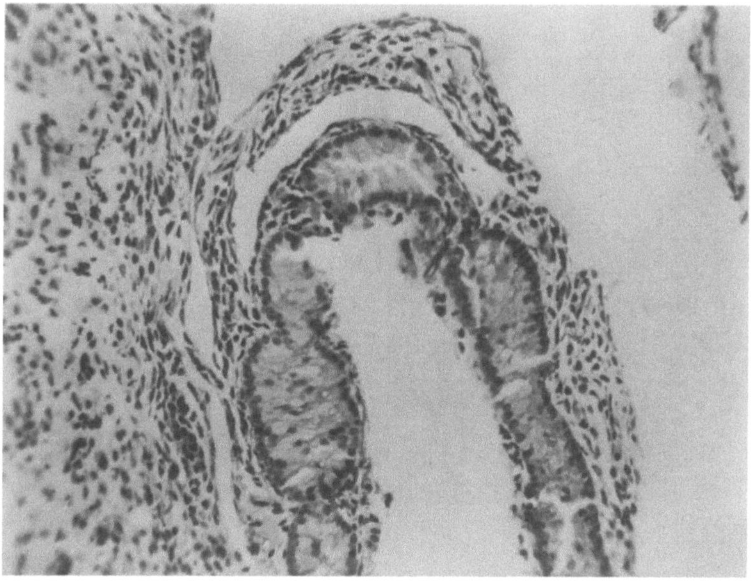

*Fig. 17. CTR.64/58 A small area of granulosa cell tumour containing tubular structures resembling those seen in Sertoli-cell tumours (H. & E. X 210)*

cyst was 8 cm in diameter and was composed of a number of locules 2 to 3 cm in diameter. The cysts were lined for the most part by columnar cells with basally situated nuclei but included numerous Call-Exner bodies. In places in the wall of the cyst more solid structures could be found (Fig. 16) which as they grew probably liquified centrally to form cysts. At one site tubular structures like those of a Sertoli cell tumour were also seen (Fig. 17). This is an unusual type of granulosa cell tumour and the question may be asked as to whether it should properly be regarded as a tumour or a large follicular cyst. The presence of the more solid structures and the focus of tubules support the view that it is a tumour.

All these tumours were benign but ANDERSON and SHELDON (1937) found a granulosa cell tumour, in a child of 3 years, with peritoneal metastases.

## Androblastomas (Sertoli-Leydig Cell Tumours)

The term androblastoma is to be preferred to the more commonly used "arrhenoblastoma" because the latter implies masculinization and a number of tumours in this category either have no overt hormonal function or are oestrogenic. It has been usual to divide them morphologically into three types (LANGLEY, 1954) - well differentiated tumours composed largely of Sertoli cells, a poorly differentiated sarcomatoid type, and those with an intermediate pattern. Leydig cells may be present in each of these types of tumour or they may form a pure Leydig cell tumour. Our material includes three androblastomas in two girls each aged 13 years and one aged 16. One girl of 13 presented a typical history. She attended hospital because of lack of breast development. Her voice had become deeper in tone during the previous 2 months and

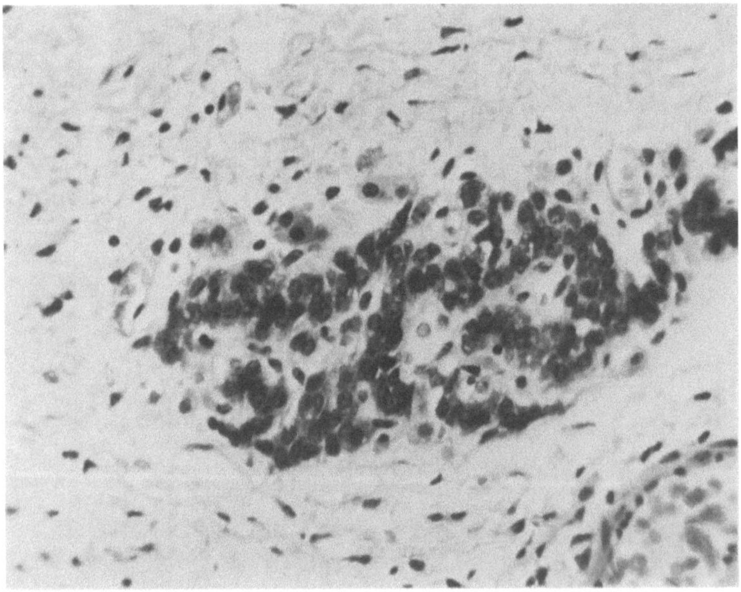

*Fig. 18. CTR.112/59 Androblastoma showing cords of rather dark cells with scanty cytoplasm. Round and intermingling with cords are cells with more abundant, eosinophilic cytoplasm and small, darker nuclei. They are Leydig-like cells (H. & E. X 120)*

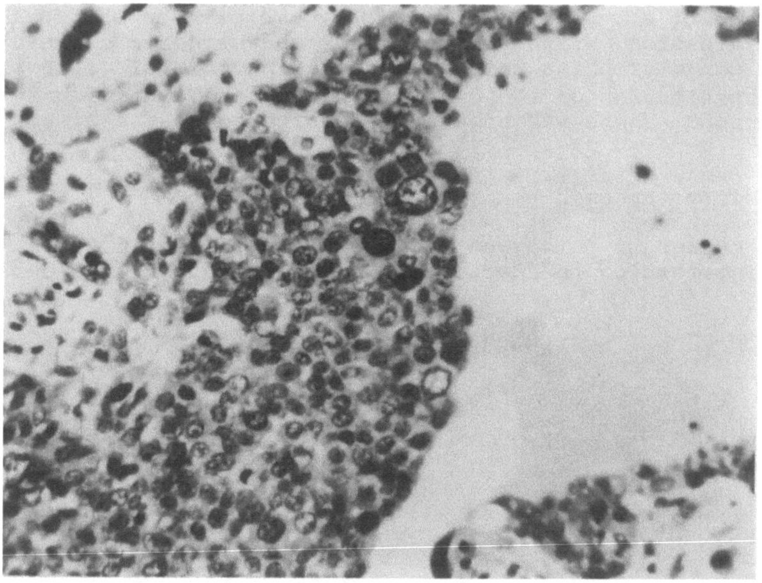

*Fig. 19. CTR.112/59 Androblastoma. Tumour cells lining one of the cystic spaces. The group is not compact and cells infiltrate adjacent stroma; there is marked nuclear pleomorphism (H. ( E. X 380)*

for 1 month abdominal swelling has been noticed. A cystic tumour about 20 cm in diameter was removed from the right ovary. Histologically, the tumour presented an intermediate pattern, cords of cells could be seen in an undifferentiated mesenchyme and occasionally groups of Leydig cells could be recognised (Fig. 18). An unusual feature was the presence of rather numerous cysts and the cells lining these often showed nuclear pleomorphism (Fig. 19). Despite this suggestion of malignancy she developed normally; she married 10 years later and was expecting her first child at the age of 24.

The second 13-year-old child showed no signs of virilism. The tumour in the 16-year-old girl contained a focus of cartilage. Heterotopic tissue has previously been described in such tumours by HUGHESDON and FRASER (1953) and by LANGLEY et al. (1972).

The Sertoli-Leydig cell tumour is more often clinically malignant than the granulosa cell tumour, but its rarity has made it difficult to estimate the malignant potential. The mortality rates cited in the literature vary from 10 to even 30 percent of cases (SCULLY, 1970 a).

## Lipoid Cell Tumours

These tumours form an ill-defined group; each tumour consisting of a single cell type which is often eosinophilic and commonly contains fat. They are usually associated with virilism but may be hormonally non-functioning. They may arise from luteinized theca or stromal cells, Leydig (hilus) cells, or from adrenal cortical rest cells. MORRIS and SCULLY (1958) referred to a Leydig cell tumour in a girl of 4 years. The 17-ketosteroid secretion fell after removal of the tumour.

We have seen bilateral tumours, microscopically similar to adrenal cortex in a girl of 16 years. The menarche occurred at the age of 13 years but she developed secondary amenorrhoea and features of masculinization. Urinary oxysteroids and oxygenic steroids were raised but gonadotrophins were low. Following removal of the tumours with reconstitution of the ovaries the steroid excretion fell and menses returned. There was however a recurrence at the age of 19 years.

Rhabdomyosarcomas

One tumour of this type was seen in a girl of 3 years (Fig. 20). It is interesting to speculate on its origin. In an older person it might

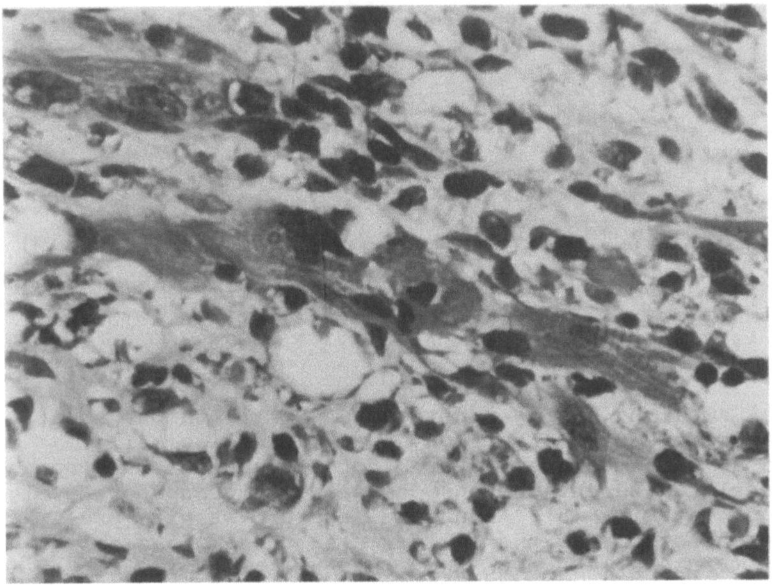

*Fig. 20. OTR.577 Rhabdomyosarcoma of ovary showing a striated muscle fibre (H. & E. X 630)*

have arisen in a focus of endometriosis but this seems unlikely at this age. Alternatively it might have arisen in a teratoma; there is no evidence of this in the tissue available which was relatively homogeneous. Nevertheless such a one-sided development of a teratoma is more likely.

Miscellaneous Tumours

Six malignant epithelial tumours in our collection were undiagnosable histologically. Each seemed to have a well-defined pattern which did not conform to any recognised type of ovarian carcinoma. ZIEGLER (1945) described bilateral ovarian carcinomas in a 30-week foetus. In parts the tumours resembled a granulosa cell tumour and in others a dysgerminoma. Opinions of a number of pathologists were sought but no firm diagnosis could be made. FORSHALL (1960) found three tumours of doubtful origin among eight non-teratoid tumours. These proportions are very similar to those of WITZBERGER and AGERTY (1937).

Disease of the reticuloendothelial system can occasionally affect the ovary although perhaps less frequently than the testis. Burkitt's lymphoma may involve the ovary in 75 percent of affected girls (WRIGHT, 1964). The Manchester Ovarian Tumour Register includes three cases of ovarian lymphoma in girls aged 15, 17, and 19 years. The first of these has been described in detail by SEED (1966). The second occurred in a Nigerian girl and a possible diagnosis of dysgerminoma was considered and rejected; in a few areas the "starry sky" appearance seen in Burkitt's tumour was seen. RAMACHANDRAN and GEORGE (1970) have described a similar case in a girl of 17 years and reviewed the literature. We found the ovary was also involved in one girl, aged 17 years, suffering from leukaemia.

## TESTICULAR TUMOURS

This account of tumours of the testis and its neighbouring structures is based on a study of material submitted during the period 1958-1973 to the Testicular Tumour Panel and Registry organised jointly by the Pathological Society of Great Britain and Ireland, The Cancer Research Campaign, and the Institute of Urology, London. Despite the rarity of testicular tumours in childhood which constituted only about 4% of the total number of tumours received, it has nevertheless been possible to collect clinical information and histological material from 127 cases of testicular neoplasm occurring in children up to the age of 15 years.

Table 5. Testicular tumours in children (Testicular tumour panel 1958-1973)

| | |
|---|---|
| Yolk sac tumour (Endodermal sinus tumours, orchioblastoma) | 53 |
| Paratesticular embryonic sarcoma | 27 |
| Differentiated teratoma | 21 |
| Malignant teratoma | 7 |
| Sertoli cell tumour | 6 |
| Seminoma | 4 |
| Malignant lymphoma | 4 |
| Miscellaneous | 5 |
| | 127 |

An analysis of these cases (Table 5) shows that three tumours - yolk sac tumour (endodermal sinus tumour), paratesticular embryonic sarcoma, and differentiated teratoma - make up the bulk of the material. Not only do these tumours account for about four-fifths of the total, but they are also extremely rarely encountered in older age-groups and can therefore be regarded as the characteristic testicular tumours of childhood. With few exceptions the other tumours listed did not differ in appearance or behaviour from similar tumours in adults. It is also interesting to observe that some types of tumour were not seen at all in children; for instance there were no examples of choriocarcinoma, interstitial cell tumour, or adenomatoid tumour in the children although numerous cases were found among the adults.

Yolk Sac Tumour (Endodermal Sinus Tumour, Orchioblastoma)

This, the commonest testicular tumour of childhood, has been described over the years under a number of different names. Following one of the earliest detailed descriptions by C. POWELL WHITE (1910) it was known for a long time as "adenocarcinoma of the infant testis" or "infantile adenocarcinoma of the testis", and was variously considered to arise from rete testis, efferent ducts, Muellerian remnants, or mesothelium, or to have a teratomatous origin, until suggestions were made (TEOH et al., 1960; WILLIS, 1962) that the tumour might have an origin from embryonic testicular tubules. By analogy with the nomenclature of other embryomas, the name orchioblastoma than began to become popular and was, in fact, used in the first edition of this book. Meanwhile, especially in the United States where the term "embryonal carcinoma" has long been popular, there arose a tendency to regard the childhood tumour as a variant of "embryonal carcinoma" and to describe it as "Embryonal carcinoma - infantile type". Gradually, however, it has become clear that these tumours of young boys are identical in histological appearance with certain ovarian tumours in girls, which, according to TEILUM (1959) arise from yolk-sac tissue and which he named Endodermal Sinus Tumour. Similar tumours can arise in the sacrococcygeal region and the mediastinum where yet another term - Mesoblastoma vitellinum - has been used (TEILMAN et al., 1967). The histogenesis of the tumour is discussed more fully in the section on tumours of the ovary and we are here concerned only with finding a suitable name for the tumour when it occurs in the testis. In spite of its slight illogicality, since no structure equivalent to the endodermal sinus of the rat seems to occur in the human placenta, the name Endodermal Sinus Tumour

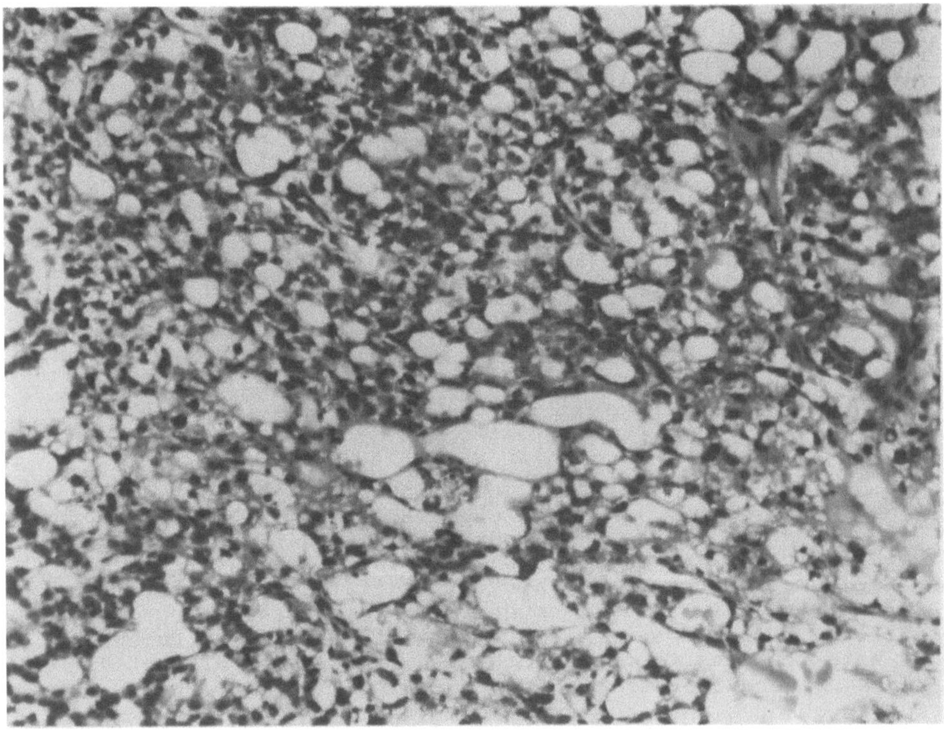

*Fig. 21. Yolk sac tumour (Endodermal sinus tumour) of testis. The pattern is that of a tubular adenocarcinoma (H. & E. X 100)*

has gained wide acceptance but the simpler term Yolk Sac Tumour has much to commend it and will be used here. Certainly, if we accept that the tumour arises from extraembryonic tissue, then any name implying an embryomatous origin, such as embryonal carcinoma or orchioblastoma, should be discarded.

Yolk sac tumour in the testis occurs in infants and young children and grows rapidly. One was found in a stillborn foetus of 39 weeks gestation and in 2 other children the tumour was noticed at birth. Of the remainder, the youngest boy was aged 2 months and the oldest 5 1/2 years when the tumour was first discovered, the mean age of presentation being 17 months. The length of time between discovery of the tumour and orchiectomy varied from a few days to 2 years, the mean being 3 months. All the tumours were unilateral and most presented as painless testicular swellings.

In gross appearance, the tumour is yellow or white and unencapsulated, replacing most of the testis and sometimes invading the epididymis and other neighbouring structures. Its texture may be firm or soft and there may be cystic or haemorrhagic areas.

Histologically (Figs. 21 and 22) it resembles a mucus-secreting adenocarcinoma composed of rounded or irregular acinar spaces and channels lined by cuboidal, columnar, or often flattened cells, one or two layers thick, and separated by a loose delicate mesenchymal stroma which may be very scanty. The epithelial cells are often vacuolated and frequently have ill-defined free borders due to active mucus secretion. Accu-

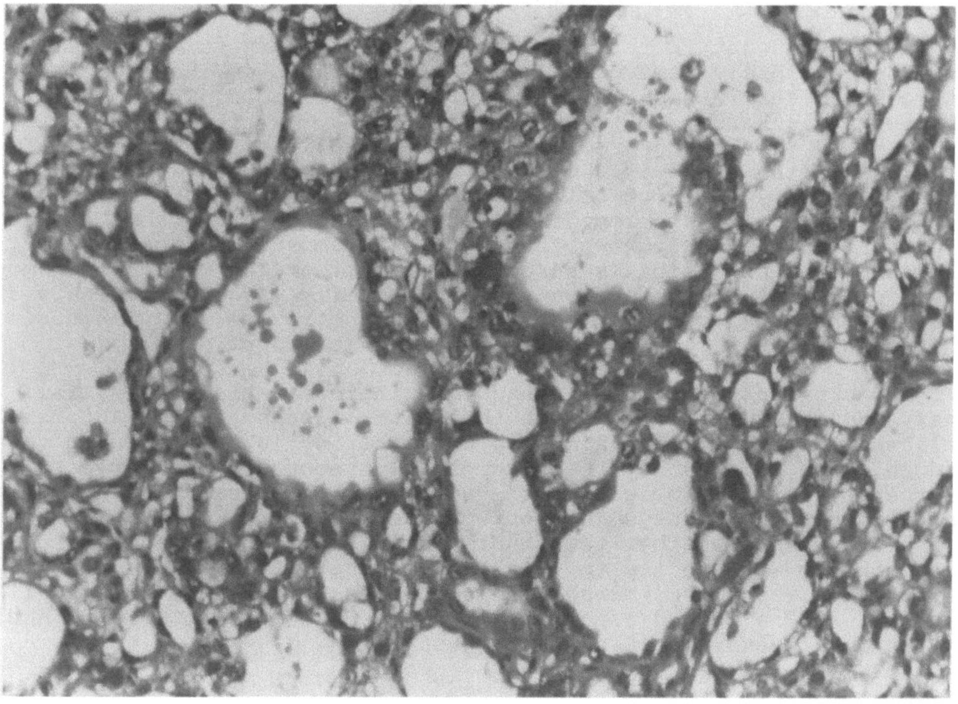

*Fig. 22. Yolk sac tumour (Endodermal sinus tumour) of testis. Irregular acini are lined by mucus-secreting cells and show cystic dilatation. Pools of mucin are also present in rather scanty mesenchymal stroma (H. & E. X 200)*

mulation of mucin may form cystic spaces and pools of mucin may be seen in the stroma. There may be papillary areas and perivascular collections of epithelial cells are frequently seen. There may also be sheets and meshworks of undifferentiated cells. Degenerative areas may be seen, but large areas of necrosis are uncommon. Mitotic figures are fairly frequent. The histological pattern is consistent throughout the tumour - in sharp contrast to the variations in structure found in a teratoma. Evidence of lymphatic invasion was found in about one-fifth of the tumours.

## Clinical Management

It is very difficult to be certain about the best methods of treating boys with this tumour because of its rarity. However certain conclusions can be drawn from the cases referred to the Testicular Tumour Panel and also those included in the Manchester Registry and treated at the Christie Hospital. All the 52 boys whose tumours were sent to the Testicular Tumour Panel were treated by orchidectomy. Only one was given postoperative radiotherapy; he is alive and well 17 years later. Seven more were given radiotherapy on the appearance of metastases; 6 of these died; 1 recent case still survives. Thirteen of the 52 children died 2-24 months after orchidectomy (mean 9 months), all with widespread metastases - to lungs, lymph nodes, liver, and peritoneum. Twelve are alive and well more than 5 years later and 5 of these children have survived for more than 10 years. Nine are alive and well 2-5 years after orchidectomy; 2 are well after less than 2 years; 2 are alive but have shown signs of metastasis within a year of operation and 13 have been lost to follow-up.

There seems no doubt therefore that when the primary tumour is small, it can be completely removed by orchidectomy which is the only treatment required and in such cases the prognosis is good. The role of radiotherapy is harder to assess. There is only 1 surviving child amongst those treated for recurrent or metastatic disease at the Chirstie Hospital. However the tumours of most of those who died responded initially to irradiation. Therefore, X-ray therapy may have some value if it is used immediately postoperatively in those cases where there is doubt about whether surgical removal was complete or where abdominal extension is suspected or proved. The value of chemotherapy cannot be assessed from the Manchester cases but in line with adult malignant teratomas actinomycin D, methotrexate, or vinblastine, either singly or in combination, may have some effect.

The most important aspects of management therefore are the initial surgery and careful investigation to exclude disease in the abdomen or elsewhere so that irradiation or chemotherapy is not given to those children whose tumours have been completely removed by surgery. If radiotherapy needs to be given, the abdominal lymph nodes should be irradiated but the kidneys left out of the treatment volume. It is not possible to assess whether the other testis should be irradiated and it is probably wise to try to shield it so that later development is not impaired. The volume irradiated should take in the groins and iliac fossae as well as the para-aortic nodes and a dose of 3000 rads should be given in 4 weeks with megavoltage radiation.

## Paratesticular Embryonic Sarcoma

The subject of embryonic sarcomas has been considered in Chapter 9. Such sarcomas of the testicular region occur throughout childhood and adolescence. The youngest child in this series was aged 1 year and the oldest 15 years, with a mean age of 7 years, but a few cases have also been seen in young adults just outside the age range being considered here. They were all unilateral and mostly appeared to arise in the spermatic cord, but since they tend early to invade the testis, epididymis, and other structures, the precise site of origin cannot always be determined; the tumour may be found attached to the tunica vaginalis.

To the naked eye the tumour is a white, yellow-brown, or pink mass, often with areas of necrosis and haemorrhage and sometimes presenting a myxoid appearance. It may reach a very large size. The histological structure is variable (Fig. 23). It is commonly composed of sheets of pleomorphic spindle-shaped polygonal, ovoid, or strap-like cells with fairly abundant eosinophilic cytoplasm. It may, however, be predominantly round-celled or composed of stellate cells with a myxomatous stroma. Longitudinal and cross-striations may be demonstrable in some cells but this feature may be absent. Nevertheless, these neoplasms are considered to be fundamentally rhabdomyosarcomatous in nature.

These tumours grow rapidly and tend to metastasize early and widely. Of the 27 children with these sarcomas, 12 died - all but 1 within 2 years and several in a few months. Four were alive and well between 2 and 5 years after operation and 5 had survived in good health for more than 5 years - one for 14 years. Five were lost to follow-up, but one of these was known to be showing signs of metastasis after 7 months. All were given postoperative radiotherapy. Despite the almost 50% mortality rate the prognosis is not entirely hopeless and it is

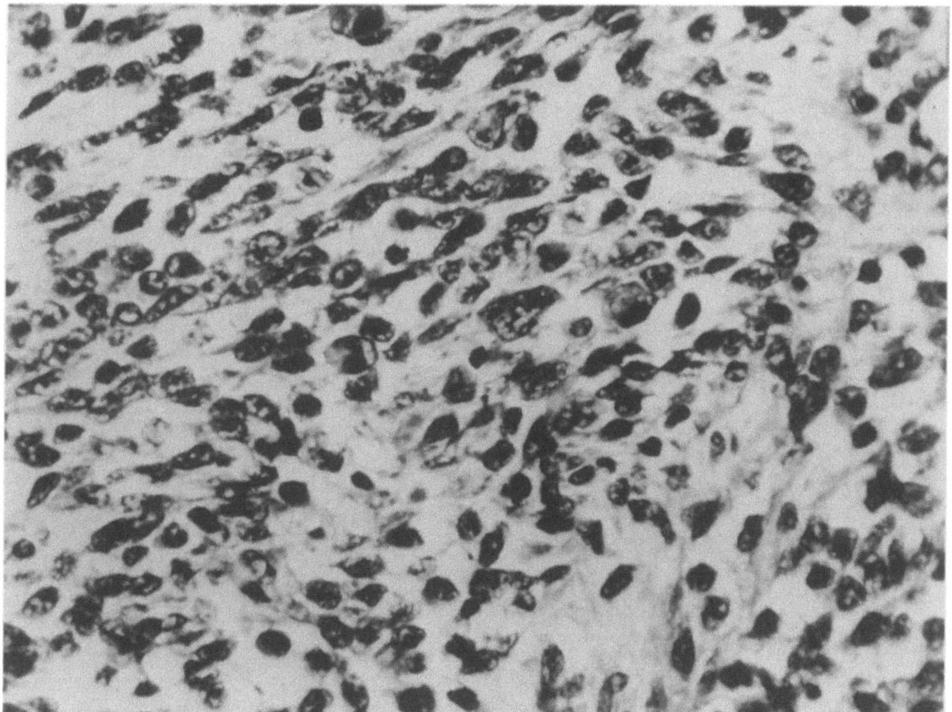

*Fig. 23. Paratesticular embryonic sarcoma. A pleomorphic sarcoma with round, ovoid, and spindle cells. Cytoplasm, which may be abundant, is eosinophilic (H. & E. X 325)*

encouraging that at least a third of the boys appear to be making promising progress.

## Testicular Teratomas

The Testicular Tumour Panel classifies testicular teratomas as:

1. Differentiated (TD) - composed of fully differentiated tissues or sometimes containing also tissues of immature, but not malignant, appearance.

2. Malignant, intermediate (MTI) - some organoid tissue present but also areas showing histological evidence of malignancy ("Terato-carcinoma" of other authors)

3. Malignant, undifferentiated (MTU) - either completely anaplastic or showing differentiation only into simple columnar or cuboidal epithelium (roughly corresponding to "embryonal carcinoma" of other authors).

4. Malignant, trophoblastic (MTT) - any teratoma containing true trophoblastic elements.

Of the 28 testicular teratomas of children studied by the Panel, three-quarters (21) were of the differentiated type (TD). These well-defined solid or cystic masses in the testis were composed of a variety of

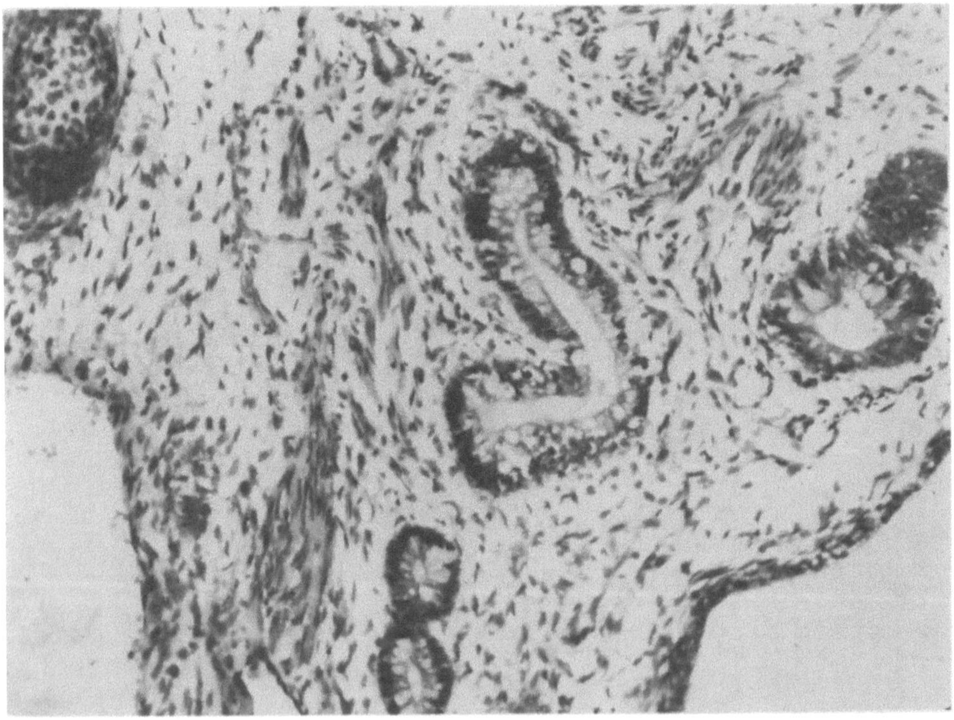

*Fig. 24. Differentiated teratoma of testis. Various types of epithelium, glandular structures, and connective tissue are present (H. & E. X 200)*

well-differentiated organoid tissues such as squamous and other epithelia, simple glandular structures, bone, cartilage and fibrous and adipose tissue, a careful search of many sections revealing no tissue which could be regarded as showing any histological evidence of malignancy. In this connection we have learned that tissues which have an immature, imperfectly formed, or atypical appearance should not necessarily be regarded as indicative of malignancy when seen in tumours of young children, their presence being merely a manifestation of immaturity

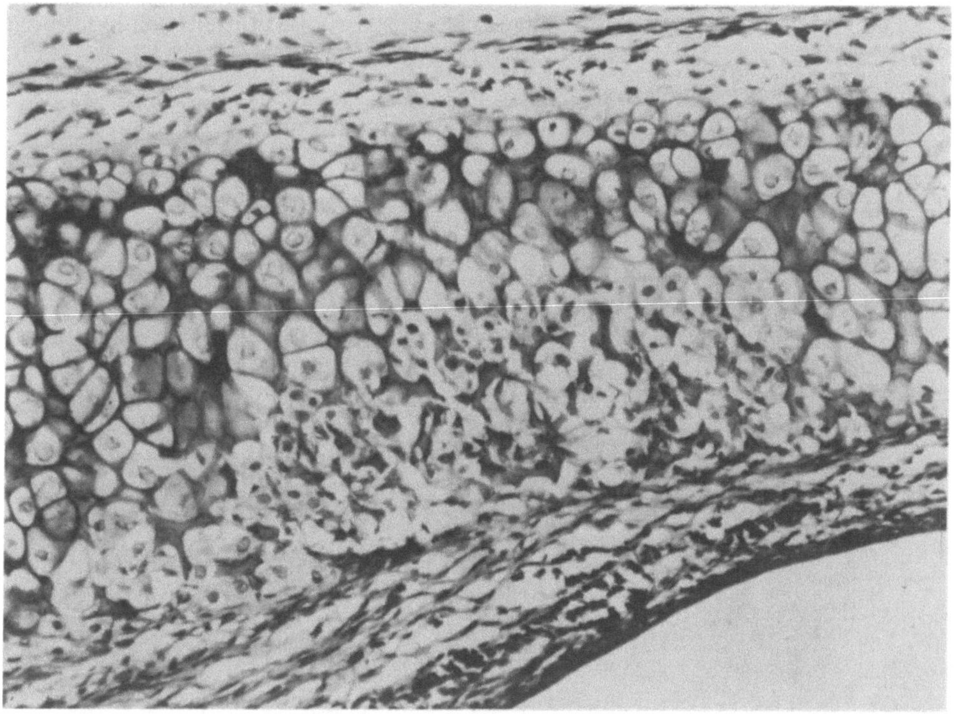

*Fig. 25. Teratoma of testis. Atypical or "immature" cartilage (H. & E. X 200)*

of tissue. This applies not only to epithelial but also mesenchymal tissues (Fig. 25). It is not always easy to make this distinction between "immature" and "malignant" tissue but it is important to attempt to do so. These differentiated teratomas occurred in children aged 3 months to 10 years (mean age 2 1/2 years) and in all the cases simple orchidectomy appears to have provided a complete cure. It is interesting that differentiated teratomas behaving in this benign manner seem to occur almost exclusively in children, virtually all the teratomas in adults being malignant; this is the reverse of the behaviour of most ovarian teratomas.

Six of the testicular teratomas in children were classified as of intermediate type (MTI). With one exception these were all in older boys aged 6 - 14 years (mean 12 years). Two (both aged 14 years) died within 18 months of orchidectomy; the others were alive and well after 10 years, 11 years, and 1 year. One tumour in a two-year-old patient deserves special mention as most of its structure was that of yolk sac tumour but it was placed in the teratoma group on account of the presence of a good deal of smooth muscle. This child died a year after operation but it could be that the youth of the patient and the bad prognosis were more the features of yolk sac tumour than of teratoma.

The remaining teratoma was classified in the undifferentiated group (MTU). This tumour occurred in a 15-year-old lad - on the very verge of adulthood - who died 1 month after operation with widespread metastases.

From our experience, therefore, it would seem that the majority of testicular teratomas in children behave in a benign manner and that it is only after the age of 12 - 14 years that a few malignant cases begin to creep in.

## Seminoma

The gross and histological features (Fig. 26) of this tumour in childhood are in no way different from the well-known pattern seen in adults.

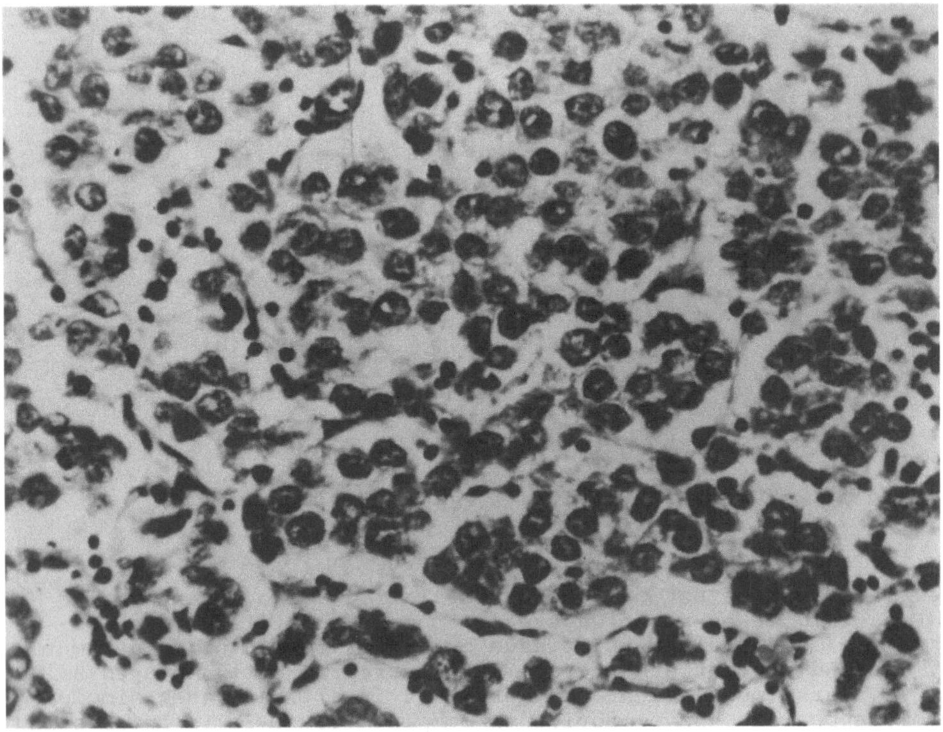

*Fig. 26. Seminoma. Clear cells with rounded nuclei and prominent nucleoli. Contrast with Fig. 28 (H. & E. X 375)*

The interest lies in the youth of some of the patients. It has commonly been believed that seminoma does not occur before puberty but this appears to be untrue. The youngest patient in the series was aged 7 years. Not only is this well before the usual age of puberty but the tubules in the residual normal testis had a typical prepubertal appearance. The ages of the other patients were 12, 13, and 15 years. In the 12-year-old the affected testis was undescended. All were given postoperative radiotherapy. Three were alive and well after 6, 7, and 10 years; the fourth was lost to follow-up.

## Sertoli Cell Tumour

Of the 6 cases observed, the youngest was aged 2 months and the oldest 9 years (mean age 5 years). The tumour was usually a firm, well-defined whitish mass within the testis. Histologically, although the picture is variable, a careful search always revealed in some part of the tu-

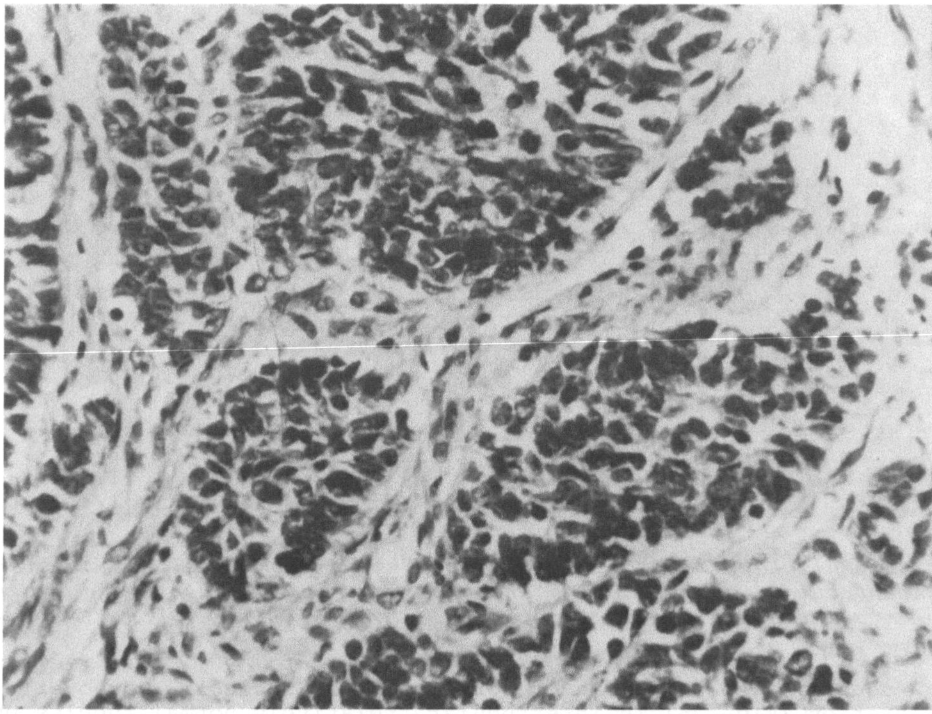

*Fig. 27. Sertoli cell tumour. Note tubular pattern with radially arranged Sertoli cells (H. & E. X 375)*

mour a tubular pattern (Fig. 27) with radially arranged cells having the appearance of Sertoli cells. The tumour grows slowly and usually behaves in a benign manner. Four of the patients were alive and well 2-10 years after operation. One was lost to follow-up and the other, who presented with gynaecomastia, recently had a recurrence of that condition about 2 years after operation.

## Malignant Lymphoma

Lymphomatous infiltration of the testis is usually a manifestation of generalised lymphomatous disease and this may present as a testicular tumour. The youngest patient was aged 1 year and the oldest 12 years although the disease is seen at all ages and is not uncommon in the elderly. Although the panel does not classify lymphomatous disease more precisely than "malignant lymphoma", the pattern in the children most closely resembled reticulum cell sarcoma. The histological appearance may be confused with seminoma but a close study of the cells shows them to have less cytoplasm than seminoma cells and darkly staining irregular compact nuclei quite unlike the round vesicular nucleus of the seminoma

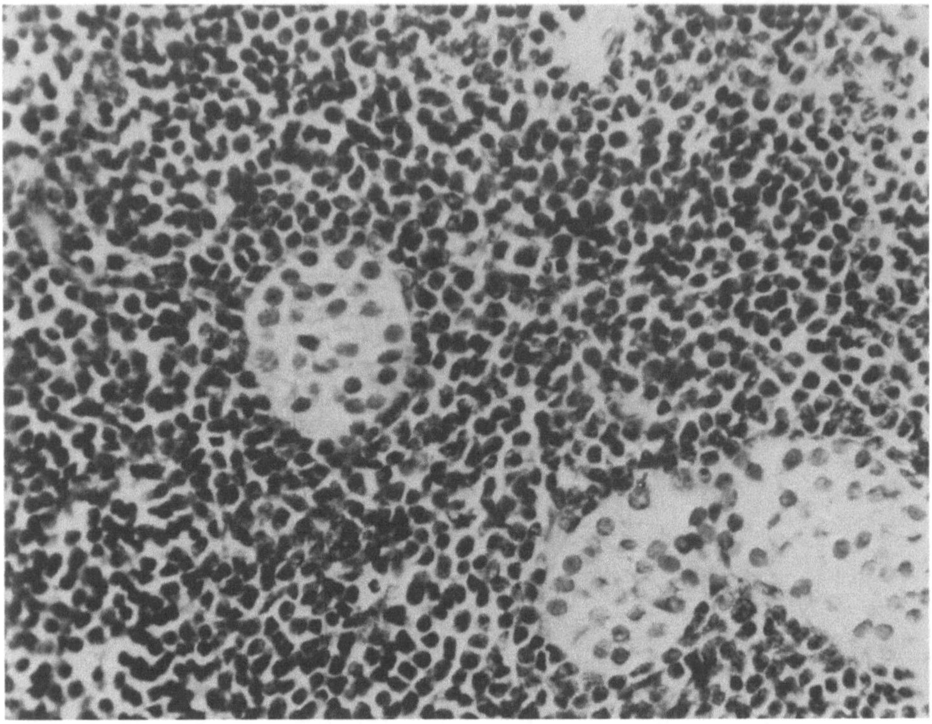

*Fig. 28. Malignant lmyphoma of testis. The lymphomatous infiltration is intertubular, tubules being preserved. Nuclei are dense and hyperchromatic and cytoplasm is scanty (H. & E. X 375)*

which usually also shows one or more prominent nucleoli. Moreover, the infiltration (Fig. 28) is intertubular, relatively normal tubules being seen widely separated by lymphoid tissue. The behaviour and prognosis are those of lymphomatous disease in general.

## Miscellaneous Tumours

There were two paratesticular sarcomas whose histological patterns were different from that of the embryonic rhabdomyosarcoma described above: one, diagnosed fibrosarcoma, had been removed from a baby aged 7 months who was known to be alive and well 25 years later, the other, regarded as a neurofibrosarcoma, came from a boy aged 3 years whose fate is unknown. From the spermatic cord of a 2-year-old child came a neuroblastoma, regarded as metastatic; the patient died of neuroblastoma 3 months later. An unusual tumour in an African boy aged 9 months consisted almost entirely of pigmented retinoblastic tissue and was regarded as a retinal anlage tumour; there was no follow-up. There was also a tumour of a dysgenetic testis - a subject fully discussed by COLLINS and SYMINGTON (1964).

## REFERENCES

ABELL, M. R., HOLTZ, F.: Am. J. Obstet. Gynec. 93, 850 (1965)

ANDERSON, M. X., SHELDON, E. A.: Am. J. Obstet. Gynec. 34, 119 (1937)

ANDERSON, W.A.D., DMYTRYK, E. T.: Am. J. Path. 22, 337 (1946)

ASKANAZY, M.: Verhandl. deutsch. path. Gesellsch. 11, 39 (1907)

BALARD, P.: J. med. Bordeaux 95, 1063 (1923)

BALE, G. F.: Am. J. Path. 26, 565 (1950)

BALLAS, M.: Am. J. Clin. Path. 57, 511 (1972)

BAUGH, C. D., O'DONOGHUE, R. T.: Arch. Dis. Childh. 30, 396 (1955)

BENTLEY, J. F. R., SMITH, J. R.: Arch. Dis. Childh. 35, 76 (1960)

BERRY, C. L., KEELING, J., HILTON, C.: J. Path. 98, 214 (1969)

BESTLE, J.: Acta path. microbiol. scand. 74, 214 (1968)

BODIAN, M., WHITE, L. L. R.: Great Ormond St. Journ. 4, 105 (1952)

BREEN, J. F., NEUBECKER, R. D.: Ann. N. Y. Acad. Science 142, 658 (1967)

BREMER, J. L.: Congenital Abnormalities of the Viscera. Cambridge, USA: Havard Univ. Press, 1957

BROWN, N. J.: Miscellaneous tumours of mainly epithelial type. In: The pathology of Testicular Tumours. D. H. COLLINS and R.C.B. PUGH (eds.). Edinburgh: Livingstone, 1964, p. 70

BUDDE, M.: Beitr. path. Anat. 75, 357 (1926)

CAMERON, A. H.: J. Path. Bact. 73, 213 (1957)

CLAIREAUX, A. E.: J. Path. Bact. 63, 743 (1951)

CLAY, R. D., SHORTER, R. G.: J. Path. Bact. 74, 162 (1957)

COLLINS, D. H., PUGH, R. C. B. (eds.): Pathology of Testicular Tumours. Edinburgh and London: Livingstone, and Supplement Brit. J. Urol. 36, (1964)

COLLINS, D. H., SYMINGTON, T.: Ibid, 57 (1964)

COSTIN, M. E., KENNEDY, R. L. J.: Amer. J. Dis. Child. 76, 127 (1948)

DAYAN, A. D., MARSHALL, A. H. E., MILLER, A. A., PICK, E. J., RANKIN, N. E.: J. Path. Bact. 92, 1 (1966)

DE CHÂTEL, A., cited by WILLIAMS, G. E. G.: Frankfurt. Z. Path. 44, 426 (1932 - 33)

DEWHURST, C. J., FERREIRA, H. P., GILLETT,.P. G.: J. Obstet. Gynec. Brit. Cwlth. 78, 1077 (1971)

FATHALLA, M. F., RASHAD, M. N., KERR, M. G.: J. Obstet. Gynaec. Brit. Cwlth 73, 812 (1966)

FINKLESTEIN, J. Z., HIGGINS, G. R., FAUST, J., KARON, M.: Cancer 30, 80 (1972)

FETTIG, O., SCHRÖTER, R., WOLF, U., SCHNEIDER, J.: Archiv. f. Gynäk. 205, 309 (1968)

FORSHALL, I.: Arch. Dis. Childh. 35, 17 (1960)

FOX, H., BUTLER-MANUEL, R.: J. Path. Bact. 88, 137 (1964)

FOX, R. A.: Amer. J. Path. 18, 223 (1942)

FUJIKURA, T., WELLINGS, S. R.: Amer. J. Obstet. Gynec. 89, 824 (1964)

GALTON, M., BENIRSCHKE, K.: Lancet 2, 761 (1959)

GORDON, A.: J. Path. Bact. 85, 441 (1963)

GROEBER, W. R.: Amer. J. Obstet. Gynec. 86, 1027 (1963)

GROSS, R. E., CLATWORTHY, H. W., MECKER, I. A.: Surg. Gynec. Obstet. 92, 341 (1951)

HAIN, A. M.: J. Clin. Endocrin. 9, 1349 (1949)

HANSMAN, G. H., BERNE, C. J.: Arch. Surg. 25, 1090 (1932)

HERBST, A. L., SULLY, R. E.: Cancer 25, 745 (1970)

HORSTEIN, B. U., HEDINGER, C.: Virchows Arch. path. Anat. 339, 83 (1965)

HUBER, R., WEBER, E., HEDINGER, C.: Virchows Arch. Abt. A. Path. Anat. 344, 40 (1968)

HUFFMAN, J. W.: Cancer and Allied Disease of Infancy and Childhood. I. M. ARIEL, G. T. PACK (eds.). London: Churchill, 1960, p. 234

HUGHESDON, P. E., FRASER, I. T.: Acta. obstet. gynec. scand. 32, Suppl. 4 (1953)

HUGHESDON, P. E., KUMARASAMY, T.: Virchows Arch. Abt. A. Path. Anat. 349, 258 (1970)

HUNTINGTON, R. W., MORGENSTERN, N. L., SARGENT, J. A., GIEM, R. N., RICHARDS, A., HANFORD, K. C.: Cancer 16, 34 (1963)

JONES, H. W., SCOTT, W. W.: Hermaphroditism, Genital Anomalies and Related Endocrine Disorders. Baltimore: Williams and Wilkins, 1971

KEEN, W. W., COPLIN, W. M. L.: Tr. Coll. Phys. Phila. 3s, 28, 197 (1906)

KIDDER, L. A.: Arch. Path. 49, 55 (1950)

KNIGHT, G., GRIFFITHS, T., WILLIAMS, I.: Brit. J. Surg. 42, 635 (1954-55)

KOOS, W. T., MILLER, M. H.: Intracranial Tumours of Infants and Children. Stuttgart: Thieme, 1971

KREYBERG, L.: J. Path. Bact. 75, 109 (1958)

LANGLEY, F. A.: J. clin. path. 7, 10 (1954)

LANGLEY, F. A., CUMMINS, P. A., FOX, H.: Acta path. microbiol. scand. Section A, 80, Suppl. 233, 76 (1972)

LEIGHTON, J., HURST, J. W., CRAWFORD, J. D.: Arch. Path. 50, 632 (1950)

LINDER, D., POWER, J.: Ann. hum. Genet. 34, 21 (1970)

LINDER, D., KAISER, B., HECHT, F.: New Eng. J. Med. 292, 63 (1975)

LYNN, J. A., VARON, H. H., KINGSLEY, W. B., MARTIN, J. H.: Amer. J. Path. 51, 639 (1967)

MAGNER, D., CAMPBELL, J. S., WIGLESWORTH, F. W.: Cancer 9, 165 (1956)

MOORE, J. C., SCHIFRIN, B. S., EREZ, S.: Am. J. Obst. Gynec. 99, 913 (1967)

MORISON, J. E.: Foetal and Neonatal Pathology, 2nd ed. London: Butterworth, 1963, p. 298

MORRIS, J. M., SCULLY, R. E.: The Endocrine Pathology of the Ovary. London: Kimpton, 1958

NICHOLSON, G. W. de P.: Studies on Tumour Formation. London: Butterworth, 1950

NORRIS, J. H., JENSEN, R. D.: Cancer 30, 713 (1972)

OVERBECK, L., PHILIP, E.: Z. Geburtsch. Gynäk. 170, 125 (1969)

PHILIP, J., TETER, S.: Acta path. microbiol. scand. 61, 543 (1964)

POTTER, E. L.: Pathology of the Fetus and Infant, 2nd ed. Chicago: Year Book Publishers, 1961, p. 189

POUND, A. W., WILLIS, R. A.: J. Path. 98, 111 (1969)

RAMACHANDRAN, P., GEORGE, G.: The Indian Journal of Cancer 7, 143 (1970)

REGISTRAR GENERAL, Statistical Review for England and Wales for 1967 Part II. London: H.M.S.O., p. 145

RHANEY, K., BARCLAY, G. P. T.: J. Path. Bact. 77, 457 (1959)

ROBBOY, S. J., SCULLY, R. E.: Human Pathology 1, 613 (1970)

RUSSELL, D. S., RUBINSTEIN, L. J.: Pathology of Tumours of the Nervous System, 2nd ed. London: Arnold, 1963, Chaps. 2, 7

SAPHIR, O.: Amer. J. Path. 5, 313 (1929)

SCULLY, R. E.: Cancer 6, 455 (1953)

SCULLY, R. E.: In The Ovary. ed. H. G. GRADY, D. E. SMITH. Baltimore: Williams and Wilkins, 1963, Chap. 9

SCULLY, R. E.: Human Pathology 1, 73 (1970 a)

SCULLY, R. E.: Cancer 25, 1340 (1970 b)

SEED, P. G.: J. Obstet. Gynaec. Brit. Cwlth. 73, 808 (1966)

SILBERMAN, R., MENDELSON, I. R.: Arch. Dis. Childh. 35, 159 (1960)

SOLOMON, R. D.: Arch. Path. 52, 561 (1951)

TAYLOR, A.: In the Early Conceptus. W. W. PARK (ed.). St. Andrews: University of St. Andrews (Publishers), 1965, p. 78

TAYLOR, H., BARTER, R. H., JACOBSON, C. B.: Amer. J. Obstet. Gynec. 96, 816 (1966)

TEILMANN, I., KASSIS, H., PIETRA, G.: Acta path. microbiol. scand. 70, 267 (1967)

TEILUM, G.: Cancer 12, 1091 (1959)

TEILUM, G.: Acta path. et microbiol. scand. 64, 407 (1965)

TEILUM, G.: Special Tumours of Ovary and Testis. Copenhagen: Munksgaard, 1971

TEILUM, G., ALBRECHTSEN, R., NØRGAARD-PEDERSEN, B.: Acta path. microbiol. scand. 82A, 586 (1974)

TEOH, T. B., STEWARD, J. K., WILLIS, R. A.: J. Path. Bact. 80, 147 (1960)

TETER, J.: Third World Congress of I.F.G.O., Vienna 43 (1961)

TETER, J.: Am. J. Obstet. Gynec. 84, 722 (1962)

TETER, J.. PHILIP, J., WEĘCEWICZ, G. R.: Amer. J. Obstet. Gynec. 90, 929 (1964)

VARANGOT, J.: Thesis. Paris: Louis Arnette, 1937

VAWTER, V. G.: Cancer 18, 1479 (1965)

WHITE, C. P.: J. Path. Bact. 14, 522 (1910)

WILLIAMS, G. E. G.: J. Path. Bact. 82, 281 (1961)

WILLIS, R. A.: J. Path. Bact. 58, 284 (1946)

WILLIS, R. A.: The Borderland of Embryology and Pathology. London: Butterworth, 1958

WILLIS, R. A.: The Pathology of Tumours of Children. Edinburgh: Oliver and Boyd, 1962

WITSCHI, E.: Carnegie Contrib. Embryol. 32, 69 (1948)
WITZBERGER, C. M., AGERTY, H. A.: Arch. Pediat. 54, 339 (1937)
WRIGHT, D. H.: Brit. J. Surg. 51, 245 (1964)
ZIEGLER, E. E.: Arch. Path. 40, 279 (1945)

# Chapter 12
# Epithelial and Other Rare Tumours

Since epithelial tumours are much less common in children than in adults, individual experience of their behaviour and management is difficult to obtain. Although a wide range of these neoplasms occurs, the number of each type included in the Registry is insufficient to provide a satisfactory picture either of their true incidence or their natural histories. This also applies to other rare non-epithelial tumours and therefore it is proposed to discuss both these groups in this chapter. Craniopharyngiomas, pituitary adenomas, pinealomas, and meningeal melanomas which are considered in Chapter 6 are not included in this section.

The neoplasms under discussion fall into four groups (Table 1).

Table 1. Epithelial and other rare tumours 1954 - 1968 assessed 1972

| | Alive | Dead | Total |
|---|---|---|---|
| Alimentary | 14 | 11 | 25 |
| Respiratory | 2 | 9 | 11 |
| Endocrine | 6 | 3 | 9 |
| Miscellaneous | 37 | 3 | 40 |
| | 59 | 26 | 85 |

## TUMOURS OF THE ALIMENTARY SYSTEM

Twenty-five children with epithelial tumours of the alimentary tract were included in the Registry and the frequencies in the various sites are shown in Table 2. In addition to these epithelial tumours, there were 6 cases of intestinal lymphosarcoma in the Registry, 4 in the ileocaecal region and 2 in the ileum. These are discussed in Chapter 5. It is important not to confuse intestinal lymphosarcoma with benign

Table 2. Alimentary Tumours 1954 - 1968, assessed 1972

| | Alive | Dead | Total |
|---|---|---|---|
| Salivary gland | 9 | 1 | 10 |
| Carcinoma floor mouth | 0 | 1 | 1 |
| Ameloblastoma | 2 | 0 | 2 |
| Hepatic | 0 | 7 | 7 |
| Carcinoid | 3 | 0 | 3 |
| Carcinoma colon | 0 | 2 | 2 |
| | 14 | 11 | 25 |

lymphoid polyp which may be large and typically occurs in the ileocaecal and rectal regions. In the latter case they may prolapse through the anus. Unnecessary abdominoperineal resections have, on occasion, been carried out on patients with benign lymphoid neoplasms.

The Manchester series, although small, seems to agree with those reported from other centres. ARIEL and PACK (1960) state that no tumours of the oesophagus or stomach have been seen in patients under 24 years old at the Memorial Hospital, New York. PELLER (1960) analysing the actual number of deaths in US white children found that a very few children had been registered as dying from tumours of the oesophagus or stomach, but most fatal children's alimentary tumours arose in the mouth, pharynx, or intestines.

## Salivary Gland Tumours

The "mixed" tumour, although much less common than in adults, is not a rare childhood neoplasm. SEIFERT (1965) discusses 20 personal cases of salivary gland tumours in childhood and reviews 77 other examples. Nearly 50% of childhood tumours in this paper were mesenchymal, i. e. haemangioma, neurofibroma, etc., compared with less than 5% in the adult. Only 25% of salivary gland tumours in childhood were malignant. SEIFERT discusses the differential diagnosis which includes cysts of the first branchial arch, accessory parotid tissue and lymphatic lesions in the parotid. In the Manchester series there were 10 children (5 boys and 5 girls) with salivary tumours. Seven were in the parotid and 3 in the submandibular gland. One patient was less than 1 year old but, in general, salivary gland tumours appear to be more common in later childhood - 6 of the patients were over 10 years old. In one case the development of a muco-epidermoid tumour of the parotid in an 8-year-old girl was followed within a few weeks by the patient's mother noticing a swelling of her own parotid which was found to contain a mixed cell adenoma.

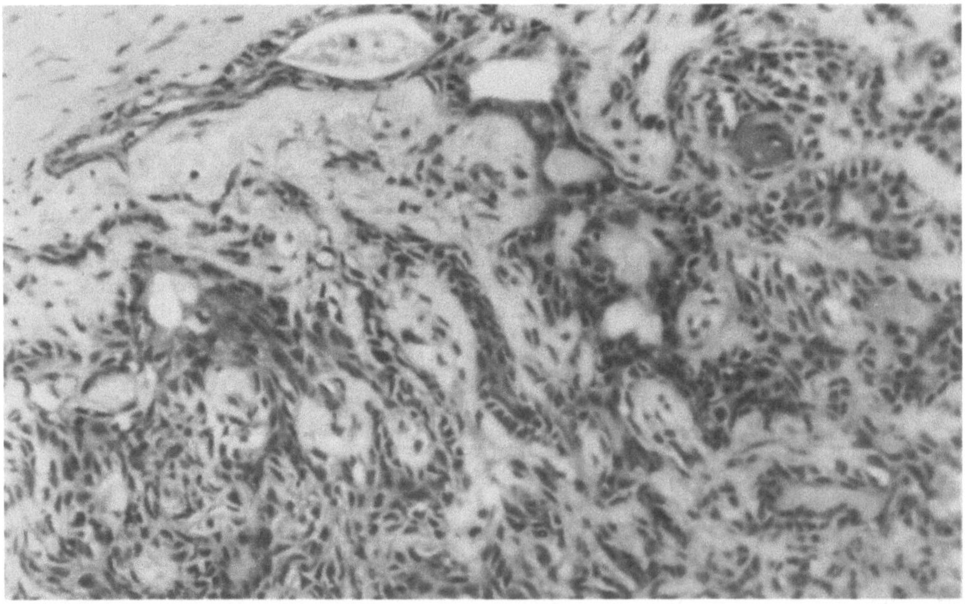

*Fig. 1. "Mixed" salivary tumour showing cords of epithelial cells and small ducts (H. & E. X 250)*

Eight of the tumours were of the "mixed salivary type". Their histogenesis has been discussed by WILLIS (1948) and EVANS (1956), who bring forward evidence that they are of purely epithelial origin. WELCH and MEYER (1968), however, following E.M. studies, contend that

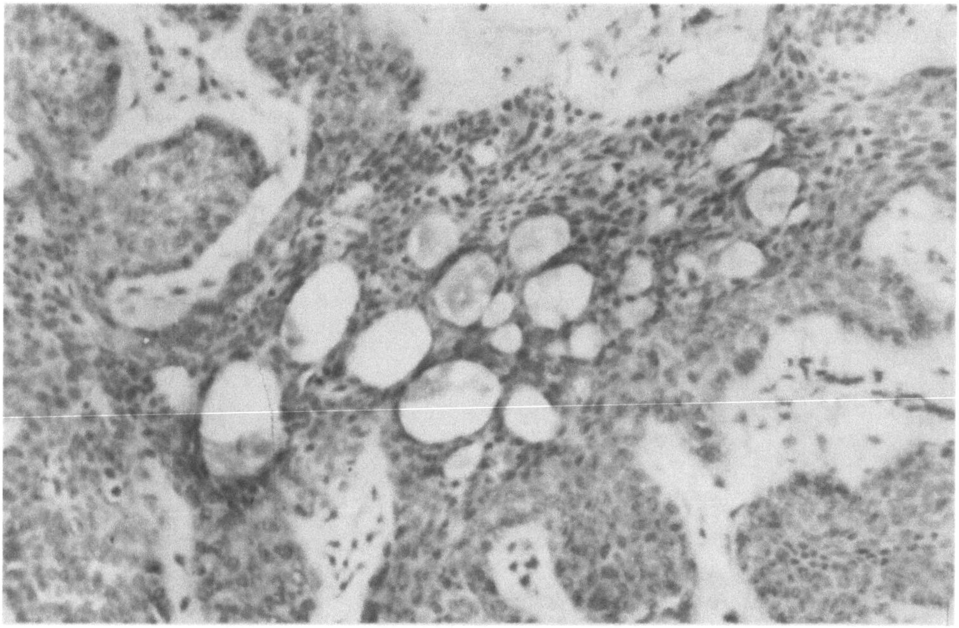

*Fig. 2. "Mixed" salivary tumour showing microcystic appearance (H. & E. X 250)*

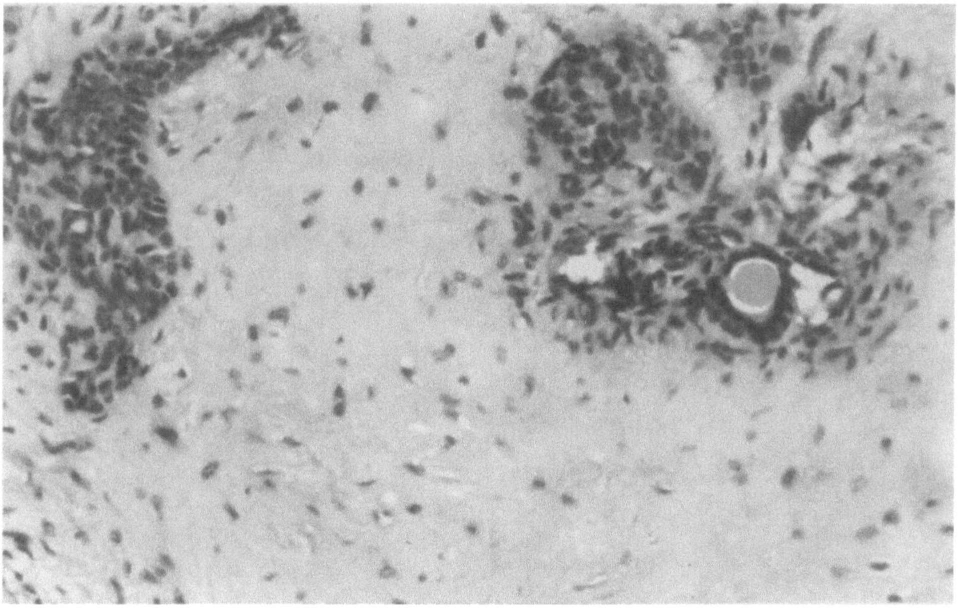

*Fig. 3. "Mixed" salivary tumour with mucinous matrix (H.&E.X250)*

true cartilage cells are present and suggest that these tumours are indeed "mixed". On gross examination these tumours were firm, white and encapsulated and occasionally cysts containing glairy fluid were noted. Microscopically, epithelial cells were present in sheets, lo-

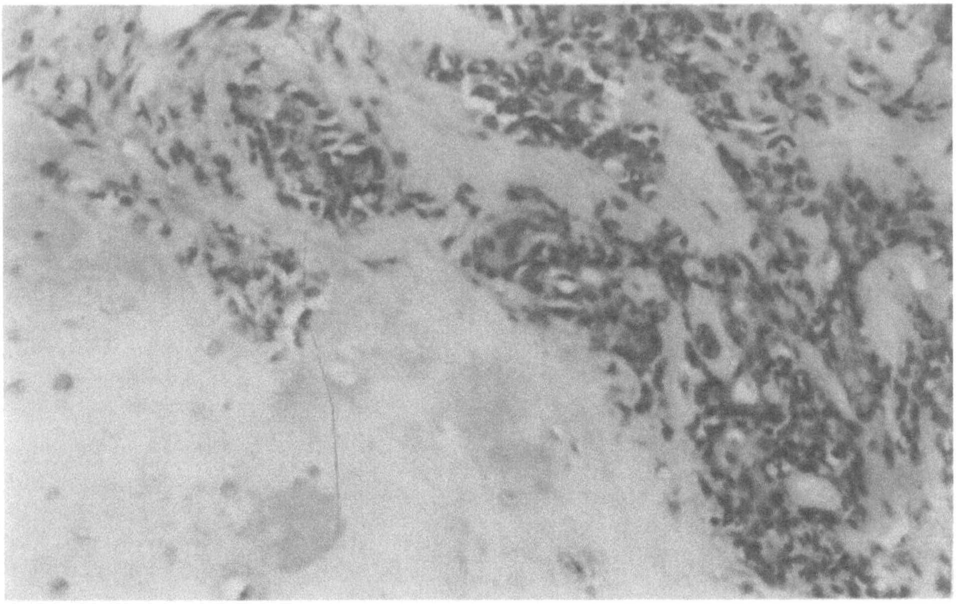

*Fig. 4. "Mixed" salivary tumour with cartilaginous appearance (H. & E. X 250)*

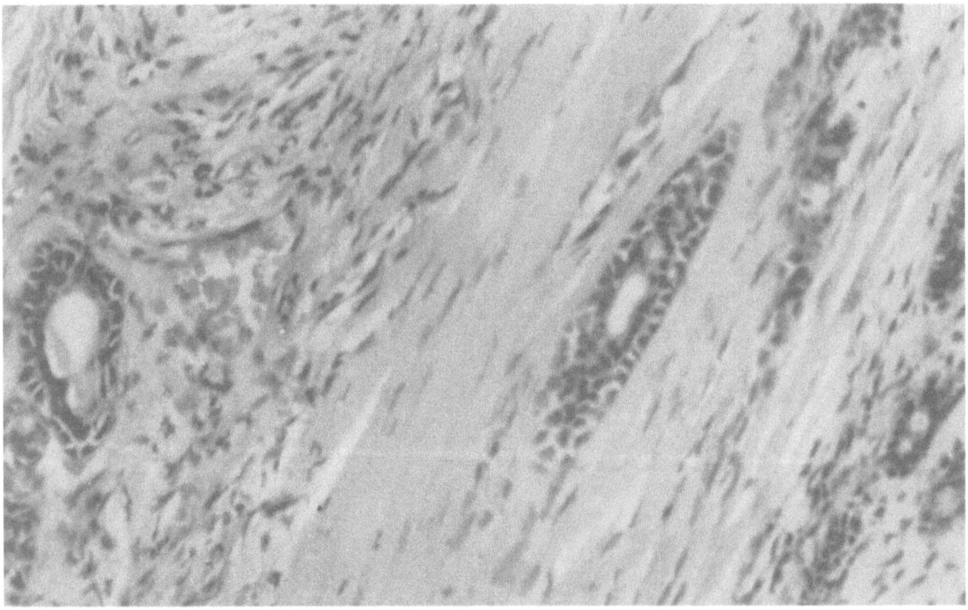

*Fig. 5. Epithelial cords extending through capsule of "mixed" tumour (H. & E. X 250)*

bules, trabeculae, or in acinar or duct formation. In addition, neoplastic epithelial cells were scattered diffusely through the stroma in some parts. Cysts with flattened lining cells were seen, sometimes relatively large and isolated and at other times giving a microcystic or honeycombed appearance, PAS positive material staining with alcian blue and metachromatic with toluidine blue being noted in the lumina. The stroma showed variations with loose chondromyxoid areas and denser fibrous portions. Small amounts of intracellular glycogen were seen, and the stromal mucins stained relatively weakly with PAS as shown by GRISHMAN (1952).

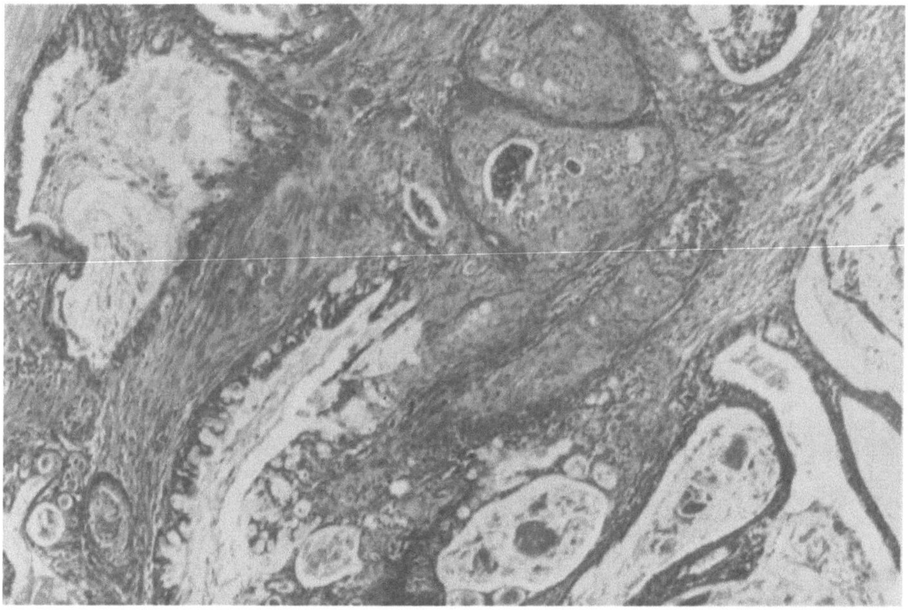

*Fig. 6. CTR.77/68. Salivary mucoepidermoid tumour with various types of epithelia and cyst formation (H. & E. X 90)*

There was one example of the more rare muco-epidermoid type (HEALEY et al., 1970) with mucus-producing, epidermoid and intermediate cells. Cyst formation was prominent and the tumour would be classified as Grade 1 according to the above authors.

The behaviour of salivary gland tumours is usually benign. All the nine survivors were treated satisfactorily by surgical excision alone. The one child who died had a carcinoma in the parotid region which responded well to radiation (4500 rads in 18 days), but lung metastases developed and the child died 7 months later. In addition, one 3-year-old boy developed a squamous carcinoma of the floor of the mouth containing small mucoid cysts. This tumour presented as a submental swelling which ulcerated into the mouth and spread to the cervical nodes with a fatal outcome after 6 months.

## Ameloblastoma

Two examples of this uncommon tumour were encountered. Both were mandibular and occurred in a boy of 10 and girl aged 13 years. Both were removed surgically and had not recurred 12 and 6 years later. Histo-

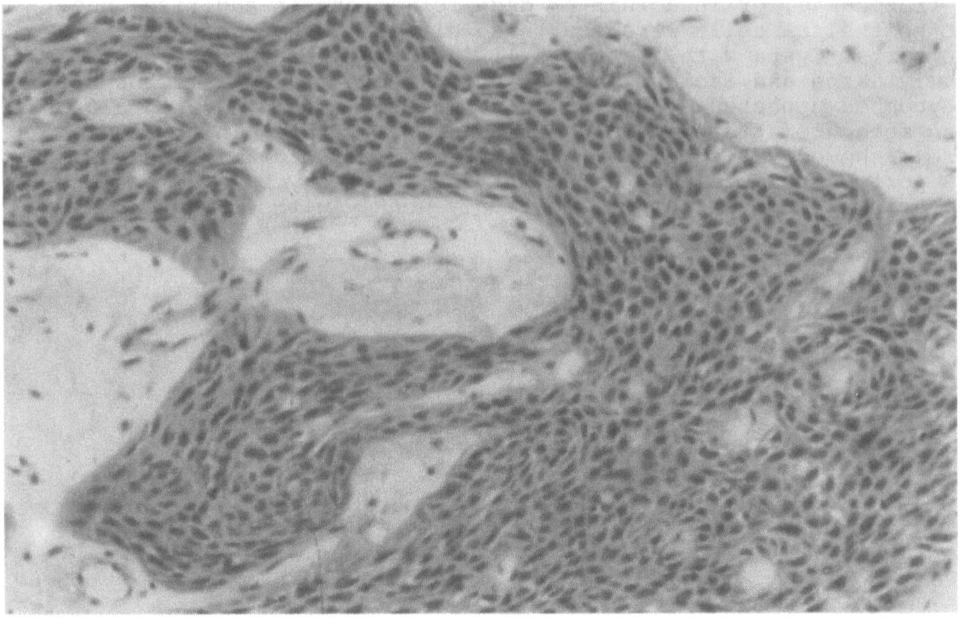

*Fig. 7. Ameloblastoma showing solid cords of epithelial cells. Peripheral columnar cells are scanty (H. & E. X 250)*

logically there were islands of "adamantinoma cells" with fluid accumulation and microcyst formation embedded in hypocellular connective tissue showing scattered psammomata.

## Tumours of the Liver

Primary hepatic tumours are rare in children. They may broadly be classified into hepatoblastomas, which show a varied histological picture and hepatic carcinomas which appear identical to similar tumours seen in adults. FRAUMENI et al. (1968) studied 282 death certificates of US children who died of hepatic tumours from 1960 to 1964 and 76 hospital charts of children with these neoplasms. They found a peak incidence in the first 5 years of life suggesting that in this early age group there was a prenatal aetiology, particularly as a few of these young patients had associated congenital abnormalities such as hemihypertrophy, haemangiomas and agenesis of the adrenal.

Although WILLIS (1962) stressed that there is no sharp histological distinction between hepatoblastomas and adult type hepatic carcinomas, ISHAK and GLUNZ (1967), MISUGI et al. (1967), KASAI and WANTANABE (1970) and KEELING (1971) have shown that hepatoblastomas occur in young children whereas adult type hepatic carcinomas present in the latter half of childhood. Although the microscopic appearance of hepatoblastomas varies in different parts of the tumour, several authors felt that hepatoblastomas could be classified according to the predominating histological picture. Thus ISHAK and GLUNZ described "embryonal" and "foetal" types while KASAI and WANTANABE added a further "anaplastic" type, The "rhabdomyoblastic" type described by WILLIS (1962) did not occur in their series and only one example has been included in the Registry since 1968, but KEELING reported three examples amongst 51 primary liver tumours seen at the Hospital for Sick Children, Great Ormond Street, London.

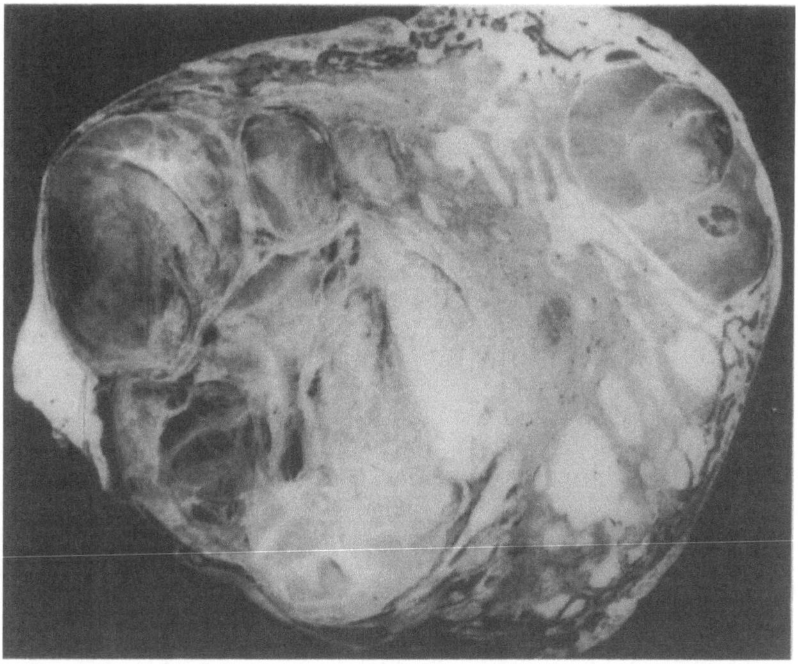

*Fig. 8. Cystic hamartoma of liver (case reported by GRIME et al., 1959)*

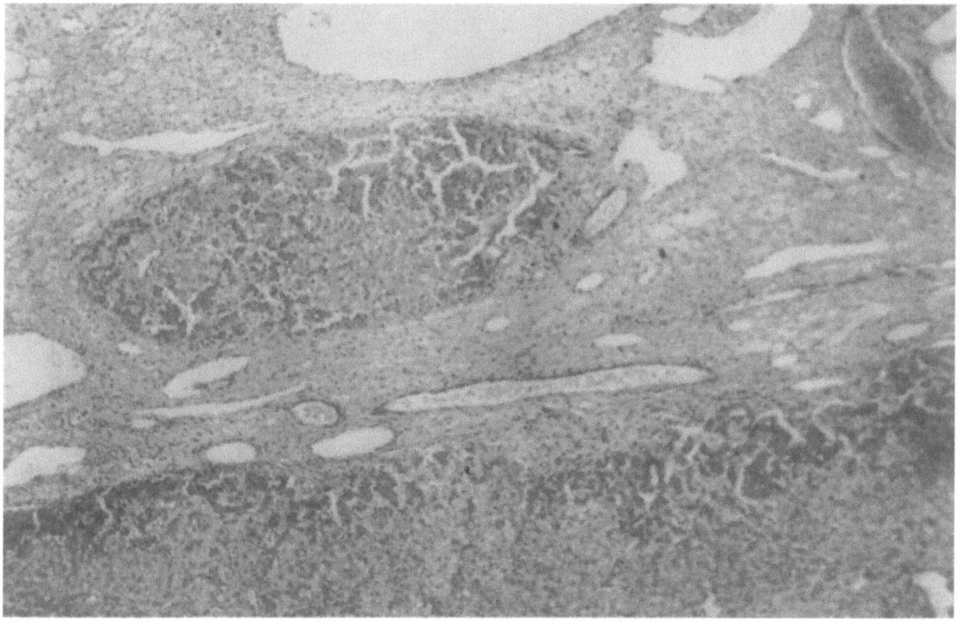

*Fig. 9. Cystic hamartoma of liver with islands of parenchymal cells and spaces lined by flattened cells (H. & E. X 60)*

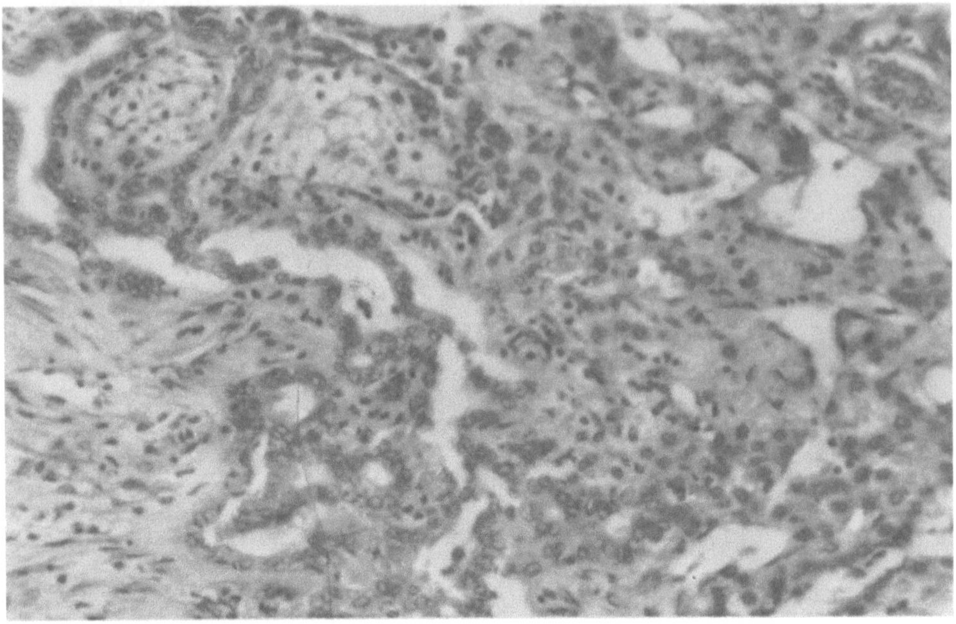

*Fig. 10. Cystic hamartoma of liver. Some of the channels are bile duct in origin (H. & E. X 250)*

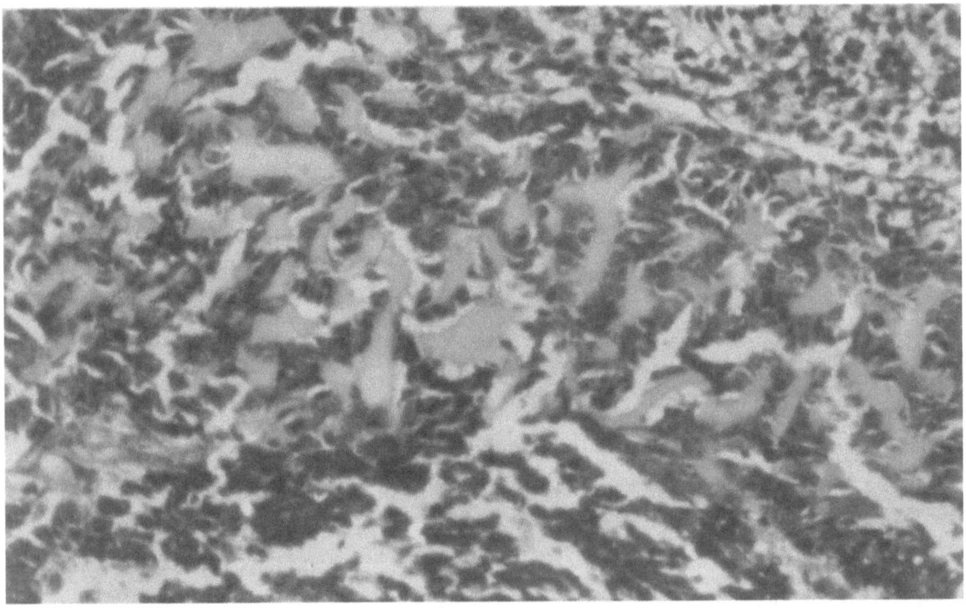

*Fig. 11. Hepatoblastoma with osteoid production (H. & E. X 250)*

There were 7 children with primary liver tumours in the Manchester series (Table 3). In 6 cases the tumour was a hepatoblastoma and in 1, the oldest, aged 11 years, a hepatocellular carcinoma. In two of the hepatoblastomas the tumours were mixed with osteoid and also car-

Table 3. Primary hepatic tumours 1954 - 1968, assessed 1972

| CTR. | Sex | Age (years) | Type of tumour | Treatment given | Metastases | Time from diagnosis to death |
|---|---|---|---|---|---|---|
| 83/58 | Boy | 1 | Hepatoblastoma | X.R.T. (875 rads in 13 days) | Nil | 3 weeks (postoperative death) |
| 112/58 | Girl | 11 | Hepatocellular carcinoma | X.R.T. (3000 rads in 27 days) | Nil | 3 1/2 years |
| 76/62 | Girl | 4 months | Hepatoblastoma | X.R.T. (2500 rads in 55 days) | Lung | 7 months |
| 123/63 | Boy | 1 | Hepatoblastoma | Hemihepatectomy Methotrexate | Lungs | 5 months |
| 72/67 | Boy | 8 | Hepatoblastoma | X.R.T. (2060 rads in 25 days) | Nil | 1 year |
| 96/68 | Boy | 2 | Hepatoblastoma | Nil | Lungs | 3 days |
| 99/68 | Boy | 9 | Hepatoblastoma | Nil | ? brain (developed Jacksonian epilepsy) | 2 months |

tilage in one case. The histological findings were sometimes limited by the amount of biopsy material available and in case CTR.99/68 the greater part of the biopsy consisted of mesenchymal tissue.

Although in one child (CTR.72/62) the tumour decreased in size following irradiation, surgical excision whenever possible is the main form of treatment in this group of tumours. ISHAK and GLUNZ reported 9 children with hepatoblastomas treated by resection who were well between 4 and 13 years later. None of the patients with adult type hepatic carcinoma in their series survived. However, FISH and McGARY (1966) reported 7 patients treated for adult-type hepatic carcinoma who survived for more than 5 years following treatment.

Although the results of treatment of the children with hepatic tumours in the Manchester Registry have been uniformly bad, there has been one child treated in Manchester (but not included in the Registry because he lived outside the Region) who has done well following surgical resection.

Boy, aged 1 1/2 years, who presented with an enlarged liver in February 1967. A large mass (7 cm in diameter) was removed from the left lobe of the liver. The tumour was a hepatoblastoma showing cords of vacuolated cells resembling foetal liver with separation into lobules

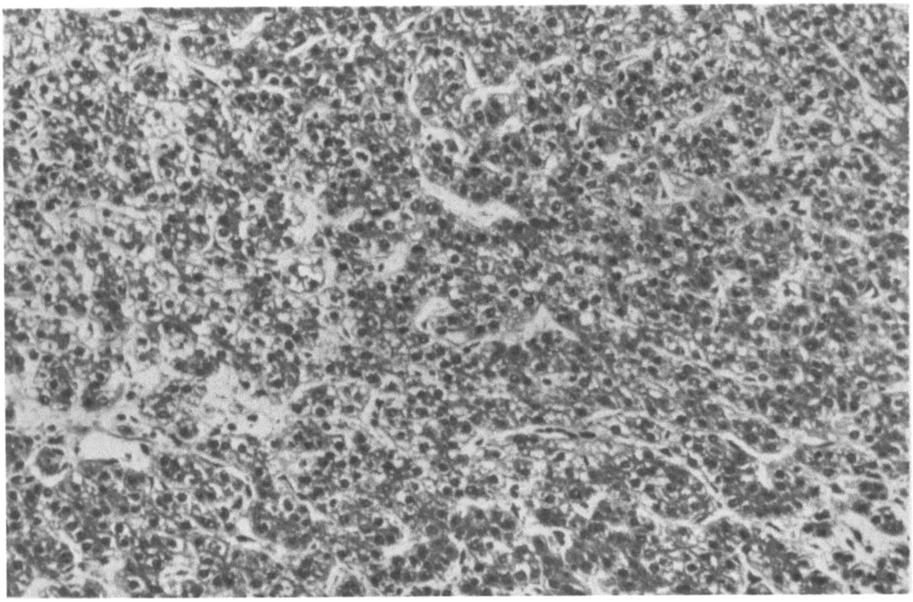

*Fig. 12. Hepatoblastoma with cords of vacuolated cells. The patient is alive 7 years after diagnosis (H. & E. X 200)*

by fibrous septa with loose mesenchyme. In addition there were more cellular areas with spheroidal and spindle cells, the latter showing a tendency to radiate round sinusoids. Cyclophosphamide 50 mg daily was given for 2 1/2 months postoperatively and the child has remained well ever since.

## Carcinoid of the Appendix and Small Intestine

Three children, aged 10, 12 and 13 years with carcinoid of the appendix were included in the Registry. In each case the tumours were small and found by chance in specimens removed at appendicectomy.

WEBSTER and WILLIAMS (1956) in a review of the world literature report that the youngest child with an intestinal carcinoid tumour was a 6-year-old boy. More than half the lesions were in the appendix and most of those in the small intestine were in the terminal ileum. FIELD et al. (1962) found 15 out of 19 non-functioning carcinoids in childhood to be situated in the appendix. It would be impossible to know the true incidence of this tumour as it is an incidental finding in the examination of specimens removed because of suspected appendicitis or intussusception. The carcinoid syndrome with an excessive production of 5-hydroxy-indoleacetic acid (5-HIAA) in the urine only occurs when the tumour has metastasized to the liver (PICKETT and BRIGGS, 1967).

## Carcinoma of the Colon

Carcinoma of the colon is an uncommon neoplasm of childhood. HOERNER (1958) collected 73 such cases in subjects under 20 years over the period 1865-1958. The youngest case is probably that of AHLFELD (1880), found in a stillborn monster although the histology is not shown. SCHILLA (1954) described adenocarcinoma in a prolapsed rectal polyp

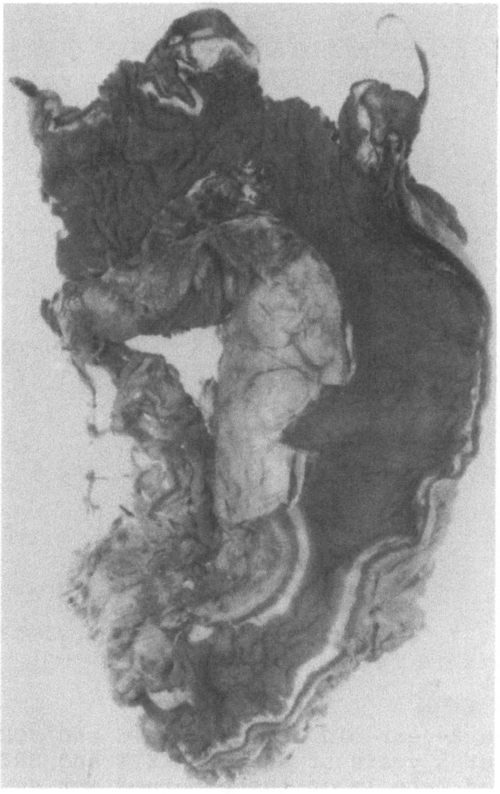

*Fig. 13. Annular carcinoma of sigmoid colon in a girl of 12 years*

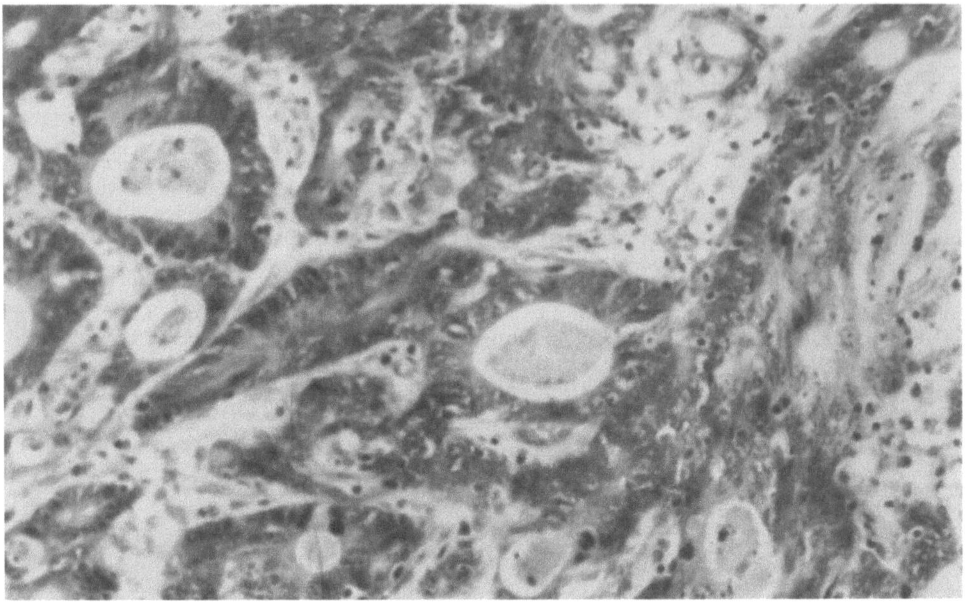

*Fig. 14. Carcinoma of colon with irregular acini (H. & E. X 250)*

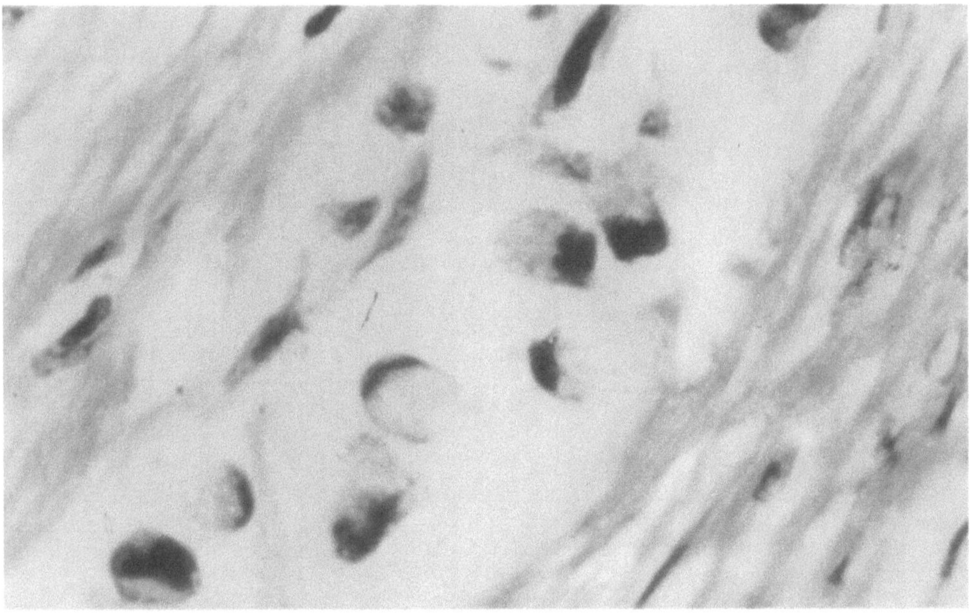

*Fig. 15. Carcinoma of colon showing "signet-ring" cells in muscle coats (H. & E. X 825)*

in a 2-year-old Mexican child and JOHNSTON (1947) collected 3 cases under 5 years of age. PICKETT and BRIGGS (1967) reviewed the literature based largely on the combined series of MIDDLEKAMP and HAFFNER (1963); CLUTTS and EMMETT (1964), ALAGHEMAND (1962) and HOERNER (1958). They found that approximately 5% of the children were under 5 years old,

15% from 5-10 years of age, and 80% were over 10 years. There appeared to be a 2 : 1 predominance of boys.

Two girls aged 12 and 13 years with carcinoma of the colon were included in the Manchester series. The tumours were both annular in type, one in the descending and the other in the sigmoid colon. One patient had symptoms for 10 months and the other a short illness thought to be due to appendicitis. At operation there was spread to lymph nodes and peritoneum. Resection was carried out in each case and radiotherapy was given to the older girl who survived 1 year, while the younger died after 4 months. Autopsy was not performed and it is not possible to say whether distant metastases occurred, but deposits have been described particularly in the brain and lungs. Histologically, the tumours were rather different, one being an anaplastic mucoid carcinoma with abundant "signet-ring" cells and the other, with the longer history, a well-differentiated adenocarcinoma. WILLIAMS (1954) and BUCHMAN and CALHOUN (1958) believe that there is a considerably greater incidence of mucoid or colloid tumours in children than in adults.

There were no children with rectal carcinomas in the Manchester series although PICKETT and BRIGGS found that there were 3 times more rectal than colon carcinomas reported in the literature.

Two diseases which predispose to carcinoma are familial polyposis and ulcerative colitis. However, these conditions usually antedate the carcinomas by at least 10 years (SACHIATELLO, 1971; DEVROEDE et al., 1971) and therefore the cancers rarely develop in childhood (KERR, 1948). DEVROEDE et al. from a follow-up of 396 children with ulcerative colitis seen at the Mayo Clinic from 1919 to 1965 found that those in whom the disease started between the ages of 5 and 10 years had the greatest risk of developing cancer.

The prognosis of carcinoma of the colon and rectum in children is very poor. PICKETT and BRIGGS only found 1 child who had survived for more than 5 years in all the series which they reviewed. However, DONALDSON et al. (1971) report 2 children who were well 28 and 23 months after surgery followed by a course of 5-fluorouracil (5-FU).

## TUMOURS OF THE RESPIRATORY SYSTEM

Eleven children with tumours of the respiratory system were included in the Registry (Table 4).

### Nasopharyngeal Carcinoma ("Lymphoepithelioma")

There were 9 Manchester children aged between 10 and 14 years with this tumour. In 8 cases the tumour presented as enlarged cervical

Table 4. Respiratory tumours 1954 - 1968, assessed 1972

| | Alive | Dead | Total |
|---|---|---|---|
| Nasopharyngeal carcinoma ("Lymphoepithelioma") | 2 | 7 | 9 |
| Carcinoma bronchus | 0 | 2 | 2 |
| | 2 | 9 | 11 |

lymph nodes which were unilateral in 6 cases and bilateral in 2. In one child there was a pharyngeal mass without any lymph node enlargement.

The fact that pharyngeal carcinomas commonly present as lymph node enlargement without the primary tumour being obvious often causes them to be misdiagnosed as lymphomas and this problem is discussed in Chapter 4. Histologically, they consist of large pale cells intermingled with small lymphocytes. The diagnosis rests on the fact that these pale cells form epithelial sheets and cords which are separated by mature lymphocytes. A good section is essential for this diagnosis since the epithelial formation may not be apparent in a small biopsy in which the picture may be indistinguishable from that of a reticulosarcoma.

The epidemiology, aetiology, pathology and clinical features of nasopharyngeal carcinoma were discussed at length at a UICC symposium in Singapore (MUIR and SHANMUGARATNAM, 1967). The disease is most common in adults over the age of 30 years and is considerably more frequent in males than in females. In the Manchester series there were seven boys and two girls. The most striking epidemiological feature of this tumour is its frequency in the Chinese, both in China and in those who have emigrated to other parts of the world. DIGBY et al. (1941) found it to be the second commonest malignant tumour admitted to Hong Kong University Hospital and YEH and COWDRY (1954) reported that it is the commonest cancer in male Formosans. The only non-Mongoloid groups with a high relative frequency are certain tribes in the Kenya highlands (CLIFFORD, 1967) although the absolute incidence in them is not great. SHANMUGARATNAM and HIGGINSON (1967) discussed many aspects of the Chinese way of life which might be aetiologically significant and were unable to find any exogenous agent which was convincingly carcinogenic. They conclude that racial or "genetic factors" probably account for the high incidence.

TEOH (1957) gave a detailed account of the necropsy findings in 31 adults and YEH (1962) described one thousand consecutive biopsies of untreated nasopharyngeal cancers in patients whose ages ranged from 3 to 78 years. Both these authors considered that the term "lymphoepithelioma" should be abandoned since this tumour is essentially a carcinoma.

Treatment is by radiotherapy (CHIA, 1967) and all the 9 Manchester children were irradiated. Temporary improvement was marked but only 2 of the children (22%) are still alive 9 and 13 years after treatment. This survival rate seems to be similar to that reported from other centres. In the large series of YEH (1962) the 5-year survival rate was 23.5% and it was 26% in the 104 patients treated at the Massachusetts General Hospital (WANG et al., 1962). The great frequency of spread to the cervical nodes has been mentioned and the tumour may invade the base of the skull. Metastases in bones are common and occurred in 5 of the 7 fatal Manchester cases. TEOH (1967) reported that 56% of his cases had bone metastases while involvement of the liver occurred in 53%, the lungs in 45% and the abdominal lymph nodes in 45%. The progress of the tumour is usually rapid (ATKINSON and SCOTT, 1967) with most of the patients with fatal disease dying within 3 years. All the deaths in the Manchester series occurred within 2 years of diagnosis.

## Carcinoma of the Bronchus

Bronchial carcinoma is a rare tumour in childhood, there being only 5 patients below 20 years of age in a large series of 1814 cases gathered from the literature by MATZ (1938). The majority of published cases up to 1954 are tabulated by ANDERSON et al. (1954). The ages of the 15 recorded cases in this paper were between 10 months and 14 years and there was an even distribution over this range. SUTER (1952) described a bronchial carcinoma in a 6 1/2-year-old girl and compared the findings with those in 12 cases up to the age of 12 years from the literature. In 7 the initial symptoms were directly attributable to the

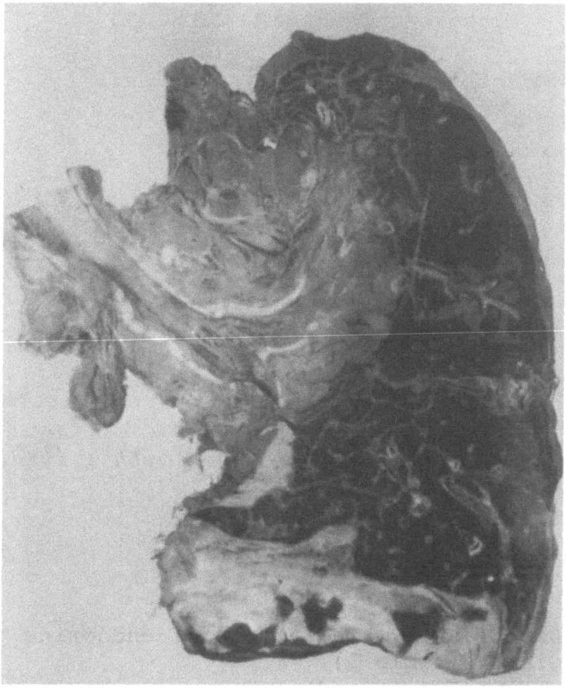

*Fig. 16. Carcinoma of bronchus in a 9-year-old boy*

primary tumour - cough, dyspnoea and pain in the chest - while in 4 the presentation was the result of metastases, in one case 16 months elapsed before lung symptoms developed. Blood-stained pleural effusion and the hardness of the tumour appear to be characteristic features.

There were 2 Manchester children with bronchial carcinoma:
CTR.74/56. Boy, aged 8 years, who presented with pain in the chest and X-ray showed an extensive opacity in the left upper lobe with a pleural effusion on that side. The effusion was found to be blood-stained, containing tumour cells, and on bronchoscopy the left upper bronchus was reduced to a slit. At thoracotomy, hard white tumour was found which on histological examination was found to be a squamous cell carcinoma mostly undifferentiated but with occasional bands and pearl formation. Radiotherapy was given but the child died a few days later, the clinical course being 4 months. At necropsy the tumour had spread to the mediastinum, opposite lung, and supraclavicular and axillary lymph nodes on the left side.
CTR.7/67. Boy, aged 14 years, who developed a swelling in the right groin. Four months later he began to spit blood and became dyspnoeic. Chest X-rays showed a bilateral hilar mass and multiple deposits throughout both lung fields. No treatment was given and the child died 2 weeks later. At autopsy there was an anaplastic carcinoma in the mediastinum, lungs and pelvis.

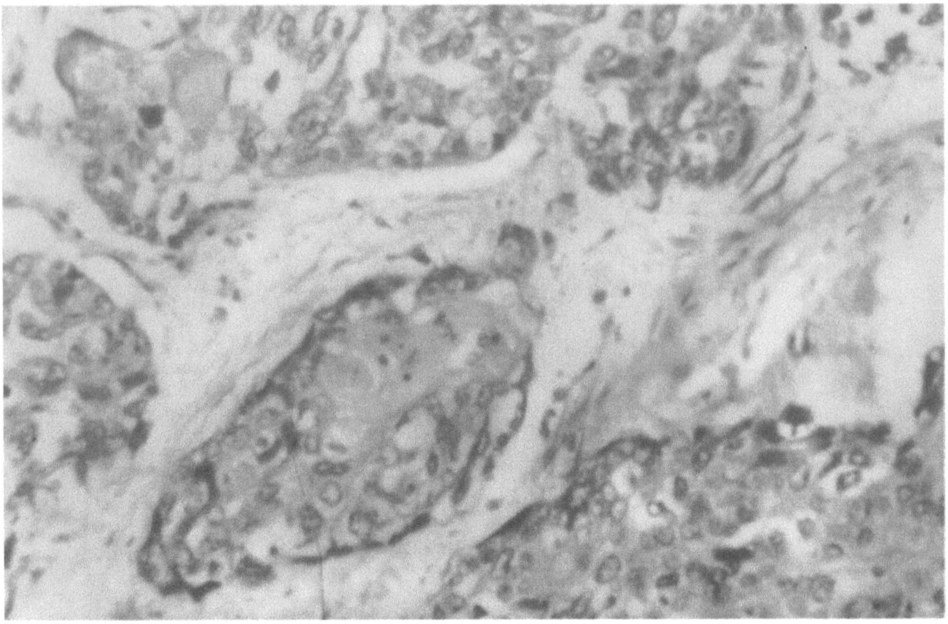

*Fig. 17. Bronchial carcinoma with epithelial islands and some pearl formation (H. & E. X 325)*

ENDOCRINE TUMOURS

Nine children with tumours of endocrine glands were included in the Registry (Table 5).

Table 5. Endocrine tumours 1954 - 1968, assessed 1972

| | Alive | Dead | Total |
|---|---|---|---|
| Adrenal cortex | 2 | 2 | 4 |
| Thyroid | 3 | 0 | 3 |
| Parathyroid | 1 | 0 | 1 |
| Islet cell tumour of pancreas | 0 | 1 | 1 |
| | 6 | 3 | 9 |

Tumours of the Adrenal Cortex

The adrenal cortex arises from the splanchnic mesoderm but in view of the histological appearance of tumours arising from it the terms "adenoma" and "carcinoma" have been retained.

In the Manchester cases the histological findings corresponded to a certain extent with the clinical behaviour but there is no sharp morphological distinction between benign and malignant tumours of the adrenal cortex. Neoplasms with a histological appearance almost identi-

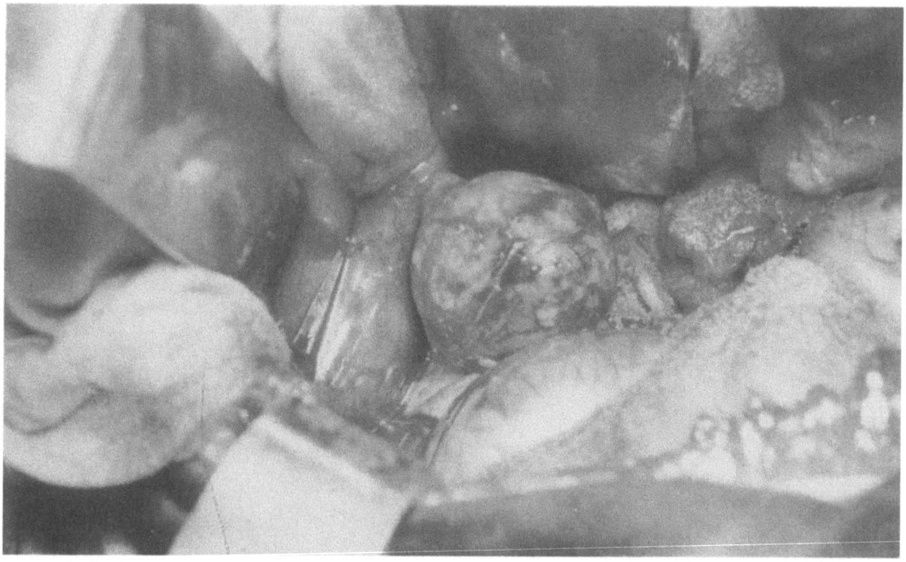

*Fig. 18. Encapsulated adrenocortical tumour during operative removal*

cal to normal adrenal cortical tissue may recur and produce metastases (EVANS, 1956).

Adrenocortical tumours may, or may not, be hormone-producing and the clinical picture which develops depends on the type of steroid produced in excess by the tumour.

The endocrine effects are usually virilism with androgen production or Cushing's syndrome due to excessive hydrocortisone. Feminization with oestrogens and hyperaldosteronism may also be encountered. Aldosteronism described by CONN (1955) usually occurs between the ages of 30 and 50 years and has only rarely been encountered in childhood. Feminization is also uncommon but such a case in a 7-year-old boy was described by MOSIER and GOODWIN (1961). Non-functioning tumours probably do occur, but it may be that in certain instances the steroids produced in excess are not biologically active.

Virilism in children is usually due to bilateral adrenal hyperplasia rather than neoplasia. During the period under review many cases of congenital virilism due to adrenal hyperplasia were encountered in Manchester. By comparison, tumours of the adrenal cortex which secrete large amounts of androgenic steroids and thus produce virilization are rare in children. Such tumours may produce signs of virilization at any age after birth including early infancy but they do not appear to function during early foetal life and do not cause pseudohermaphroditism in the female infant. Virilization commencing after birth in a female infant is generally due to an adrenal tumour.

Urinary 17-oxosteroids are usually raised in functional adrenal tumours causing virilism and very high values are sometimes found. There is quite often an excess of dehydroepiandrosterone (but this is not invariably so) and other $C_{19}$ steroids with the $\Delta^5$-3-$\beta$-hydroxy configuration. There would appear to be a deficiency of the enzyme 3$\beta$-hydroxysteroid dehydrogenase in the tumour tissue. This pattern is similar to that found in congenital adrenal hyperplasia due to the deficiency of this enzyme but in tumour cases there is no accompanying salt-losing

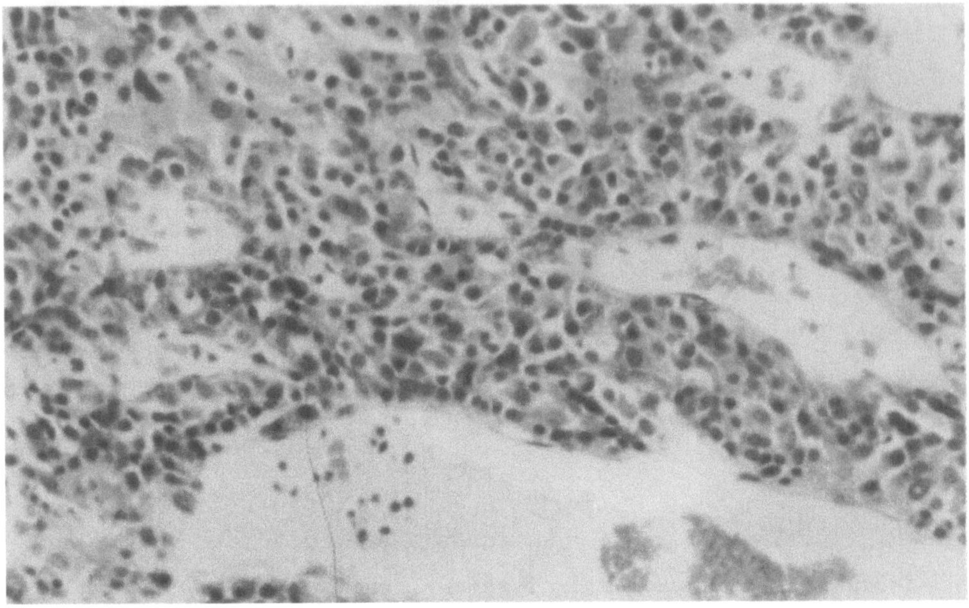

*Fig. 19. Adrenocortical carcinoma showing pleomorphism, hyperchromatic nuclei, and large vascular sinusoids (H. & E. X 250)*

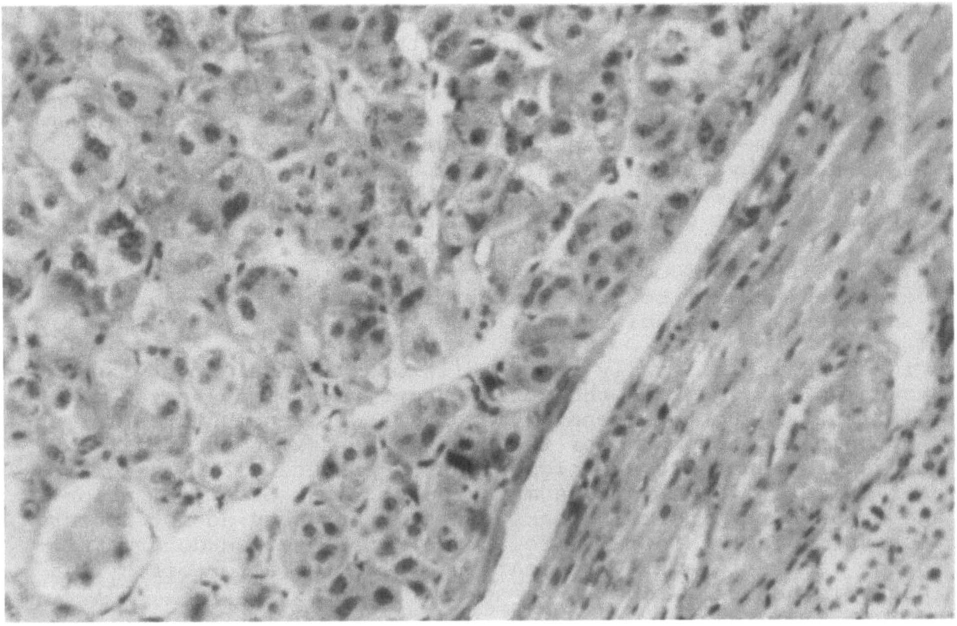

*Fig. 20. Encapsulated adrenocortical tumour showing relative uniformity of cells (H. & E. X 250)*

tendency nor do the urinary steroid levels fall in response to cortisol administration. An increase in the excretion of 17-oxosteroids is also found in congenital adrenal hyperplasia and in interstitial cell tumours of the testis. Other enzyme deficiencies may be present in tumour cases and a deficiency of 11-β-hydroxylase will result in an increased secretion of 11-desoxycortisol (compound S) and the urinary excretion of total 17-oxogenic steroids will be raised. The pattern will be similar to that found in conditions of congenital adrenal hyperplasia due to a deficiency of 11-β-hydroxylase. Pregnane -3α, 17α, 20α-triol excretion is usually low in tumour cases and an elevated level is suggestive of congenital adrenal hyperplasia.

It is important to distinguish between hyperplasia and a tumour of the adrenal cortex. A marked increase in the excretion of 17-oxosteroids is suggestive of a neoplasm but there is considerable overlap and the excretion is increased in hyperplasia and other conditions. The presence of considerable amounts of dehydroepiandrosterone is highly suggestive of a tumour. Suppression tests may be useful in the differential diagnosis. Cortisol quickly suppresses the excretion of 17-oxosteroids in congenital adrenal hyperplasia but not so in the case of a virilizing tumour. The administration of the potent steroid dexamethasone usually has no effect on the steroid excretion in tumour cases, since in most patients there is an autonomy of the neoplastic tissue to suppression or stimulation.

It is not usually possible to distinguish between an adrenocortical adenoma and carcinoma on the basis of steroid assay.

One of the children in the Manchester series from whom a carcinoma was removed at the age of 3 years had a urinary 17-oxosteroid excretion of 13 mg per 24h (normal value at this age being less than 2 mg per day) and a 17-oxogenic steroid excretion of 10 mg per 24 h (normal value at this age less than 4 mg per day). Following the successful removal of the tumour these levels fell below 1 mg per 24h. More recently a further patient who presented with virilism due to an adrenal carcinoma was found at the age of 9 months to have markedly elevated 17-oxosteroid excretion (33 mg/24h) and a total 17-oxogenic steroid excretion of 7 mg/ 24 hours.

Cushing's syndrome results from the prolonged hypersecretion of cortisol. In addition, other steroids, e. g. androgens, oestrogens and mineral corticoids, may be produced in excess giving rise to a spectrum of disorders including virilism. Cushing's syndrome is rare in children but has been reported at all ages. WILKINS (1957) reports 26 cases under the age of 10 years. Cushing's syndrome in a child who is not receiving steroids or ACTH is usually due to a tumour which is malignant rather than benign (HOLT et al., 1962), but cases due to bilateral adrenal hyperplasia have been reported.

Consistently elevated plasma cortisol levels together with the loss of diurnal rhythm are strong evidence in favour of a diagnosis of Cushing's syndrome. There is increased urinary excretion of cortisol and its metabolites but the urinary excretion of these compounds and the fasting level of blood cortisol may also be raised in conditions of stress and the diagnosis should not be based on single estimations. Several 24h collections of urine should be examined to eliminate errors in collection and timing and also to minimise the effect of stress on adrenocortical function. Simple obesity may cause a moderate increase in total 17-oxogenic steroid excretion.

The estimation of urinary free cortisol levels is said to be the most sensitive index for the diagnosis of Cushing's syndrome, or alternatively, 11-hydroxycorticosteroid estimations may be more readily available (BURKE, 1974).

The measurement of plasma ACTH is the best method in determining the aetiology of Cushing's syndrome, with negative results in adrenal tumours.

Suppression tests may be of value in distinguishing between adrenal hyperplasia and neoplasia giving rise to Cushing's syndrome and stimulation tests using ACTH have also been used.

An 11-year-old patient in the Manchester series excreted 41 mg of 17-oxosteroids per 24h and 53 mg of total 17-oxogenic steroids per day (normal values less than 10 mg and 12 mg per 24h, respectively).

There were 4 children with adrenocortical tumours in the Manchester series. The 2 who have survived were both girls who presented with virilism. In one the signs started at the age of 18 months. A low-grade encapsulated carcinoma was removed when she was 3 years old and she is well 12 years later. The other survivor developed a deep voice, an enlarged clitoris and pubic hair when she was 10 months old. She had a poorly encapsulated carcinoma with local lymph node enlargement. The tumour was removed and postoperative irradiation given (3000 rads in 34 days), and the child had no sign of recurrence 5 years later. Both the children who died were older. One was a 9-year-old girl with a very anaplastic tumour which presented as an abdominal mass without any endocrine abnormality. At laparotomy the tumour was biopsied and irradiation given (3000 rads in 27 days). There was some shrinkage of the tumour but it did not disappear and she was readmitted to hospital 8 months later. She was given cyclophosphamide orally but died 2 weeks later.

The other fatal adrenocortical tumour was in a boy who had been diagnosed as a cretin when he was 2 weeks old and had been given thyroid up to the age of 7 years. He progressed normally up to the age of 11 years when he developed Cushing's syndrome. A large carcinoma of the left adrenal was found at laparotomy but it had burst through the capsule and could only be incompletely removed. Apart from being given cortisone and a small dose of irradiation terminally he received no other treatment and died 9 months later. At autopsy there were metastases in the left kidney, the para-aortic lymph nodes and the hila of both lungs.

## Thyroid Tumours

Carcinoma of the thyroid in children has attracted considerable attention largely due to the studies of WINSHIP (1951) who collected records of a large series of cases from many parts of the world. Ten years later WINSHIP and ROSVOLL (1961) were able to publish an account of 562 cases of thyroid carcinoma in children, approximately 80% of whom lived in the United States. There was an increased incidence in the years 1945 to 1957 and 80% of the patients questioned were found to have received irradiation previously for "enlarged thymus", hypertrophied tonsils or adenoids, naevi or angiomas. There seems little doubt that irradiation of children for these non-neoplastic conditions can play a part in the production of thyroid carcinomas. In the absence of such irradiation these tumours are rare and in the Manchester series only one example was encountered.

CTR.29/58. Boy aged 8 years who developed a lump on the right side of the neck in November 1957. There was no history of previous exposure to X-rays. A biopsy showed the mass to be a papillary carcinoma of the thyroid which had spread to a cervical lymph node. Subtotal thyroidectomy was performed and postoperative irradiation was given (2000 rads MV in 20 days). Over the next 8 months a total of 500 mCs of radio-

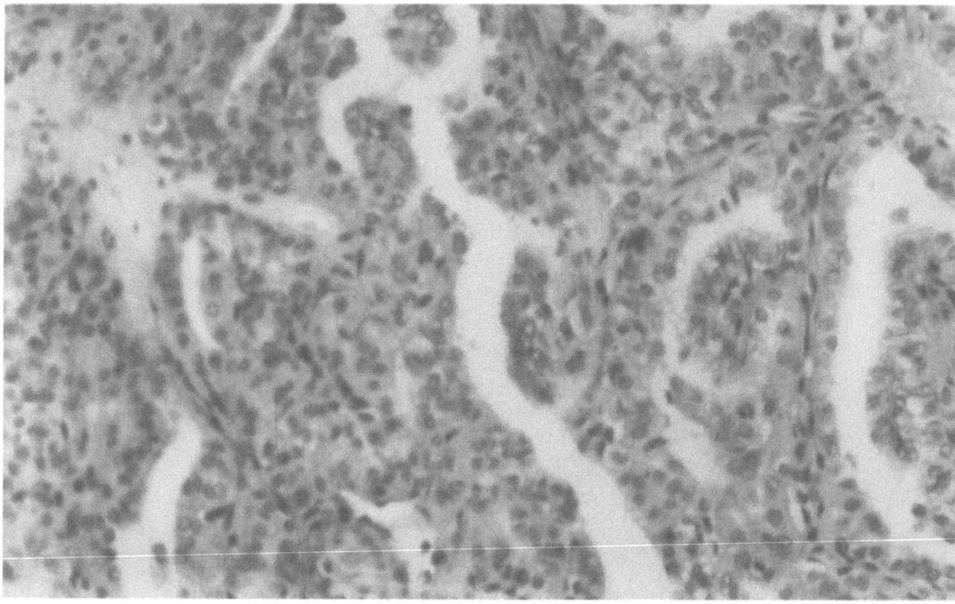

*Fig. 21. Carcinoma of thyroid with predominantly papillary structure (H. & E. X 250)*

iodine was given. Since then he has needed to take thyroxine and has remained well except that in 1971 he was found to have paralysis of his right vocal cord presumably due to fibrosis following the XRT. He is now married and has a son and a daughter both of whom are normal.

HORN and RAVDIN (1951) describe papillary, adenomatous and solid types in a survey of 22 patients up to the age of 25 years. Metastases in the lungs were described in 2 cases only, one adenomatous and one papillary tumour. These authors point out that the neoplasms were not, however, of pure type. Cervical metastases sometimes present for several years before a primary tumour of the thyroid became apparent, occurred in 77%. Thyroid cancer in childhood in spite of the frequent incidence of metastases would appear to be relatively benign and even with pulmonary deposits HORN and RAVDIN regard the outlook as by no means hopeless. HARE and NEWCOMB (1950) suggest that carcinoma of the thyroid is less malignant in children than adults. In the large series of WINSHIP and ROSVOLL (1961) 76% of the children presented with cervical lymph node involvement which was bilateral in almost one-third. Most of the tumours were papillary carcinomas but some children had follicular or undifferentiated tumours. Almost 18% of the patients died from their disease, mostly during the first postoperative year. However, 24 died having had the disease for more than 10 years.

Medullary carcinoma from the parafollicular or calcitonin-producing cells may occur in childhood in association with other endocrine tumours and multiple neuromas, the association being now known as multiple endocrine adenoma syndrome type II (leading article Brit. Med. J. 1974). The familial aspect is referred to in chapter 2, and the variety of hormonal effects of medullary carcinoma is discussed by STANBURY and DE GROOT (1973).

In the Manchester series there were 2 children with thyroid adenomas. In one, there were several partly solid and partly microfollicular

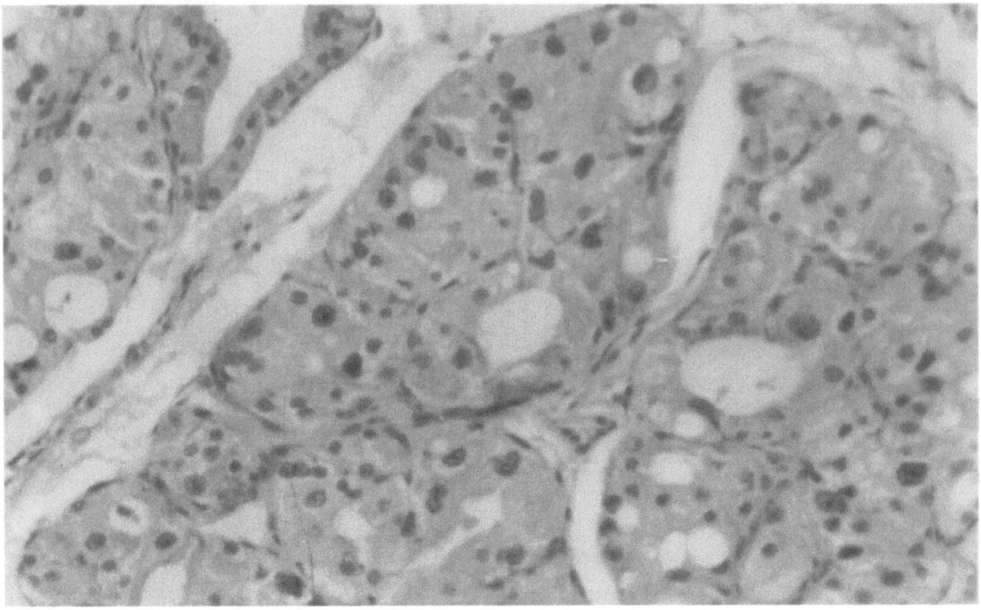

*Fig. 22. Thyroid adenoma with swollen degenerate cells having Hürthle-cell appearance (H. & E. X 250)*

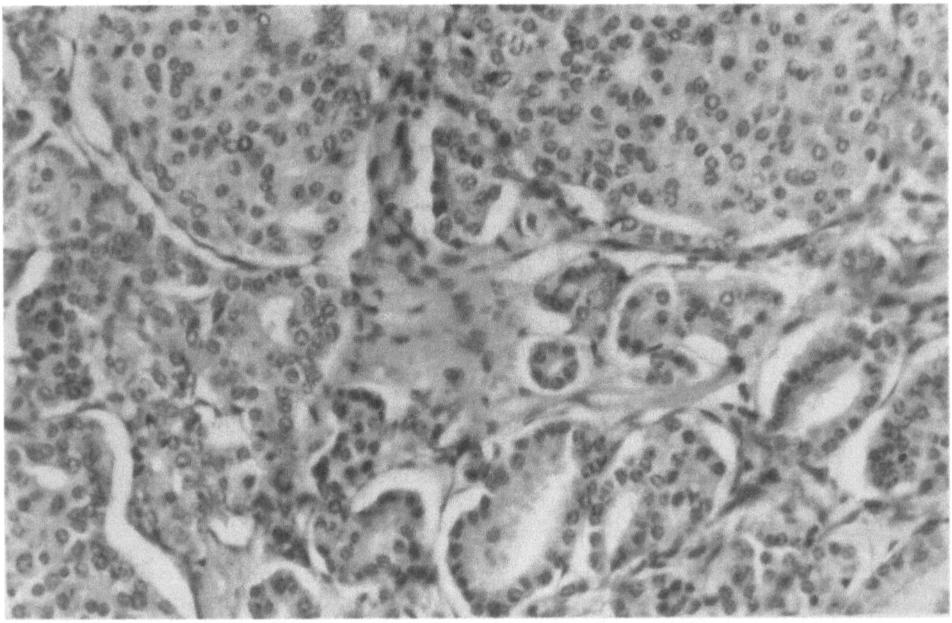

*Fig. 23. Thyroid adenoma with solid and microfollicular areas (H. & E. X 250)*

encapsulated adenomata in the thyroid of a girl of 7 years. The gland had been swollen from birth and her growth in height was slow. Clinical evidence of hypothyroidism was confirmed by a low protein bound iodine and the gland apart from the adenomata showed swollen, granular cells with nuclear pleomorphism and irregular follicle formation. There were three siblings but no evidence of thyroid disease was detected in the family. The other patient with multiple adenomata was a 13 1/2-year-old boy who was deaf and mentally defective.

## Parathyroid Adenoma

A 2 cm diameter encapsulated tumour weighing 2.8 g was removed from below the lower pole of the left lobe of the thyroid in a 14-year-old boy who had nocturnal enuresis, lassitude, muscular wasting and pain in the heels. On several occasions there had been fainting attacks. His serum calcium was 20.5 mg %, phosphorus 4.3 mg %, alkaline phosphatase 25 King-Armstrong units/100 ml. The blood urea was 90 mg %. X-rays showed osteoporosis, subperiosteal absorption in the phalanges and lower end of the radius and ulna together with a cyst in the latter. The tumour was clinically palpable and was homogeneous, yellow brown

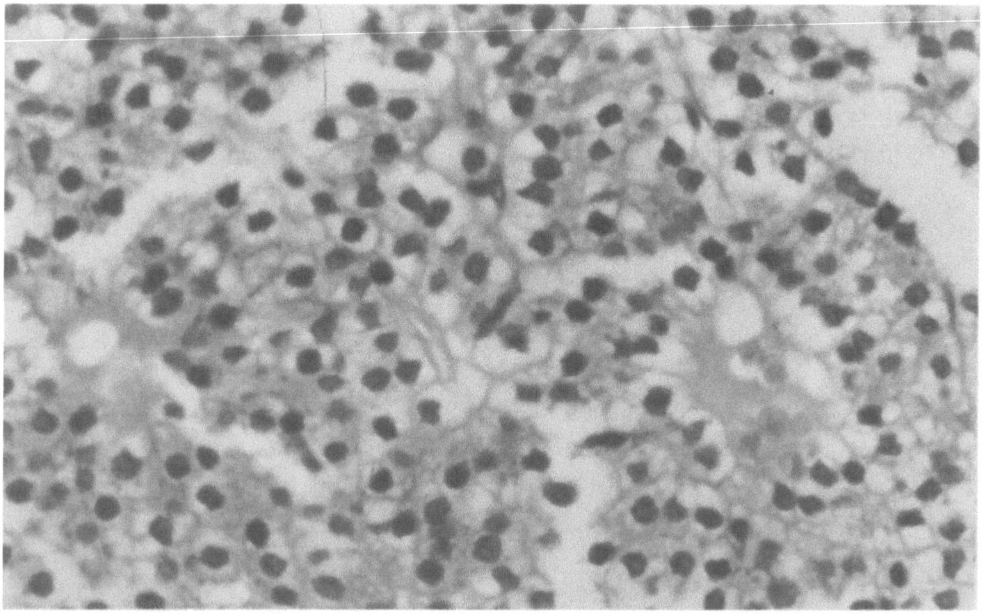

*Fig. 24. Parathyroid adenoma with large water-clear cells (H.&E.X625)*

with clefts and cystic spaces. Microscopically, clear cuboidal and larger cells with enlarged nuclei and finely granular eosinophilic cytoplasm were grouped into small acini by fine trabeculae. Postoperative recovery was excellent, accompanied by marked increase in the height of the patient but calcification of the tendons of the feet caused some inconvenience.

Parathyroid adenomata may be associated with other endocrine tumours which show familial features (WILLIAMS, E. D., 1965), as may islet cell tumours of the pancreas. This association is known as the multiple endocrine adenoma syndrome type I.

## Islet Cell Tumour of the Pancreas

There was one example of this tumour in the Registry. A 9-month-old boy became comatose and was admitted to hospital. Two days later he

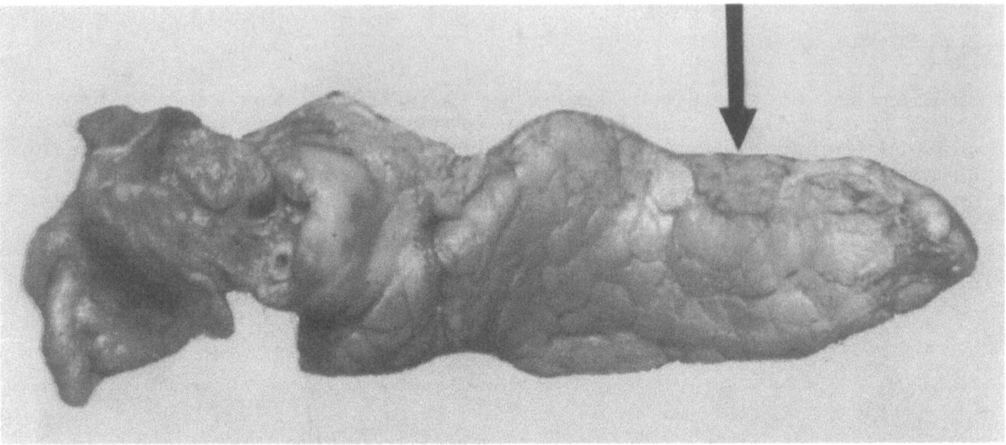

*Fig. 25. CTR.48/65. Islet cell adenoma in superior aspect of pancreas of a 9-month-old boy*

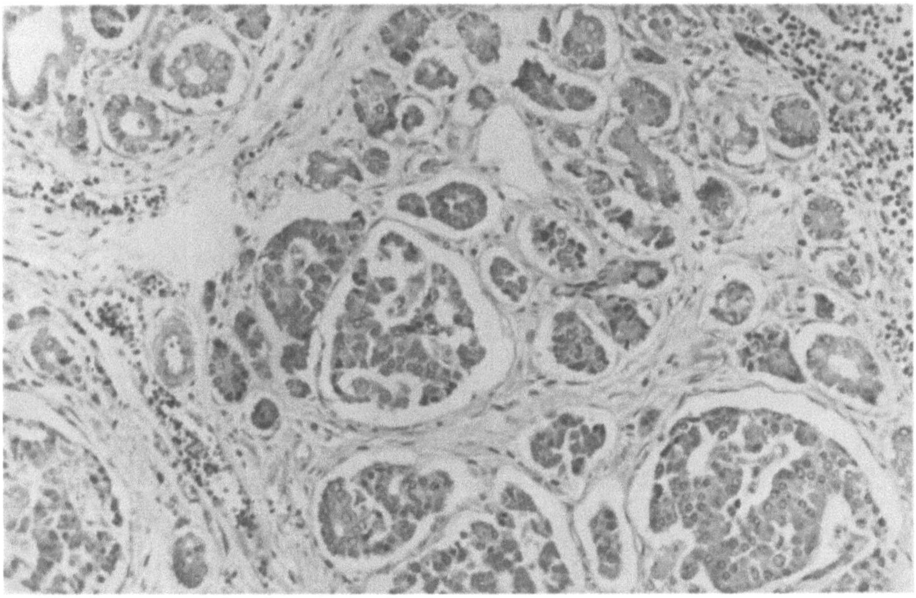

*Fig. 26. CTR.48/65. Islet cell adenoma with islands of cells and tubule formation (Aldehyde-fuchsin X 225)*

was found to have a blood sugar of 12 mg /100 ml and was given hydrocortisone, glucagon and intravenous glucose. Although his blood sugar rose to 200 mg /100 ml it could not be maintained and the child died 2 days later. At autopsy an islet cell tumour of the pancreas was found.

ROBINSON et al. (1971) describe islet cell adenomas in 2 newborn infants, one of whom was cured by removal of 75% of the pancreas. They were able to find reports of 7 other cases in the literature. They point out that severe symptomatic hypoglycaemia in the newborn is most frequently seen in infants whose birth weights are low compared with the period of gestation. They suggest that severe hypoglycaemia of obscure origin persisting beyond the age of 3 weeks in a newborn infant of normal birth weight and not responding to medical treatment justifies exploration of the pancreas.

## MISCELLANEOUS TUMOURS

Forty cases in the Registry were in this group (Table 6).

Table 6. Miscellaneous tumours 1954 - 1968, assessed 1972

| | Alive | Dead | Total |
|---|---|---|---|
| Neural sheath | 18 | 1 | 19 |
| Breast | 2 | 0 | 2 |
| Granular myoblastoma | 5 | 0 | 5 |
| "Benign calcifying epithelioma" (Pilomatrixoma) | 3 | 0 | 3 |
| Malignant melanoma | 1 | 1 | 2 |
| Sweat glands | 2 | 0 | 2 |
| Thymus | 0 | 1 | 1 |
| Chordoma | 1 | 0 | 1 |
| Carotid body tumour | 1 | 0 | 1 |
| Alveolar soft part sarcoma | 1 | 0 | 1 |
| "Malignant haemangioma" | 1 | 0 | 1 |
| Pigmented neuroectodermal tumour of infancy | 1 | 0 | 1 |
| Uncertain | 1 | 0 | 1 |
| | 37 | 3 | 40 |

### Neural Sheath Tumours

Tumours of the sheaths of peripheral nerves may be single or multiple. Depending on the histological appearance, these lesions may be divided into neurofibromas and neurilemmomas. However, this division is not absolute since in the fully formed (plexiform) neurofibroma there is a proliferation of Schwann cells and in patients with multiple neurofibromatosis (von Recklinghausen's disease) some of the lesions may be neurofibromas and others neurilemmomas. The gross and microscopic appearances of tumours of the peripheral nervous system are fully described by HARKIN and REED (1968).

There were 19 children (11 boys and 8 girls) with nerve sheath tumours in the Manchester series. The excised tumours were neurofibromas in 15 cases, neurilemmomas in 3 cases, and one tumour consisted of gang-

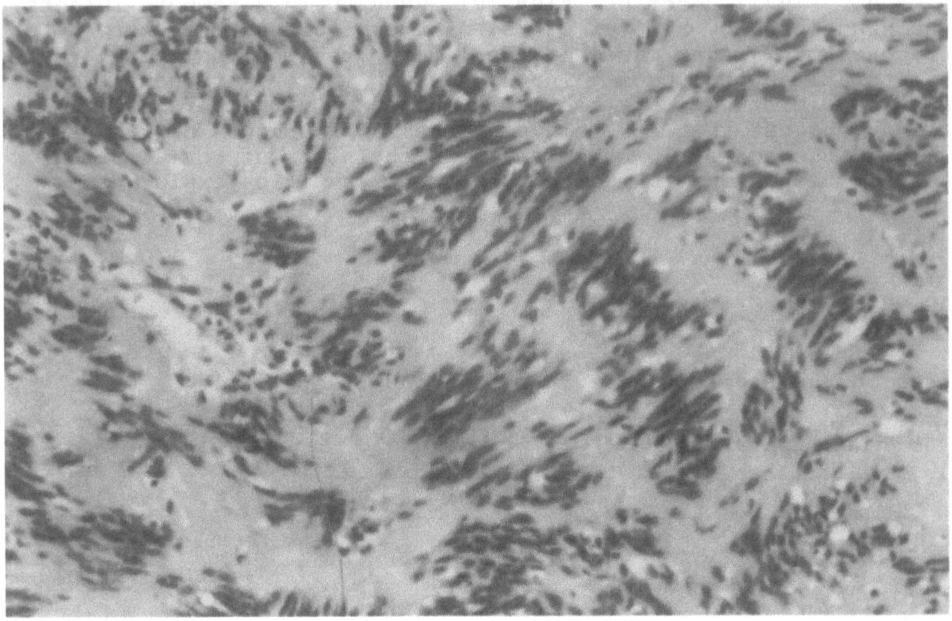

*Fig. 27. Neurilemmoma with regimentation of nuclei (H. & E. X 250)*

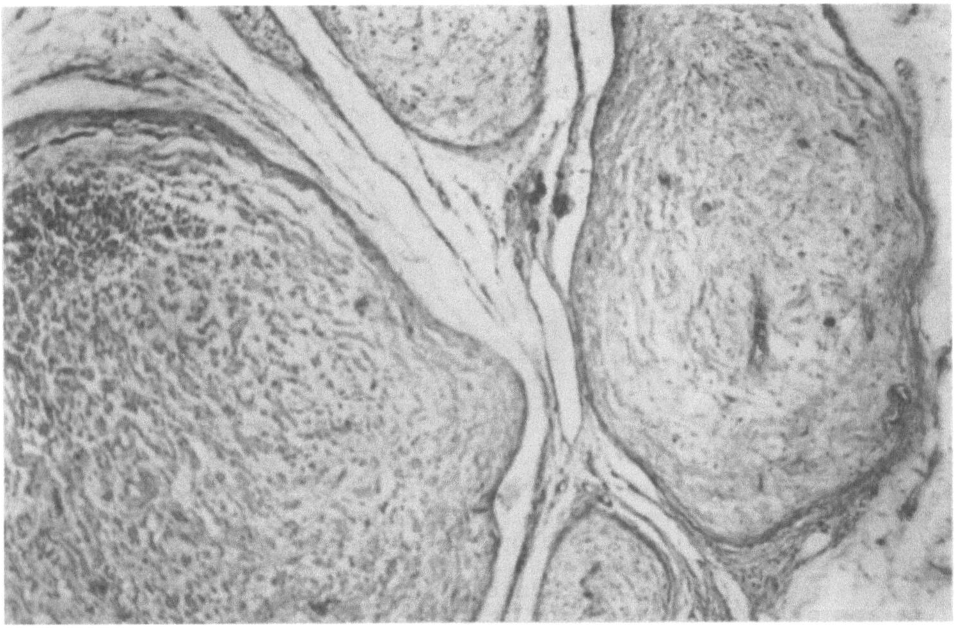

*Fig. 28. Plexiform neurofibroma with oedematous bundles (H.&E.X60)*

lion cells and neurofibromatous tissue. Neurofibromas, even when small, are particularly dangerous in the larynx. They may involve the tongue or intestine and have caused congenital megacolon in the latter situation (TERNBERG and WINTERS, 1965). Megacolon has also been seen in

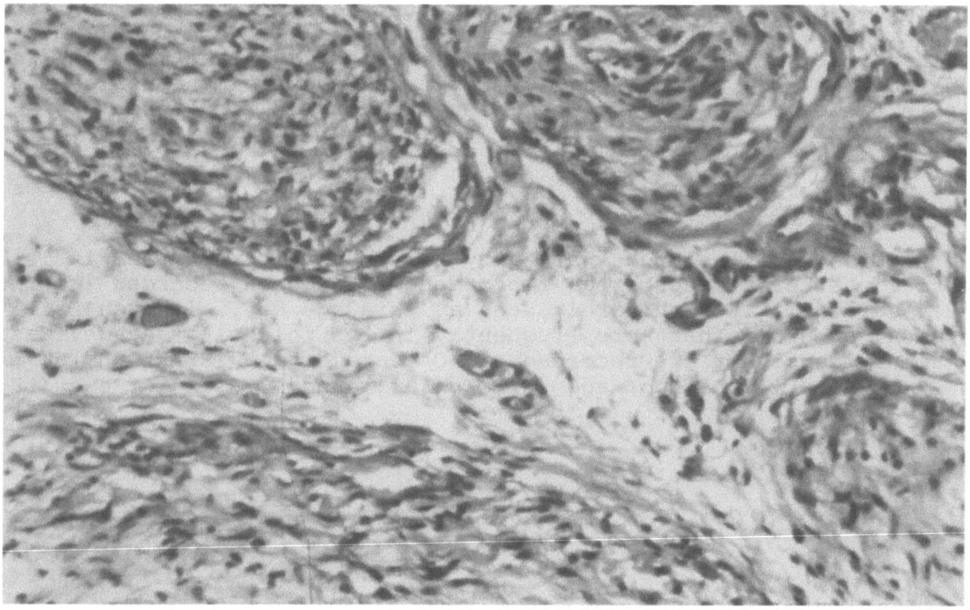

*Fig. 29. Neurofibromatous bundles separated by loose connective tissue (H. & E. X 250)*

the multiple endocrine adenoma syndrome Type II. Neurofibromas may be extensive as in the following case:
CTR.8/68. Boy who attended hospital in November 1964 with a lump in the side of his neck. Biopsy showed it to be a plexiform neurofibroma. During the next 7 years the mass had grown so that it extended from the external auditory meatus to the shoulder, pressed against the pharyngeal wall and caused facial palsy and Horner's syndrome.

Although the widespread nature may cause considerable problems in the surgical treatment of these lesions, few patients die from the tumours unless there is malignant transformation. This has been reported in 5 - 16% of cases but more usually in adults (CROWE et al., 1956). Malignant features have not been encountered in some series (RAFFENSPERGER and COHEN, 1972).

In the Manchester series all except one of the children are still alive. The one child who died was a boy who presented at the age of 6 years with weakness of the right leg which had been first noticed 8 months previously. Laminectomy revealed multiple neurofibromas of the nerve roots of L5 and S1. A second operation was carried out 10 months later and this time the whole cauda equina was found to be matted together in a sarcomatous mass. The child died 11 months later.

Most of the lesions in the Manchester series presented as subcutaneous nodules. The tumours were orbital in 2 children; they were extradural in 3 children and one child had a neurilemmoma of the auditory nerve. The extradural and acoustic tumours have been discussed in Chapter 6.

Multiple neurofibromatosis is a familial disease, being transmitted as an autosomal dominant. It is not certain whether the discovery of a single tumour in a child should be regarded as indicating that the patient is suffering from a mild form of the generalised disease. HARKIN and REED (1968) reject this view unless the neurofibroma is found to be plexiform which they consider to be found only in von Recklinghausen's disease. In the Manchester cases 9 children had multiple lesions and 5 of the remaining 10 children had plexiform neurofibromas. On this evidence 14 of the 19 children had von Recklinghausen's disease.

## Tumours of the Breast

True neoplasms of the breast are very rare before puberty and it is doubtful whether a prepubertal fibroadenoma has been recorded (WILLIS, 1962). Carcinoma is very rarely seen at this age but, although still uncommon, occurs rather more frequently in the following decade. Cases of mammary carcinoma are recorded at 10 years of age (SEARS and SCHLESINGER, 1940), 11 years of age (ELIOT, 1911) and 12 years of age (LEVINGS, 1917).

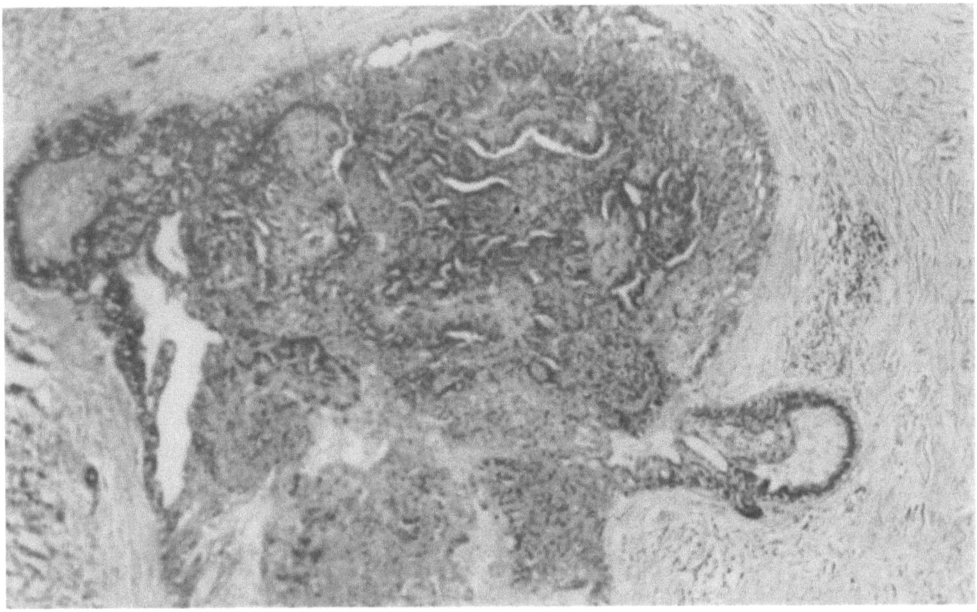

*Fig. 30. Intraduct carcinoma of the breast in 11-year-old girl (H. & E. X 60)*

Localised hyperplasia in the prepubertal age group may suggest a fibroadenoma but in this case the duct proliferation is less active and the fibrous stroma is less cellular without a neoplastic appearance.

In the present series one true fibroadenoma was seen in a girl of 14 years who began to menstruate at 13 years. The mass was firm, pale and grey, measuring 3.5 x 2.5 x 2 cm.

A carcinoma was encountered in a girl of 11 years who had a history of blood-stained discharge from the nipple for some months. The patient had a mass in the axillary quadrant of the right breast. The tumour was excised and was firm and lobulated, measuring 5.5 x 2.5 x 2 cm. There was irregular intraductal proliferation of epithelium with moderate mitoses. The basement membrane was mostly intact but was penetra-

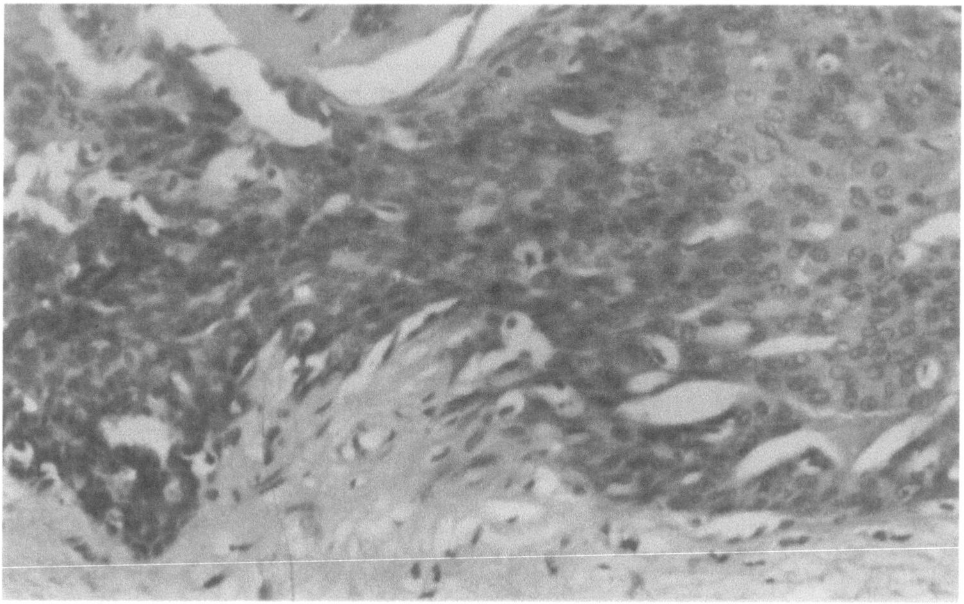

*Fig. 31. Detail of Fig. 3C showing disruption of the basement membrane (H. & E. X 250)*

ted in some places. The tumour was regarded as an intraduct carcinoma which had not yet invaded lymphatics. Radiotherapy was not given and the patient is alive and well 17 years later. McDIVITT et al. (1966) in an analysis of 7 cases of breast carcinoma in childhood regard the tumour as being less aggressive than in the adult.

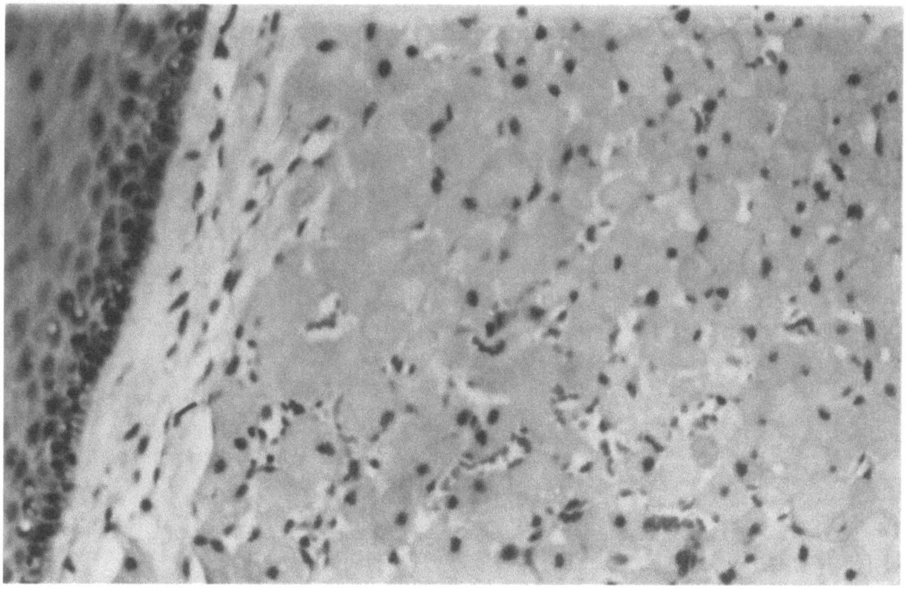

*Fig. 32. Granular cell myoblastoma with swollen granular cells (H. & E. X 250)*

## Granular Cell Myoblastoma

There were 5 tumours in this group. Three were congenital epulides including 2 in the upper and 1 in the lower jaws detected in the neonatal period. One tumour was present at the side of the anus in a 3 1/2-year-old girl and another was excised from the left axilla in a 5-year-old girl. Large eosinophilic, granular, polyhedral cells with small nuclei were present in all cases. Similar cells have been found in tumours of the tongue where cross striations and transition to muscle fibres have, on occasion, been noted. They have also been found in tumour masses in the skin, breast, uterus, respiratory tract and, in about 5% of cases, in striated muscle.

ABRIKOSSOFF (1926 and 1931) used the term "myoblastoma" but the muscle origin has been doubted and WILLIS (1948) suggests that they are degenerative lesions of muscle fibres rather than neoplasms. ABRIKOSSOFF himself felt that some myoblastomas were derived from damage to muscle

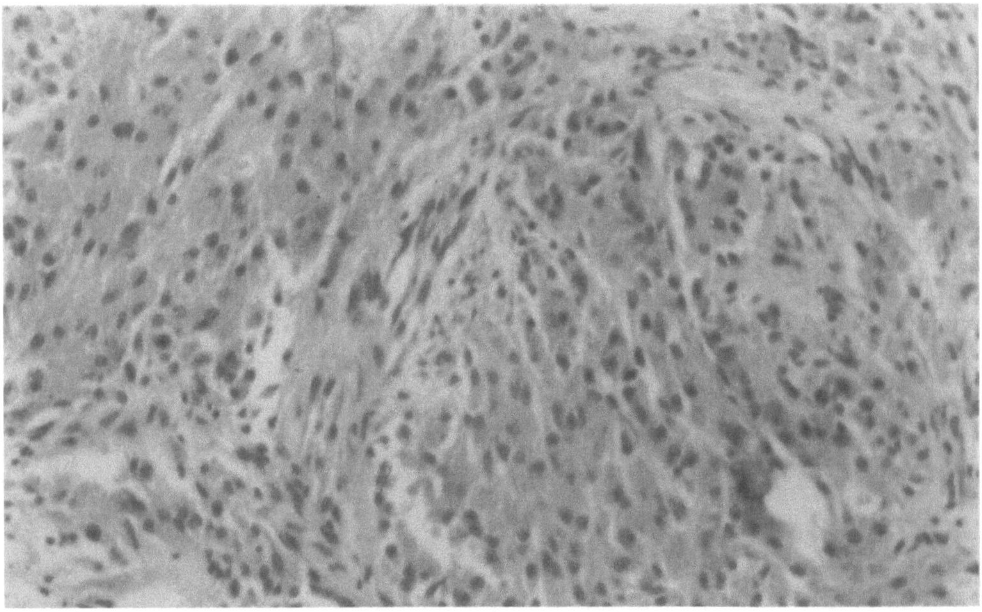

*Fig. 33. Granular cell myoblastoma with spindle-celled fibroblasts blending with large granular cells (H. & E. X 250)*

and that others were embryonic in origin. FUST and CUSTER (1949) considered the granular cell myoblastoma to be of neurogenic origin while WEGELIN (1947) believed it to be histiocytic.

It is probable that the term "granular-cell myoblastoma" includes a variety of lesions, some possibly non-neoplastic. The tumour is benign. Support for a connective or perineural fibroblastic histogenesis in some cases was seen in the tumour of the axilla in the present series. There were spindle-celled areas with transition to swollen granular cells, a feature not seen in any of the other 4 cases.

## "Benign Calcifying Epithelioma" (Pilomatrixoma)

This has been suggested as arising from stem or hair matrix cells and the term "pilomatrixoma" was introduced by FORBIS and HELWIG (1961). BINGUL et al. (1962) discuss this lesion in childhood and an association with myotonica atrophica has been suggested (CANTWELL and REED, 1965). The Manchester series contains 3 children with this condition. One.was a girl of 1 year 11 months in whom a subcutaneous swelling had been noted behind the angle of the jaw on the left side at the age of 6 months and had increased in size since then. Another was a 1-year-old girl with a lump in front of the right ear which had been growing for the previous 3 months. The third child was a 7-year-old boy with a

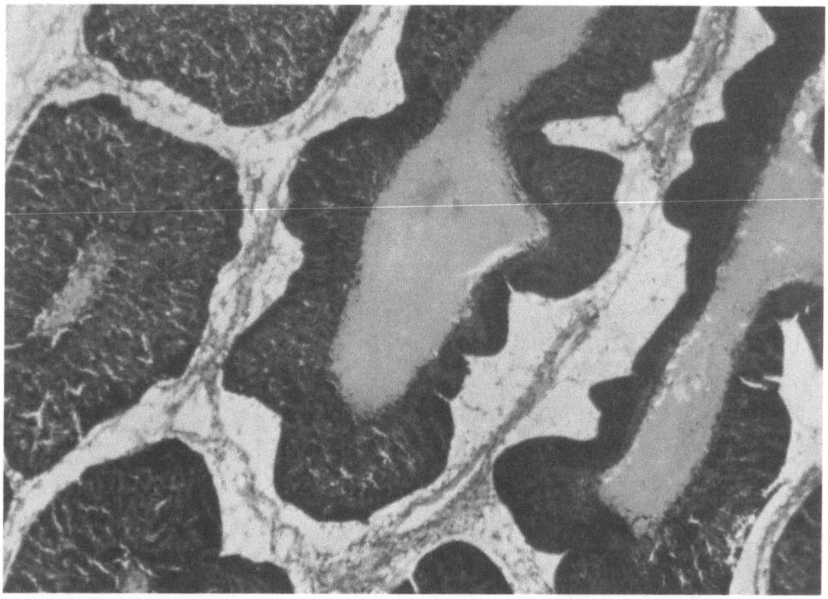

*Fig. 34. "Benign calcifying epithelioma" (pilomatrixoma) with basophilic and "ghost" epithelia (H. & E. X 60)*

lump on the shoulder for 6 months. All three lesions were excised and they have not recurred subsequently.

The histological appearances were typical with dark, epithelial bands showing numerous mitoses, "ghost" epithelium, foreign-body reaction, fibrous tissue and calcification.

## Malignant Melanoma

There has been a considerable increase in the understanding of naevi, juvenile melanomas and malignant melanomas of childhood since the publication of SPITZ (1948). McWHORTER and WOOLNER (1954) review the literature and include 13 cases to which they add 5 of their own, all under the age of 13 years. The histological diagnosis of a melanoma which will metastasize is still difficult in childhood. Fortunately, such tumours are rare and only 14 children died from malignant melanomas in England and Wales during the ten years 1955 - 1964 (Reg. Gen.). In earlier papers on melanoma of childhood many of the cases were probably juvenile melanomas.

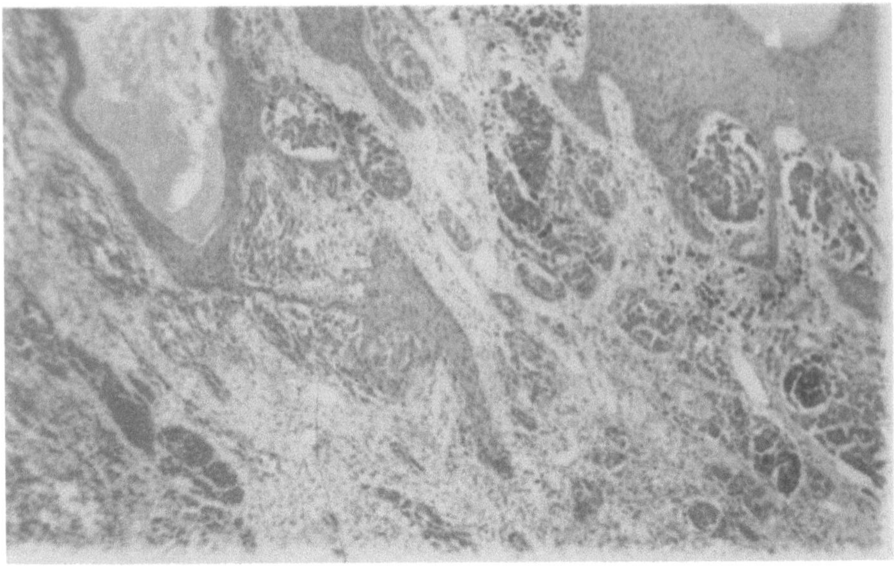

*Fig. 35. Malignant melanoma with abundant pigment production (H. & E. X 60)*

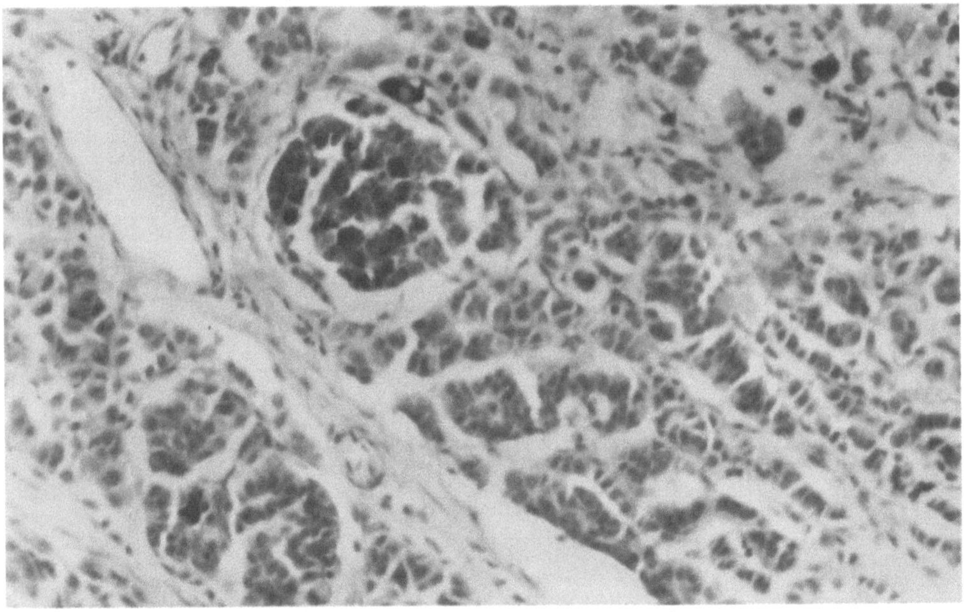

*Fig. 36. Malignant melanoma showing bands of cuboidal and polygonal cells (H. & E. X 250)*

Malignant melanoma has been reported in the newborn as in the case of COE (1925) where such a tumour was found in the scalp and spread to lymph nodes causing death at 4 months. Placental transfer has also been described (HOLLAND, 1949).

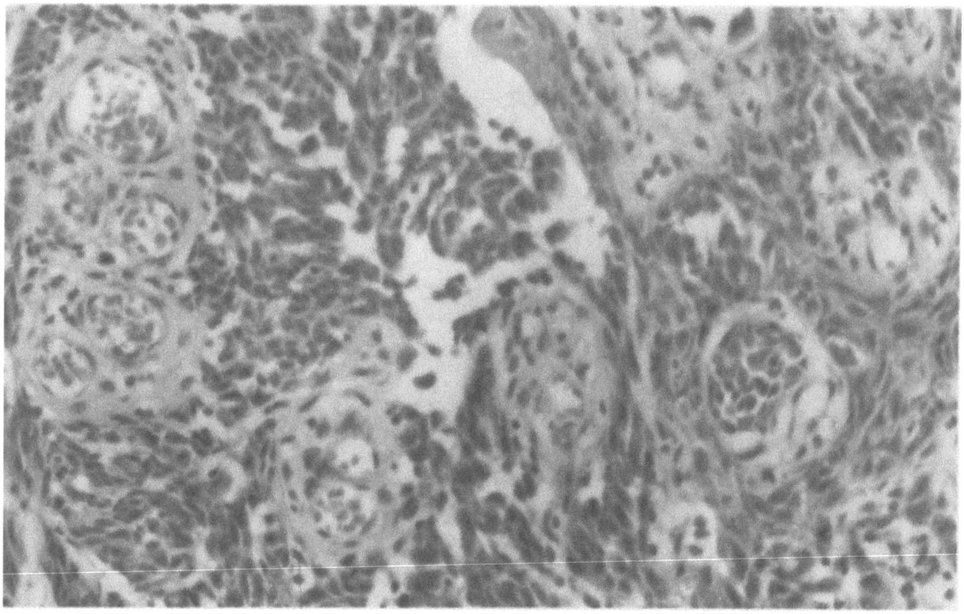

*Fig. 37. Malignant melanoma showing spindle cells and marked vascularity (H. & E. X 250)*

The spread of malignant melanoma is initially to lymph nodes and only later are widespread blood-borne metastases seen. It is possible that tumours in childhood are less malignant than those occurring in later life, although SKOV-JENSEN et al. (1966) regard the prognosis in cases with local or regional lymph node metastases as similar to that in adults. WEBSTER et al. (1944) record a case of an 8-year-old child with malignant melanoma of the shoulder. Metastases in skin and lymph nodes developed which were resected, the patient remaining well 12 years up to the time of publication. As pointed out by SPITZ, spread to lymph nodes does not necessarily mean a fatal outcome. SKOV-JENSEN et al. draw attention to the relatively high likelihood of malignant melanomas arising in pre-existing naevus pigmentosus giganticus.

There were 2 children with malignant melanomas in the Registry. One was an 8-year-old girl who was born with a pink mark on the left buttock. The area became larger and darker over the 15 months prior to consultation. There had also been some bleeding and suppuration. A pedunculated, warty lesion about 4 cm in diameter was excised with an adequate margin. Metastases to the groin glands developed and were excised 3 months later. The tumour spread to the lungs and brain, causing death 1 year after the initial excision. Histologically, there was junctional involvement with pleomorphic cuboidal polygonal cells showing alveolar grouping. Sheaves of spindle cells and occasional giant cells were noted. The tumour was very vascular with interstitial polymorphonuclear infiltration. Mitotic figures were scanty.

The other patient was a boy who developed an infected spot on his right cheek when he was 2 years old. Six months later it was 3/4" in diameter and the cervical nodes were enlarged. The lesion was excised and a lymph node removed. Sections showed pleomorphic naevus cells with scanty melanin and a moderate number of mitoses in the skin lesion and lymph node. XRT to the whole involved area was then given (4000 rads in 11 days). An extensive block dissection of the neck was then performed and the primary lesion was re-excised. Both skin and lymph nodes were shown to be infiltrated with tumour cells. The child is alive and well 5 years later.

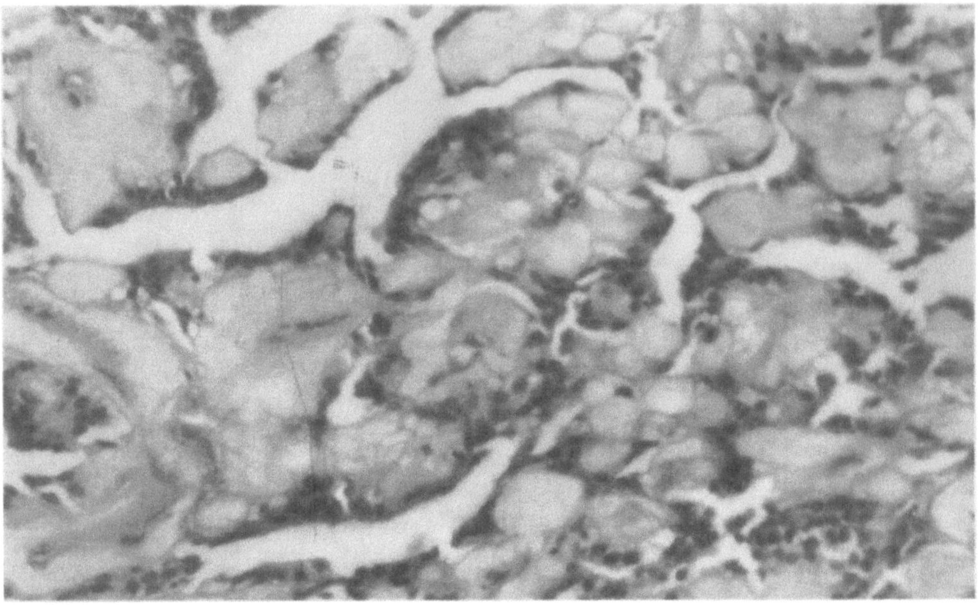

*Fig. 38. Sweat gland adenoma with swollen mucoid cells in papillary arrangement (H. & E. X 250)*

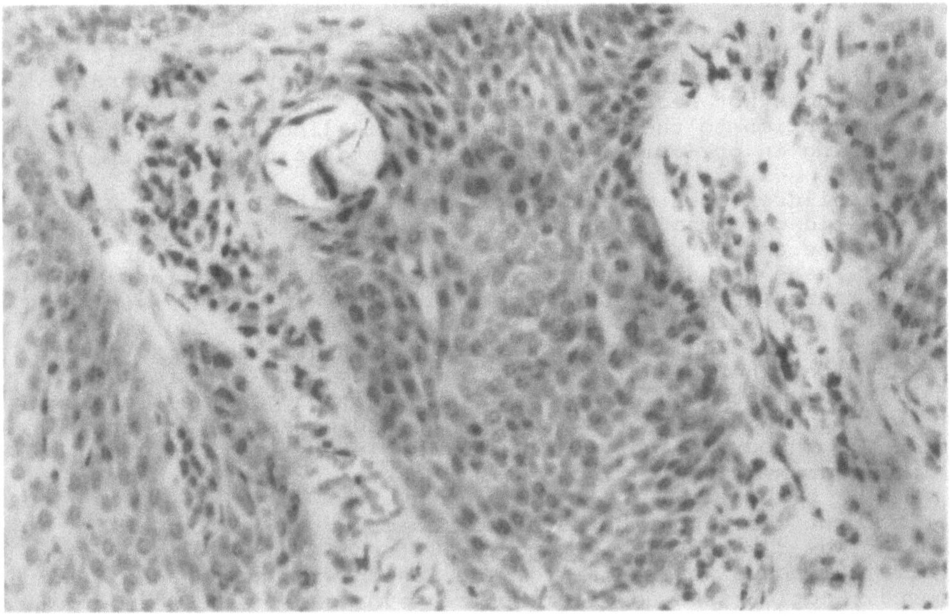

*Fig. 39. Sweat gland carcinoma with epithelial sheets and inflammatory cell reaction (H. & E. X 275)*

The diagnosis of malignant melanoma in childhood is, as already stated, difficult, but some of the features seen in these cases may be significant pointers. These include vascularity of the lesion, interstitial infiltration, pleomorphism of cells with prominence of nucleoli and irregular sheaves of spindle cells. Mitoses were not numerous but the presence of abnormal figures is important.

The malignant melanoma is described as brown or black to the naked eye whereas the juvenile melanoma may be light brown or even yellow or red. WINKELMANN (1961) suggests that histochemical demonstration of enzymes including dopa, tyrosinase, and cholinesterase may be of value.

## Tumours of Sweat Glands

Two tumours were regarded as being of sweat gland origin. One was seen over the lower back in a boy of 8 years. The tumour consisting of a yellow nodule with fibrous bands and microscopically showing a papillary structure with swollen mucoid cells was classified as a cystadenoma. The other lesion occurred as a papule of the face in a 9 1/2-year-old girl. There was acanthosis with sheets of spindle cells having an epitheliomatous appearance. The tumour was circumscribed and in view of its relationship to sweat ducts was classified as a carcinoma of sweat gland origin. There has been no recurrence in either child more than 10 years after excision.

## Thymoma

CTR.88/68. Boy aged 10 years who presented with marked clubbing of the fingers and toes with bilateral periosteal new bone formation of the distal bones of the arms and legs. X-rays showed a mass in the thymic region which was biopsied and treated with irradiation (3000 rads in 21 days). During the following months multiple bone metastases appeared in spite of vincristine and cyclophosphamide and the child died 2 years later. At autopsy no thymic tumour remained but in addition to the bone metastases there were deposits in the lungs, liver and spleen. The tumour in this case was of lymphoepitheliomatous type but spindle-celled neoplasms also occur in the thymus in childhood and more recently such a case has been included in the Registry.

## Chordoma

CTR.136/68. Boy aged 8 years who suddenly developed headache and 6th nerve palsy. Air encephalography showed a space-occupying lesion in the region of the pons. A chordoma arising from the base of the skull was removed. The child remains well 5 years later.

## Carotid Body Tumour

CTR.137/66. Girl aged 11 years who started with difficulty in speaking and having attacks of unconsciousness which were thought to be epileptic. A few months later a lump in the right side of the neck was noted. Three years later she developed atrophy of the tongue and Horner's syndrome on the right side. Surgical exploration revealed a malignant chemodectoma which had eroded the base of the skull. The tumour could only be partially removed. Six months later the residual tumour was enlarging and it was therefore irradiated (4000 rads in 20 days). The tumour resolved and the child was well and without any palpable masses 2 years after being irradiated and 7 years after the illness started.

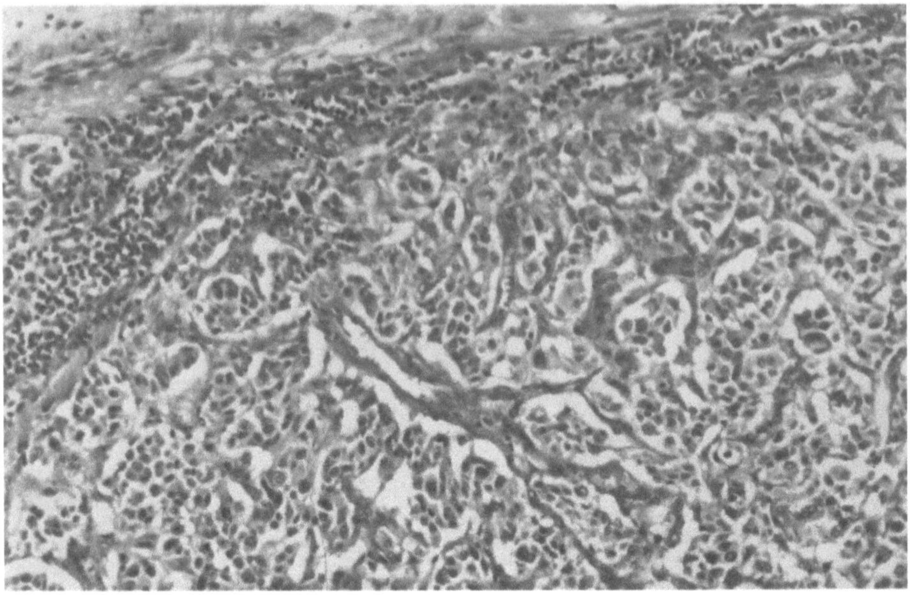

*Fig. 40. CTR.137/66. Chemodectoma in lymph node showing groups of eosinophilic cells separated by fibrous septa (H. & E. X 250)*

Alveolar Soft Part Sarcoma

SMETANA and SCOTT (1951) described a rare group of tumours found particularly in the thigh and retroperitoneum. These authors regarded them

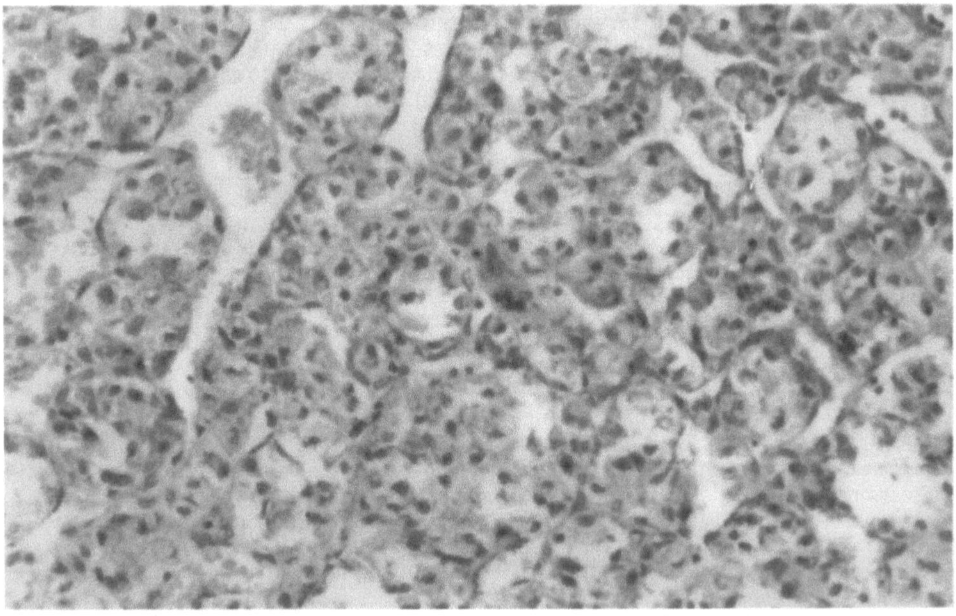

*Fig. 41. Alveolar soft part sarcoma with grouping of cells, vascular sinusoids, and fine septa (H. & E. X 250)*

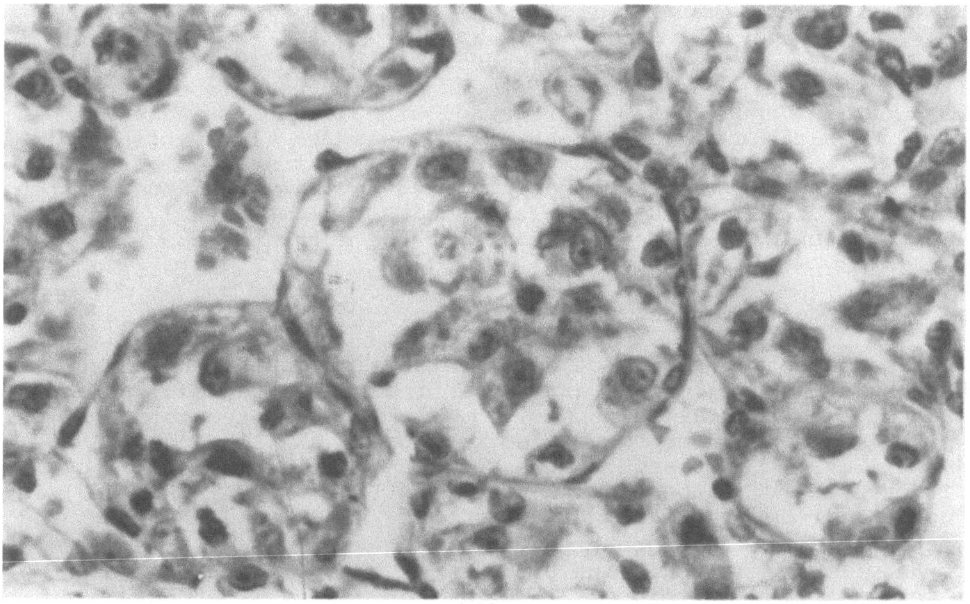

*Fig. 42. Detail of Fig. 41 (H. & E. X 625)*

as malignant tumours of nonchromaffin paraganglia. CHRISTOPHERSON et al. (1952) doubted such an origin and introduced the descriptive term of "alveolar soft part sarcoma". Certain resemblances to alveolar rhabdomyosarcoma, cerebellar haemangioblastoma, and malignant granular cell myoblastoma have also been considered although the last term is itself open to question.

One such case was encountered in this series, the patient being a 10-year-old girl in whom a painless swelling had been noticed in the left leg 2 weeks earlier. A mobile mass 3.5 x 3.5 cm was found on the outer aspect of the thigh and a highly vascular, yellow and white encephaloid tumour was excised from the vastus lateralis. There was no sign of spread for 6 years but then lung metastases became apparent. Thoracotomy revealed that the lungs were studded with many nodules of tumour. These caused no symptoms and no treatment has been given. The patient remains well 11 years after the primary first appeared and is married.

The histological appearance of the tumour was typical with polygonal, granular, eosinophilic cells showing prominent nucleoli and arranged in alveolar or tubular pattern. There were thin-walled vascular sinusoids. The tumour was circumscribed with a fibrous capsule and satellite areas possibly due to vascular spread.

MARSHALL and HORN (1961) showed histochemical differences in these tumours from haemangioblastoma, alveolar rhabdomyosarcoma and tumours of paraganglia. FISHER and REIDBORD (1971) found cytoplasmic crystalloids on electron microscopy which were similar to the rods in rhabdomyoma, nemaline myopathy, z-band material and tropomysin B. The clinical features and the histological appearance indicate a specific neoplasm for which it is suggested that the term alveolar soft part sarcoma be retained at the present time.

The alveolar soft part sarcoma occurs more commonly in girls than in boys, although the sex difference is not so apparent in older patients (G. D'ANGIO, personal communication, 1975).

## "Malignant Haemangioma"

CTR.145/66. A 12-year-old boy attended hospital in April 1966 with a warty growth on his back which had been present for 6 months. It was excised but in January 1973 he returned with a lump, 2 inches in diameter in his right axilla. The axillary mass was also excised. Histologically the 2 tumours were very similar, consisting of angiomatous tissue, but the axillary mass was confined to the lymph node. Although a multifocal origin could not be excluded, it seemed likely that the axillary lesion was a late metastasis of the original tumour.

## Pigmented Neuroectodermal Tumour of Infancy

There are pigmented tumours of infancy the histogenesis of which is rather obscure. Such lesions arising in the maxilla have been regarded as melanotic epithelial odontomas. The terms "pigmented teratoma" and "atypical melanoblastoma" have also been used. BRATTON and ROBINSON (1946) believed that these tumours contained glial tissue in addition to differentiating into rods and cones. HALPERT and PATZER (1947) introduced the term "retinal anlage tumour". CLARKE and PARSONS (1951) reported the first instance of a tumour elsewhere than in the facial bones, namely in the scalp and BLANC et al. (1958) described a similar lesion in the deltoid of a 5-month-old infant. They have also been found in the scapular region (LURIE and ISAACSON, 1961), and even the epididymis (EATON and FERGUSON, 1956). To account for the widespread distribution and because the odontogenic and retinal anlage theories did not seem entirely satisfactory, STOWENS (1957) introduced the term melanotic progonoma, implying sensory neuroectodermal origin with atavism. LURIE (1961) fully discusses this theory which is supported by the electron-microscope studies of MISUGI et al. (1965) and the report of BORELLO and GORLIN (1966) of high VMA excretion in a patient with this tumour.

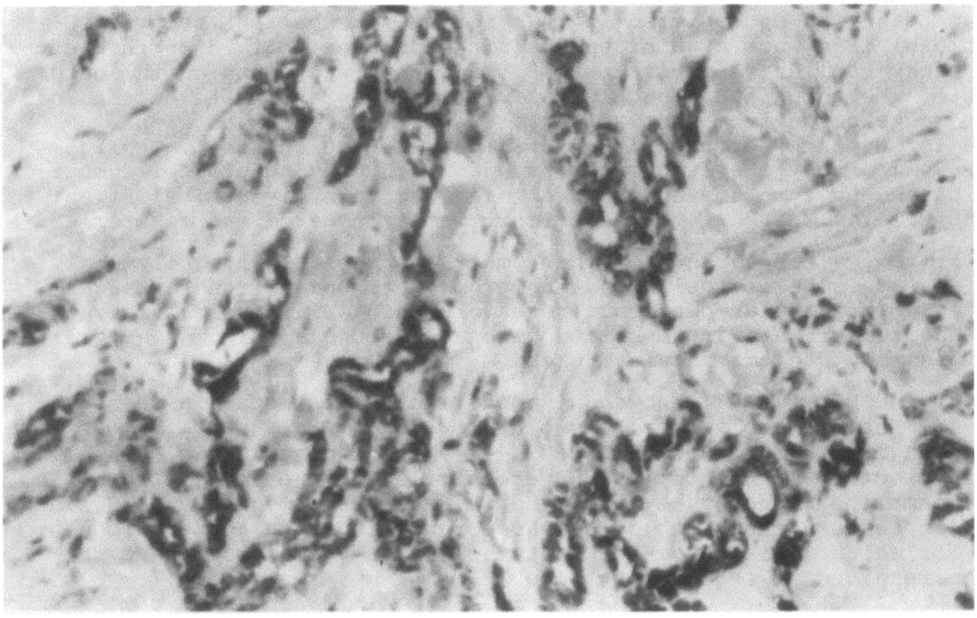

*Fig. 43. Pigmented neuroectodermal tumour of infancy with rudimentary tubules and pigment (H. & E. X 250)*

There was one pigmented tumour having similar histological features to the above cases in the Manchester series. This was found in a 4 1/2-month-old girl and consisted of a firm mass 5.5 x 4 cm behind the right ear. It appeared to be encapsulated and showed primitive tubule formation and clefts with solid masses of small spheroidal cells and fibrous tissue. Rather large, pale cells were noted and there was abundant pigment. No evidence of dental structures was detected and glial tissue could not be shown with certainty. These tumours appear to be benign but may recur if excision is inadequate. Treatment in the Manchester case consisted of an initial biopsy followed by irradiation and subsequent surgical excision. The patient is well 13 years after treatment.

## Tumour of Uncertain Origin

CTR.100/64. Boy who had a subcutaneous swelling of the scalp at birth. The mass was excised when the child was 4 months old. It was found to be attached to the dura. The child is well 8 years later. The histological appearance showed pale vacuolated cells with rather small, uniform nuclei separated into groups by capillaries. There was a well-developed capsule but clumps of tumour cells were noted outside this capsule. A glomus origin was suggested for the tumour. Glomus tumours in children are discussed by KOHOUT and STOUT (1961) who record 57 cases.

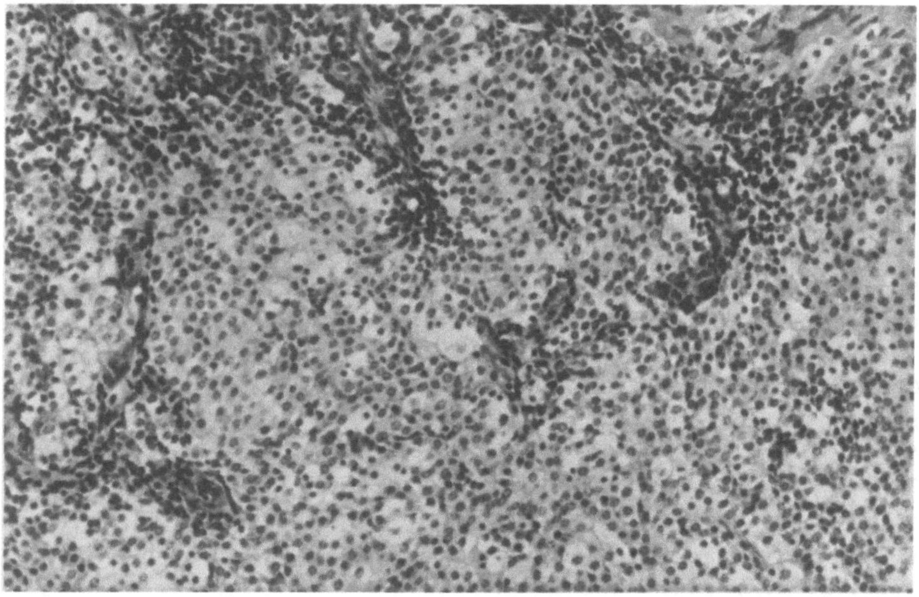

*Fig. 44. CTR.100/64. Scalp tumour in newborn infant referred to in text, showing groups of pale vacuolated cells (H. & E. X 250)*

## REFERENCES

ABRIKOSSOFF, A. I.: Virchow's Arch. 260, 215 (1926)

ABRIKOSSOFF, A. I.: Virchow's Arch. 280, 723 (1931)

AHLFELD, F.: Arch. Gynäk. 16, 135 (1880)

ALAGHEMAND, A.: Amer. Surgeon 28, 784 (1962)

ANDERSON, A. E., BUECHNER, H. A., YAGER, I., ZISKIND, M. M.: Amer. J. Med. 16, 404 (1954)

ARIEL, I. M., PACK, G. T.: Cancer and Allied Disorders of Infancy and Childhood. London: Churchill, 1960

ATKINSON, L., SCOTT, G. C.: Cancer of the Nasopharynx. C. S. MUIR and K. SHANMUGARATNAM (eds.). Copenhagen: Munksgaard, 1967

BINGUL, O., GRAHAM, J. H., HELWIG, E. B.: Pediat. 30, 233 (1962)

BLANC, W. A., ROSENBLATT, P., WOLFF, J. A.: Cancer 11, 959 (1958)

BORELLO, E. D., GORLIN, R. J.: Cancer 19, 196 (1966)

BRATTON, A. B., ROBINSON, S. H. G.: J. Path. Bact. 58, 643 (1946)

BUCHMAN, J. A., CALHOUN, J. D.: Amer. Surg. 24, 280 (1958)

BURKE, C. W.: Brit. J. Hosp. Med. 11, 759 (1974)

CANTWELL, A. R., REED, W. B.: Acta. derm. and Vener. (Stockholm) 45, 387 (1965)

CHIA, K. B.: Cancer of the Nasopharynx. C. S. MUIR and K. SHANMUGARATNAM (eds.). Copenhagen: Munksgaard, 1967

CHRISTOPHERSON, W. M., FOOTE, F. W., STEWART, F. W.: Cancer 5, 100 (1952)

CLARKE, B. E., PARSONS, H.: Cancer 4, 78 (1951)

CLIFFORD, P.: Cancer of the Nasopharynx. C. S. MUIR and K. SHANMUGARATNAM (eds.). Copenhagen: Munksgaard, 1967

CLUTTS, G. R., EMMETT, J. M.: Amer. Surgeon 30, 671 (1964)

COE, H. E.: Northwest Med. 24, 181 (1925)

CONN, J. W.: J. Lab. Clin. Med. 45, 3 (1955)

CROWE, F. W., SCHULL, W. J., NEED, J. U.: A Clinical Study of Multiple Neurofibromatosis. Springfield, Ill.: Thomas, 1956

DEVROEDE, G. J., TAYLOR, W. F., SAUER, W. G., JACKMAN, R. T., STICKLER, G. B.: New Eng. J. Med. 285, 17 (1971)

DIGBY, K. H., FOOK, W. L., CHE, Y. T.: Brit. J. Surg. 28, 517 (1941)

DONALDSON, M. H., TAYLOR, P., RAWITSCHER, R., SEWELL, J. B.: Pediatrics 48, 307 (1971)

EATON, W. L., FERGUSON, J. P.: Cancer 9, 718 (1956)

ELIOT, E.: Ann. Surg. 53, 726 (1911)

EVANS, R. W.: Histological Appearances of Tumours. London: Livingstone 1956, p. 392, 525

FIELD, J. L., ADAMSON, L. F., STOECKLE, H. E.: Pediatrics 29, 953 (1962)

FISH, J. C., McGARY, R. G.: Arch. Surg. 93, 355 (1966)

FISHER, E. B., REIDBORD, H.: Cancer 27, 150 (1971)

FORBIS, R. Jr., HELWIG, E. B.: Arch. Dermat. 83, 606 (1961)

FRAUMENI, J. F. Jr., MILLER, R. W., HILL, J. A.: J. Nat. Canc. Inst. 40, 1087 (1968)

FUST, J. A., CUSTER, R. P.: Amer. J. Clin. Path. 19, 522 (1949)

GRIME, R. T., MOORE, T., NICHOLSON, A., WHITEHEAD, R.: Brit. J. Surg. 47, 307 (1959)

GRISHMAN, E.: Cancer 5, 700 (1952)

HALPERT, B., PATZER, R.: Surgery 22, 837 (1947)

HARE, H. F., NEWCOMB, R. V.: Radiology 54, 401 (1950)

HARKIN, J. C., REED, R. J.: Tumors of the Peripheral Nervous System, Atlas of Tumor Pathology, Fascicle 3, Second series: Armed Forces Institute of Pathology, Washington, D. C. 1968

HEALEY, W. V., PERZIN, K. H., SMITH, L.: Cancer 26, 368 (1970)

HOERNER, M. T.: Amer. J. Surg. 96, 47 (1958)

HOLLAND, E.: J. Obst. and Gyn. Brit. Emp. 56, 539 (1949)

HOLT, L. E., McINTOSH, R., BARNETT, H. L.: Pediatrics. 13th ed. New York: Appleton - Century - Crofts Inc., 1962

HORN, R. C., RAVDIN, I. S.: J. Clin. Endocrin. 11, 1166 (1951)

ISHAK, K. G., GLUNZ, P. R.: Cancer 20, 396 (1967)

JOHNSTON, J. H.: Amer. J. Surg. 73, 703 (1947)

KASAI, M., WANTANABE, I.: Cancer 25, 551 (1970)

KEELING, J. W.: Jour. Path. 103, 69 (1971)

KERR, J. G.: Amer. J. Surg. 76, 667 (1948)

KOHOUT, E., STOUT, A. P.: Cancer 14, 555 (1961)

Leading Article, Brit. Med. J. 2, 461 (1974)

LEVINGS, A. H.: Amer. J. Surg. 31, 29 (1917)

LURIE, H. I.: Cancer 14, 1090 (1961)

LURIE, H. I., ISAACSON, C.: Cancer 14, 1088 (1961)

McDIVITT, R. W., STEWART, F. W.: J. A. M. A. 195, 388 (1966)

McWHORTER, H. E., WOOLNER, L. B.: Cancer 7, 564 (1954)

MARSHALL, R. B., HORN, R. C.: Cancer 14, 779 (1961)

MATZ, P. B.: J. A. M. A. 111, 2086 (1938)

MIDDELKAMP, J. N., HAFFNER, H.: Pediatrics 32, 558 (1963)

MISUGI, K., OKAJIMA, H., MISUGI, N., NEWTON, W. A.: Cancer 20, 1760 (1967)

MISUGI, K., OKAJIMA, H., NEWTON, W. A., KMETZ, D. R., De LORIMIER, A.A.: Cancer 18, 477 (1965)

MOSIER, H. D., GOODWIN, W. E.: Pediatr. 27, 1016 (1961)

MUIR, C. S., SHANMUGARATNAM, K.: Cancer of the Nasopharynx. A symposium organised by the International Union against Cancer. Copenhagen: Munksgaard, 1967

PELLER, S.: Cancer in Childhood and Youth. Bristol: John Wright and Sons Ltd., 1960

PICKETT, L. K., BRIGGS, H. C.: Ped. Clin. North America 14, 223 (1967)

RAFFENSPERGER, J., COHEN, R.: J. Ped. Surg. 7, 144 (1972)

ROBINSON, M. J., CLARKE, A. M., GOLD, H., CONNELLY, J. F.: Pediatrics 48, 232 (1971)

SACHIATELLO, C. R.: Cancer 28, 581 (1971)

SCHILLA, F. W.: Amer. J. Surg. 88, 759 (1954)

SEARS, J. G., SCHLESINGER, M.J.: New Eng. J. Med. 223, 760 (1940)

SEIFERT, G.: Z. Kinderchir. 2, 285 (1965)

SHANMUGARATNAM, K., HIGGINSON, J.: Cancer of the Nasopharynx. C. S. MUIR and K. SHANMUGARATNAM (eds.). Copenhagen: Munksgaard, 1967

SKOV-JENSEN, T., HASTRUP, J., LAMBRETHSEN, E.: Cancer 19, 620 (1966)

SMETANA, H. F., SCOTT, W. F.: Mil. Surg. 109, 330 (1951)

SPITZ, S.: Amer. J. Path. 24, 591 (1948)

STANBURY, J. B., De GROOT, L. J.: Cancer of the Thyroid. In: Methods of Cancer Research. Harris BUSCH (ed.). New York: Academic Press 10, 143, 1973

STOWENS, D.: J. Path. Bact. 73, 43 (1957)

SUTER, L.: Ann. Pediat. 179, 361 (1952)

TEOH, T. B.: J. Path. Bact. 73, 451 (1957)

TEOH, T. B.: Cancer of the Nasopharynx. C. S. MUIR and K. SHANMUGARATNAM (eds.). Copenhagen: Munksgaard, 1967

TERNBERG, J. L., WINTERS, K.: Amer. J. Surg. 109, 663 (1965)

WANG, C. C., LITTLE, J. B., SCHULZ, M. D.: Cancer 15, 921 (1962)

WEBSTER, J. P., STEVENSON, T. W., STOUT, A. P.: Surg. Clin. North Amer. 24, 319 (1944)

WEBSTER, R., WILLIAMS, A.: Med. J. Australia 2, 553 (1956)

WEGELIN, C.: Schweiz. Z. Allg. Path. 10, 631 (1947)

WELCH, R. A., MEYER, A. T.: Arch. Path. 85, 433 (1968)

WILKINS, L.: The Diagnosis and Treatment of Endocrine Disorders in Childhood and Adolescence. Oxford: Blackwell Scientific Publications, 1957

WILLIAMS, C.: Ann. Surg. 139, 816 (1954)

WILLIAMS, E. D.: J. Clin. Path. 18, 288 (1965)

WILLIS, R. A.: Pathology of Tumours. London: Butterworth and Co. Ltd., 1948

WILLIS, R. A.: Pathology of the Tumours of Children. Edinburgh: Oliver and Boyd, 1962

WILLIS, R. A.: Pathology of Tumours. 2nd ed. London: Butterworth and Boyd, 1962

WINKELMANN, R. K.: Cancer 14, 1001 (1961)

WINSHIP, T.: Trans. Amer. Goiter Ass. 3, 64 (1951)

WINSHIP, T., ROSVOLL, R. V.: Cancer 14, 734 (1961)

YEH, S.: Cancer 15, 895 (1962)

YEH, S., COWDRY, E. V.: Cancer 7, 425 (1954)

# Chapter 13
# Ewing's Tumours

JAMES EWING (1922) selected a small-celled non-osteogenic tumour of bone with a number of clinical features, including slow growth rate, and classified it as an endothelial myeloma or diffuse endothelioma of bone. All the patients in his series were under 20 years old and in 7 of the 10 cases the long bones of limbs were affected. PARKER and JACKSON (1939) described a somewhat similar tumour occurring mainly in adults, called it reticulum cell sarcoma of bone, and noted that, in contrast with EWING's cases, it appeared to have a good prognosis.

Up to the end of 1968 there were 30 children in the Manchester Children's Tumour Register with small-celled non-osteogenic tumours of bone. The presenting sites are shown in Table 1.

Table 1. Ewing's tumours - primary sites

| | |
|---|---|
| Tibia | 6 |
| Femur | 4 |
| Humerus | 5 |
| Fibula | 5 |
| Pelvis | 5 |
| Rib | 2 |
| Ulna | 1 |
| Vertebra | 2 |
| | 30 |

By far the commonest initial symptom was pain, which was present in 26 patients and sometimes appeared worse at night. Swelling was noted in 17 cases. One child had a history of vague malaise which was probably due to a pleural effusion caused by a tumour in a rib.

Because the tumours in the Register more closely resembled those described by EWING than those of PARKER and JACKSON, and also because, in the present stage of knowledge, it would be unwise to speculate on their histogenesis, they have all been called EWING's tumours. The difficulty in diagnosing such tumours on histological grounds, particularly when only a small biopsy is available, has led to confusion between EWING's tumours and metastatic neuroblastoma in bone.

## Comparison Between Ewing's Tumours and Neuroblastomas

There were 30 children with EWING's tumours and 101 with neuroblastomas in the Register. Twenty-eight of those with Ewing's tumours have died - all with active tumour present at death. Fifty of those with neuroblastoma developed bone metastases and all except one of these died. Autopsies were performed on 8 of those with Ewing's tumour and 24 with neuroblastoma metastatic to bone.

## Primary Sites

Tumour was detected in the pararenal or paravertebral region at some point along the spinal column in all the cases of neuroblastoma. There were masses in the pararenal or paravertebral areas in only 5 of the children with Ewing's tumour.

## Age Incidence

The patients with neuroblastoma were younger than those with Ewing's tumours. There was no case of the latter in children under 2 years old (Table 2).

Table 2. Neuroblastomas and Ewing's tumours - age at diagnosis

| Age (years) | -1 | 1 | 2 | 3 | 4 | 5 | 6 | 7 | 8 | 9 | 10 | 11 | 12 | 13 | 14 |
|---|---|---|---|---|---|---|---|---|---|---|---|---|---|---|---|
| Ewing's tumours | 0 | 0 | 1 | 2 | 0 | 3 | 4 | 5 | 1 | 2 | 3 | 2 | 2 | 3 | 2 |
| All neuroblastomas | 29 | 21 | 11 | 15 | 9 | 2 | 2 | 5 | 2 | 1 | 0 | 1 | 2 | 0 | 1 |
| Neuroblastomas with bone metastases | 5 | 13 | 5 | 12 | 6 | 1 | 2 | 3 | 2 | 0 | 0 | 0 | 0 | 0 | 1 |

## Progress of the Disease

Ewing's tumours progress much more slowly than neuroblastomas. Seventy percent of cases with Ewing's tumours survived for more than 1 year after diagnosis whereas 94% of the children with neuroblastomas died within 1 year of the first sign of bone involvement (Fig. 1).

The slow progress of the Ewing's tumour may result in children who die of the disease becoming extremely emaciated (Fig. 2).

## Spread

In order to obtain a complete picture of the spread of neuroblastomas and Ewing's tumours it would be necessary to investigate these patients in much greater detail than was the practice in Manchester prior to 1969. It was before the era of isotope scanning, bone marrow examinations were seldom performed, and skeletal X-ray surveys were not carried out regularly. However, even with the somewhat limited investigations performed, several differences between the modes of spread of neuroblastomas and Ewing's tumours were obvious.

Neuroblastomas and Ewing's tumours appear to have an equal tendency to metastasize in bones but there is a marked difference in the frequency of lung metastases in the two tumours (Table 3).

Bones were the most frequent metastatic sites in the neuroblastoma cases. Lymph nodes were the second most frequent sites of secondary involvement encountered in neuroblastoma, whereas this mode was seldom apparent in the Manchester patients with Ewing's tumour. This feature has been remarked upon by LICHTENSTEIN (1959). Hepatic involvement could not be excluded in patients dying without post-mortem examina-

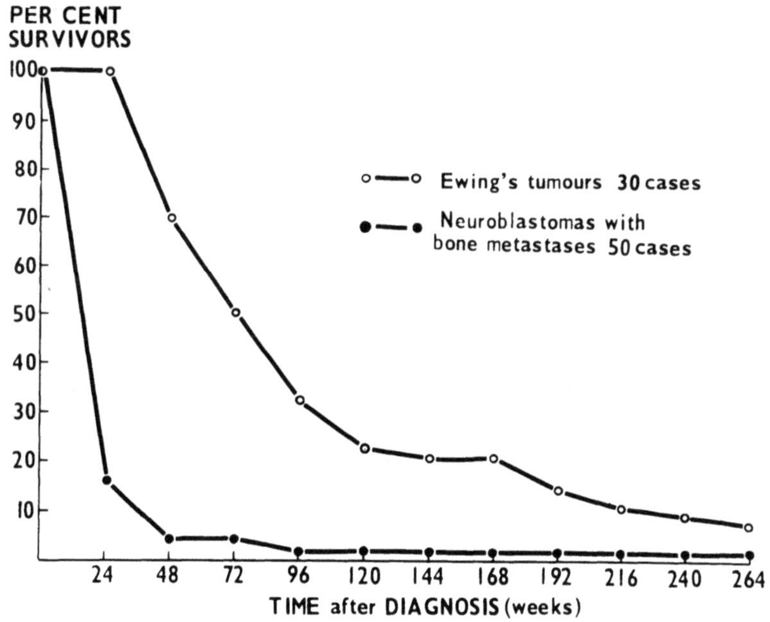


*Fig. 1. Curves showing the difference in length of survival of children with Ewing's tumours and neuroblastomas metastatic in bone*

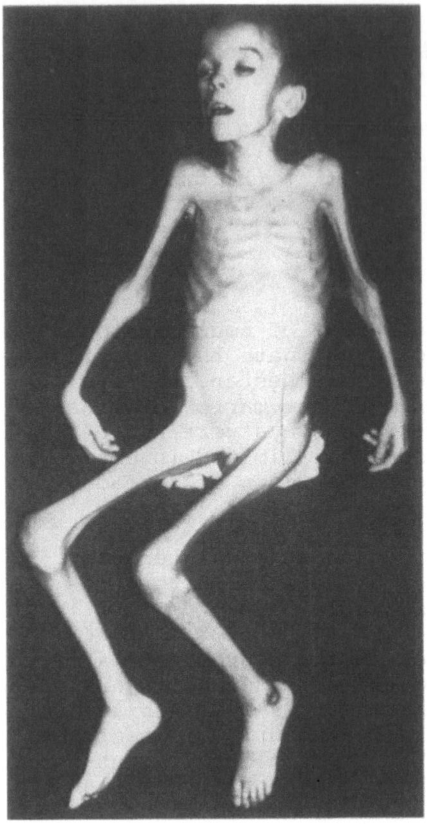

*Fig. 2. Boy aged 8 years with metastases from Ewing's tumour of left ulna. Primary had not recurred following irradiation. Slow progress of disease may cause extreme emaciation*

Table 3. Metastases of Ewing's tumours and neuroblastomas

| | Ewing's tumours (percent) | Neuroblastomas (percent) |
|---|---|---|
| Bone | 57 | 50 |
| Lungs | 70 | 8 |

tion, but a liver deposit was detected in only 1 of the 8 children with Ewing's tumours who had autopsies. Hepatic invasion was relatively frequent in neuroblastoma. No example of widespread liver invasion was seen in any case of Ewing's tumour such as may be found in the so-called Pepper syndrome (PEPPER, 1901). The lungs were the most frequently encountered site of metastasis in the cases of Ewing's tumour. The deposits were multiple, subpleural and intrapulmonary and could sometimes be readily separated from the surrounding lung parenchyma. By contrast, neuroblastomas seldom spread to the lungs - there was pulmonary involvement in only 8 of the 50 children with the Hutchison syndrome and in 6 of them this was probably due to direct spread from a thoracic tumour. Only 2 Manchester children had definite blood-borne neuroblastoma deposits in the lungs.

## Pattern of Skeletal Involvement

In children with neuroblastoma one bone deposit was nearly always rapidly followed by many others so that the children became riddled with metastases within a few weeks. As judged by clinical and radiological examinations the behaviour of the 30 Ewing's tumours was quite different. Twenty-eight of the children appeared to have single lesions at the time of diagnosis and in over 60% no other bone tumours were detected for more than a year. The 2 survivors have been kept under observation for 11 and 15 years without further skeletal involvement.

Although this shows the difference between Ewing's tumours and neuroblastomas, the Manchester experience prior to 1969 underestimates the extent of the tendency of Ewing's tumours to spread to other bones. Modern isotope scanning has shown that bone deposits may be present without any radiological change and at autopsy microscopic medullary foci of Ewing's tumour have been seen in bones which appear normal to the naked eye (Fig. 3).

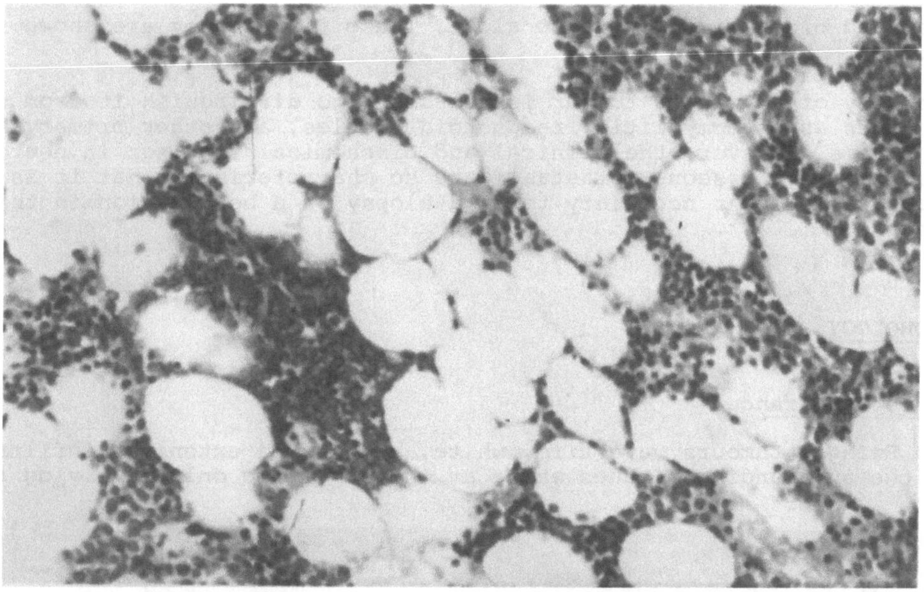

*Fig. 3. Microscopic Ewing's tumour metastasis in bone which appeared normal on naked eye examination (H. & E. X 400)*

## Biochemical Findings

In chapter 7 it was pointed out that children with neuroblastomas nearly always had an increased excretion of catecholamines and their metabolites. Sixteen Manchester children with Ewing's tumours were examined biochemically and showed no evidence of increased excretion of catecholamines or their metabolites. Six of these patients had started treatment but in some this was just prior to examination of the urine. In 10 children there was extensive and active tumour present.

In summary, therefore, there is such a sharp contrast between the clinical and metabolic behaviour of the Ewing's tumours and the secondary neuroblastomas in bone that the distinction should be made on the clin-

Table 4

| Ewing's tumour | Secondary neuroblastoma in bone |
|---|---|
| Paravertebral or pararenal (secondary) deposits very rarely present | Paravertebral or pararenal primary tumours present |
| Slowly progressive | Rapidly progressive |
| Rarely seen in young children | Common age incidence 1-5 years |
| Commonly spreads to lungs | Commonly spreads to lymph nodes and liver, but very rarely spreads to lungs |
| No detectable secretory activity | Abnormal catecholamine excretion in nearly all patients |

ical and biochemical evidence alone. These differences are shown in Table 4.

A biopsy of a Ewing's tumour is necessary to distinguish it from such diseases as osteomyelitis, rheumatoid nodules, and other primary bone neoplasms. However, the clinical and biochemical findings in neuroblastoma with osseous metastases are so characteristic that it is practically never necessary to do a biopsy of a bone lesion in this disease.

## PATHOLOGY

### Gross Appearance

The Ewing's tumours were firm, white, and showed extensive infiltration of the surrounding tissues while at the same time only involving the

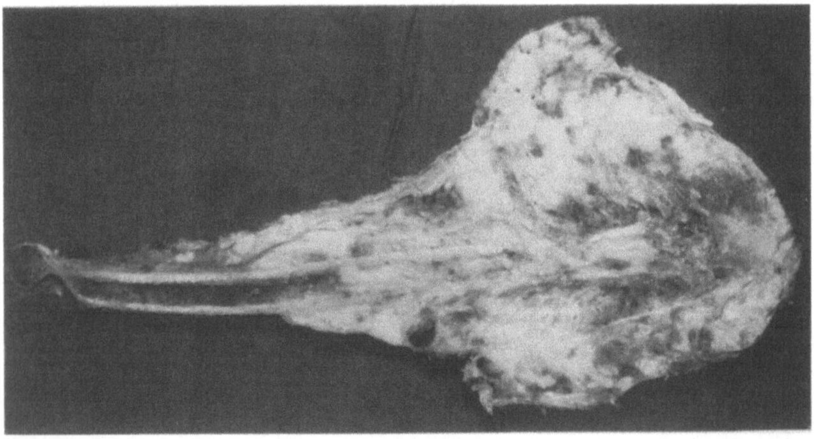

*Fig. 4. Ewing's tumour in upper end of humerus showing firm white structure. Extensive extraosseous spread with limited involvement of medullary cavity*

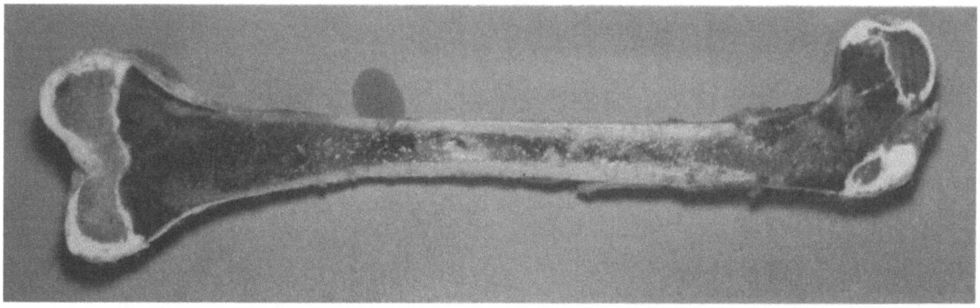

*Fig. 5. Metastatic neuroblastoma in bone, showing extensive vascular medullary tumour with limited intracortical and subperiosteal spread*

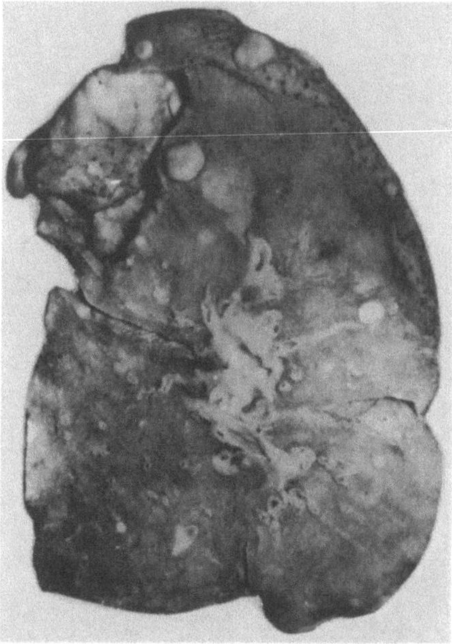

*Fig. 6. Lung metastases in Ewing's tumour*

medullary cavity to a limited extent. This contrasted with the neuroblastoma which was red, vascular, and with scattered involvement of the marrow space. In the lungs, Ewing's tumour deposits could sometimes be readily separated from the surrounding parenchyma.

## Microscopic Appearance

The Ewing's tumours in the Manchester series were made up of closely packed cells. In the bone deposits these had only a small rim of cytoplasm but in metastases in soft tissue a variable amount of eosinophilic cytoplasm was visible. Groups of cells were frequently separated by broad bands of fibrous tissue. Sometimes tumour cells grouped themselves along fibrous trabeculae giving a somewhat ill-defined rosette appearance. True endothelial spaces were not seen although their presence was occasionally suggested, probably due to degeneration and liquefaction of tumour cells. These tumours lacked the neuroblastoma's histological

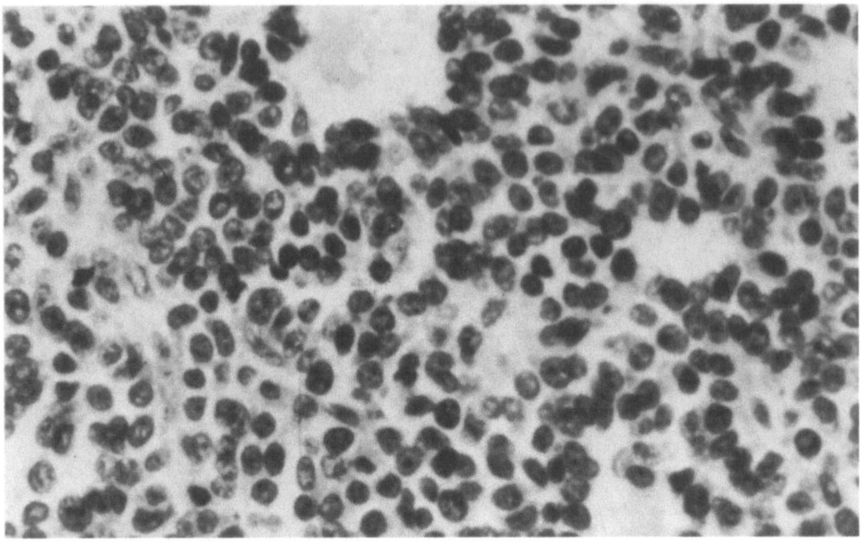

*Fig. 7. Ewing's tumour in bone showing uniform small cells with endothelial appearance possibly due to liquefaction (H. & E. X 500)*

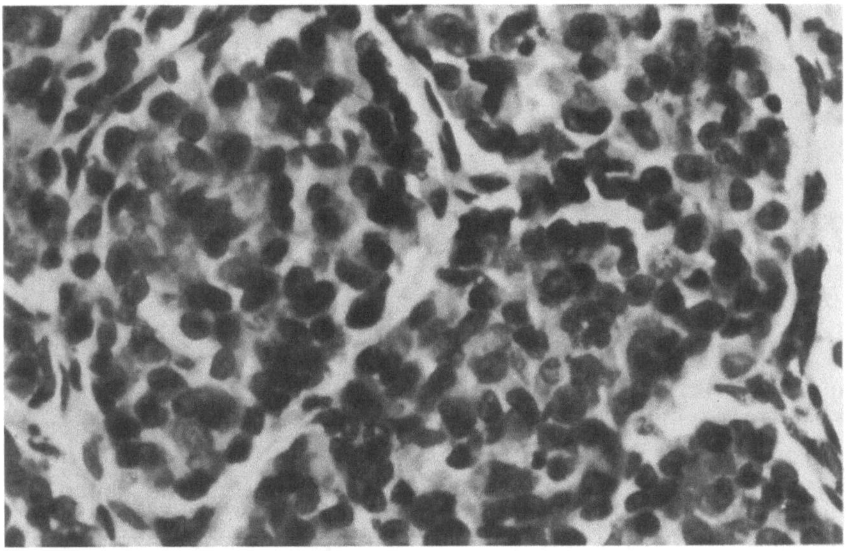

*Fig. 8. Metastatic Ewing's tumour in lung showing more abundant cytoplasm (H. & E. X 500)*

characteristics as described in chapter 7. Eosinophilic fibrils, true rosettes, maturation towards neurones and giant cells were not seen in Ewing's tumours. PARKER and JACKSON (1939) stated that in reticulosarcoma of bone the reticulin surrounded individual cells, whereas in Ewing's tumour it is confined to the septa between cell groups. In the Manchester sections studied, the reticulin in the Ewing's tumours was only seen in the septa, but it is felt that a much larger series of these neoplasms, both in adults and children, needs to be studied before any definite statement can be made on this point.

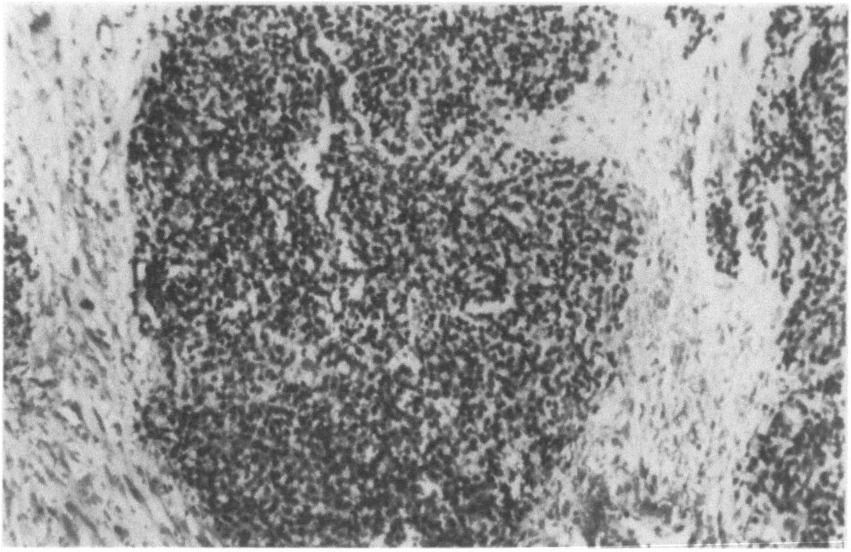

*Fig. 9. Ewing's tumour showing fibrous trabeculae (H. &. E. X 125)*

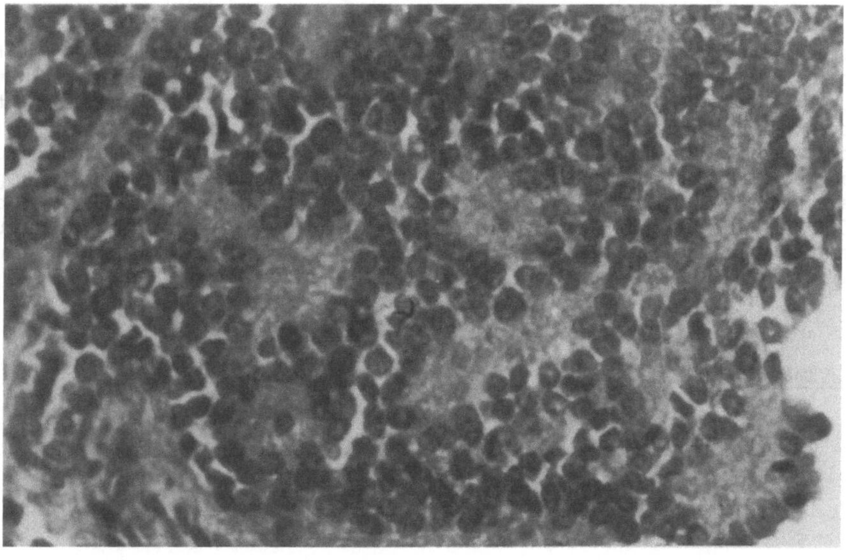

*Fig. 10. Imperfect rosettes in Ewing's tumour (H. & E. X 500)*

The presence of glycogen has been used to differentiate Ewing's tumour from neuroblastoma and reticulosarcoma of bone. In some series glycogen has not been detected in neuroblastoma (SCHAJOWICZ, 1973). However, in his material, PRICE (1973) found that 5 out of 27 neuroblastomas contained glycogen. In the Manchester series suitable fixation and systematic study has not been carried out on all cases but glycogen, as shown by PAS staining and electron microscopy, has occasionally been seen in neuroblastomas. The amounts were less than those commonly encountered in Ewing's tumours. It is considered that, although it is a useful marker, the presence of glycogen cannot be regarded as an infallible criterion for distinguishing a neuroblastoma from a Ewing's tumour.

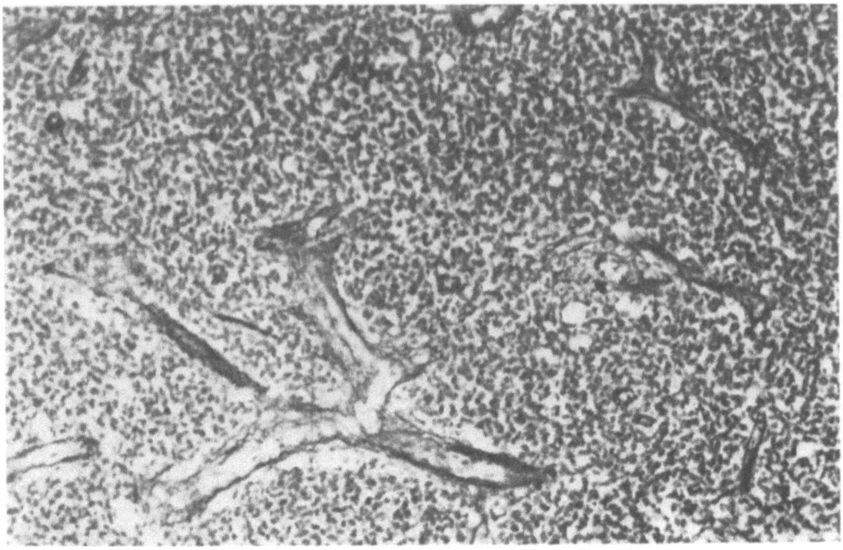

*Fig. 11. Reticulin confined to perivascular regions in Ewing's tumour (Gomori X 125)*

The electron microscopic findings in the Manchester Ewing's tumours agree with those of FRIEDMAN and GOLD (1968). Two main cell types are encountered. One has an electrontranslucent ovoid nucleus with a fine chromatin pattern and relatively few cytoplasmic organelles. In the other type, the nucleus has coarser chromatin blocks and a more irregular outline with more mitochondria and vacuoles in the cytoplasm. Transitional forms between these two cell types may occur and FRIEDMAN and GOLD suggest that the darker cells are the result of maturation. These authors also draw attention to the similarities between the darker cells and both normal and neoplastic reticulum cells.

## TREATMENT

The initial treatment given to the Manchester children is shown in Table 5.

Table 5. Initial treatment given to children with Ewing's tumours

| Alive | | Dead | |
|---|---|---|---|
| X-rays | 1 | X-rays | 19 |
| X-rays and chemotherapy | 1 | X-rays and chemotherapy | 5 |
| | | Amputation | 3 |
| | | Chemotherapy | 1 |

All the 28 children who died had active tumour present at death and in 26 of these there was definite evidence of blood-borne metastases. On the other hand, local recurrence developed in only 14 patients.

Thus the treatment given to control the primary tumours was reasonably satisfactory since in over half the children there was no recurrence at the primary site. Radiotherapy seemed just as effective as amputation for this purpose. The main therapeutic problem was that, although these tumours were radiosensitive, distant metastases appeared months or years after the initial treatment.

Therefore, for practical purposes, it should be assumed that every case of Ewing's tumour is metastatic at the time of diagnosis and a combination of irradiation and chemotherapy should be given from the beginning. Co-operative study groups in the USA began treating children with Ewing's tumours with combination chemotherapy in the early 1960's and since then there has been evidence of prolonged survival without metastatic spread (JOHNSON et al., 1970; HUSTU et al., 1972; FREEMAN et al., 1972). However, because the number of cases remains small and metastatic spread may be delayed, assessment of any treatment method is prolonged.

Radiotherapy. It has been known for many years that small celled non-osteogenic tumours of bone showed rapid response to radiation therapy with an early decrease in local swelling and relief of pain after one or two treatments. Before megavoltage therapy became available, the dose which could be given to these patients was limited mainly by skin reaction. Since megavoltage was introduced it has been possible to give a higher biological dose to the whole bone than could be given using orthovoltage.

In the treatment of the 30 children in this series, an attempt was made where possible to give at least 4500 rads in 3 weeks to the whole bone.

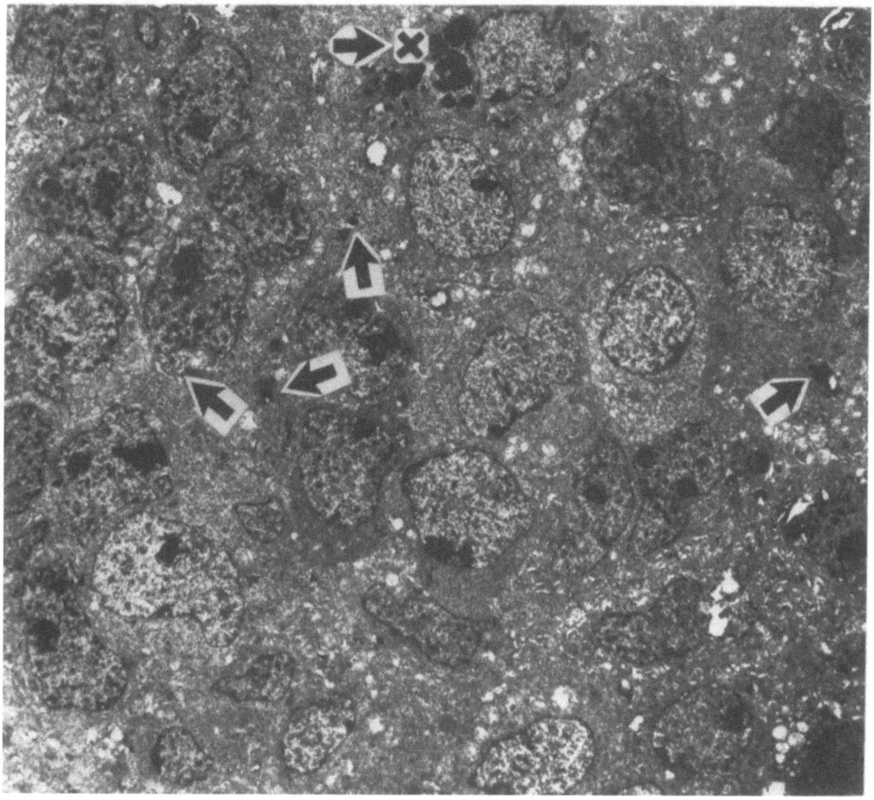

Fig. 12 a

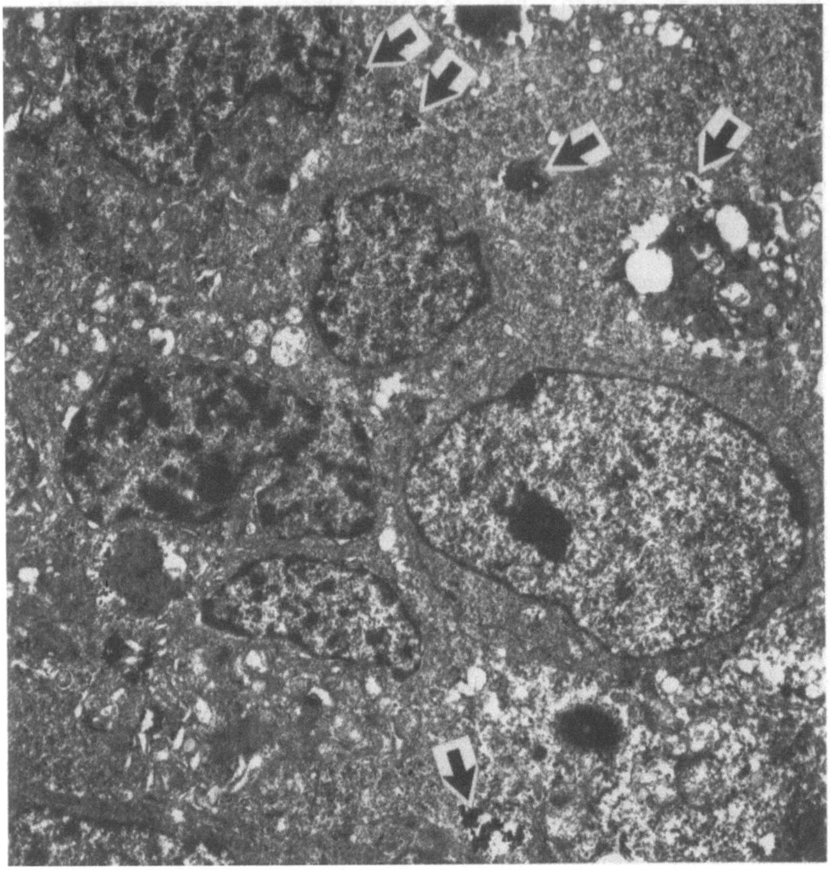

Fig. 12 b

*Fig. 12. Electron microscopic appearance of Ewing's tumour. The nuclei have 2 different patterns of chromatin - one pale and delicate with a single large nucleolus, the other darker and with random clumping. There are intermediate forms*
*-----------X  bizarre inclusions, probably lysosomes*
*-----------→  glycogen deposits*
*Uranyl acetate - lead citrate stain*
*a) x 2500  b) x 6250*

Lower doses had to be given on occasion because of the position of the primary in the trunk, and where tolerance was dictated by such vital structures as the bowel, lungs, and spinal cord. In some other patients a full course of therapy to the primary was not given because metastases were present at the time of the initial diagnosis or developed during the treatment of the primary.

In Manchester 4500 rads in 3 weeks seemed to be the highest tolerated dose, as at 5000 rads gross soft tissue fibrosis occurred with distal oedema. Other centres quote higher doses, but in longer overall times, and probably these are biologically similar to the dose given in 3 weeks. In this series it is possible to see how important this level of dose is in controlling the primary tumour. Eleven patients received 4500 rads or more to the whole bone and only 3 of them showed recurrence of the primary. On the other hand, there was local recurrence in 8 of the 15 patients who received less than 4500 rads. Therefore, for primary control it is important to try to achieve this 4500 rads dose in all patients. For limb bones this is easily achieved using parallel opposed fields and 4 MeV radiation. In the vertebrae the cord will be the limiting factor, but providing there is not too great a volume of soft tissue involvement, this same dose can be given to the involved vertebrae and the one above and below, using a 4 MeV radiation and two wedged fields from the back, thereby avoiding a high dose to tissues anterior to the spine. Pelvic bones and ribs need treatment to half the pelvis or chest, and the dose which can be given depends on bowel and lung tolerance. For the former, probably 4000 rads can be given, and reinforced by an extra 500 rads or 1000 rads to the area

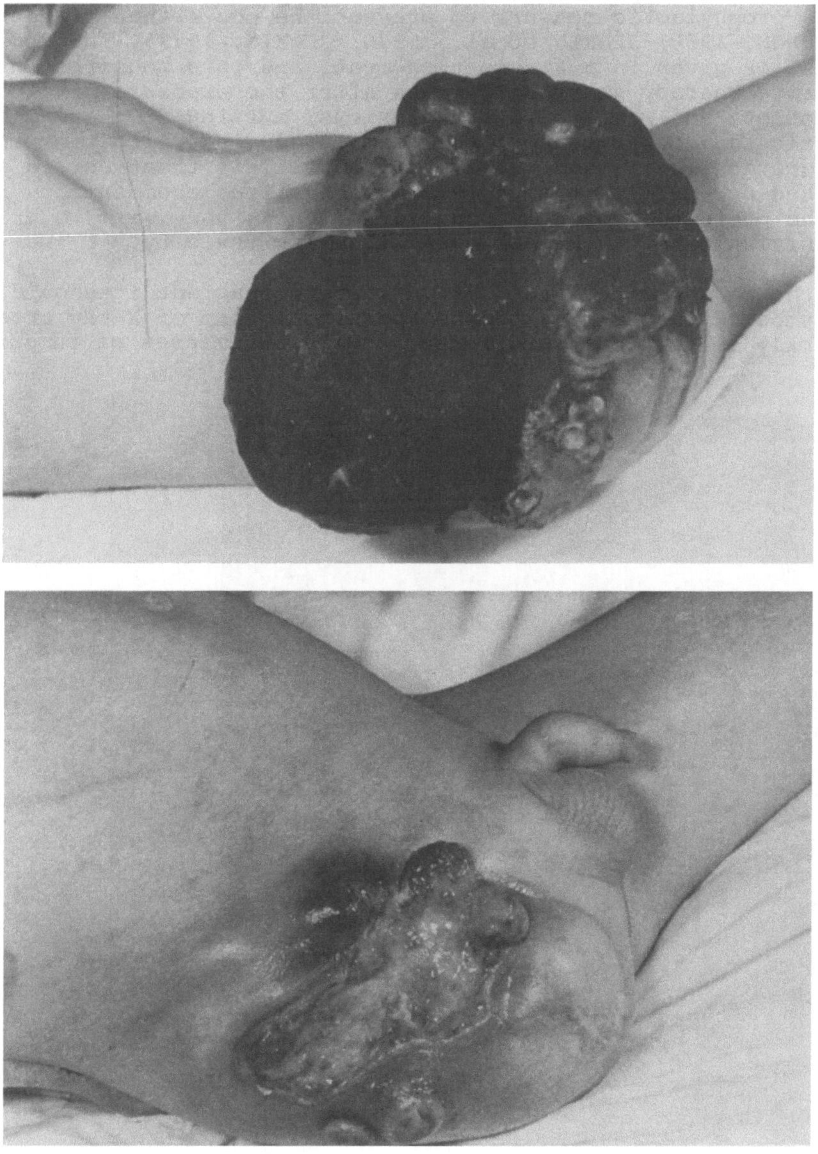

*Fig. 13. Effect of vincristine on local recurrence of Ewing's tumour. a) 4 February 1963; b) 26 March 1963*

of the small remaining tumour. A simple parallel pair of 4 MeV fields is the usual technique. In the chest in order to treat a whole rib a considerable proportion of lung has to be included in the field, and it is probable that no more than 3000 rads can be tolerated in 3 weeks. Again an extra 1500 or 2000 rads in a further week should be added to the primary tumour.

X-ray therapy for metastatic disease has rarely produced cures, although chest metastases may well disappear and even be controlled for a long time by a chest bath which consists of treating both lungs (whole chest) to a midline dose of 2500 rads in 4 weeks with megavoltage radiation.

Some radiotherapists have recommended the use of whole body radiation as a prophylactic measure to prevent the occurrence of metastases (JENKIN, 1966; JENKIN et al., 1970; JENKIN, 1973). The dose used, 300 rads, is given in a single treatment, and this requires intensive supportive therapy starting 2 weeks after the exposure, including blood, platelet and white cell transfusions, nursing in a sterile unit, antibiotics and other supportive measures, during which time the patient is critically ill and could easily die. This treatment is also described by MILLBURN et al. (1968). The various chemotherapy regimes are to be preferred to whole body radiation as they seem to produce as good a survival and can be achieved with less toxicity.

In the management of the late metastatic patient it should always be remembered that a modest dose and simple form of X-ray treatment can quickly relieve pain and reduce unpleasant masses of tumour.

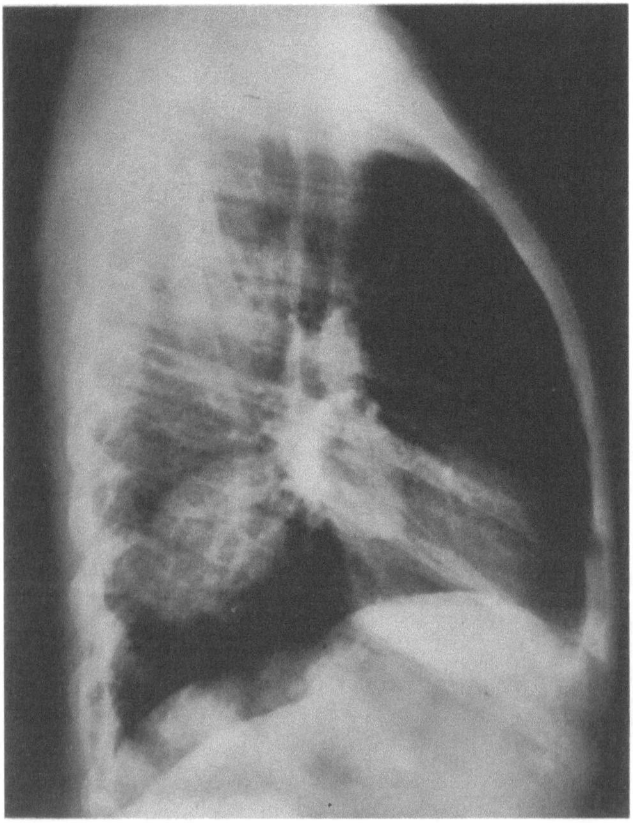

Fig. 14 a

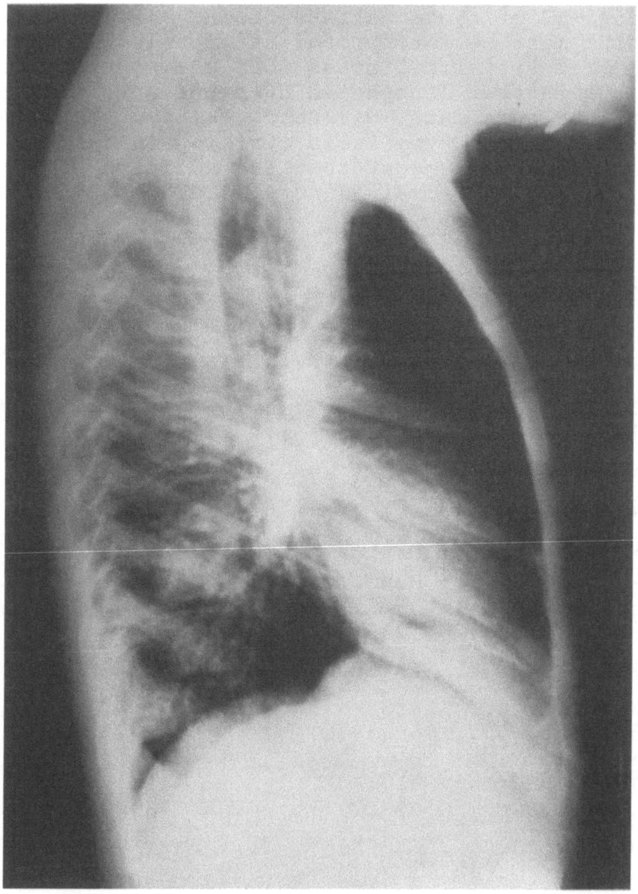

Fig. 14 b

*Fig. 14. Effect of vincristine on lung metastases of Ewing's tumour. a) 10 October 1966; b) 7 November 1966*

Chemotherapy. Only 7 of the 30 Manchester children received chemotherapy as part of their initial treatment. In 6 children this consisted of adenopterin 1 mg daily for 3 weeks, while one boy presenting with multiple secondaries was given vincristine and cyclophosphamide. Terminal chemotherapy was given in several cases and in 2 patients the effect of vincristine was very striking (see Figs. 13 and 14).

In recent years in Manchester new cases of Ewing's tumours have been treated with a combination of vincristine and cyclophosphamide in the schedule outlined below:

| | |
|---|---|
| Surgery<br>(biopsy only) | (Radiotherapy<br>(Cyclophosphamide 400 mg/m$^2$ weekly for 6 weeks<br>(Vincristine 2.0 mg/m$^2$ weekly for 6 weeks<br>(maximum dose 2.0 mg) |

The chemotherapy is started at the onset of radiotherapy. After 6 weeks the drugs are given alternately at weekly intervals for a total period of 1 year and then at fortnightly intervals for the second year. To date, experience has been very similar to other reported series and metastatic rates so far in a series followed for 6 months to 4 years is 25% - 2 of these patients being alive with disease. However, these results must be interpreted cautiously. The delay seen in the appearance of metastatic disease when chemotherapy has not been used, may only be further lengthened by drugs and it is too early to assume an increased cure rate. Nevertheless, the improvement seen with chemotherapy of this type is so striking that it is essential to continue. Recent reports suggest that the addition of adriamycin to the regime may improve the survival rate (ROSEN et al., 1974).

## REFERENCES


EWING, J.: Arch. Surg. 4, 485 (1922)

FREEMAN, A. I., SACHATELLO, C., GAETA, J., SHAH, N. K., WANG, J. J., SINKS, L. F.: Cancer 29, 1563 (1972)

FRIEDMAN, B., GOLD, H.: Cancer 22, 307 (1968)

HUSTU, H. O., PINKEL, D., PRATT, C. B.: Cancer 30, 1552 (1972)

JENKIN, R. D. T.: Clinical Radiology 17, 97 (1966)

JENKIN, R. D. T.: Bone - Certain Aspects of Neoplasia. Colston Papers No. 24. C. H. G. PRICE and F. G. M. ROSS (eds.). London: Butterworths, 1973, p. 236

JENKIN, R. D. T., RIDER, W. D., SONLEY, M. J.: Radiology 96, 151 (1970)

JOHNSON, R. E., SENZSZYN, J. J., RABSON, A. S., PETERSON, K. A.: Radiology 95, 195 (1970)

LICHTENSTEIN, L.: Bone tumours, 2nd ed. St. Louis: Mosby, 1959, p. 239

MILLBURN, L. F., O'GRADY, L., HENRICKSON, F. R.: Cancer 22, 919 (1968)

PARKER, F. Jr., JACKSON, H. Jr.: Surg. Gynec. Obstet. 68, 45 (1939)

PEPPER, W.: Amer. J. Med. Sci. 121, 287 (1901)

PRICE, C. H. G.: Bone - Certain Aspects of Neoplasia. Colston Papers No. 24. C. H. G. PRICE and F. G. M. ROSS (eds.). London: Butterworths, 1973, p. 177

ROSEN, G., WOLLNER, N., TAN, C., WU, S. J., HAJDU, S. I., CHAM, W., D'ANGIO, G. J., MURPHY, M. L.: Cancer 33, 384 (1974)

SCHAJOWICZ, F.: Bone - Certain Aspects of Neoplasia. Colston Papers No. 24. C. H. G. PRICE and F. G. M. ROSS (eds.). London: Butterworths, 1973, p. 189

# Chapter 14
# Tissue Culture and Immunological Studies

It was pointed out in Chapter 1 that an essential requirement of any service for children with tumours is to attract research workers to the problems of these patients. Clinical, epidemiological, and laboratory research are complementary and, largely due to the efforts of MILLER, FRAUMENI and DAVIES in America and STEWART in Britain, much epidemiological success has been achieved in paediatric oncology. However, closer collaboration between paediatric oncologists and basic laboratory cancer research is desirable to enable children to obtain full advantage from developments in the latter field. Based on the experience in Manchester the following ways of improving collaboration are suggested:

1. The wards where the children are treated must be within easy walking distance of the research laboratories so that there is a continual interchange of ideas and support.

2. Ideally, the paediatric oncologist would want to know of any technique which could be applied to children. However, basic cancer research is progressing at such a rate that it is difficult for anyone to keep up with more than a small part of it. A possible way of overcoming this difficulty would be for some sections (e. g. immunology, virology) in a research institute to have one member permanently assigned to paediatric oncology. There should also be career prospects for medically qualified paediatric oncologists who are academically minded and have received the training which makes them capable of spending much of their time in laboratory research.

3. The paediatric oncologist is at an enormous disadvantage in competing for the interest of research workers because of the great difficulty of assembling sufficient material from children, compared with the ease with which tumours can be obtained from animals or from adult humans. Clinical centralisation of children with cancer is an essential first step in solving this difficulty but it does not automatically provide a complete solution. In an area such as Manchester where 100 children develop tumours each year, acute lymphatic leukaemia is the only children's neoplasm which is sufficiently common for fresh material to be readily available. It is necessary, therefore, to be continually building up a store of non-leukaemic tumours in ways which will allow them to be used in tissue culture, immunological, biochemical and electron microscopical investigations. This tissue bank needs to be established without any precise idea of the projects for which it will be used, but in the knowledge that material stored will provide information beyond the scope of the ordinary histological examination of fixed stained sections.

## Tissue Culture

A tumour consists of different clones of neoplastic cells with a framework of non-neoplastic connective tissue containing blood vessels.

In vivo these elements form an organised whole, but in vitro this organisation is upset. The non-neoplastic stromal fibroblasts often grow more vigorously in cultures than the neoplastic cells and after a few weeks they may be the only cells remaining. Sometimes, by repeated subculture, a line of neoplastic cells can be established which retains some of the characteristics of the original tumour. However, the frequent manipulation required to keep such a line going always carries the risk that it may be contaminated and ultimately replaced by other cells which are being used in the laboratory. Thus, the longer cells are grown in vitro, the less chance they have of resembling the original neoplasm in vivo and there is much to be said for using short-term cultures of tissues either freshly removed from the patient or stored immediately after surgical excision. Such a storage of living cells has been made possible by the advances of cryobiology and the use of liquid nitrogen as a refrigerant. Metabolic processes are temperature-dependent and at -180°C in liquid nitrogen cellular metabolism virtually ceases. The tissues can be protected from freezing damage by impregnation by dimethyl sulphoxide, the addition of serum and controlling the rate of cooling. Thawing causes least damage if it is done rapidly. For a more detailed discussion of freezing techniques the reader is referred to STOWELL, 1965; FARRANT and SMITH, 1966; MERYMAN, 1966, 1970; MAZUR et al., 1970; ASHWOOD-SMITH et al., 1973.

Since 1965 fragments of 197 children's tumours removed in Manchester have been stored in liquid nitrogen and after being thawed out, even after several years, they grow well in culture. The following description of the short-term cultural behaviour of children's tumours is based largely on observations made on this material. There has been no obvious difference in viability between the stored tissues and those cultured immediately after surgical removal.

Methods. The tumours were grown on rectangular coverslips placed in the wells of Leighton tubes in a medium consisting of TC 199 + 20% serum. In some cases tumour explants were cultured in cockerel plasma or on coverslips coated with collagen (EHRMAN and GEY, 1956), while in other cases the cells were dispersed on collagen-coated coverslips or directly on glass. In general, renal and glial tumours were friable and could be easily dispersed, while neuroblastomas and connective tissue tumours often had to be grown initially as explants and trypsinized later. The cultures were inspected frequently with an inverted microscope. When a more accurate view was needed the coverslip was removed and the cultures were fixed and stained. Alternatively, the movement of the living cells could be followed by incorporation of the coverslip into a chamber which was mounted on a warm stage of a phase contrast microscope. Growth was measured by autoradiography (BASSERGA and MALAMUD, 1969) after labelling with $^3$H-TdR.

## Growth Characteristics of 197 Children's Tumours Cultured in Manchester

Apart from the neoplastic cells, two non-neoplastic elements are seen in a cultured tumour. There is often an initial wave of macrophages which move rapidly away from the tumour and usually die within 48h. There are also mesodermal cells derived from the fibrous stroma and blood vessels. These are larger cells, with coarsely staining cytoplasm. Their nuclei contain several nucleoli and the cells move more slowly than do the macrophages. They are often spindle-shaped and are loosely referred to as "fibroblasts" although they are not necessarily derived from fibroblasts as recognised by histologists.

In spite of inevitable changes occurring in culture, the differences in the growth patterns of tumours of different histological types were often obvious. It was usually possible to predict the cell types which would grow from tumours of a particular histological diagnosis and this information was occasionally helpful when the histological diagnosis was in doubt. It is recognized that a great deal of work needs to be done before it is possible to know the ideal cultural conditions for the growth of children's tumours. It is felt that this investigation has at least provided a base line for future research along these lines.

Neural Tumours. Neuroblastomas and ganglioneuromas have such a characteristic growth pattern in vitro that MURRAY and STOUT (1947) suggested that tissue culture might be useful for their rapid diagnosis. Usually, within 24h of setting up the culture, neurites start to grow out from the edge of the explant. These neurites have nodal varicosities, branch dichotomously and possess a flattened swelling with multiple processes at the tip. As the cultures grow older, clumps of cells and occasionally single cells may be seen lying in between the well-formed neurite network. Whereas the neurites grow to considerable lengths, the cells themselves have little ability to move in culture. Thus, they often remain buried in the explant where they cannot be seen.

Glial Tumours. Many successful studies of the tissue culture of glial tumours have been made and there are comprehensive reviews of the subject by KERSTING (1961) and LUMSDEN (1971). Usually, within 48h of setting up the culture, individual cells or fringes of fine processes are seen to emerge radially from the explants. More malignant tumours have shorter and plumper processes. The length of the processes increases

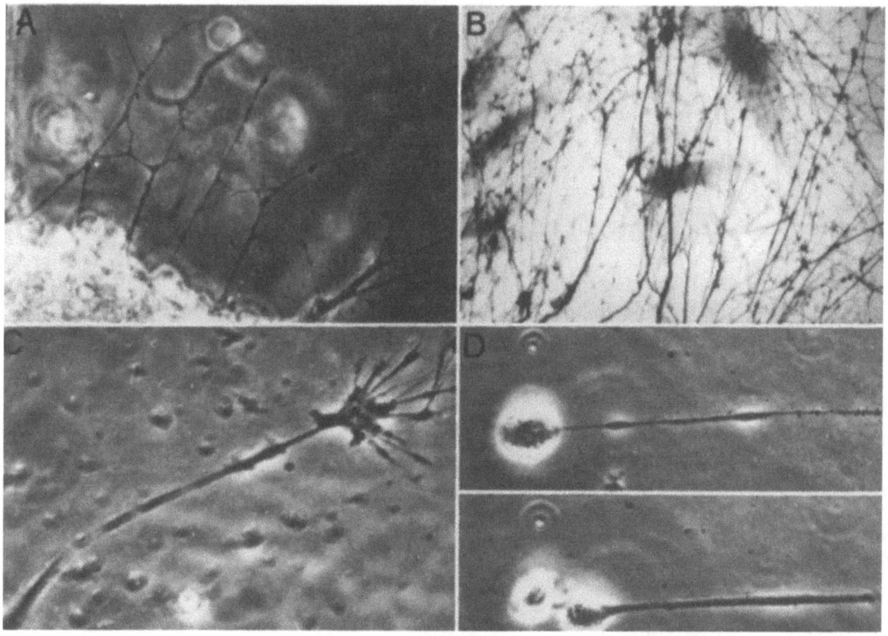


*Fig. 1. Neuroblastoma. A) 24h plasma clot culture showing neurite outgrowths which are much thinner and longer than those seen in gliomas (see Fig. 2). Phase x 400. B) 8 days' culture on collagen showing dense neurite network with varicosities, a characteristic feature. Bodian X 100. C) 6 days' culture in plasma clot showing characteristic swelling at the tip of neurite with brushlike processes ("end-plate"). Phase X 400. D) 7 days' culture on collagen showing mitosis. Note: neuroblast can divide without withdrawing the neurite. Phase X 400*

during the next few days and sometimes the cells become trapped in the criss-crossing processes. Fine intracytoplasmic fibres may be seen in some of the glial cells. Glial tumours tend to lyse the plasma clot and are therefore best grown either on bare glass or collagen. Although the different types of gliomas have certain cultural similarities, there are also certain differences between them.

Astrocytomas. Since the cells from an astrocytoma migrate away from the explant and become separated from each other, their morphology in culture can be easily studied. The cell bodies are, on the whole, polygonal but may be fusiform and they have a variable amount of cytoplasm. Their

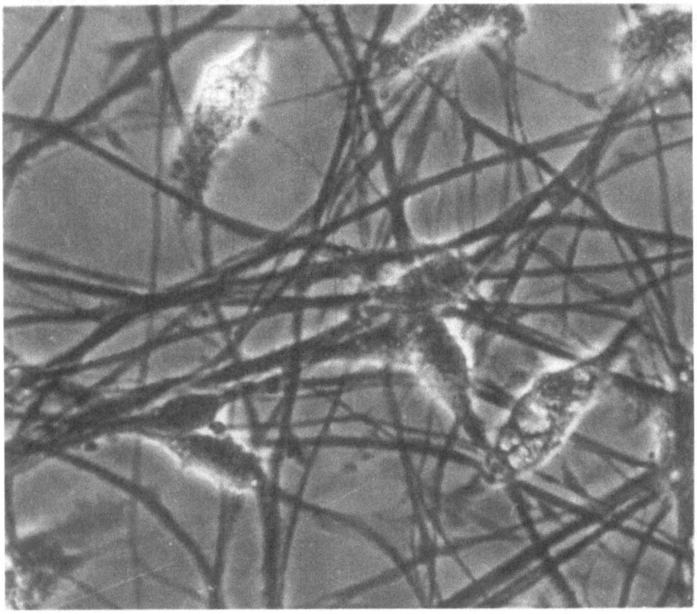

*Fig. 2. Astrocytoma. 8 days' culture on collagen showing multipolar and polygonal cells with long processes which form an anastomosing network. Phase X 600*

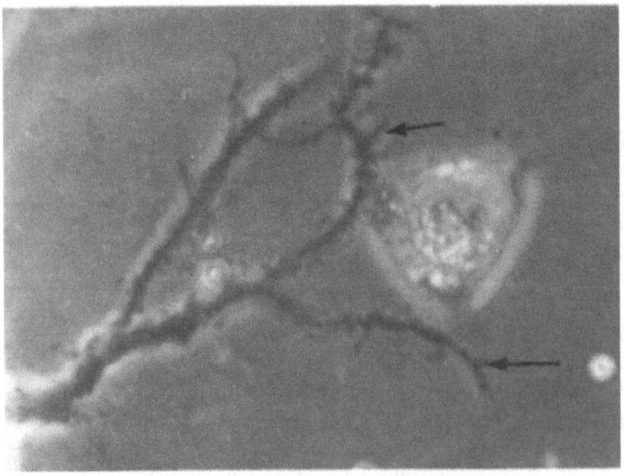

*Fig. 3. Mixed glioma. 5 days' culture in plasma clot showing lateral buddings, "gliosomes". Phase X 600*

characteristic feature is that they have a number of cytoplasmic processes so that they resemble astrocytes as seen in sections of brain stained by the metallic impregnation methods of GOLGI, CAJAL, and HORTEGA. In tissue culture these processes occasionally have lateral buds or gliosomes (LUMSDEN, 1971) which may represent abortive attempts of rapidly growing neoplastic cells to produce further processes. These astrocytes may be easily distinguished from the non-neoplastic mesodermal stromal cells since they appear small and do not have the characteristic sharply defined nuclear membrane and coarse cytoplasm of "fibroblasts" in culture. They also differ from neuroblasts which have very scanty cytoplasm and are much less mobile than astrocytes. The neurites growing from neuroblasts are longer and thinner than the processes from astrocytes and have characteristic varicosities along their length and also have end-plates.

Ependymomas. Two types of growth from ependymomas have been observed. COSTERO and POMERAT (1955) describe a glial-like growth while KERSTING (1961) reported a more epithelial-like appearance. The 5 ependymomas cultured in Manchester produced outgrowths of each type. The epithelial type appeared earlier than the glial fibres. Within 24h sheets of poly-

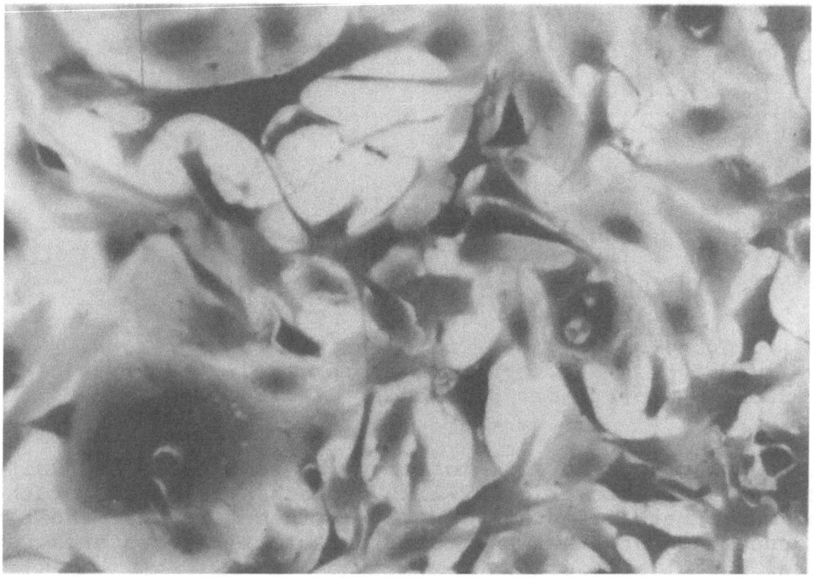

*Fig. 4. Ependymoma culture showing cells of different sizes and shapes, including giant cell in lower left hand corner. Giemsa X 150*

gonal cells appeared which migrated out to form characteristic fronds. By the fourth or fifth day some of the cells abandoned the others and lay individually or in groups. A striking feature during the later stages was the appearance of a network of glial fibres.

Oliogodendrogliomas. No example of this tumour was cultured in the Manchester series. KERSTING (1961) described 16 cases and found outgrowths ranging from astrocytes to small cells with chromatin rich nuclei and 3-4 delicate processes.

Medulloblastomas. A description of the tissue culture behaviour of the medulloblastoma was included in Chapter 6. It was pointed out that early workers reported varying growth patterns (KREDEL, 1929; RUSSELL and BLAND, 1933; KERSTING, 1961; NAGAI et al., 1967). LUMSDEN (1971) contends from his own observation and KERSTING's description that the medulloblastoma's behaviour in culture indicates that it is a purely neural and not a glial tumour. From our own experience of culturing 9 medulloblastomas in Manchester we would not agree entirely with LUMSDEN's conclusion. Admittedly these tumours contained cells with scanty cytoplasm and neurite-like fibres. However, they differed from neuroblastomas and resembled gliomas in the following respects: a) the

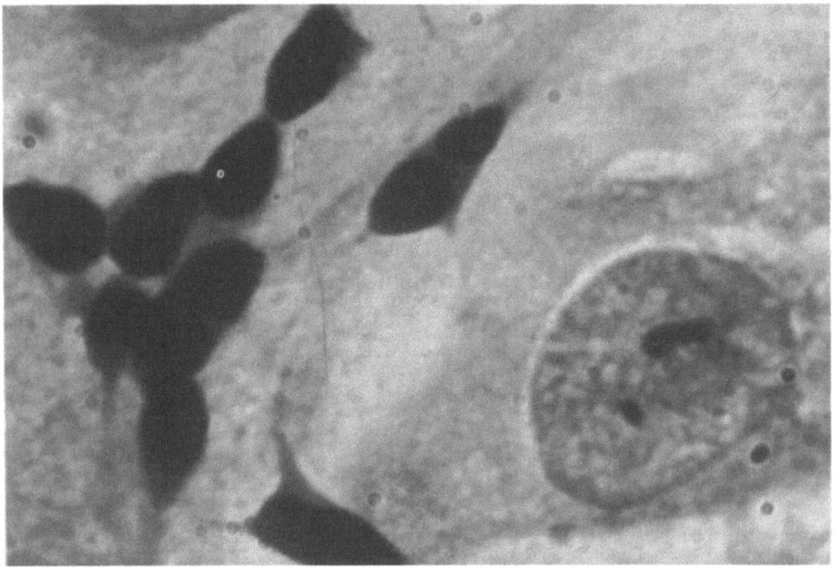

*Fig. 5. Medulloblastoma. 9 days' culture on collagen. A large fibroblast is clearly distinguishable from small, darkly stained medulloblasts which have short processes. Giemsa X 600*

cells showed considerable motility; b) some cells had quite a lot of cytoplasm and thicker glial-like processes; c) lysis of the plasma clot was a marked feature. We think therefore that the tissue culture evidence suggests that the medulloblastoma has features resembling both neural and glial tissue.

Retinoblastomas. Three Manchester retinoblastomas were cultured - 2 from the primary in the eye and the other taken at autopsy from a metastasis. KERSTING reported 12 cases in which the growth resembled to a certain extent that seen in medulloblastomas. The characteristic cell was round with a slender branching process. He regarded these cells as more primitive than those in his medulloblastomas. Two of the 3 Manchester retinoblastomas grew poorly in culture but one from the primary in the eye developed a glio-epithelial type of growth.

Wilms' Tumours. These are very easy to grow in culture. Usually they are friable and the tissue can be dispersed mechanically without trypsinization. Within a few hours of setting up the culture there is often a wave of macrophages followed by two types of cells which migrate across the coverslip: a) fusiform cells which resemble fibroblasts and b) polygonal cells 25 - 35 μ in diameter lying either by themselves or in epithelial-like sheets. Because the cells from a Wilms' tumour have

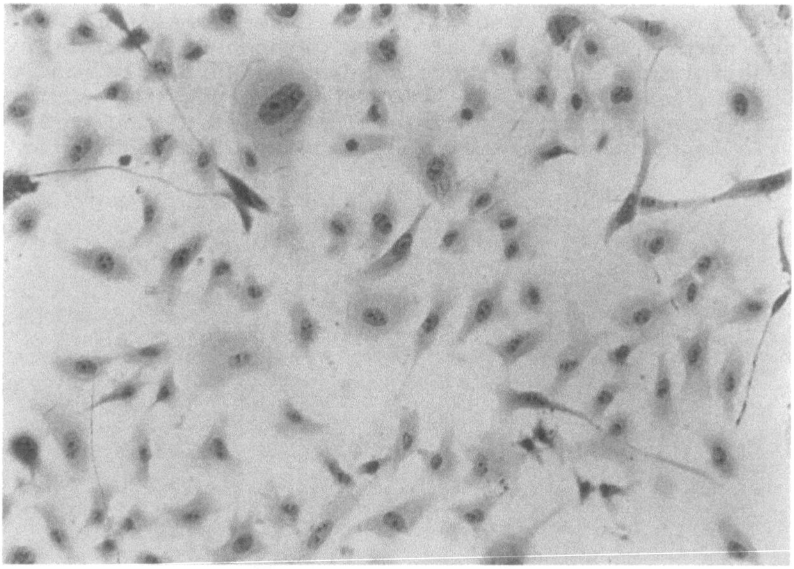

*Fig. 6. Retinoblastoma. 9 days' culture on collagen, showing glio-epithelial type of cells. Bodian X 150*

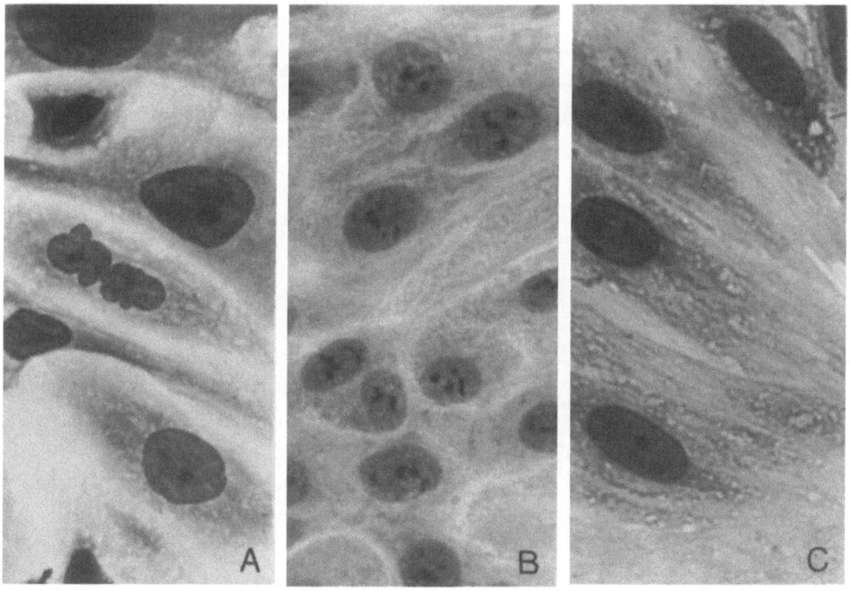


*Fig. 7. Typical appearance of cultured cells A) Wilms' tumour. Giemsa X 500. B) Normal kidney. Giemsa X 500. C) Skin fibroblast. Giemsa x 500*

a certain mesenchymal appearance in their nuclear and cytoplasmic pattern it is impossible to distinguish with certainty the stromal from the neoplastic elements. However, there is considerable variation in nuclear size suggesting that most of the outgrowth is neoplastic. Lysis of the clot is a marked feature. Also in plasma clot cultures, but not on collagen or bare glass, polykaryocytes containing up to 100 nuclei are a marked feature of Wilms' tumours.

Mesoblastic Nephroma. One mesoblastic nephroma in the Manchester series was cultured. The predominant outgrowth was fibroblastic but besides the fusiform cells there were some which were polygonal with little cytoplasm. As in the Wilms' tumour, polykaryocytes occurred in plasma clot which also underwent lysis. The nuclei of the cells of a mesoblastic nephroma were more regular than those of a Wilms' tumour.

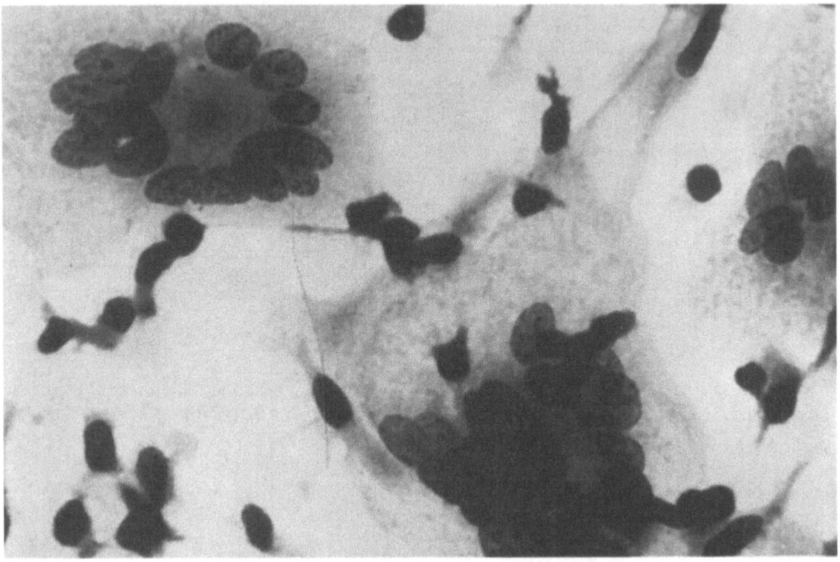

*Fig. 8. Mesoblastic nephroma. 4 days' culture in plasma clot, unlike collagen culture (Fig. 9), showing multinucleated cells. Giemsa X 600*

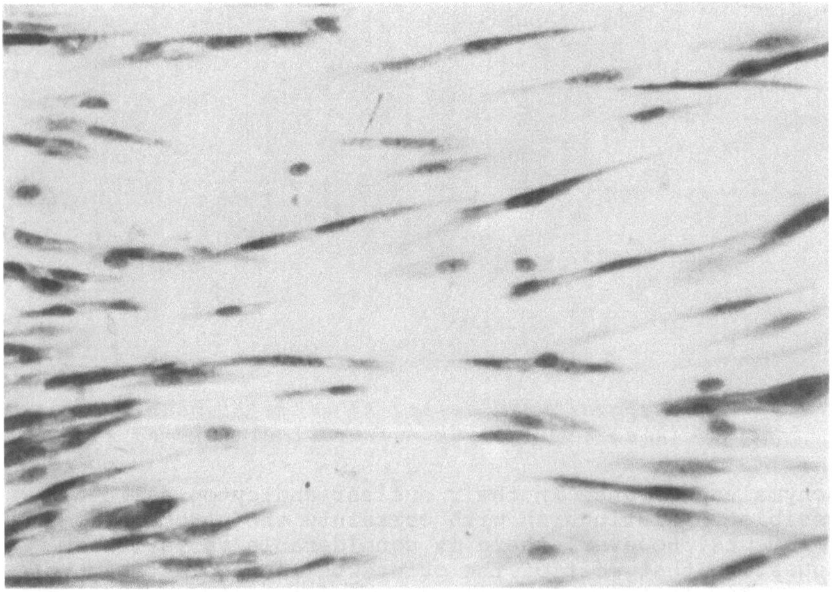

*Fig. 9. Mesoblastic nephroma. 4 days' culture on collagen. Predominant cells were fibroblast-like. Giemsa X 150*

Hepatoblastoma. Two hepatoblastomas were cultured. They produced an outgrowth of polygonal and cuboidal, epithelial-like cells within 24h. These formed themselves into sheets. Fibroblast-like cells made their appearance after 4 days. Polykaryocytes were rare but many of the tu-

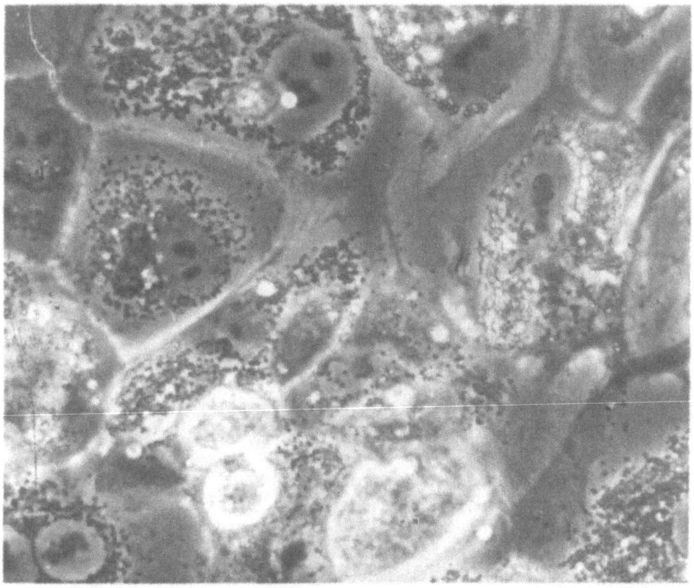

*Fig. 10. Hepatoblastoma. 5 days' culture on collagen. Mainly epithelial-type cells with nuclear polymorphism. Phase X 600*

mour cells had two or three nuclei. Lysis of the plasma clot was marked. The behaviour of the hepatoblastoma was very different from that of normal liver. A piece of liver adjacent to the tumour was removed and in culture produced a scanty growth of fibroblasts and small clusters of round and polygonal cells which began to degenerate on the fifth day.

Yolk Sac Tumour. One yolk sac tumour from the testis of an 11-month-old boy was cultured. Within 24h a few isolated sprouts were seen extending from the explant and a day later spindle-shaped granular cells migrated out. Within 4-5 days small round or oval bipolar or multipolar cells with slender processes appeared. There were some fusiform cells with vacuolated cytoplasm. Occasional binucleate forms were seen. The cells were motile. Mitotic figures were very few and there was moderate lysis of the clot. The tumours were friable and could be grown on bare glass. On the whole, the collagen cultures were better than those on bare glass or in plasma clots.

Embryonic Sarcomas. Within 24h polygonal cells 30 - 50 μ in diameter migrated out of the explants. Within a few days the cells moved a considerable distance and some assumed a fusiform shape. The polygonal cells usually had one or two nuclei but in a few there were up to five nuclei. They had a granular cytoplasm and the nuclei had one or two cleoli. There was moderate lysis of the plasma clot. In one of the 13 Manchester embryonic sarcomas which were cultured there were strap cells containing many nuclei arranged either centrally or along the periphery like striped muscle. Embryonic sarcomas resemble Wilms' tumours in the motility of the cells in culture and the difficulties of distinguishing stromal from neoplastic elements.

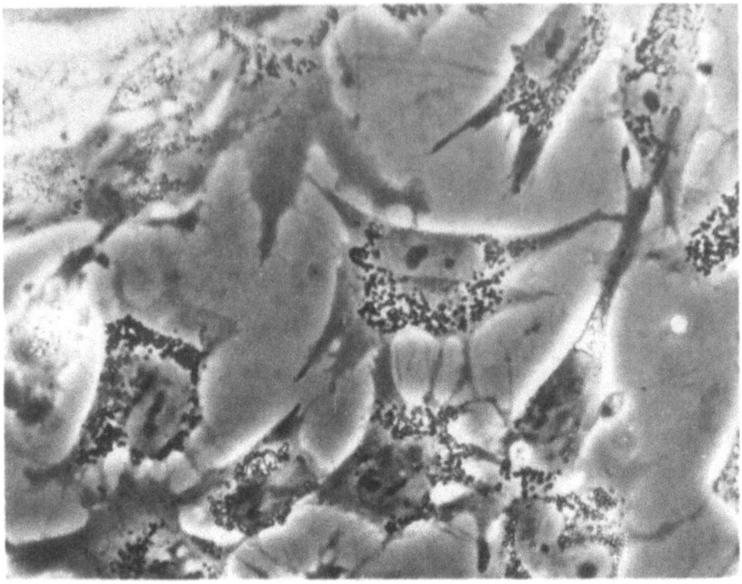

*Fig. 11. Embryonic sarcoma. 13 days' culture on collagen. Most of cells are polygonal or fusiform with granular cytoplasm. Phase X 600*

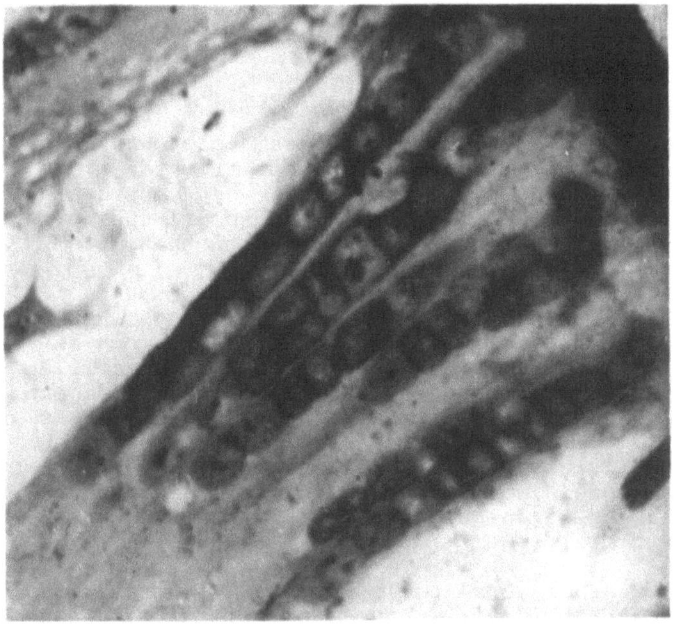

*Fig. 12. Embryonic sarcoma. 5 days' culture on collagen showing strap-cells with centrally aligned nuclei. Giemsa X 600*

Osteosarcoma. Three osteosarcomas were cultured, one of which was a second tumour in a child who previously had a retinoblastoma. Within 48h of culture, ramified cells were noticed in all the 3 tumours. These cells were very mobile and mitotic figures among them were frequent.

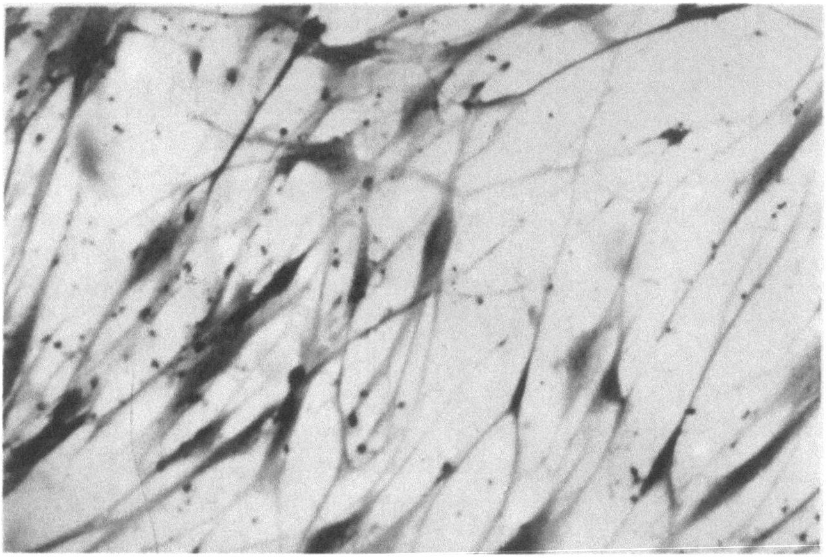

*Fig. 13. Osteosarcoma. 15 days' culture on collagen. Main type of cell was fibroblastic in character, which after a week in culture had an elongated bipolar shape and a single branched process. Giemsa X 150*

Ewing's Tumour. One Ewing's tumour was tissue-cultured and it grew very rapidly. The cells were small, polygonal in shape and contained numerous mitoses. The cell-cycle time was found to be 41h. Cytogenetic studies revealed 50 chromosomes in every cell. This implied that the tumour mass was made of cells which had originated from a single clone.

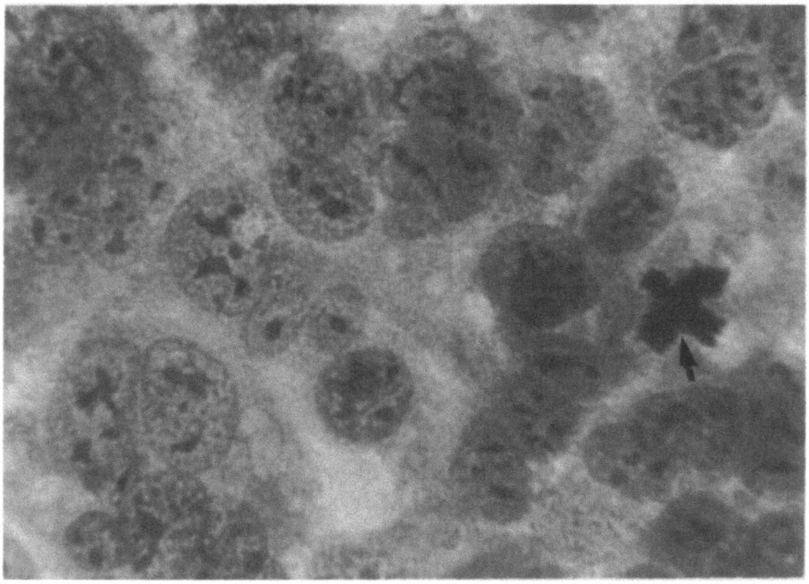

*Fig. 14. Ewing's tumour. 7 days' culture on glass. Predominantly epithelial type of growth with numerous abnormal mitotic figures. Bodian X 700*

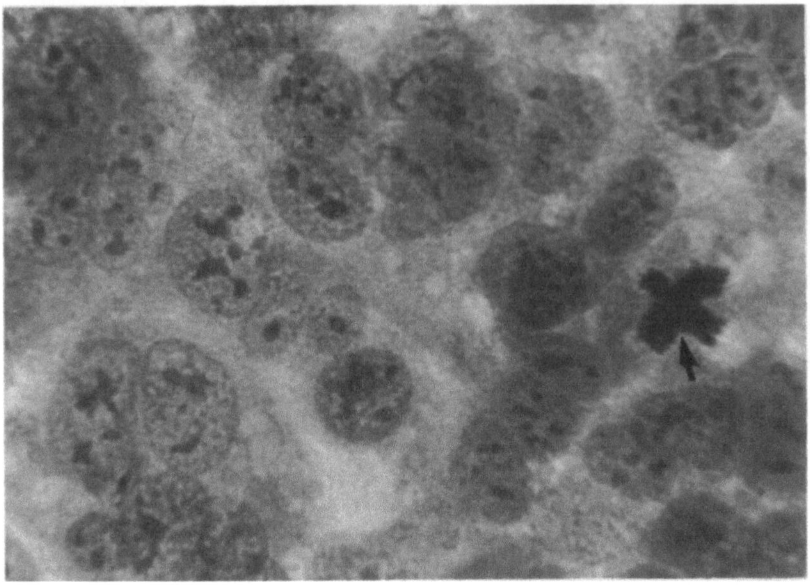

*Fig. 15. Melanoma. Autoradiograph of a 7 days' culture on collagen. Elongated bipolar cells, with darkly $^{3}H$-TdR labelled nuclei. Giemsa X 600*

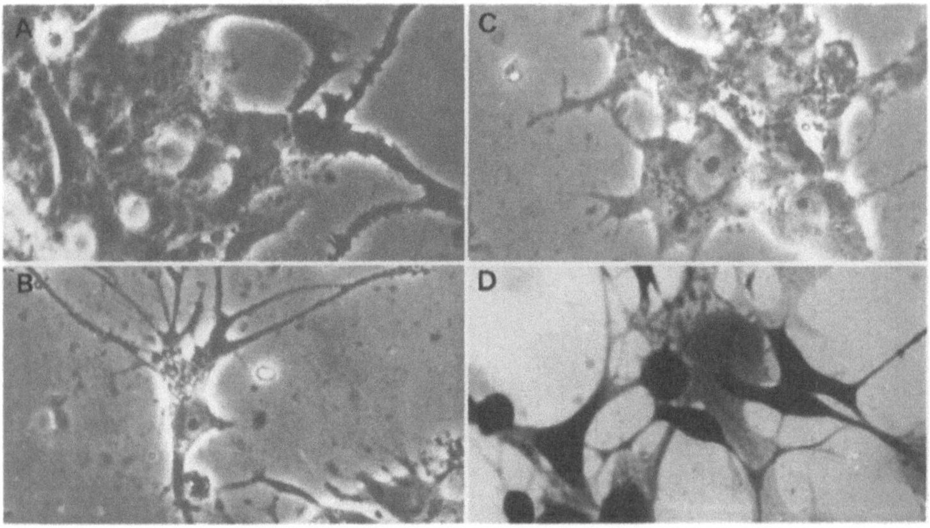


*Fig. 16. Extradural tumours A) Case 1, 5 day culture. Cells with several protoplasmic processes bearing "gliosome"-like structure (see also Fig. 3). Phase X 400. B) and C) Case 1, multipolar cells with polygonal morphology. Unlike neuroblastoma cultures no neurite network was seen. B) Phase X 400, and C) Phase X 800. D) Case 2, 7 days' culture. 2 types of cells can be seen, one darkly stained with short processes and the other with relatively light staining. Giemsa X 800*

Malignant Melanoma. One malignant melanoma derived from a block dissection of a child's cervical node, after it had failed to respond to X-ray treatment, was cultured. Examination of sections stained with Masson-Fontana and electron microscopy failed to reveal melanin granules in this material. Within 24 - 48h of incubation, a fringe of fine processes was observed around the explant. After about a week, cells which were either uni- or bipolar or oligodendritic or, rarely, polydendritic were seen. The presence of these dendritic cells tended to confirm the neuroectodermal origin of melanomas. The other type of cells that were present was spindle-shaped. Masson-Fontana staining of cultures showed the presence of melanin granules in the dendritic type of cells only. Acquisition of melanin granules by tumour cells, after in vitro growth, corroborates similar earlier reports (LEIGHTON, 1968).

Extradural Tumours. Histological examination of 2 extradural tumours from 2 children of 5 and 9 years failed to provide a definite diagnosis. The morphology of the cells grown from these 2 cases suggested that they may be of glial origin.

Growth Rate in Culture - Thymidine Indices. Autoradiographic studies of cultures of tumours labelled with $^{3}$H-TdR from 41 Manchester children were used to calculate the rate of growth as indicated by the percentage of labelled cells (thymidine indices). It was found that the thymidine indices of cultures of fragments stored in liquid nitrogen were roughly the same as those of freshly removed tumours and repeated experiments on different fragments of the same tumour gave very similar results irrespective of the age of the cultures; i. e. it was roughly the same on the 5th and 14th day. Most of the autoradiographs were done on collagen cultures 16h after a medium change, although on this substrate changing the medium had little effect on the thymidine index.

In interpreting the results the tumours were divided into two groups:

1. Wilms' tumour, embryonic sarcoma, mesoblastic nephroma, hepatoblastoma, yolk sac tumour and osteosarcoma in which the distinction between neoplastic and stromal cells could not be made with certainty. The indices of the mesoblastic nephroma and yolk sac tumour were each 8% but in general the Wilms' tumours, embryonic sarcomas, osteosarcomas and hepatoblastoma ranged from 10% to 30%.

2. Glial and neural tumours in which it was possible to distinguish neoplastic from stromal cells. The striking feature about this group was that the thymidine indices of the stromal cells were much higher than those of the neoplastic cells. Between 18% and 39% of the stromal cells were labelled, whereas the highest readings of the neoplastic cells was 21% in a medulloblastoma and 18% in a neuroblastoma. The neoplastic astrocytoma and ependymoma cells gave values ranging from 0 to 8%. The high thymidine indices of stromal cells in cultures of gliomas lends support to the suggestion of LUMSDEN (1971) that the stroma was being stimulated by the glial cells. Many of these stromal cells must be derived from the blood vessels of the tumour and there is a great deal of evidence to show that in animal experiments tumour fragments cannot grow more than a few millimetres in diameter unless they stimulate an outgrowth of their host's blood vessels. FOLKMAN et al. (1971) and FOLKMAN (1975) have shown that an extract of tumours can be made which causes very rapid proliferation of capillaries in vivo. This tumour angiogenic factor (TAF) may be the cause of the high thymidine index of the stromal cells in cultured gliomas. However, PHILLIPS et al. (1976) were unable to demonstrate any increase in the uptake of thymidine in fibroblast cultures derived from the white matter of rat brains after the addition of TAF to the medium.

## Immunological Studies

Tumour immunology rests on the concept that neoplastic cells possess antigens which are absent from normal cells. Experiments in tumour immunology before 1943 were inadequately controlled and therefore could not be used as evidence that transplantable animal tumours possess tumour specific transplantation antigens (TSTA). Some of the tumours were transplanted among xenogeneic (one species to another) and allogeneic (genetically incompatible individuals of the same species) rather than among syngeneic (genetically compatible) animals and in such situations it was not possible to determine whether rejection was the result of a response to TSTA or to histocompatibility antigens. Modern tumour immunology dates from the experiments of GROSS (1943) and FOLEY (1953) who showed that methylcholanthrene-induced tumours in mice were antigenic in syngeneic animals and since then it has been demonstrated by transplantation techniques that many experimental tumours contain TSTA. In general, TSTA of chemically induced tumours are individually distinct for each neoplasm, while tumours of viral aetiology possess TSTA which are common to all neoplasms induced by the same virus and different from those induced by other viruses. During the past 20 years a vast amount of work in animals has been carried out in attempting to elucidate the mechanism and importance of these immune reactions and the literature has been reviewed many times (CURRIE, 1974; HELLSTRÖM and HELLSTRÖM, 1974; HERBERMAN, 1974).

Although only a limited literature has been published on the sequential evaluation of immune parameters in man, it is generally accepted that immunological reactions offer some degree of resistance against the establishment and progression of malignant tumours. BURNET (1970) has called this policing action "immune surveillance". For the reasons given at the beginning of the chapter there has been very little investigation of the role of immune surveillance in paediatric oncology. However, there are several features about children's tumours which could have an immunological explanation:

1. It is known that individuals with congenital or drug-induced immunodeficiency have an increased liability to tumour formation (see Chapter 2). Might it not be that these are not just rare curiosities but that many children develop tumours because they suffer from undetected inborn immunodeficiencies? If these immunodeficiencies were the result of low frequency genetic mutations it would account for the constant incidence of some children's tumours in widely separated communities (STEWARD, 1974).

2. Spontaneous regression of neuroblastomas (EVERSON and COLE, 1966) and retinoblastomas (STEWARD et al., 1956) may have an immunological basis.

3. The liability of children with familial retinoblastoma to develop other cancers later in life (see Chapter 8) may be due to inborn immunodeficiency.

Too little is known about tumour immunology in children to allow any comprehensive account of the subject to be given. All that can be attempted is a discussion of the following aspects of tumour immunology which may be relevant to paediatric oncology.

1. In vivo evidence for the presence of tumour specific antigens in man.
2. Tests for immunocompetence.
3. In vitro tests for cell-mediated and humoral immunity.
4. Xenogeneic antibodies.

5. Foetoproteins.
6. Immunotherapy.

In Vivo Studies. The in vivo experiments which have been done in humans have consisted either of inoculating living tumour cells into autologous hosts (SOUTHAM, 1967) or else performing skin tests with tumour extracts on patients with cancer (OREN and HERBERMAN, 1971; CHAR et al., 1973). However, the number and interpretation of these experiments have been limited not only by ethical considerations but also by the non-specific depression of immunity caused by generalized neoplasia and the irradiation and chemotherapy which the patient requires.

Tests for Immunocompetence in Cancer. Most workers have been unable to demonstrate significant depression of the humoral responses in cancer patients to a variety of microbial antigens. Impairment of cell-mediated responses is, however, well documented in lymphoreticular neoplasia as determined by cutaneous reactivity to various microbial antigens as well as homograft survival (SOKAL, 1966; YOUNG et al., 1972). Although one group of workers (SOLOWEY and RAPAPORT, 1965) reported some impairment of reactivity to a battery of skin test reagents in patients with localized disease, depression of cell-mediated immunity has been reported mainly in patients with "active" or advanced cancer. There is some evidence that the recording of cellular and humoral immune responses may be of some prognostic value. Thus, EILBER and MORTON (1970) reported that cancer patients who failed to develop cutaneous hypersensitivity to DNCB were likely to be inoperable or develop early recurrences, while most patients who reacted to DNCB were free of disease for a significantly longer period of time. Reactivity to recall antigens was less valuable in predicting prognosis.

In vitro lymphocyte response to phytohaemagglutinin (PHA) has been widely used as a test for cell-mediated immunity. The PHA responses in 100 patients (adults and children) with solid tumours and 31 normal children undergoing minor surgery have been examined (KUMAR and TAYLOR, 1973). There was frequently a delay in the peak of lymphocyte transformation in the cancer patients before operation but there was a tendency to show more normal responses within a year after operation. Inhibition of PHA-induced lymphocyte transformation by the sera of a proportion of these cancer patients was observed. As with the studies of childhood solid tumours serum inhibitors in leukaemia of PHA-induced blastogenesis and mixed leucocyte reactions have also been described (WALKER et al., 1973).

Current methods of treatment of acute leukaemia demand not only prompt initiation of chemotherapy but also the long-term administration of cytotoxic drugs when in remission, and in the case of acute lymphoblastic leukaemia additional phophylactic CNS irradiation. Most investigations of immune competence of acute leukaemia have therefore been performed in patients on treatment, and in such cases it is impossible to dissociate the immunological incompetence produced by drugs and radiotherapy from that associated with the disease itself. Marked immunosuppression may frequently occur following chemotherapy and X-irradiation (OGRA et al., 1971; HERSH and OPPENHEIM, 1967; BAKKARA et al., 1972; HUMPHREY et al., 1972; CAMPBELL et al., 1973) but a general depression of immunity has not been demonstrated conclusively in untreated acute leukaemia (LARSON and TOMLINSON, 1953; ASTALDI et al., 1966; DUPUY et al., 1971). HERSH et al. (1971) however, using a battery of in vitro tests that included delayed hypersensitivity skin reactions and in vitro lymphocyte blastogenic response to PHA and streptolysin "O", found that many of the patients were immunoincompetent to these tests and further that patients recovering from immunoincompetence during therapy or maintaining immunocompetence throughout were more likely to achieve remission than those converting from immunocompetence to incompetence.

Tests for Cell-Mediated Immunity

A. Lymphocytotoxicity Tests. Colony inhibition (CI) assay and its modification ("micro" method) have been extensively used to study the inhibitory action of patient's lymphocytes on tissue-cultured tumour cells and the serum factors which influence this cytotoxicity (HELLSTRÖM and HELLSTRÖM, 1974). Among childhood tumours HELLSTRÖM et al. (1968) have shown that the lymphocytes of children with neuroblastoma and those of their mothers inhibit the growth of neuroblasts in tissue culture. In general, the results using these two methods are in agreement, but the "micro" method has the advantage of economy of tumour cells and lymphocytes. In both these assays, the target cells are grown overnight in either Petri dishes or in the wells of microplates. The following day, patient's or normal donor's lymphocytes are added and after 48 - 72h incubation the number of surviving cells is counted. The results are considered positive when the patient's lymphocytes cause a significant reduction in the number of target cells, compared with controls that have received either no lymphocytes or normal donor's lymphocytes. The exact mechanism of tumour cell killing is not known. In Manchester, studies with time-lapse cinematography have shown that contact between lymphocytes and tumour cells is necessary but lymphocyte transformation or multiplication is not essential for the tumour cell killing (KUMAR et al., 1973). The nature of the effector cytotoxic cells is not definite, thymus-dependent (T), thymus-independent (B), and killer (K) cells having been implicated (for details see HELLSTRÖM and HELLSTRÖM, 1974; HERBERMAN, 1974).

In both these lymphocytotoxic systems, a number of cells are killed by lymphocytes derived from whatever source, but the proportion is very much higher if lymphocytes from a patient suffering from that tumour type are used, as compared with the proportion killed by either lymphocytes from patients with other tumour types or from normal volunteers. However, cytotoxicity varies considerably from combination to combination. It is likely that this represents immunity against non-specific tumour antigens, and as such, this "background" cytotoxicity must be accepted. The additional cytotoxicity above "background" is likely to be tumour-specific, because autologous and allogeneic combinations were equally highly effective in killing tumour cells. Furthermore, lymphocytes from children with neuroblastoma, whilst being highly cytotoxic to allogeneic neuroblasts, produced only "background" levels of cytotoxicity against normal kidney cells from the same patient who provided the neuroblasts. In contrast to the lack of cross-reactivity observed between tumours of different histology, lymphocytes from patients with hypernephroma proved to be highly cytotoxic to cultures of Wilms' tumour cells and vice versa. This implies that there are antigenic determinants in common between embryonic and adult types of renal tumours. Lymphocytotoxicity against CNS tumours was also observed (KUMAR et al., 1973), and here an interesting feature was that the higher the lymphocytotoxicity against autologous tumour, the lower was the reactivity against allogenic tumour cells of the same histological type. This could be explained by assuming that a particular histological type of tumour possesses multiple tumour-associated antigenic determinants, some of which are commonly shared and some of which are peculiar to an individual tumour.

The main problem in the interpretation of lymphocytotoxicity results is that cells cultured from all tumours consist of a mixture of neoplastic and stromal cells. Against which cell type is the cytotoxicity directed? In cultures of neuroblastoma it is relatively easy to distinguish neoplastic from stromal cells since neuroblasts have a characteristic morphology, contain acetylcholinesterase and take up $^{3}$H-dopamine (KUMAR et al., 1972). The disappearance of recognizable neuroblasts from cultures to which lymphocytes from patients with neuroblastoma are added suggests that it is the neoplastic cells which are selectively destroyed. Similarly, tissue-cultured cells from glial tumours have a distinct morphology and are easily distinguishable from the fibroblast-like ones. The distinction between neoplastic and stromal cells in cultured tumours of mesenchymal origin in man is more difficult, although the fact that many cells exhibit loss of contact inhibition, tend to have bizarre or multinucleate cells and abnormal chromosome patterns suggests that many of them are neoplastic. It is these cells in mesenchymal tumours having the stigmata of neoplasia that disappear when confronted with immune lymphocytes and this suggests that lymphocytotoxicity is directed against tumour-specific antigens which are shared within the tumour type.

A great disadvantage of cell and colony inhibition tests is the labour involved in reading the results. Therefore, lymphocytotoxicity has also been evaluated by measuring the release of radioactivity from cells labelled with isotope. The commonly employed radioactive compounds are chromium, thymidine, iodine, proline (BEAN et al., 1973; BRUNNER et al. 1968; COHEN et al., 1972; JAGARLAMOODY et al., 1971). This technique has been particularly useful in the study of lymphoid tumours where cells grow in suspension and not in monolayers. Mixtures of tumour cells and lymphocytes are incubated for various lengths of time, after which the release of radioactivity into the medium is measured. The drawbacks of this method are that there is often a significant spontaneous release of an isotope (especially chromium) and, for meaningful results, one needs a very large number of lymphocytes and target cells. The problem of spontaneous release has been reported to have been overcome in animal tumours by the use of technetium-99m (BARTH et al., 1972) which binds firmly to the cell. It will be worthwhile to assess the usefulness of technetium-99m in human tumour systems.

B. Lymphocyte Stimulation by Tumour Cells. Incubation of intact tumour cells or their extracts with peripheral blood lymphocytes may lead to enhanced DNA synthesis in the latter. Autologous and allogeneic non-neoplastic cells have no such stimulatory effect. This difference has been interpreted as a demonstration of cellular immunity when in vivo sensitized lymphocytes are stimulated by the recall antigens present on the surface of tumour cells. STJERNSWÄRD et al. (1973) have shown that 31 of 85 tumours in adults induced statistically significant stimulation of autologous lymphocytes compared with 3 of 51 non-neoplastic cell types. Several other workers have confirmed the above findings but the clinical relevance of these findings remains uncertain (BACH et al., 1969; FRIDMAN and KOURILSKY, 1969; GUTTERMAN et al., 1973a; MAVLIGIT et al., 1973; NAGEL et al., 1971; TAYLOR et al., 1971; VIZA et al., 1969).

Blocking and Unblocking Factors. The paradox that patients die from their tumours even in the presence of a high degree of in vitro lymphocytotoxicity may be at least partially explained by the presence of tumour-specific blocking factors (HELLSTRÖM et al., 1971). The nature of the "blocking factor" is not known, but dissociable tumour-specific antigen-antibody complexes (HELLSTRÖM and HELLSTRÖM, 1974), IgG (JOSE and SKVARIL, 1974), and antigen alone (BALDWIN et al., 1973) have been suggested. Blocking factors tend to disappear when a patient becomes clinically free of disease. Serum samples from 33 of 59 patients with active disease had blocking factors, compared with 11 of 42 patients with inactive disease. Since the absence of blocking factor would seem to some extent to be associated with inactivity of the tumour, it is possible that the regular follow-up of lymphocytotoxicity and the alterations in the blocking activity may provide an index of prognosis. In later studies the HELLSTRÖM group reported that the sera of patients who were clinically free from tumours could "unblock" the blocking effect of sera from patients bearing tumours of the same histological types (HELLSTRÖM et al., 1971). Again the exact nature and mechanism of the "unblocking" factors has not been resolved.

Tests of Humoral Immunity. Two methods were used in Manchester in the search for evidence of humoral immunity to children's tumours: a) immunofluorescence and b) complement-dependent serum cytotoxicity.

A. Immunofluorescence (IF). This can be done by the direct method (COONS et al., 1941) using immunoglobulins which have been conjugated

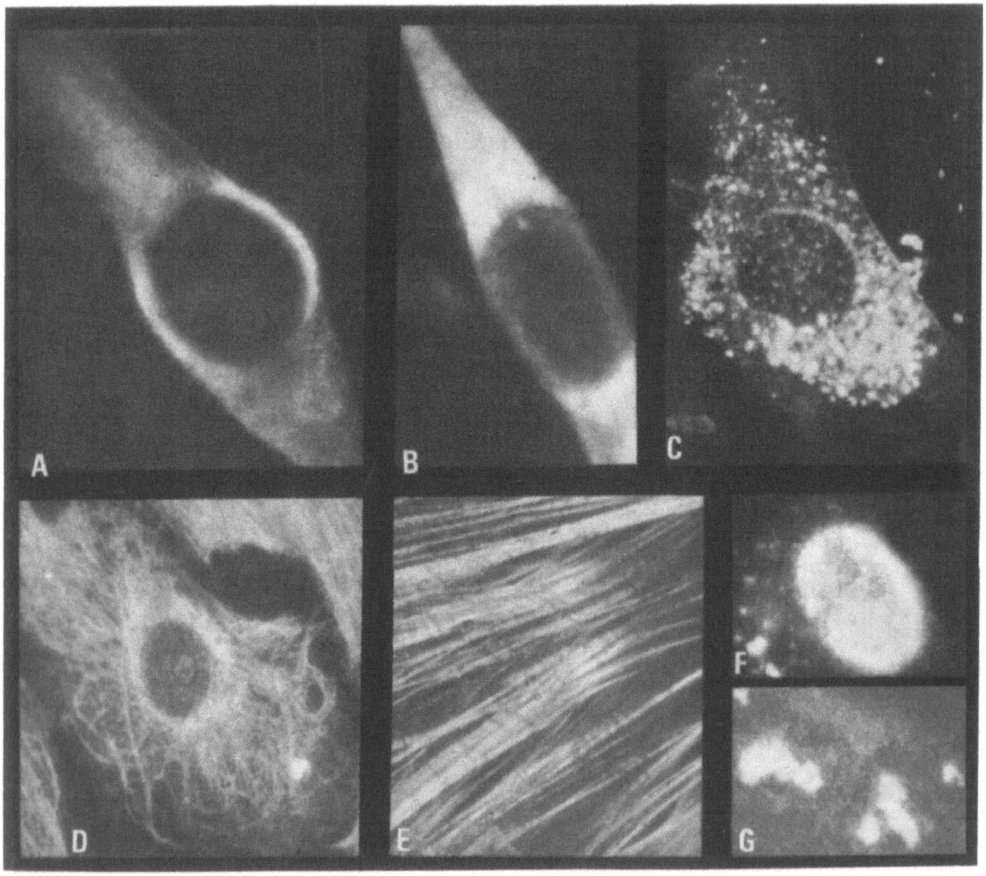


*Fig. 17. Indirect immunofluorescence. Sera of children with Wilms' tumour produced the following intracytoplasmic staining patterns of tissue cultured Wilms' tumour cells: a) crescentic; b) diffuse cytoplasmic; c) granular cytoplasmic; d) microfilamentous; e) microtubular; f) nuclear; g) nucleolar*

with a fluorescent dye. Alternatively an indirect method may be used in which the tissue containing the antigen is first treated with the patient's serum (unconjugated immunoglobulins) and then with fluorescent anti-human serum raised in animals (NAIRN, 1969). The test can be done on unfixed fresh tissue in which case antigens on the cell membranes will be stained, or in fixed tissue when antigens within the cell can be detected.

In Manchester this technique has been applied mainly to study humoral responses in children with renal tumours (KUMAR and TAYLOR, 1975). Sera from 45 children with Wilms' tumours were tested against 18 renal tumours (16 Wilms', 1 kidney carcinoma, 1 mesoblastic nephroma). Forty-two produced one of the following types of IF staining pattern: diffuse, granular, crescentic, microfilamentous, microtubular, nuclear or nucleolar. In order to test the tumour specificity of this staining, all the sera were absorbed with tissue-cultured normal skin fibroblasts and normal kidney cells. After absorption these sera were again tested against cells from 6 different Wilms' tumours. The number of positives fell from 42 to only 1. The implication of this finding is that a very high percentage of children with renal tumours have autoantibodies which are not tumour-specific. It is only possible to speculate on why these children frequently produce non-specific antibody. Possibly the antibodies arise as a result of the liberation of non-specific antigens from the tumour or are due to an adjuvant-like property derived from the tumour; alternatively, they may precede the tumour and indicate an abnormal immune state predisposing to tumour formation. If antibodies resulted simply from release of cellular components, a higher incidence might be expected in children with active disease rather than those who clinically appeared free of tumour after therapy. Comparing the incidence of antibody in these two groups, 8 of 19 children with active disease were positive as opposed to 13 of 26 with inactive disease. This difference is not statistically significant. Only a prospective study can resolve the question of whether non-specific antibodies precede tumour formation.

KLEIN and his colleagues at the Karolinska Institute, Stockholm, have extensively investigated the immunological aspects of the Burkitt lymphoma (BL). Using the "IF" technique they found that the sera of BL patients reacted more frequently than African control sera from donors with other neoplastic and non-neoplastic diseases. The reactivity of the BL sera was not due to isoantibodies as autologous serum-cell combinations were found to give positive "IF" (KLEIN, 1971).

B. Complement dependent serum cytotoxicity. Tumour-specific antibodies in the sera of patients with tumours can inhibit the growth of tumour cells in the presence of complement (HAKALA et al., 1974). In Manchester, none of 27 sera obtained from children undergoing minor surgery (healthy group) produced significant reductions in the numbers of tissue-cultured Wilms' cells. Serum samples from 4 of 44 children (9 percent) with Wilms' tumours and 2 of 24 children (8 percent) with other solid non-renal tumours caused a significant inhibition of tumour target cells derived from renal tumours. The 6 sera which showed a significant inhibition of tumour target cells were absorbed with tissue-cultured human skin fibroblasts and normal kidney cells and again tested for cytotoxicity. After absorption, sera from 3 of the 4 Wilms' patients and both of the non-Wilms' patients were cytotoxic to the Wilms' target cells. Further absorption of these 5 cytotoxic sera with a pool of 3 different tissue-cultured Wilms' tumour cells completely removed the inhibitory activity of the 3 Wilms' sera and one of the 2 sera from the non-renal group. The clinical state of the disease ("active" or "inactive") did not appear to influence the serum cytotoxicity results.

Xenogeneic antibodies. A different approach which is used in the demonstration of tumour specific antigens in human cancer is by the immunization of animals (rabbits, goats, pigs, etc.) with crude or partially purified homogenates of tumours (GOLD and FREEDMAN, 1965; VIZA et al., 1969). Appropriately controlled studies which included careful absorption of the antisera with normal tissues have confirmed the existence of antigens that are specific for some tumours. One such example is the W-antigen which was shown to be present in 27 of 31 Wilms' tumour extracts (BURTIN and GENDRON, 1973). It is conceivable that small amounts of W-antigen are present in the sera of children with Wilms' tumours and their detection by radioimmunoassay would be of considerable diagnostic and prognostic value.

Foetoproteins. In the sera of children with tumours the following 4 foetoproteins (FP) have been demonstrated by immunological methods: $\alpha_1$-FP, $\alpha_2$-H, and 2 $\beta$-proteins (BUFFE and RIMBAUT, personal communication). Alpha$_1$-FP has been shown to be present in 90% of sera of children with hepatoma and teratoma. After surgery and during efficient chemotherapy it disappears from serum and reappears in cases of metastasis and recurrence of disease. This protein is not absolutely tumour-specific since it has also been recorded in some hepatopathies of young children, tyrosinemia and Indian cirrhosis.

Although $\alpha_2$-H is not tumour-specific, its demonstration may be of some clinical value. Regardless of the histological type and location, $\alpha_2$-H ferroprotein has been found in all extracts of livers obtained from children with malignant tumours. Similarly, 80% of 452 children with tumours have been reported to contain a significant level of $\alpha_2$-H ferroprotein. In contrast, only 9% of 177 healthy children or children with benign disease contained this protein.

The clinical value of the other 2 $\beta$-proteins has not yet been clearly elucidated.

Immunotherapy. The recognition that the immune system may play a role in the defence against human malignant disease raised the possibility that immunological procedures might be used in treatment. Depending on whether antibodies or immunocompetent cells are administered, or whether the body's own immune defences are stimulated, immunotherapy is called respectively, passive, adoptive or active. This rather simple classification to some extent reflects the crudity of immunotherapeutic techniques, but a more sophisticated approach will depend upon a better understanding of the immune mechanisms involved in tumour rejection. Because of this lack of understanding and because most treated patients had widely disseminated cancer, it is hardly surprising that immunotherapy has not been very successful. In recent years, however, more encouraging results have been reported, particularly in malignant melanoma and acute leukaemia.

Several agents are available that can produce a non-specific stimulation of immunological reactivity in man and animals, e.g. oleic acid, zymosan, Corynebacterium parvum and BCG. Administration of BCG has been shown to be valuable in the prevention and retardation of growth of some experimental animal tumours. The dosage as well as the timing in relation to chemotherapy are important and indeed there are circumstances when it may be either ineffective or even cause tumour enhancement (BLUMING et al., 1972). BCG is a potent stimulator of the reticulo-endothelial system but its precise mechanism of action is not certain (OLD et al., 1959). It appears to be most effective when given directly into the tumour tissue and is thought to act there by encouraging the infiltration of the area by macrophages and perhaps other immunocompetent cells which are then capable of destroying the tumour cells.

GUTTERMAN et al. (1974) have been treating patients with disseminated malignant melanoma with a combination of chemotherapy and intradermal injections of BCG. They reported a greater response rate, compared with an historical control where patients were treated with chemotherapy only. In view of the lack of concurrent controls and the inevitable subjectivity in the grading of these patients, it is necessary to keep an open mind about these results.

Recent results in acute leukaemia using specific and non-specific active immunisation are perhaps more impressive. MATHÉ et al. (1968, 1969) showed in certain transplanted leukaemias that treatment of animals with irradiated leukaemic cells or BCG, given even after the challenge with non-irradiated cells, could delay and reduce mortality. These results formed the basis of a clinical trial of active immunisation in patients suffering from acute lymphoblastic leukaemia (ALL) (MATHÉ et al., 1969). The patients first received chemotherapy to induce a remission and then complementary chemotherapy designed to reduce the number of residual leukaemic cells. The patients completing the above courses were then randomised to 4 groups receiving either no treatment, BCG alone, pooled irradiated allogeneic leukaemia cells alone or BCG plus cells. Patients receiving no further treatment did significantly worse than those on immunotherapy. The number of patients involved in this trial was small and doubts have been expressed as to their selection. A multicentre randomised controlled clinical trial was held in this country by the Medical Research Council (Concord trial). After initial chemotherapy, children in remission were randomised to receive BCG alone, twice weekly methotrexate or no further treatment. In contrast to MATHÉ's findings there was no significant difference between the groups receiving BCG alone or no treatment, whereas the patients receiving methotrexate did significantly better (Preliminary report MRC. 1971). A similar trial in the United States by the Children's Cancer Study Group A (HEYN et al., 1973) also showed the BCG to be without effect. However, the BCG used in both these studies was different from the one used by the MATHÉ group, who continue to use immunotherapy for the maintenance of remission in ALL. Since all their patients receive this treatment it is impossible to assess whether the results that this group is achieving are due to the immunotherapy or to the initial chemotherapy and CNS irradiation. In acute myeloid leukaemia (AML) where the prognosis is still extremely poor, the median duration of remission in many centres being no more than 6 months, CROWTHER et al. (1973) have reported from London that intermittent combination chemotherapy + immunotherapy achieve longer remission than the same chemotherapy given alone. Based on the work of the London group, in Manchester 7 adult patients with AML who had achieved remission following initial chemotherapy were maintained on immunotherapy alone (FREEMAN et al., 1973). The median duration of remission was not significantly greater than in comparable trials using chemotherapy for maintenance. However, a reinduction rate with 5 out of 6 patients was achieved and one patient achieved a total of 6 remissions. Four out of the 7 patients are still alive, the median survival being 2 3/4 years. This high reinduction rate has been confirmed in a larger group of 20 adult patients maintained with immunotherapy alone as part of the MRC 6th trial.

Although one may be cautiously optimistic on surveying the results of immunotherapy in malignant melanoma and acute leukaemia, it is too early to be certain that this form of treatment is effective in these diseases. In spite of considerable progress in tumour immunology, there are so many unanswered questions that it would be surprising if any trial were to produce dramatic results at the present time. Possibly it will be necessary to tailor the techniques to a particular patient. In future it will be of vital importance to devise precise quantitative in vitro tests to assess the responses of individual patients; only then will it become possible to provide a rational basis for the treatment of malignant disease by immunotherapy.

At the beginning of this chapter an attempt was made to analyse the factors which have got in the way of laboratory research in paediatric oncology. Our lack of knowledge of the immunology of children's tumours is largely due to these factors, but there is another special difficulty. The success of chemotherapy has not only made clinicians much more interested in the development of new chemotherapeutic regimes than in immunology, but it has also increased the difficulties of analysing the significance of any abnormality in the immunological state of a patient. However, it is no more likely that cytotoxic drugs will provide all the answers to paediatric oncology than antibiotics have in infectious diseases. In spite of all the practical difficulties, the hope that it may be possible to enhance host resistance makes the study of tumour immunology worthwhile.

## REFERENCES


ASHWOOD-SMITH, M. J., VOSS, W. A. G., WARBY, C.: Cryobiol. 10, 502 (1973)

ASTALDI, E., MASSIMO, L., AIRO, R., MARI, P. G.: Lancet 1, 1265 (1966)

BACH, M. L., BACH, F. H., JOO, P.: Science 166, 1520 (1969)

BAKKERA, J. A. J. M, DeVAAN, G. A. M., SCHRETTER, E. D. A. M., SCAND, J.: Haemat. 9, 36 (1972)

BALDWIN, R. W., PRICE, M. R., ROBINS, R. A.: Int. J. Cancer 11, 527 (1973)

BARTH, R. F., GILLESPIE, G. Y., III, GOBUTY, A.: Nat. Cancer Inst. Monogr. 35, 39 (1972)

BASSERGA, R., MALAMUD, D.: Autoradiography, Techniques and Application, New York: Harper and Row, 1969

BEAN, M. A., PEES, H., ROSEN, G., OETTGEN, H. F.: Nat. Cancer Inst. Monogr. 37, 41 (1973)

BLUMING, A. L., VOGEL, C. L., ZIEGLER, J. L., MODY, N., KAMYA, G.: Ann. Intern. Med. 76, 405 (1972)

BRUNNER, K. T., MAUEL, J., CEROTTINI, J. C., CHAPUIS, B.: Immunology 14, 181 (1968)

BURNET, F. M.: Immunological Surveillance. London: Pergamon Press, 1970

BURTIN, P., GENDRON, M. C.: Proc. Nat. Acad. Sci. USA 70, 2051 (1973)

CAMPBELL, A. C., HERSEY, P., MacLENNAN, I. C. M., KAY, H. E. H., PIKE, M. C.: BMJ 2, 383 (1973)

CHAR, D. H., LEPOURHIET, A., LEVENTHAL, B. G., HERBERMAN, R. B.: Int. J. Cancer 12 (2), 409 (1973)

COHEN, A. M., MILLAR, R. C., KETCHAM, A. S.: Cancer REs. 32, 2421 (1972)

COONS, A. H., CREECH, H. J., JONES, R. N.: Proc. Soc. Exp. Biol. N. Y. 47, 200 (1941)

COSTERO, I., POMERAT, C. M.: Cellular Protypes of central gliomata, Proc. 2nd Int. Cong. Neuropaths. London: Excerpta Medica, 1955, p. 273

CROWTHER, D., POWLES, R. L., BATEMAN, C. J. T., BEARD, M. E. J., GAUCI, C. L., WRIGLEY, P. F. M., MALPAS, J. S., HAMILTON-FAIRLEY, G., BODLEY SCOTT, R. B.: BMJ 1, 131 (1973)

CURRIE, G. A.: Cancer and Immune Response, London: Edward Arnold, 1974

DUPUY, J. M., KOURILSKY, F. M., FRADELIZZI, D., FEINGOLD, N., JACQUILLAT, C. E., BERNARD, J., DAUSSET, J.: Cancer 27, 323 (1971)

EHRMANN, R. L., GEY, G. O.: J. Nat. Cancer Inst. 16, 1375 (1956)

EILBER, F. R., MORTON, D. L.: Cancer 25, 362 (1970)

EVERSON, T. C., COLE, W. H.: Spontaneous Regression of Cancer. Philadelphia: W. B. Saunders Co., 1966, Chap. 3

FARRANT, J., SMITH, A.: Progress in Low Temperature Biology. Penguin Science Survey, B. A. Allison (ed.). Harmondsworth: Penguin Books, 1966

FOLEY, E. J.: Cancer Res. 13, 835 (1953)

FOLKMAN, J. L.: Advances in Cancer Research 19, 331 (1974)

FOLKMAN, J.: Ann. Int. Med. 82, 96 (1975)

FOLKMAN, J., MERLER, E., ABERNATHY, C., WILLIAMS, G.: J. Exp. Med. 133, 275 (1971)

FREEMAN, C. B., HARRIS, R., GEARY, C. G., LEYLAND, M. J., MacIVER, J. E., DELAMORE, I.: BMJ 4, 571 (1973)

FRIDMAN, W. H., KOURILSKY, F. M.: Nature (LOND.) 224, 277 (1969)

GOLD, P., FREEDMAN, S. O.: J. Exp. MEd. 122, 467 (1965)

GROSS, L.: Cancer Res. 3, 326 (1943)

GUTTERMAN, J. U., MAVLIGIT, G., GOTTLIEB, J. A., BURGESS, M. A., McBRIDE, C. E., EINHORN, L., FREIREICH, E. J., HERSH, E. M.: New Eng. J. Med. 291, 592 (1974)

GUTTERMAN, J. U., ROSEN, R. D., BUTLER, W. J., McCREDIE, K. B., BODEY, G. P., FREIREICH, E. J., HERSH, E. M.: New Eng. J. Med. 288, 169 (1973)

HAKALA, T. R., CASTRO, A. E., ELLIOT, A. Y., FRALEY, E. E.: Invest. Urol. 11, 405 (1974)

HELLSTRÖM, K. E., HELLSTRÖM, I.: Advances in Immunology 18, 209 (1974)

HELLSTRÖM, I., HELLSTRÖM, K. E., PIERCE, G., BILL, A. H.: Proc. Nat. Acad. Sci. U. S. 60, 1231 (1968)

HELLSTRÖM, I., SJOGREN, H. O., WARNER, G. A., HELLSTRÖM, K. E.: Int. J. Cancer 7, 226 (1971)

HERBERMAN, H. R.: Fed. Proc., Fed. Amer. Soc. Exp. Biol. 32, 160 (1973)

HERBERMAN, R. B.: Advances in Cancer Res. 19, 207 (1974)

HERSH, E. M.. OPPENHEIM, J. J.: Cancer Res. 27, 98 (1967)

HERSH, E. M., WHITECAR, J. P., McCREDIE, W. B., BODEY, G. P., FREIREICH, E. J.: New Eng. J. Med. 285, 1211 (1971)

HEYN, R., BORGES, W., JOO, P., KARAN, M., NESBITT, M., SHORE, N.: Proc. Amer. Assoc. for Cancer Res. 14, 45 (1973)

HUMPHREY, E. B., NESBITT, J. M. E., CHARY, K. K. N., KRIVIT, W.: Cancer 29, 402 (1972)

JAGARLAMOODY, S. M., AUST, J. C., TEW, R. H., McKHANN, C. F.: Proc. Nat. Acad. Sci. U. S. 68, 1346 (1971)

JOSE, D. G., SKVARIL, F.: Int. J. Cancer 13, 173 (1974)

KERSTING, G.: Die Gewebszüchtung Menschlicher Hirngeschwulste, Berlin: Springer Verlag, 1961

KLEIN, G.: Israel J. Med. Sci. 7, 111 (1971)

KREDEL, F. E.: Arch. Surg. 18, 2008 (1929)

KUMAR, S., TAYLOR, G.: J. Clin. Path. 26, 476 (1973)

KUMAR, S., TAYLOR, G.: Int. J. Cancer 16, 448 (1975)

KUMAR, S., TAYLOR, G., STEWARD, J. K., WAGHE, M. A., JONES, P. H. M.: Int. J. Cancer 12, 194 (1973)

KUMAR, S., TAYLOR, G., STEWARD, J. K., WAGHE, M. A., PEARSON, D.: Int. J. Cancer 10, 36 (1972)

LARSAN, D. L., TOMLINSON, L. J.: J. Clin. Invest. 32, 317 (1953)

LEIGHTON, N. J.: Invasive Growth and Metastasis in Tissue Culture Systems. Methods in Cancer Research IV. H. Busch (ed.), New York: Academic Press, 1968, p. 85

LEVENTHAL, B. G., HALTERMAN, R. H., ROSENBERG, E. B., HERBERMAN, R. B.: Cancer Res. 32, 820 (1972)

LUMSDEN, C. E.: Tissue Culture in Relation to Tumours of the Nervous System. Pathology of Tumours of the Nervous System. D. S. RUSSELL and L. J. RUBINSTEIN (eds.). London: E. Arnold, 1971, p. 281

MATHÉ, G.: Rev. Franc. Etud. Clin. Biol. 13, 881 (1968)

MATHÉ, G.: Strategy for the treatment of acute leukaemia. In: Immunology. XIII. Int. Cong. Ped., Wien, 1971. Weiner Med. Akad., p. 21

MATHÉ, G., AMIEL, J. L., SCHWARZENBERG, L., SCHNEIDER, M., CATTAN, A., SCHLUMBERGER, J. R., HAYAT, M., De VASSAL, F.: Lancet 1, 697 (1969)

MAVLIGIT, G., AMBUS, U., GUTTERMAN, J. U., HERSH, E. M.: Nature (Lond.) New Biol. 243, 188 (1973)

MAZUR, P., LEIBO, S. P., FARRANT, J., CHU, E. H. Y., HANNA, M. G. Jr., SMITH, L. H.: The Frozen Cell. A Ciba Foundation Symposium. Wolstenholme and O'Connor (eds.). London: Churchill, 1970, p. 69

MERYMAN, H. T.: Cryobiology. London: Academic Press, 1966

MURRAY, M. R., STOUT, A. P.: Amer. J. Path. 19, 429 (1947)

NAGAI, M., HOSHINA, T., TSUCHIDA, T., SATO, F., SANO, K.: Brain nerve (Tokyo) 19, 1055 (1967)

NAGEL, G. A., PIESSENS, W. F., STILLMANT, M. M., LEJEUNE, F.: Europ. J. Cancer 7, 41 (1971)

NAIRN, R. C.: Fluorescent Protein Tracing. Edinburgh: E. & S. Livingstone Ltd., 1969

OGRA, P. L., SINKS, L. F., KARZAN, D. T.: J. Ped. 79, 444 (1971)

OLD, L. J., CLARK, D. A., BENACERRAF, B.: Nature 184, 291 (1959)

OREN, M. E., HERBERMAN, R. B.: Clin. Exp. Immunol. 9, 45 (1971)

PHILLIPS, P., STEWARD, J. K., KUMAR, S.: Int. J. Cancer (1976 in press)

POMERAT, C. M.: J. Neuropath. 14, 28 (1955)

Preliminary report of Medical Research Council on leukaemia in childhood (Concord trial). BMJ 4, 189 (1971)

ROSE, N. R., BONSTEIN, H. S.: Clin. Exp. Immunol. 7, 355 (1970)

RUSSELL, D. S., BLAND, J. D. W.: J. Path. Bact. 36, 273 (1933)

SOKAL, J. E.: Cancer Res. 26, 1161 (1966)

SOLOWEY, A. C., RAPAPORT, F. T.: Surg. Gynecol. Obstet. 121, 756 (1965)

SOUTHAM, C. M.: Progr. Exp. Tumour Res. 9, 1 (1967)

STEWARD, J. K.: In: Malignant Diseases in Children. T. DEELEY (ed.). London: Butterworth's, 1974, Chap. 3

STEWARD, J. K., SMITH, J. L. S., ARNOLD, E. L.: B. J. Ophthalm 40, 449 (1956)

STOWELL, R. E.: Fed. Proc. 24, 5324 (1965

TAYLOR, J. F., JUNGE, U., WOLFE, L.: Int. J. Cancer 8, 468 (1971)

VIZA, D. C., BERNARD-DEGANI, O., BERNARD, C., HARRIS, R. C.: Lancet 2, 493 (1969)

WALKER, J. S., DAVIS, D., FREEMAN, C. B., HAM, R.: Br. J. Cancer 27, 703 (1973)

YOUNG, R. C., CORDER, M. P., HAYNES, H. A., De VITA, U. T.: Amer. J. Med. 52, 63 (1972)

# Subject Index*



*Italic page numbers refer to illustrations

# Recent Results in Cancer Research

Sponsored by the Swiss League against Cancer. Editor in Chief: P. Rentchnick, Genève

**For information about Vols. 1—9, please contact your bookseller or Springer-Verlag.**

10 NELSON, R. S.: Radioactive Phosphorus in the Diagnosis of Gastrointestinal Cancer.
11 FREEMAN, R. G. and J. M. KNOX: Treatment of Skin Cancer.
12 LYNCH, H. T.: Hereditary Factors in Carcinoma.
13 Tumours in Children, 2nd Edition. Edited by H. B. MARSDEN and J. K. STEWARD.
14 ODARTCHENKO, N.: Production Cellulaire Erythropoïétique.
15 SOKOLOFF, B.: Carcinoid and Serotonin.
16 JACOBS, M. L.: Malignant Lymphomas and Their Management.
17 Normal and Malignant Cell Growth. Edited by R. J. M. FRY, M. L. GRIEM, and W. H. KIRSTEN (Symposium).
18 ANGLESIO, E.: The Treatment of Hodgkin's Disease.
19 BANNASCH, P.: The Cytoplasm of Hepatocytes during Carcinogenesis. Electron- and Lightmicroscopical Investigations of the Nitrosomorpholine-intoxicated Rat Liver.
20 Rubidomycin. A new Agent against Cancer. Edited by J. BERNARD, R. PAUL, M. BOIRON, C. JACQUILLAT, and R. MARAL.
21 Scientific Basis of Cancer Chemotherapy. Edited by G. MATHÉ (Symposium).
22 KOLDOVSKÝ, P.: Tumor Specific Transplantation Antigen.
23 FUCHS, W. A., J. W. DAVIDSON, and H. W. FISCHER: Lymphography in Cancer. With contributions by G. JANTET and H. RÖSLER.
24 HAYWARD, J.: Hormones und Human Breast Cancer. An Account of 15 Years Study.
25 ROY-BURMAN, P.: Analogues of Nucleic Acid Components. Mechanisms of Action.
26 Tumors of the Liver. Edited by G. T. PACK and A. H. ISLAMI.
27 SZYMENDERA, J.: Bone Mineral Metabolism in Cancer.
28 MEEK, E. S.: Antitumour and Antiviral Substances of Natural Origin.
29 Aseptic Environments and Cancer Treatment. Edited by G. MATHÉ (Symposium).
30 Advances in the Treatment of Acute (Blastic) Leukemias. Edited by G. MATHÉ (Symposium).
31 DENOIX, P.: Treatment of Malignant Breast Tumors. Indications and Results.
32 NELSON, R. S.: Endoscopy in Gastric Cancer.
33 Experimental and Clinical Effects of L-Asparaginase. Edited by E. GRUNDMANN and H. F. OETTGEN (Symposium).
34 Chemistry and Biological Actions of 4-Nitroquinolin 1-Oxide. Edited by H. ENDO, T. ONO, and T. SUGIMURA.
35 PENN, I.: Malignant Tumors in Organ Transplant Recipients.
36 Current Concepts in the Management of Lymphoma and Leukemia. Edited by J. E. ULTMANN, M. L. GRIEM, W. H. KIRSTEN, and R. W. WISSLER (Symposium).
37 CHIAPPA, S., R. MUSUMECI, and C. USLENGHI: Endolymphatic Radiotherapy in Malignant Lymphomas. With contributions by G. BONADONNA, B. DAMASCELLI, G. FAVA, F. PIZZETTI, U. VERONESI.
38 KOLLER, P. C.: The Role of Chromosomes in Cancer Biology.
39 Current Problems in the Epidemiology of Cancer and Lymphomas. Edited by E. GRUNDMANN and H. TULINIUS (Symposium).
40 LANGLEY, F. A. and A. C. CROMPTON: Epithelial Abnormalities of the Cervix Uteri.
41 Tumours in a Tropical Country. A Survey of Uganda (1964—1968). Edited by A. C. TEMPLETON.
42 Breast Cancer: A Challenging Problem. Edited by M. L. GRIEM, E. V. JENSEN, J. E. ULTMANN, and R. W. WISSLER (Symposium).
43 Nomenclature, Methodology and Results of Clinical Trials in Acute Leukemias. Edited by G. MATHÉ, P. POUILLART, L. SCHWARZENBERG (Symposium).

MIX
Papier aus verantwortungsvollen Quellen
Paper from responsible sources
FSC® C105338

If you have any concerns about our products,
you can contact us on
**ProductSafety@springernature.com**

In case Publisher is established outside the EU,
the EU authorized representative is:
**Springer Nature Customer Service Center GmbH**
**Europaplatz 3, 69115 Heidelberg, Germany**

Printed by Libri Plureos GmbH
in Hamburg, Germany